KU-539-333

Skin Cancer – A World-Wide Perspective

Reinhard Dummer · Mark R. Pittelkow
Keiji Iwatsuki · Adele Green
Nagwa M. Elwan
(Editors)

Skin Cancer - A World-Wide Perspective

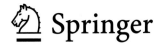
Springer

ALISTAIR MACKENZIE LIBRARY
Barcode: 3690289157
Class no: WR 500 DUM

Editors

Prof. Reinhard Dummer
Department of Dermatology
University Hospital of Zürich
Gloriastrasse 31
8091 Zürich
Switzerland
reinhard.dummer@usz.ch

Prof. Mark R. Pittelkow
Department of Dermatology
Department Biochemistry and Molecular Biology
Mayo Clinic College of Medicine
Mayo Medical School
Rochester, MN 55905
USA
pittelkow.mark@mayo.edu

Prof. Keiji Iwatsuki
Department of Dermatology
Okayama University
Graduate School of Medicine
Dentistry and Pharmaceutical Sciences
2-5-1 Shikata-cho
Okayama, 700-8558
Japan
keijiiwa@cc.okayama-u.ac.jp

Prof. Adele Green
Cancer and Population Studies
The Queensland Institute of Medical Research
Royal Brisbane Hospital
Brisbane, Queensland 4029
Australia
adele.green@qimr.edu.au

Prof. Nagwa M. Elwan
Department of Medicine
Tanta University
Tanta-Egypt
elwan2egy@yahoo.com

Assistant Editor
Dr. med. Marie C. Zipser
University Hospital of Zürich
Department of Dermatology F2
Gloriastrasse 31
8091 Zürich
Switzerland
marie.zipser@usz.ch

ISBN 978-3-642-05071-8   e-ISBN 978-3-642-05072-5
DOI 10.1007/978-3-642-05072-5
Springer Heidelberg Dordrecht London New York

© Springer-Verlag Berlin Heidelberg 2011

This work is subject to copyright. All rights are reserved, whether the whole or part of the material is concerned, specifically the rights of translation, reprinting, reuse of illustrations, recitation, broadcasting, reproduction on microfilm or in any other way, and storage in data banks. Duplication of this publication or parts thereof is permitted only under the provisions of the German Copyright Law of September 9, 1965, in its current version, and permission for use must always be obtained from Springer. Violations are liable to prosecution under the German Copyright Law.

The use of general descriptive names, registered names, trademarks, etc. in this publication does not imply, even in the absence of a specific statement, that such names are exempt from the relevant protective laws and regulations and therefore free for general use.

Product liability: The publishers cannot guarantee the accuracy of any information about dosage and application contained in this book. In every individual case the user must check such information by consulting the relevant literature.

Cover design: eStudioCalamar, Figueres/Berlin

Printed on acid-free paper

Springer is part of Springer Science+Business Media (www.springer.com)

Preface

Alistair Mackenzie Library
Wishaw General Hospital
50 Netherton Street
Wishaw
ML2 0DP

Dear reader

Is it still necessary to print a book?

Is it an anachronism to nowadays read print at all?

In the present era, the electronic equivalent of entire libraries of information is routinely distributed via the internet. This has led some to question the future relevance of print. However, it is our conviction that books still have their place in the world, and it is not merely because books preserve the information of generations with a security that electronic media cannot match. There is also great pleasure to be derived from lifting a text down from the shelf, repairing to a place of comfort, and wandering among pages of print thoughtfully collected and edited.

This book reviews the current state of the art among various aspects of skin cancer biology, diagnosis, and treatment. We have engaged five skin cancer experts as editors from five continents to collect information on the spectrum of cutaneous malignancies as it is described by the WHO classification. Furthermore, we have motivated the best researchers and clinicians to contribute their extensive knowledge base to the endeavor. This has resulted in the compilation of a unique reflection of medical and molecular knowledge about skin cancers. It is anticipated that this book will remain a basic reference for many years to come.

We invite you to take the time to go through this work.

In the name of all authors

Reinhard Dummer, MD
Mark R. Pittelkow, MD
Keiji Iwatsuki, MD
Adele Green, MD
Nagwa M. Elwan, MD

Contents

3   Disease Entities

     Michael B. Colgan, Mark A. Cappel, Mark R. Pittelkow,
     Kazuyasu Fujii, Dorothea Terhorst, and Eggert Stockfleth

     3.1.1 **Basal Cell Carcinoma**. 89
            Michael B. Colgan, Mark A. Cappel, and Mark R. Pittelkow

     3.1.2 **Squamous Cell Carcinoma**. 100
            Mark A. Cappel, Michael B. Colgan, and Mark R. Pittelkow

     3.1.3 **Bowen's Disease**. 109
            Kazuyasu Fujii

     3.1.4 **Actinic keratosis** 112
            Dorothea Terhorst and Eggert Stockfleth

3.2 **Non-Melanoma Skin Cancer: Appendageal Tumours** 121
     Jivko A. Kamarashev and Steven Kaddu

     3.2.1 **Tumours with Apocrine and Eccrine Differentiation** 121
            Jivko A. Kamarashev

     3.2.2 **Tumours with Follicular Differentiation**. 141
            Steven Kaddu

     3.2.3 **Tumours with Sebaceous Differentiation** 153
            Steven Kaddu

3.3 **Melanocytic Tumors** 169
     Jivko A. Kamarashev, Leo Schärer, Marie C. Zipser,
     Lauren L. Lockwood, Reinhard Dummer, and Sven Krengel

     3.3.1 **Disease Entities: Malignant Melanoma**. 169
            Jivko A. Kamarashev, Leo Schärer, Marie C. Zipser,
            Lauren L. Lockwood, and Reinhard Dummer

     3.3.2 **Benign Melanocytic Tumors**. 186
            Sven Krengel

3.4 **Cutaneous Lymphoma, Leukemia and Related Disorders** 197
     Günter Burg, Werner Kempf, Reinhard Dummer, and Mirjana Urosevic-Maiwald

     3.4.1 **Mature T-Cell and NK-Cell Neoplasms** 197
            Günter Burg, Werner Kempf, and Reinhard Dummer

     3.4.2 **Mature Cutaneous B-Cell Neoplasms (CBCL)**. 214
            Günter Burg, Werner Kempf, and Reinhard Dummer

     3.4.3 **Immature Hematopoietic Malignancies** 222
            Mirjana Urosevic-Maiwald

3.5 **Histiocytoses** 233
     Keiji Iwatsuki

3.6 **Mastocytosis, Vascular, Muscular and Fibrohistiocytic Tumors**. 241
     Naohito Hatta, Nagwa M. Elwan, L. Weibel, Luis Requena,
     Davide Donghi, Jürg Hafner, Beata Bode-Lesniewska, and Kenji Asagoe

     3.6.1 **Mastocytosis**. 241
            Naohito Hatta

Epidemiology of Basal Cell and Squamous Cell Carcinoma of the Skin

Jolieke C. van der Pols

1.1.1 Introduction

Although often collectively named "keratinocyte skin cancers" or less specifically "non-melanoma skin cancers", basal cell carcinoma (BCC) and squamous cell carcinoma (SCC) are two quite different skin cancer types each with distinct epidemiological features, ranging from different typical age of onset, to different mortality rates, to different causal pathways.

BCC and SCC do have in common that most of the information about their occurrence and risk factors is obtained from ad hoc research studies, because most cancer registries do not routinely report skin cancers apart from melanoma. This chapter summarises the epidemiological features of BCC and SCC and briefly discusses the main factors associated with occurrence of these skin cancers.

Treatment costs of keratinocyte skin cancers are very high in countries with predominantly white-skinned populations, with an annual cost of US $13 billion in the USA alone [53]. Although fatality from BCC and SCC is low, the many patients affected by these cancers may experience discomfort and scarring and require follow-up to detect recurrence or spread. Thus the disproportionately large medical costs associated with treatment of BCC and SCC warrant continued research to increase understanding of their natural history, for better treatment, and to identify cost-effective prevention measures.

1.1.2 Basal Cell Carcinoma Epidemiology

1.1.2.1 Geographic Variation

BCC predominantly occurs in white-skinned individuals, and the strong correlation between latitude and incidence of this cancer reflects the important role of sunlight exposure in its aetiology. Incidence of BCC in the USA is almost 14 times higher in whites than in Hispanics [45], but highest incidence rates of all are reported in Australia, a country with a mostly Caucasian population living at relatively low latitudes (close to the equator). The risk of Caucasian Australians developing a BCC before age 70 is more than 50%, with an age-standardised incidence rate of 884 per 100,000 [80]. Within Australia the incidence rates show a threefold gradient between the tropical and sub-tropical northern regions of Australia compared to southern regions [98] and data from the USA show similar patterns [45, 61]. In Western Europe, BCC incidence rates are higher in mainland Europe compared to Scandinavia, and higher still in the UK (reviewed in [23]), probably due to regional differences in skin colour within Caucasians.

1.1.2.2 Temporal Trends

Many countries that are commonly affected by BCC have reported large increases in BCC incidence over the past decades, and these increases often vary by age-group. In parts of Western Europe, BCC incidence rates have increased by as much as two to threefold during the last three decades (reviewed in [23]), while BCC incidence in the North-East of the USA nearly doubled in a 15-year period [61]. In the Netherlands [23] and USA [13], BCC incidence has particularly risen in young women in the last three decades.

In Australia, age-standardised incidence rates of BCC have increased only by a third in the last two decades [80] and this increase was greatest for persons aged 60 years and older. Incidence rates in younger age groups had stabilised, possibly due to intensive skin cancer prevention efforts in that country [98].

1.1.2.3 Age and Sex Distributions

Incidence of BCC increases steadily with age, with BCC rarely occurring in persons younger than 30 years, even in high-risk

J.C. van der Pols
Cancer and Population Studies, The Queensland Institute
of Medical Research, Post Office Royal Brisbane Hospital, Brisbane,
QLD 4029, Australia
e-mail: jolieke.vanderpols@qimr.edu.au

R. Dummer et al. (eds.), *Skin Cancer – A World-Wide Perspective*,
DOI: 10.1007/978-3-642-05072-5_1.1, © Springer-Verlag Berlin Heidelberg 2011

populations such as Australia [80]. Peak BCC incidence is achieved in the seventh to eighth decade of life [23, 61].

In most affected populations there is a different age-related incidence pattern between males and females. Below the fifth decade of life, women tend to be affected more often by BCC than men, but in older ages men are more commonly affected [5, 13, 23, 98].

1.1.2.4 Incidence by Anatomical Site

In both sexes, BCCs occur most commonly on the head or neck, followed by the trunk, and upper limbs and lower limbs [30, 87]. When the body surface area is taken into account, highest rates in men and women are found on the head, especially the eyelid, lip and nasolabial fold, followed by ears, nose and cheek and neck [11, 30].

In terms of the distribution of different BCC sub-types on body sites, the evidence is inconsistent. Studies from the Netherlands [3], France [94] and Southern Australia [76] showed that superficial BCC has a predilection to occur on the trunk (49% on the trunk vs. 23% on head and neck in the South Australian study) and that nodular BCC predominantly occurred on the head and neck. However, data from Italy [85] and lower-latitude locations in Northern Queensland [89] have shown more equal distributions of superficial BCC between trunk and head/neck.

Interpretation of these site distributions is further complicated by the observation that despite the possible predilection of the superficial BCC sub-type for the trunk, nodular BCCs predominated over superficial BCCs on the trunk in the South Australian series [76], and they occurred in similar proportions on the trunk in the Dutch series [3]. In a recent cohort study, BCCs of the trunk had a relatively strong association with sunburns and truncal lentigines, but they were not associated with sun sensitivity compared with BCCs of the head and neck [81]. These findings were thought to suggest that truncal BCCs result from acute, intense sun exposure, sufficient to cause sunburn among people whose ability to tan makes the skin of their face less susceptible to ultraviolet (UV) carcinogenesis. In one study, patients with an initial superficial BCC on the trunk seemed to experience a faster increase in the number of subsequent BCC (number of subsequent BCC per year) than those with other site and histology combinations [70], but further evidence is needed to confirm this.

When interpreting studies of the site distribution of BCC sub-types it is important to keep in mind that most of these have been based on retrospective reviews of hospital records. Such results can be biased by dependency of referral patterns on histological sub-types and body site of occurrence. Also, bias may be caused by differential management of different body sites and lesion types and subsequent opportunities for histological identification. Thus further evidence from population series and from molecular investigations is needed to elucidate the biology of the different BCC sub-types.

1.1.2.5 Repeated Occurrence

Patients affected by BCC are at high risk of subsequent BCCs. Based on a meta-analysis of 17 studies it was estimated that a person has a 44% risk of a subsequent BCC within 3 years after a first BCC, about ten times the incidence rate expected in the general population [71], although this is dependent on age and geographic location. For example, the relative risk of a second BCC after a first BCC is higher in those affected at a younger age compared to those first affected in older age [67]. The risk of developing a BCC after an initial SCC is similar to the risk among persons with a prior BCC [71].

1.1.3 Squamous Cell Carcinoma Epidemiology

1.1.3.1 Geographic Variation

Like BCC, SCC is predominantly a cancer that occurs in white-skinned people, with incidence rates varying strongly between countries. At a population level, SCC tumors occur less frequently than BCC tumors. Incidence rates can also vary strongly between population sub-groups according to skin colour. For example, SCC incidence rates in the USA are almost 11 times higher in whites than in Hispanics [45].

Lifetime risk of SCC is high particularly in high-risk countries such as Australia, where the estimated risk of developing an SCC by age 70 is 28% and age-standardised incidence rate for SCC is 387 per 100,000 [80]. By comparison, the estimated lifetime risk of SCC in Canada is 5% [47]. Occurrence of SCC is closely related to ambient hours of sunlight and proximity to the equator. For example, in Australia the SCC incidence rates are more than three times higher in those living in sub-tropical and tropical latitudes compared to those living at higher latitudes (>37°S) [98]. Within the USA, high ambient UV levels at the location of residence throughout the life course is also a strong predictor of increased SCC risk [88].

1.1.3.2 Temporal Trends

Many countries in Europe [10], North America [47] and Oceania [98] have reported significant increases in SCC incidence in the last decades. Doubling or tripling of SCC incidence rates over the past 2–3 decades has been reported in the USA [61] and Australia [98] with large increases also reported in Europe [10, 20]. Secular trends in ageing of populations may be an underlying reason for this increase, as well as changed sun-exposure behaviours and improved skin cancer awareness and detection. Most studies that have reported changes in SCC incidence rates have explicitly excluded in situ SCC or other lesions, thus minimising the possibility that increases are inflated by changed inclusion criteria. Data from Switzerland suggest that SCC incidence (but not BCC or melanoma incidence) rates may have levelled off since the late 1980s [68] and data from Scotland showed a stabilising of SCC incidence in men older than 60 years [10], but such a declining trend is not seen in data from other countries.

1.1.3.3   Age and Sex Distributions

As for BCC, the incidence of SCC increases with increasing age. Up to the fifth decade of life, women tend to be more commonly affected by SCC than men, but in older age incidence rates of SCC are generally much higher in men than in women [61, 97]. The difference in SCC incidence between males and females is less in the north of Australia, closer to the equator, than in central and southern regions [80], suggesting that any difference in sun-exposure behaviour that may underlie these sex differences plays less of a role in very high compared to lower sunlight environments.

1.1.3.4   Incidence by Anatomical Site

The head and neck are the most common sites of occurrence for SCC in both men and women, followed by the neck and upper and lower limbs [20, 30]. When the body surface area is taken into account, the highest SCC incidence in both men and women is found on the face, especially the lip region, ears, nose, cheek and eyelid, with neck, dorsa of hands and forearms next most affected [11].

1.1.3.5   Repeated Occurrence

Patients affected by SCC are at high risk of subsequent SCC lesions. The general risk of a subsequent SCC after a first diagnosis has been estimated from published studies to be about 18% after 3 years, at least a tenfold increase in incidence compared with the incidence of

first tumors in a comparable general population [71]. The risk of developing an SCC within 3 years after a BCC is also high [71].

1.1.3.6   Actinic Keratoses

Actinic keratoses (AKs) are benign keratotic tumors, with only a very small proportion progressing to become SCC. Over time, actinic keratoses can clear spontaneously, persist [31] or progress into invasive skin cancer [74].

There are no published population-based incidence rates of people who develop actinic keratoses and this would be difficult to calculate given the lability of these lesions. However, in a follow-up study of adults in southern Australia who were initially lesion-free, 19% had a prevalent actinic keratosis at 12 months follow-up [72]. In a population-based prevalence study in the sub-tropical Australian town of Nambour, Queensland (26°S), 44% of men and 37% of women between the ages of 20 and 69 years had at least one actinic keratosis on examination of head, neck, hands and arms [39], the most common sites of occurrence. Prevalence of AKs is strongly age-dependent [51], reflecting incidence and recurrence rates that exceed rates of regression as people age [51].

Definitive evidence from long-term, closely monitored studies on the progression rates from actinic keratosis to SCC is lacking. The general rate of progression has been estimated at 0.025–16% per year [34]. In a medium-term (5-year) study in southern Australia [74], the rate of malignant transformation was estimated to be less than 1:1,000 (though without histological confirmation of the initial lesion the possibility remains that the lesion was an SCC at the outset) [51]. In another Australian study in a high-risk sub-tropical population not one of more than 1,000 AKs in 200 affected persons who were followed up every 2–6 months for 18 months underwent malignant transformation [31]. A spontaneous remission rate of 26% has been reported based on follow-up after 12 months [72], though with more intense lesion surveillance, substantially higher rates of remission are seen [31].

Higher rates of progression to invasive cancers have been reported for Bowen's disease and SCC in situ, with an estimated 3–5% of patients developing invasive carcinomas from such lesions [60]. Such estimates may be biased, however, due to differential follow-up patterns [17].

The probability that an individual SCC has arisen from solar keratosis is high. However, 60% of incidental SCCs in the study in southern Australia arose from a lesion diagnosed previously as an actinic keratosis [74] while another study reported that 72% of SCCs were contiguous with actinic keratoses [19].

In summary, the chances that an individual actinic keratosis will develop into an SCC are extremely small. However, when one encounters an SCC, the chance that it has arisen in association with actinic keratoses is very high.

1.1.4 Risk Factors for Basal Cell Carcinoma

1.1.4.1 Genetic Factors

1.1.4.1.1 Patched Mutations and the Sonic Hedgehog Pathway

Studies of patients with Gorlin's syndrome (nevoid BCC syndrome), an autosomal dominant disorder characterised by the development of multiple BCCs at an early age, have helped obtain much important knowledge about the pathogenesis of BCC [36]. Affected patients carry mutations in the *patched* gene, a tumor suppressor gene: one defective copy of this gene is inherited but tumors arise after inactivation of the remaining allele [102]. They develop BCCs as early as 2 years of age, with the highest incidence between puberty and 35 years of age [36]. Almost all white-skinned Gorlin's syndrome patients develop BCC, but only about half of affected black patients develop these cancers [35], indicating the important role of UV exposure in addition to the genetic component in the aetiology of BCC.

The *patched* gene product is part of the Sonic Hedgehog (Shh) protein receptor, which is involved in embryonic development. When Sonic Hedgehog binds to the patched, it releases smoothened, a transmembrane signalling protein. Mutations of the *patched* and *smoothened* genes result in upregulation of the Hedgehog signalling pathway and activation of downstream target genes that are associated with cell growth and differentiation [27], including the Gli family of transcription factors [50]. Evidence for the importance of Shh pathway activation in BCC carcinogenesis comes from transgenic human-skin models in which Shh-expressing human keratinocytes formed BCC-like lesions when grafted onto the skin of immune-deficient mice [28]. Also, *patched* heterozygous knockout mice develop BCC-like lesions when exposed to UV or ionising radiation [2]. Only around 0.5% of all BCC cases arise in individuals with Gorlin's syndrome but up to 90% of sporadic BCC show *patched* mutations [101] and approximately 10% show *smoothened* mutations [92]. It is now thought that upregulation of the Shh pathway is the pivotal abnormality in all BCCs, and that little more than Shh upregulation is needed for BCC carcinogenesis [27].

1.1.4.1.2 DNA Repair Defects

Another rare disorder which has helped gain insights in the pathogenesis of BCC is xeroderma pigmentosum (XP), a rare autosomal recessive disorder which is part of a family of nucleotide excision repair diseases [14]. BCC is common in XP patients and manifests as an extreme photosensitivity to UV radiation as the result of a deficiency in the enzyme that permits excisional repair of UV-damaged DNA. XP occurs in approximately 1 in 250,000 people in the USA and Europe and 1 in 40,000 in Japan [52].

Skin cancer is a characteristic of XP but not of some other nucleotide excision repair diseases such as Cockayne syndrome, despite the sun sensitivity in both disorders. It has, therefore, been suggested that the increased mutation rates in both XP and Cockayne syndrome patients may be necessary but not sufficient for carcinogenesis. Chromosome instability as seen in XP may, therefore, be an additional requirement for cancer development in these patients [14].

Skin tumors in XP patients commonly show *ras* oncogene activation, *Ink4a-Arf* and *p53* tumor suppressor gene modifications, and aberrations of the Sonic Hedgehog pathway [21]. UV-specific mutations of the *smoothened* gene are three time higher in XP patients as in normal sporadic BCCs, confirming the high rate of UV-induced mutations in these DNA-repair deficient persons [16].

The observation that BCCs commonly develop in XP patients has raised the question whether other genetic variants that affect DNA repair capacity may be involved in sporadic BCC formation in persons without XP. Until now results of studies of single gene polymorphisms with such effects have been conflicting and associations weak, but combined effects of multiple polymorphisms remains a possibility [27].

1.1.4.1.3 Detoxifying Proteins

One of the mechanisms by which UV induces skin cancer is through formation of free radicals that cause oxidative stress in the skin. Members of the enzyme family glutathione-*S*-peroxidase are known to utilise the toxic products produced by UV light-induced oxidative stress. Polymorphisms in GSTM1, GSTM3, GSTT1, and GSTP1 in particular appear to be associated with increased occurrence of BCC [66, 90].

1.1.4.1.4 The *p53* Tumor Suppressor Gene

Around half of all BCC tumors carry mutations in the *p53* tumor suppressor gene. However, people who suffer from the Li–Fraumeni syndrome, which is characterised by germline mutations in the *p53* gene, do not show increased incidence of BCC. It is thus assumed that *p53* mutations are secondary events in BCC pathogenesis [102].

1.1.4.2 Solar Radiation

Numerous epidemiological studies have consistently shown that populations who receive low ambient sun exposure or those with dark skin colour at high latitudes, rarely develop BCC [40, 56]. The predominant role of solar UV radiation in the aetiology of BCC is evidenced by the consistent observation that clinical signs of chronic sun damage to the skin are the strongest predictors of BCC, despite an overall lack of association between BCC and self-reported chronic sun exposure [65] which may be due to some extent to people with sun-sensitive skin being underrepresented in outdoor occupations due to self-selection [38]. The particular increase in BCC incidence in young women in the Netherlands and USA in the last three decades is thought to be due partly to increased sun-seeking behaviour among young females [13, 23].

The "intermittent UV" exposure theory proposes that it is not the total amount of sun exposure but rather the pattern of sun exposure that determines the risk of BCC [65]. In particular, it has been hypothesised that a certain dose of solar UV delivered in infrequent, intense increments will increase the risk of BCC more than the same total dose delivered continuously over the same period [65, 109]. However, the intermittent pattern theory does not explain all the epidemiologic evidence of BCC's UV dose dependence. The predilection of BCCs for occurrence on the head and neck [30] as well as the association between age at migration from low-UV to high-UV country of residence and BCC [64] risk indicate that total UV dose is an important risk factor.

There is suggestive evidence from a couple of case-control studies that sunlight exposure early in life, as well as freckling and sunburn in childhood are independent predictors of BCC risk [15, 33], but more data on this, in particular from prospective study, are needed.

UV dose-dependence may also vary among the commonest BCC sub-types as suggested by their clinical and histological differences. Patients with superficial BCC tend to be younger than those with other BCC sub-types [3, 69, 76, 89], suggesting that superficial BCC has a lower threshold for UV carcinogenesis than the nodular sub-type. Also, the increase in incidence with age is gradual for superficial BCC in contrast to a progressive and dramatic age-related increase in incidence of nodular BCC [89].

1.1.4.2.1 Sunscreen Use

Exposure to sunlight is the single-most important environmental risk factor for BCC and sun avoidance both in childhood and adulthood is the most effective strategy to prevention. There is little firm evidence that use of sunscreens provides additional benefit in BCC prevention. In a community-based randomised-trial of daily sunscreen use for some 5 years, BCC incidence was not affected [41]. However, the time between a first and subsequent BCCs was reduced in those who had used sunscreen daily during this trial [84], and 8 years after cessation of the trial there was a tendency for BCC incidence to be lower in participants who had used sunscreen daily compared to discretionary use [105], though this finding could have been due to chance.

1.1.4.3 Dietary Factors

There is some evidence that dietary factors may be associated with skin cancer risk in humans, supported by a large body of evidence from animal models. The mechanisms underlying such associations may relate to the role of anti-oxidant nutrients in the skin's defence against UV-induced genetic and cellular damage, and the effect of dietary fats on the UV-induced inflammatory response through modification of prostaglandin production [95].

A large American cohort study showed a small (13%) but significant increase in risk of BCC for men with a high intake of long chain n-3 fatty acids and an inverse association with intake of total and monounsaturated fat [104]. In a randomised trial, a low fat intake (~20% of energy from fat) compared to normal fat intake (~40% of energy from fat) was shown to reduce the incidence of skin cancers [6], but since BCC and SCC were combined in the analyses of this study, it does not provide evidence for BCC per se. Other studies have not found clear evidence for an association between dietary fat and BCC risk [77]. The small number of studies of BCC risk and intake of antioxidant nutrients have thus far not shown firm evidence for associations between retinol, carotenoids, vitamin E, vitamin C, or selenium and BCC risk [48, 77]. Randomised trials of beta-carotene [41, 42] and selenium supplementation [24] have not shown an effect on BCC incidence.

1.1.4.4 Other Risk Factors

A number of other risk factors are known to affect BCC risk in population sub-groups.

Persons exposed to ionising radiation therapy are at increased risk of BCC occurrence, in particular in persons who received radiation treatment for acne [63]. Radiation-exposure-related BCCs tend to arise within the radiation treatment field [63]. BCC tumors can also be associated with scars, such as those from smallpox vaccination [18].

Inorganic arsenic is a human carcinogen that occurs in high concentrations in groundwater of some regions around the world, in particular affecting populations in the West Bengal region of India and Bangladesh, but also affecting regions in other parts of the world including Europe and USA [107]. Chronic arsenic exposure is associated with increased BCC occurrence [108].

Immunocompromised patients such as organ transplant recipients have an increased risk of developing skin cancers, including BCCs [57]. The incidence of BCC in Dutch transplant patients was ten times higher than the general population [46]. Use of immune-suppressing glucocorticoids, is also associated with increased BCC risk [96].

1.1.5 Risk Factors for Squamous Cell Carcinoma

1.1.5.1 Genetic Factors

SCC occurs commonly in XP patients (see Sect. 1.1.4). Also, the rare Ferguson–Smith syndrome predisposes to the development of lesions that are indistinguishable from SCC, although they tend to resolve spontaneously. Gene mapping has excluded *patched* as a causative gene but has shown loss of heterozygosity, suggesting that the gene for this syndrome is likely a tumor-suppressor gene [7].

The majority of SCCs carry mutations of the *p53* tumor-suppressor gene [1]. These mutations are often "UV-signature mutations" which indicates that they are the result of damage caused by exposure to UV radiation or sunlight. Mutations in the *p53* gene can cause uncontrolled cell proliferation and loss of apoptosis, which supports cancerous growth. Immunohistochemically detectable clusters of epidermal cells with accumulated nuclear p53 protein ("p53 patches") are found in normal skin before tumors arise. It is thought that these patches are an early step in the development of actinic keratoses and subsequent SCC, though the progression rate is probably very small [91].

Variants of the melanocortin-1 receptor (MC1R) gene are associated with phenotypic features such as red hair, light skin colour and tanning ability of the skin. A number of MC1R variants are also independently associated with risk of BCC and SCC [4, 8], with carriers of certain variants carrying an up to threefold increased risk of SCC compared to other individuals with the same skin type [93].

1.1.5.2 Solar Radiation

The strongest environmental risk factor for SCCs and SCC precursor lesions actinic keratoses is cumulative sun

exposure. Epidemiological evidence for this comes from observations that (1) SCC risk is increased in those living at relatively low latitudes with higher ambient UV exposure [98], (2) indicators of skin ageing, in particular presence of solar keratoses, are predictors of SCC risk [25, 38], (3) SCC incidence is lower in immigrants from low to high sunlight locations [26], and (4) relatively high self-reported sunlight exposure is associated with increased SCC risk [25]. Furthermore, the distribution of anatomic sites on which SCC occurs reflects sites of maximal sun exposure (see Sect. 1.1.3.4).

Actinic keratoses (AKs) can progress to become SCC and their occurrence is strongly associated with cumulative sunlight exposure. While AKs share many of the same determinants as SCC, they are a more sensitive indicator of intense sunlight exposure [73]. In sub-tropical Queensland, high levels of occupational exposure and sunburns were strongly and significantly associated with AK prevalence, especially in those people with multiple AKs [32]. Also in the Italian population, presence of actinic keratosis was strongly associated with signs of skin ageing and past sunlight exposure, while AK prevalence (0.3%) was much lower in Italy than that expected from data from the USA or Australia [79].

1.1.5.2.1 Sunscreen Use

The strong correlation between chronic sun exposure and SCC risk suggests that avoidance of sunlight exposure both in childhood and adulthood should be an effective strategy to prevention. Furthermore, there is evidence that regular use of sunscreens provides additional benefit in SCC prevention. In a community-based randomised-trial of daily sunscreen use, the incidence of SCC tumors in those randomised to daily sunscreen use for some 5 years was 40% lower than in those randomised to continuation of their normal sunscreen use habits [41]. In addition, 8 years after cessation of this trial the rate at which persons were affected by SCC continued to be significantly lower in persons who had used sunscreen daily for over about a 5 year period compared to discretionary users [105].

1.1.5.3 Human Papilloma Virus

Infection with certain cutaneous HPV types is associated with increased cutaneous SCC risk. In particular the beta-types of papilloma viruses, which were originally identified in studies of patients with epidermodysplasia verruciformis [22], are associated with skin cancer risk [83]. Infection with HPV is very common among the general population [86].

Studies that have assessed HPV positivity through measurement of beta-HPV antibodies, as well as those that have assessed the presence of beta-HPV DNA, have shown that beta-HPVs are associated with actinic keratoses and SCC [9, 29, 62, 99]. If etiologically involved it is likely that beta-HPV acts to potentiate the effect of UV radiation. This could take place possibly via viral inhibition of DNA repair or prevention of apoptosis following UV radiation [44, 75]. This was shown by in vitro studies in which certain beta-HPV types reduced the apoptotic responses upon UV irradiation in human keratinocytes and thus may augment the carcinogenic effect of UV radiation in the skin [100].

1.1.5.4 Dietary Factors

There is some evidence that a diet high in antioxidant-rich foods may help prevent SCC, independent of sun exposure. A prospective study of food intake and SCC tumor risk in an Australian sub-tropical population showed a 55% reduced SCC risk for relatively high intake of green-leafy vegetables in adults with a history of skin cancer [54]. Results from this observational study were fully adjusted for past UV-exposure, and skin type. The protective association of green-leafy vegetables in this study was most likely due to intake of lutein and zeaxanthin, two carotenoids commonly found in green-leafy vegetables [48]. The same study showed a doubling of SCC tumor risk associated with high intake of unmodified dairy products (e.g. full-cream dairy milk and cheese) in adults with a history of skin cancer [54]. Further study of this sub-tropical Australian population extended this finding to show that a "meat and fat" dietary pattern, characterised by components such as processed meat, discretionary fat, and white bread, had an additional association over and above the association with the high-fat dairy food group alone with the development of subsequent SCC tumors [55].

Because intervention studies that tested specific antioxidants in the form of a dietary supplements have generally not shown an effect on skin cancer risk [41, 42] or even negative effects [24], it may be the integration of nutrients in whole foods that modify skin cancer risk rather than individual nutrients, though more evidence for this is needed.

1.1.5.5 Other Risk Factors

A number of other risk factors are known to affect SCC risk in population sub-groups.

SCCs are among the most common malignancies occurring in immunosuppressed organ transplant recipients [103]. Such patients develop more aggressive and more numerous SCCs than immunocompetent individuals [49], at an incidence about 65 times higher than in the normal population [58].

Smoking was associated with a 50% increased risk of SCC in the US Nurses Health Study [43], but other studies have not shown an increased risk in smokers [38, 82]. SCC on the lip is often associated with a history of smoking [78].

Chronic arsenic exposure is associated with increased incidence of keratinocyte skin cancers including SCC, in particular in association with hyperkerotsosis [108] SCCs can be also be associated with scars such as those from smallpox vaccination [106], as well as chronic ulcers and sinus tracts [59]. There is some evidence that use of non-steroidal anti-inflammatory drugs may reduce the risk of SCC [12, 37] and actinic keratosis [12].

References

1. Ahmadian, A., Ren, Z.P., Williams, C., et al.: Genetic instability in the 9q22.3 region is a late event in the development of squamous cell carcinoma. Oncogene 17(14), 1837–1843 (1998)
2. Aszterbaum, M., Epstein, J., Oro, A., et al.: Ultraviolet and ionizing radiation enhance the growth of BCCs and trichoblastomas in patched heterozygous knockout mice. Nat. Med. 5(11), 1285–1291 (1999)
3. Bastiaens, M.T., Hoefnagel, J.J., Bruijn, J.A., et al.: Differences in age, site distribution, and sex between nodular and superficial basal cell carcinoma indicate different types of tumors. J. Invest. Dermatol. 110(6), 880–884 (1998)
4. Bastiaens, M.T., ter Huurne, J.A., Kielich, C., et al.: Melanocortin-1 receptor gene variants determine the risk of nonmelanoma skin cancer independently of fair skin and red hair. Am. J. Hum. Genet. 68(4), 884–894 (2001)
5. Bath-Hextall, F., Leonardi-Bee, J., Smith, C., et al.: Trends in incidence of skin basal cell carcinoma. Additional evidence from a UK primary care database study. Int. J. Cancer 121(9), 2105–2108 (2007)
6. Black, H.S., Thornby, J.I., Wolf Jr., J.E., et al.: Evidence that a low-fat diet reduces the occurrence of non-melanoma skin cancer. Int. J. Cancer 62(2), 165–169 (1995)
7. Bose, S., Morgan, L.J., Booth, D.R., et al.: The elusive multiple self-healing squamous epithelioma (MSSE) gene: further mapping, analysis of candidates, and loss of heterozygosity. Oncogene 25(5), 806–812 (2006)
8. Box, N.F., Duffy, D.L., Irving, R.E., et al.: Melanocortin-1 receptor genotype is a risk factor for basal and squamous cell carcinoma. J. Invest. Dermatol. 116(2), 224–229 (2001)
9. Boxman, I.L., Russell, A., Mulder, L.H., et al.: Case-control study in a subtropical Australian population to assess the relation between non-melanoma skin cancer and epidermodysplasia verruciformis human papillomavirus DNA in plucked eyebrow hairs. The Nambour Skin Cancer Prevention Study Group. Int. J. Cancer 86(1), 118–121 (2000)
10. Brewster, D.H., Bhatti, L.A., Inglis, J.H., et al.: Recent trends in incidence of nonmelanoma skin cancers in the East of Scotland, 1992-2003. Br. J. Dermatol. 156(6), 1295–1300 (2007)
11. Buettner, P.G., Raasch, B.A.: Incidence rates of skin cancer in Townsville, Australia. Int. J. Cancer 78(5), 587–593 (1998)

12. Butler, G.J., Neale, R., Green, A.C., et al.: Nonsteroidal anti-inflammatory drugs and the risk of actinic keratoses and squamous cell cancers of the skin. J. Am. Acad. Dermatol. **53**(6), 966–972 (2005)

13. Christenson, L.J., Borrowman, T.A., Vachon, C.M., et al.: Incidence of basal cell and squamous cell carcinomas in a population younger than 40 years. JAMA **294**(6), 681–690 (2005)

14. Cleaver, J.E.: Cancer in xeroderma pigmentosum and related disorders of DNA repair. Nat. Rev. Cancer **5**(7), 564–573 (2005)

15. Corona, R., Dogliotti, E., D'Errico, M., et al.: Risk factors for basal cell carcinoma in a Mediterranean population: role of recreational sun exposure early in life. Arch. Dermatol. **137**(9), 1162–1168 (2001)

16. Couve-Privat, S., Bouadjar, B., Avril, M.F., et al.: Significantly high levels of ultraviolet-specific mutations in the smoothened gene in basal cell carcinomas from DNA repair-deficient xeroderma pigmentosum patients. Cancer Res. **62**(24), 7186–7189 (2002)

17. Cox, N.H., Eedy, D.J., Morton, C.A.: Guidelines for management of Bowen's disease: 2006 update. Br. J. Dermatol. **156**(1), 11–21 (2007)

18. Curry, J.L., Goulder, S.J., Nickoloff, B.J.: Occurrence of a basal cell carcinoma and dermatofibroma in a smallpox vaccination scar. Dermatol. Surg. **34**(1), 132–134 (2008)

19. Czarnecki, D., Meehan, C.J., Bruce, F., et al.: The majority of cutaneous squamous cell carcinomas arise in actinic keratoses. J. Cutan. Med. Surg. **6**(3), 207–209 (2002)

20. Dal, H., Boldemann, C., Lindelof, B.: Trends during a half century in relative squamous cell carcinoma distribution by body site in the Swedish population: support for accumulated sun exposure as the main risk factor. J. Dermatol. **35**(2), 55–62 (2008)

21. Daya-Grosjean, L., Sarasin, A.: The role of UV induced lesions in skin carcinogenesis: an overview of oncogene and tumor suppressor gene modifications in xeroderma pigmentosum skin tumors. Mutat. Res. **571**(1–2), 43–56 (2005)

22. de Villiers, E.M., Fauquet, C., Broker, T.R., et al.: Classification of papillomaviruses. Virology **324**(1), 17–27 (2004)

23. de Vries, E., Louwman, M., Bastiaens, M., et al.: Rapid and continuous increases in incidence rates of basal cell carcinoma in the southeast Netherlands since 1973. J. Invest. Dermatol. **123**(4), 634–638 (2004)

24. Duffield-Lillico, A.J., Slate, E.H., Reid, M.E., et al.: Selenium supplementation and secondary prevention of nonmelanoma skin cancer in a randomized trial. J. Natl. Cancer Inst. **95**(19), 1477–1481 (2003)

25. English, D.R., Armstrong, B.K., Kricker, A., et al.: Case-control study of sun exposure and squamous cell carcinoma of the skin. Int. J. Cancer **77**(3), 347–353 (1998)

26. English, D.R., Armstrong, B.K., Kricker, A., et al.: Demographic characteristics, pigmentary and cutaneous risk factors for squamous cell carcinoma of the skin: a case-control study. Int. J. Cancer **76**(5), 628–634 (1998)

27. Epstein, E.H.: Basal cell carcinomas: attack of the hedgehog. Nat. Rev. Cancer **8**, 743–754 (2008)

28. Fan, H., Oro, A.E., Scott, M.P., et al.: Induction of basal cell carcinoma features in transgenic human skin expressing Sonic Hedgehog. Nat. Med. **3**(7), 788–792 (1997)

29. Feltkamp, M.C., Broer, R., di Summa, F.M., et al.: Seroreactivity to epidermodysplasia verruciformis-related human papillomavirus types is associated with nonmelanoma skin cancer. Cancer Res. **63**(10), 2695–2700 (2003)

30. Franceschi, S., Levi, F., Randimbison, L., et al.: Site distribution of different types of skin cancer: new aetiological clues. Int. J. Cancer **67**(1), 24–28 (1996)

31. Frost, C., Williams, G., Green, A.: High incidence and regression rates of solar keratoses in a queensland community. J. Invest. Dermatol. **115**(2), 273–277 (2000)

32. Frost, C.A., Green, A.C., Williams, G.M.: The prevalence and determinants of solar keratoses at a subtropical latitude (Queensland, Australia). Br. J. Dermatol. **139**(6), 1033–1039 (1998)

33. Gallagher, R.P., Hill, G.B., Bajdik, C.D., et al.: Sunlight exposure, pigmentary factors, and risk of nonmelanocytic skin cancer. I. Basal cell carcinoma. Arch. Dermatol. **131**(2), 157–163 (1995)

34. Glogau, R.G.: The risk of progression to invasive disease. J. Am. Acad. Dermatol. **42**(1 pt 2), 23–24 (2000)

35. Goldstein, A.M., Pastakia, B., DiGiovanna, J.J., et al.: Clinical findings in two African-American families with the nevoid basal cell carcinoma syndrome (NBCC). Am. J. Med. Genet. **50**(3), 272–281 (1994)

36. Gorlin, R.J.: Nevoid basal cell carcinoma (Gorlin) syndrome. Genet. Med. **6**(6), 530–539 (2004)

37. Grau, M.V., Baron, J.A., Langholz, B., et al.: Effect of NSAIDs on the recurrence of nonmelanoma skin cancer. Int. J. Cancer **119**(3), 682–686 (2006)

38. Green, A., Battistutta, D., Hart, V., et al.: Skin cancer in a subtropical Australian population: incidence and lack of association with occupation. The Nambour Study Group. Am. J. Epidemiol. **144**(11), 1034–1040 (1996)

39. Green, A., Beardmore, G., Hart, V., et al.: Skin cancer in a Queensland population. J. Am. Acad. Dermatol. **19**(6), 1045–1052 (1988)

40. Green, A., Whiteman, D., Frost, C., et al.: Sun exposure, skin cancers and related skin conditions. J. Epidemiol. **9**(6 suppl), S7–S13 (1999)

41. Green, A., Williams, G., Neale, R., et al.: Daily sunscreen application and betacarotene supplementation in prevention of basal-cell and squamous-cell carcinomas of the skin: a randomised controlled trial. Lancet **354**(9180), 723–729 (1999)

42. Greenberg, E.R., Baron, J.A., Stukel, T.A., et al.: A clinical trial of beta carotene to prevent basal-cell and squamous-cell cancers of the skin. The Skin Cancer Prevention Study Group. N. Engl. J. Med. **323**(12), 789–795 (1990)

43. Grodstein, F., Speizer, F.E., Hunter, D.J.: A prospective-study of incident squamous-cell carcinoma of the skin in the Nurses Health Study. J. Natl. Cancer Inst. **87**(14), 1061–1066 (1995)

44. Hall, L., Struijk, L., Neale, R.E., et al.: Re: Human papillomavirus infection and incidence of squamous cell and basal cell carcinomas of the skin. J. Natl. Cancer Inst. **98**(19), 1425–1426 (2006)

45. Harris, R.B., Griffith, K., Moon, T.E.: Trends in the incidence of nonmelanoma skin cancers in southeastern Arizona, 1985-1996. J. Am. Acad. Dermatol. **45**(4), 528–536 (2001)

46. Hartevelt, M.M., Bavinck, J.N., Kootte, A.M., et al.: Incidence of skin cancer after renal transplantation in The Netherlands. Transplantation **49**(3), 506–509 (1990)

47. Hayes, R.C., Leonfellner, S., Pilgrim, W., et al.: Incidence of nonmelanoma skin cancer in New Brunswick, Canada, 1992 to 2001. J. Cutan. Med. Surg. **11**(2), 45–52 (2007)

48. Heinen, M.M., Hughes, M.C., Ibiebele, T.I., et al.: Intake of antioxidant nutrients and the risk of skin cancer. Eur. J. Cancer **43**(18), 2707–2716 (2007)

49. Herman, S., Rogers, H.D., Ratner, D.: Immunosuppression and squamous cell carcinoma: a focus on solid organ transplant recipients. Skinmed **6**(5), 234–238 (2007)

50. High, A., Zedan, W.: Basal cell nevus syndrome. Curr. Opin. Oncol. **17**(2), 160–166 (2005)

51. Holmes, C., Foley, P., Freeman, M., et al.: Solar keratosis: epidemiology, pathogenesis, presentation and treatment. Australas. J. Dermatol. **48**(2), 67–74 (2007). quiz 75–76

52. Horenstein, M., Diwan. A.: Xeroderma pigmentosum. E-medicine. http://www.emedicine.com/DERM/topic462.htm (2005)

53. Housman, T.S., Feldman, S.R., Williford, P.M., et al.: Skin cancer is among the most costly of all cancers to treat for the Medicare population. J. Am. Acad. Dermatol. **48**(3), 425–429 (2003)

54. Hughes, M.C., van der Pols, J.C., Marks, G.C., et al.: Food intake and risk of squamous cell carcinoma of the skin in a community: the Nambour skin cancer cohort study. Int. J. Cancer **119**, 1953–1960 (2006)

55. Ibiebele, T.I., van der Pols, J.C., Hughes, M.C., et al.: Dietary pattern in association with squamous cell carcinoma of the skin: a prospective study. Am. J. Clin. Nutr. **85**(5), 1401–1408 (2007)

56. International Agency for Research on Cancer: IARC Monographs on the Evaluation of Carcinogenic Risks to Humans, vol. 55. Solar and Ultraviolet Radiation. IARC, Lyon (1992)

57. Jemec, G.B., Holm, E.A.: Nonmelanoma skin cancer in organ transplant patients. Transplantation **75**(3), 253–257 (2003)

58. Jensen, P., Hansen, S., Moller, B., et al.: Skin cancer in kidney and heart transplant recipients and different long-term immunosuppressive therapy regimens. J. Am. Acad. Dermatol. **40**(2 pt 1), 177–186 (1999)

59. Johnson, T.M., Rowe, D.E., Nelson, B.R., et al.: Squamous cell carcinoma of the skin (excluding lip and oral mucosa). J. Am. Acad. Dermatol. **26**(3 pt 2), 467–484 (1992)

60. Kao, G.F.: Carcinoma arising in Bowen's disease. Arch. Dermatol. **122**(10), 1124–1126 (1986)

61. Karagas, M.R., Greenberg, E.R., Spencer, S.K., et al.: Increase in incidence rates of basal cell and squamous cell skin cancer in New Hampshire, USA. New Hampshire Skin Cancer Study Group. Int. J. Cancer **81**(4), 555–559 (1999)

62. Karagas, M.R., Nelson, H.H., Sehr, P., et al.: Human papillomavirus infection and incidence of squamous cell and basal cell carcinomas of the skin. J. Natl. Cancer Inst. **98**(6), 389–395 (2006)

63. Karagas, M.R., Nelson, H.H., Zens, M.S., et al.: Squamous cell and basal cell carcinoma of the skin in relation to radiation therapy and potential modification of risk by sun exposure. Epidemiology **18**(6), 776–784 (2007)

64. Kricker, A., Armstrong, B.K., English, D.R., et al.: Pigmentary and cutaneous risk factors for non-melanocytic skin cancer–a case-control study. Int. J. Cancer **48**(5), 650–662 (1991)

65. Kricker, A., Armstrong, B.K., English, D.R., et al.: Does intermittent sun exposure cause basal cell carcinoma? A case-control study in Western Australia. Int. J. Cancer **60**(4), 489–494 (1995)

66. Lear, J.T., Heagerty, A.H., Smith, A., et al.: Multiple cutaneous basal cell carcinomas: glutathione *S*-transferase (GSTM1, GSTT1) and cytochrome P450 (CYP2D6, CYP1A1) polymorphisms influence tumor numbers and accrual. Carcinogenesis **17**(9), 1891–1896 (1996)

67. Levi, F., Randimbison, L., Maspoli, M., et al.: High incidence of second basal cell skin cancers. Int. J. Cancer **119**(6), 1505–1507 (2006)

68. Levi, F., Te, V.C., Randimbison, L., et al.: Trends in skin cancer incidence in Vaud: an update, 1976-1998. Eur. J. Cancer Prev. **10**(4), 371–373 (2001)

69. Lovatt, T.J., Lear, J.T., Bastrilles, J., et al.: Associations between UVR exposure and basal cell carcinoma site and histology. Cancer Lett. **216**(2), 191–197 (2004)

70. Lovatt, T.J., Lear, J.T., Bastrilles, J., et al.: Associations between ultraviolet radiation, basal cell carcinoma site and histology, host characteristics, and rate of development of further tumors. J. Am. Acad. Dermatol. **52**(3 pt 1), 468–473 (2005)

71. Marcil, I., Stern, R.S.: Risk of developing a subsequent nonmelanoma skin cancer in patients with a history of nonmelanoma skin cancer: a critical review of the literature and meta-analysis. Arch. Dermatol. **136**(12), 1524–1530 (2000)

72. Marks, R., Foley, P., Goodman, G., et al.: Spontaneous remission of solar keratoses: the case for conservative management. Br. J. Dermatol. **115**(6), 649–655 (1986)

73. Marks, R., Rennie, G., Selwood, T.: The relationship of basal cell carcinomas and squamous cell carcinomas to solar keratoses. Arch. Dermatol. **124**(7), 1039–1042 (1988)

74. Marks, R., Rennie, G., Selwood, T.S.: Malignant transformation of solar keratoses to squamous cell carcinoma. Lancet **1**(8589), 795–797 (1988)

75. McBride, P., Neale, R., Pandeya, N., et al.: Sun-related factors, betapapillomavirus, and actinic keratoses: a prospective study. Arch. Dermatol. **143**(7), 862–868 (2007)

76. McCormack, C.J., Kelly, J.W., Dorevitch, A.P.: Differences in age and body site distribution of the histological subtypes of basal cell carcinoma. A possible indicator of differing causes. Arch. Dermatol. **133**(5), 593–596 (1997)

77. McNaughton, S.A., Marks, G.C., Green, A.C.: Role of dietary factors in the development of basal cell cancer and squamous cell cancer of the skin. Cancer Epidemiol. Biomark. Prev. **14**(7), 1596–1607 (2005)

78. Moore, S., Johnson, N., Pierce, A., et al.: The epidemiology of lip cancer: a review of global incidence and aetiology. Oral Dis. **5**(3), 185–195 (1999)

79. Naldi, L., Chatenoud, L., Piccitto, R., et al.: Prevalence of actinic keratoses and associated factors in a representative sample of the Italian adult population: results from the Prevalence of Actinic Keratoses Italian Study, 2003-2004. Arch. Dermatol. **142**(6), 722–726 (2006)

80. NCCI Non-Melanoma Skin Cancer Working Group: The 2002 National Non-Melanoma Skin Cancer Survey, p. 51. Carlton, National Cancer Control Initiative (2003)

81. Neale, R.E., Davis, M., Pandeya, N., et al.: Basal cell carcinoma on the trunk is associated with excessive sun exposure. J. Am. Acad. Dermatol. **56**(3), 380–386 (2007)

82. Odenbro, A., Bellocco, R., Boffetta, P., et al.: Tobacco smoking, snuff dipping and the risk of cutaneous squamous cell carcinoma: a nationwide cohort study in Sweden. Br. J. Cancer **92**(7), 1326–1328 (2005)

83. Orth, G., Favre, M., Breitburd, F.: Epidermodysplasia verruciformis: a model for the role of papillomaviruses in human cancer. In: Essex, M., Todaro, G., ZurHausen, H. (eds.) Viruses in Naturally Occurring Cancers, pp. 259–282. Cold Spring Harbor Laboratory, Cold Spring Harbor (1980)

84. Pandeya, N., Purdie, D.M., Green, A., et al.: Repeated occurrence of basal cell carcinoma of the skin and multifailure survival analysis: follow-up data from the Nambour Skin Cancer Prevention Trial. Am. J. Epidemiol. **161**(8), 748–754 (2005)

85. Pelucchi, C., Di Landro, A., Naldi, L., et al.: Risk factors for histological types and anatomic sites of cutaneous basal-cell carcinoma: an italian case-control study. J. Invest. Dermatol. **127**(4), 935–944 (2007)

86. Pfister, H.: Chapter 8: Human papillomavirus and skin cancer. J. Natl. Cancer Inst. Monogr. **31**, 52–56 (2003)

87. Plesko, I., Severi, G., Obsitnikova, A., et al.: Trends in the incidence of non-melanoma skin cancer in Slovakia, 1978-1995. Neoplasma **47**(3), 137–142 (2000)

88. Qureshi, A.A., Laden, F., Colditz, G.A., et al.: Geographic variation and risk of skin cancer in US women. Differences between melanoma, squamous cell carcinoma, and basal cell carcinoma. Arch. Intern. Med. **168**(5), 501–507 (2008)

89. Raasch, B.A., Buettner, P.G., Garbe, C.: Basal cell carcinoma: histological classification and body-site distribution. Br. J. Dermatol. **155**(2), 401–407 (2006)

90. Ramachandran, S., Hoban, P.R., Ichii-Jones, F., et al.: Glutathione *S*-transferase GSTP1 and cyclin D1 genotypes: association with numbers of basal cell carcinomas in a patient subgroup at high-risk of multiple tumors. Pharmacogenetics **10**(6), 545–556 (2000)

91. Rebel, H., Kram, N., Westerman, A., et al.: Relationship between UV-induced mutant p53 patches and skin tumors, analysed by mutation spectra and by induction kinetics in various DNA-repair-deficient mice. Carcinogenesis **26**(12), 2123–2130 (2005)

92. Reifenberger, J., Wolter, M., Knobbe, C.B., et al.: Somatic mutations in the PTCH, SMOH, SUFUH and TP53 genes in sporadic basal cell carcinomas. Br. J. Dermatol. **152**(1), 43–51 (2005)

93. Scherer, D., Bermejo, J.L., Rudnai, P., et al.: MC1R variants associated susceptibility to basal cell carcinoma of skin: interaction with host factors and XRCC3 polymorphism. Int. J. Cancer **122**(8), 1787–1793 (2008)

94. Scrivener, Y., Grosshans, E., Cribier, B.: Variations of basal cell carcinomas according to gender, age, location and histopathological subtype. Br. J. Dermatol. **147**(1), 41–47 (2002)

95. Sies, H., Stahl, W.: Nutritional protection against skin damage from sunlight. Annu. Rev. Nutr. **24**, 173–200 (2004)

96. Sorensen, H.T., Mellemkjaer, L., Nielsen, G.L., et al.: Skin cancers and non-hodgkin lymphoma among users of systemic glucocorticoids: a population-based cohort study. J. Natl. Cancer Inst. **96**(9), 709–711 (2004)

97. Stang, A., Ziegler, S., Buchner, U., et al.: Malignant melanoma and nonmelanoma skin cancers in Northrhine-Westphalia, Germany: a patient- vs. diagnosis-based incidence approach. Int. J. Dermatol. **46**(6), 564–570 (2007)

98. Staples, M.P., Elwood, M., Burton, R.C., et al.: Non-melanoma skin cancer in Australia: the 2002 national survey and trends since 1985. Med. J. Aust. **184**(1), 6–10 (2006)

99. Struijk, L., Hall, L., van der Meijden, E., et al.: Markers of cutaneous human papillomavirus infection in individuals with tumor-free skin, actinic keratoses, and squamous cell carcinoma. Cancer Epidemiol. Biomark. Prev. **15**(3), 529–535 (2006)

100. Struijk, L., van der Meijden, E., Kazem, S., et al.: Specific beta-papillomaviruses associated with squamous cell carcinoma of the skin inhibit UVB-induced apoptosis of primary human keratinocytes. J. Gen. Virol. **89**, 2303–2314 (2008)

101. Teh, M.T., Blaydon, D., Chaplin, T., et al.: Genomewide single nucleotide polymorphism microarray mapping in basal cell carcinomas unveils uniparental disomy as a key somatic event. Cancer Res. **65**(19), 8597–8603 (2005)

102. Tilli, C.M., Van Steensel, M.A., Krekels, G.A., et al.: Molecular aetiology and pathogenesis of basal cell carcinoma. Br. J. Dermatol. **152**(6), 1108–1124 (2005)

103. Ulrich, C., Kanitakis, J., Stockfleth, E., et al.: Skin cancer in organ transplant recipients–where do we stand today? Am. J. Transplant. **8**(11), 2192–2198 (2008)

104. van Dam, R.M., Huang, Z., Giovannucci, E., et al.: Diet and basal cell carcinoma of the skin in a prospective cohort of men. Am. J. Clin. Nutr. **71**(1), 135–141 (2000)

105. van der Pols, J.C., Williams, G.M., Pandeya, N., et al.: Prolonged prevention of squamous cell carcinoma of the skin by regular sunscreen use. Cancer Epidemiol. Biomark. Prev. **15**(12), 2546–2548 (2006)

106. Walling, H.W., Persichetti, G.B., Scupham, R.K.: Squamous cell carcinoma in situ arising in a smallpox vaccination scar. Int. J. Dermatol. **47**(6), 599–600 (2008)

107. World Health Organization. and International Agency for Research on Cancer: Some Drinking-Water Disinfectants and Contaminants, Including Arsenic. IARC, Lyon (2004)

108. Yu, H.S., Liao, W.T., Chai, C.Y.: Arsenic carcinogenesis in the skin. J. Biomed. Sci. **13**(5), 657–666 (2006)

109. Zanetti, R., Rosso, S., Martinez, C., et al.: Comparison of risk patterns in carcinoma and melanoma of the skin in men: a multi-centre case-case-control study. Br. J. Cancer **94**(5), 743–751 (2006)

Epidemiology of Malignant Melanoma

1.2

David Whiteman and Adele Green

1.2.1 Introduction

Melanomas are common cancers arising from the pigment cells of the skin. While in situ and locally invasive melanomas are curable by surgery, advanced disease is difficult to treat and can be lethal, as reflected in the rising mortality rates for these cancers [1]. Population-based strategies to control the disease have largely focused on primary prevention and early detection. For such strategies to be implemented, it is imperative that the underlying epidemiology of melanoma is understood. Emerging evidence from diverse disciplines suggests that melanomas may arise through several different causal pathways; characterizing these pathways is crucially important to developing rational approaches for preventing and treating cutaneous melanoma. The aim of this chapter is to briefly describe the patterns of melanoma occurrence, before reviewing recent discoveries that have changed our understanding of the way in which melanoma arises.

1.2.2 Patterns of Melanoma Incidence and Mortality

1.2.2.1 Geographic Variation

Cutaneous melanoma is a cancer mostly afflicting fair-skinned Caucasian populations; however, the incidence of the disease varies enormously depending upon the geographic location of the population under study. Indeed, the variation in melanoma incidence across populations is among the greatest observed for any cancer [2], and this single fact remains the most

persuasive evidence regarding the role of the environment (notably, sunlight) in the causation of this cancer.

The "latitude gradient" for melanoma was first reported by Lancaster [3, 4], and has been a consistently observed feature of melanoma since reliable cancer registrations commenced around the world. Summaries of national melanoma notifications provided to the International Agency for Research on Cancer (IARC) (2002) demonstrate that the highest reported national incidence rates for melanoma occurred in the populations of Australia (39:100,000 per year) and New Zealand (34:100,000 per year). The next highest national melanoma rates were observed in the USA (17:100,000 per year) followed by the Scandinavian countries with rates around 12–15:100,000 per year. Other European populations (e.g., the UK, Germany, Netherlands, Austria, France) reported melanoma rates in the range 4–10:100,000 per year. The predominantly non-Caucasian populations of Africa, Asia, and the Pacific and the mixed populations of Central and South America consistently reported melanoma rates less than 3:100,000 per year.

National figures provide a basis for global comparisons of melanoma incidence, but do not reveal the extremes in melanoma incidence within populations having large subgroups that are heterogeneous for melanoma risk (e.g., within the USA, New Zealand, Israel, and South Africa), nor do they reveal variations in melanoma incidence observed in those nations that span many degrees of latitude (e.g., Australia). In all such jurisdictions, melanoma rates are the highest among the fair-skinned residents with European ancestry (e.g., "non-Hispanic whites" in the USA; "Europeans" in New Zealand) and considerably lower among those with darker skin (e.g., "Hispanics" and "Blacks" in the USA; "Maoris" in New Zealand) [5, 6]. With respect to latitude, those residing at low latitudes tend to experience higher rates of melanoma than those residing at higher latitudes. For example, within Australia, residents of predominantly tropical Queensland (capital city Brisbane, latitude 27°S) have higher melanoma rates (65:100,000 per year) than those residing in New South Wales (capital city Sydney, latitude 34°S; 47:100,000 per year) or Victoria (capital city Melbourne, latitude 38°S, 36:100,000 per year)

D. Whiteman (✉) and A. Green
Cancer and Population Studies, The Queensland Institute
of Medical Research, Royal Brisbane Hospital,
Brisbane, Queensland 4029, Australia
e-mail: david.whiteman@qimr.edu.au; adele.green@qimr.edu.au

R. Dummer et al. (eds.), *Skin Cancer – A World-Wide Perspective*,
DOI: 10.1007/978-3-642-05072-5_1.2, © Springer-Verlag Berlin Heidelberg 2011

[7]. Similar gradients have been observed within the USA, New Zealand, Scandinavia, and other nations [8–10].

A latitude gradient for melanoma is not observed in all regions however; for example, the Caucasian populations of southern Europe (southern Spain, Italy, the Balkans) experience lower rates of melanoma than those prevailing in northern Europe. This phenomenon has been described and explored previously [11], and is widely assumed to reflect the overall darker pigmentary characteristics that predominate within the populations of southern compared with northern Europe.

1.2.2.2 Temporal Trends

1.2.2.2.1 Incidence

During recent decades, the incidence of melanoma has risen rapidly around the world, with increases in the age-standardized incidence of at least 4–6% per annum reported in many fair-skinned populations including Queensland [12], New South Wales [13], the USA [14], Canada [15], Scotland [16], Germany [17], Finland [18], France [19], and most other European nations [20].

The rates of increase have not been uniform across populations however, and even within populations, there have been notable differences in rates of change across anatomical sites, age groups, and birth cohorts. These changes potentially mask some important developments that may herald a turning point in the "epidemic" of melanoma. Thus, in many populations the rates of melanoma have risen more rapidly in men than in women, particularly in older age groups [14, 16, 17]. There are encouraging signs, however, that the incidence of melanoma among young people (<40 years) has stabilized or even declined in several high-incidence populations.

An analysis of US SEER data reported annual percentage changes (APC) for melanoma of +2.4% for men younger than 40 years in the period 1974/75 through to 1988/89, but −2.1% in the period 1990/91 through to 1996/97 [14]. By way of comparison, for men aged more than 60 years, the changes in melanoma incidence for the corresponding periods were +7.0% per annum and +5.2% per annum respectively. These data indicate that while melanoma continues to increase in older men, it would appear that the incidence may be declining in younger men. Notably, melanoma incidence in young US women increased in both time periods.

Melanoma incidence rates across Europe have changed markedly during the past five decades. Recent analyses of European data have identified up to tenfold increases in melanoma incidence in the Scandinavian countries in the five decades since the 1950s, with lesser but still sizeable increases in western European nations [20]. It appears that these trajectories have now leveled off in most northern and western European nations, particularly among more recent birth cohorts. In contrast, while the countries of southern and eastern Europe have experienced relatively small increases in incidence during the past five decades, there is no evidence that the rate of increase has stabilized [20].

Similar to the recent experiences reported from the USA and western Europe, registry data from Queensland and New South Wales in Australia suggest that melanoma incidence has plateaued among young people of both sexes [12, 21], and may be declining [13].

Another notable feature of recent melanoma trends has been the widespread observation of rapid rises in the incidence of in situ, thin, and early-stage melanomas [12, 14, 16, 17, 19, 22]. Such increases have raised concerns about the "over-diagnosis" of melanoma and resurrected the hypothesis that much of the observed increase is due to the increasing rates of diagnosis of a prevalent pool of "non-metasizing" or clinically indolent melanomas [19, 23] (for a full discussion of the concept, see Burton et al. [24, 25]).

1.2.2.2.2 Mortality

As melanoma incidence has risen rapidly in many parts of the world, so has melanoma mortality, albeit at a slower pace. For example, in the USA, melanoma incidence increased by about fivefold between 1950 and 1990, whereas mortality increased by slightly less than twofold during the same period [26]. Similar observations have been made in western and northern Europe [20, 27, 28].

There are data to suggest that melanoma mortality may have peaked in the USA and parts of Europe [20, 26]. In Australia, an analysis conducted in the mid-1990s demonstrated that melanoma mortality was still climbing overall, but that among the youngest birth cohorts, there were early signs of a decline in mortality [29]. The most recent data [30] suggest that between 1989 and 2002, overall melanoma mortality stabilized in Australian males and declined in females (−0.8% per annum). When examined by age, it was found that mortality had declined significantly among those less than 54 years and had stabilized among those aged 55–79 years, but continued to rise among those aged 80 years and older.

1.2.2.3 Age and Sex Distributions

In all populations, melanoma is uncommon before the age of 40 years; thereafter the age-specific incidence climbs steadily and peaks in the seventh and eighth decades [12, 14, 16, 31, 32]. When examined according to the anatomical site of the melanoma, consistent differences emerge, the implications of which are discussed in more detail in Sect. 1.2.4.1 below. In summary, most studies reveal that the peak incidence of melanomas on the trunk occurs at younger ages (fifth to sixth decades) than melanomas arising on the head and neck (eighth decade) [31–35].

The sex distribution of melanoma has varied by population, with high-latitude, low-incidence populations (e.g., Scotland, Canada) historically reporting substantially higher rates among females (of up to twofold in Scotland) [15, 36]. Recently, the patterns of occurrence of melanoma have undergone striking change (see below), and the excess of melanomas observed among females in previous generations in these populations has been ameliorated owing to rapid increases in melanoma incidence among men [15, 16]. In contrast, in most mid- to low-latitude populations (e.g., Australia, the USA), melanoma incidence appears always to have been higher among men and remains so in spite of recent increases in both sexes. In New Zealand, however, melanoma incidence among women was previously higher than men [37], but rapid rises in melanoma incidence among men have resulted in similar rates for men and women.

1.2.2.4   Incidence by Anatomical Site

Early studies reporting on the anatomical distribution of melanoma reported an excess of melanomas on the back and shoulders in men and the lower limbs in women [38–41]. These data were often interpreted as evidence that melanoma was associated predominantly with intermittent patterns of sun exposure. Another approach to compare the incidence of melanoma at different body sites is to adjust for the surface areas of the sites being compared. In so doing, one is comparing the propensity for melanomas to arise *per unit area of skin*. When this is done, the area-adjusted incidence of melanoma is found to be highest on the face in both sexes, and then on the shoulders and back in males and the shoulders, upper arms, and back in females [42]. Negligibly low rates of melanoma are observed on the buttocks and the female scalp [38, 43].

1.2.3   Analytical Epidemiology: Risk Factors for Melanoma

During more than three decades of epidemiologic research, investigators have identified a range of factors that have been associated consistently with melanoma. For comparative

purposes, these are classified as environmental factors and host factors.

1.2.3.1   Environmental Factors

Sunlight (and most particularly the ultraviolet (UV) spectrum of sunlight) is the only environmental factor that has been compellingly implicated as a cause of melanoma. Data from human studies may be summarized as follows:

1. Melanoma incidence is 10–20-fold higher among the fair-skinned than the dark-skinned people [44].
2. Among fair-skinned people, melanoma incidence generally increases with proximity to the equator (some exceptions occur, particularly in continental Europe, where the association is confounded by pigmentation).
3. Fair-skinned migrants from high- (e.g., the UK) to low-latitude countries (e.g., Australia) have lower melanoma rates than native-born residents, and vice versa [45].
4. People with xeroderma pigmentosum (XP) (a disorder in which sufferers have a single gene mutation that abolishes their ability to repair sunlight-induced DNA damage) have 1,000-fold higher risks of melanoma than the average population [46].
5. People with a past history of other types of skin cancer (basal cell carcinomas and squamous cell carcinomas) caused by high doses of solar UV radiation have threefold higher risks of melanoma than the average population [47, 48].
6. Phenotypic measures of sun sensitivity (such as fair skin, freckling, and tendency to burn) confer approximately twofold raised risks of melanoma in all populations [49].

In addition, there is mounting evidence from animal studies that UV radiation is intimately involved in melanoma development ([50]).

1.2.3.1.1   Opposition to the Sunlight Hypothesis

Despite these persuasive findings, the question continually arises as to whether sunlight plays a role in melanoma development (reviewed by Tucker [51]), with some concluding that sunlight plays little, if any, role [52]. Opponents of the "sunlight hypothesis" cite two observations which they claim negate the role of sunlight in melanoma.

Firstly, opponents argue that since the majority of melanomas develop on body sites that are habitually covered by clothing (such as the back and shoulders in males and the lower limb in females), as opposed to sun-exposed sites (such as the face or hands), it follows that most melanomas cannot be caused by sunlight. As described above, the rank order and magnitude of area-adjusted incidence rates for melanoma at specific anatomical sites (see Sect. 1.2.2.4 above) would affirm rather than preclude a role for sunlight in their causation.

The second line of argument against sun exposure as a cause of melanoma has been that case–control studies have typically reported modest associations between measures of past sun exposure and melanoma risk, and a number of meta-analyses have reported inverse associations between measures of chronic or occupational sun exposure and melanoma risk [53].

To interpret the findings of case–control studies, it is important to acknowledge that participants in such studies need to be sampled from within a defined geographic area, which implicitly matches cases and controls on their background level of exposure to ambient solar UV radiation. Thus each separate case–control study is constrained to discriminate across limited ranges of sun exposure when assessed on a global scale (the only exception being if the population has a very high incidence of migration into the study area from other latitudes). This problem is compounded by the lack of reliable, objective methods to assess past exposure to the sun, with consequent misclassification.

Because of these design limitations, a strong argument can be made that ecological studies (demonstrating, for example, the five to tenfold higher rates of melanoma in Queensland than in the ethnically similar population of Scotland [54], or that migrants from low to high solar environments have substantially higher rates of melanoma than pertain in their place of origin [55, 56]) constitute higher-quality evidence than case–control studies for assessing the relationship between sunlight and melanoma. In summary, the case–control method is a strong design for identifying markers of *susceptibility* for melanoma, but it has limited utility for assessing those factors which are strongly determined by the geographic location of the study. (Analogous observations regarding the limitations of the case–control design have been made for studies attempting to identify dietary factors associated with cancer. As for sunlight, the dietary range within each population is small relative to the range across populations [57].)

Accepting that solar UV is a determinant of melanoma, several issues have been the subject of recent inquiry and debate. These include the question of a "critical period" for the development of melanoma, the role of different patterns of sun exposure, and the role of artificial sources of UV radiation.

1.2.3.1.2 The "Critical Period" Hypothesis for Sun Exposure

There has been longstanding speculation that children may be particularly susceptible to the carcinogenic effects of sunlight, and that UV exposure during this time may have more potent effects on the cells of origin for melanoma than sun exposure at older ages. A recent systematic review of the literature assessed the issue of childhood sun exposure by compiling data on two separate groups of studies, ecological (or descriptive) studies and analytical studies [45]. In the former, 20 studies were identified that assessed melanoma risk in relation to measures of ambient sun exposure at different ages; the latter comprised 13 case–control studies that assessed melanoma risk according to recall of sun exposure patterns at different ages. The two groups of studies yielded strikingly different conclusions. Those studies comparing measures of ambient sun exposure consistently reported that the incidence of melanoma was significantly lower among those whose childhoods were spent in environments of low ambient insolation.

Most informative were the studies of fair-skinned migrants from areas of high to low solar irradiance (e.g., from Africa or Pacific Islands to northern Europe). For these migrants, lifetime risks of melanoma remained significantly higher than for native-born residents, despite decades of residence in a low solar environment [58]. In contrast to the consistent and clear findings from the ambient exposure studies, case–control studies relying on recall of individual sun exposure habits differed widely in their findings, and no consistent associations with childhood sun exposure were observed. These discrepant sets of results highlight the difficulties that can arise when interpreting epidemiologic data from different types of studies. In this instance, the studies of ambient exposure were considered more reliable, and hence more likely to reflect a true association, than the studies which measured sun exposure through recall of time outdoors.

While these findings were compatible with childhood being a period of particular susceptibility to sunlight, they could not rule out an independent effect of adult sun exposure. Indeed, adult migrants to Australia still develop melanoma at higher rates than if they had remained in their place of birth. Moreover, melanoma incidence is higher among migrants settling in low-latitude environments (such as Queensland, Australia) compared with higher latitudes (such as Victoria, Australia), and their risk of melanoma continues to increase with longer durations of residence [59]. Each of these observations suggests that sun exposure during adulthood confers additional melanoma risks, over and above any risks accrued through childhood exposure.

1.2.3.1.3 Patterns of Exposure

A prevailing view in the melanoma literature is that "intermittent" exposure to sunlight confers higher risks of melanoma than "chronic" (or occupational) sun exposure [11, 60, 61]. At least three high-quality systematic reviews have addressed this issue, each deriving summary estimates of melanoma risk associated with measures of intermittent and chronic sun exposure [53, 62, 63] Nelemans et al. [62] reviewed 25 published case–control studies and calculated pooled odds ratios of 1.57 (95% CI 1.29–1.91) and 0.73 (95% CI 0.60–0.89) for "intermittent" and "chronic" sunlight exposures respectively. Elwood and Jopson [53] reviewed 29 case–control studies, and calculated an adjusted summary odds ratio of 1.87 (95% CI 1.67–2.09) for "intermittent" sun exposure and 1.18 (95% CI 1.02–1.38) for total sun exposure.

The most recent meta-analysis [63] separately estimated summary relative risks for melanoma associated with measures of "intermittent," "chronic," and "total" sun exposure, and sunburn. Importantly, the authors identified significant heterogeneity of risk estimates for each of these measures of sun exposure, with differences in risk estimates variously associated with country, latitude, and choice of controls. In particular, there was an inverse correlation between latitude and the magnitude of the risk estimate for chronic sun exposure, indicating that chronic patterns of sun exposure are more strongly associated with melanoma risk with increasing proximity to the equator. Given the inherent limitations of retrospective assessments of solar exposure, the heterogeneity of study findings, and the absence of experimental data, definitive statements about the relative carcinogenicity of different patterns of sun exposure cannot be made. Moreover, newly emerging evidence suggests that the relationship between sun exposure and melanoma differs by anatomical site and genotype [64–67], raising new questions about the mechanisms through which sunlight causes melanoma. Since very few individual studies (and no meta-analyses) have assessed the site-specific risk of particular patterns of sun exposure, the epidemiological evidence for a specific effect of exposure pattern must be considered inconclusive at this time.

1.2.3.1.4 Artificial Sources of Ultraviolet Radiation

Because of the ecological and analytical studies linking sun exposure to melanoma and the conclusion that the carcinogenic component of sunlight is UV radiation, one would infer that artificial sources of UV radiation exposure (such as sunbeds and tanning lamps) are also potential causes of melanoma [68]. In a recent systematic review, ten studies were identified (nine case–control; one cohort) that addressed this hypothesis and provided relevant estimates of risk [69]. While there were differences in methodology, the simplest measure of exposure (ever/never exposed) was associated with a summary relative risk of 1.25 (95% CI 1.05–1.49). Young age at first use of sunbeds was associated with significantly increased risk of melanoma (summary OR 1.69, 95% CI 1.32–2.18).

A similar exercise was undertaken by The IARC Working Group on Artificial Sources of Ultraviolet Radiation [70]. That review identified 23 informative studies including 1 cohort study, 14 population-based case–control studies, and 8 hospital-based case–control studies. Similar to the earlier review, the summary risk estimate for ever/never use of sunbeds was 1.15 (95% CI 1.00–1.31), although significant heterogeneity in the risk estimates was noted. Sunbed use before the age of 35 years was associated with a 75% increased risk of melanoma (OR 1.75, 95% CI 1.35–2.26). On the basis of these findings, the IARC Working group concluded that there was evidence of a causal relationship between sunbed exposure and melanoma of sufficient strength to merit changes in policy regarding public access to these sources of UV exposure.

1.2.3.2 Host Factors for Melanoma

Epidemiological studies have consistently shown that a suite of host characteristics are associated with significantly increased risks of melanoma, including numbers of nevi (systematically reviewed by Gandini et al. [71]), tanning ability (systematically reviewed by Bliss et al. [49]), red hair or freckling (systematically reviewed by Bliss et al. [49]), and family history (systematically reviewed by Ford et al. [72]).

Of these factors, the numbers of nevi on the skin confer the highest relative risks for melanoma, with risks increased by up to sevenfold for people with >100 nevi compared with <15 nevi [71]. The role of nevi as risk markers, and possible precursors, for melanoma is discussed in more detail below (Sect. 1.2.4.3).

1.2.3.3 Genes and Melanoma

A brief discussion of the genetic determinants of melanoma is warranted in this chapter since much new information has been generated recently which has direct relevance to our understanding of the interplay of causal factors of this cancer. What follows is a brief account of notable developments and the current state of play with respect to epidemiological risk assessment.

1.2.3.3.1 High-Risk Genes

The clinical observation that up to 10% of people with melanoma had a family history of the disease hinted at an underlying genetic cause and prompted initial efforts to identify kindreds in which melanoma occurred in multiple family members. Using such approaches, genetic epidemiologists identified a region on the short arm of chromosome 9 associated with melanoma [73–75] which was found to map to a region that was also commonly deleted in cancer cell lines (9p21). The deleted locus was later identified as harboring the *CDKN2A* gene. Germline mutations in this gene have since been reported in "melanoma-prone" families worldwide [76–78]. Two other genes have since been identified within the same locus, one of which, *P14ARF*, overlaps *CDKN2A* and shares some coding regions, albeit in a different reading frame. The other candidate high-risk gene, *CDKN2B*, lies very close to *CDKN2A* and shares a similar mechanism of action. The three proteins encoded by these genes (namely, p16^{INK4a}, p14^{ARF}, and p15^{INK4b}) are each potential tumor suppressors, and each plays a role in cell-cycle arrest [79]. Another, very rare, high-penetrance familial melanoma gene, *CDK4* [80], encodes the primary target of p16^{INK4a}. Currently, it appears that each of these genes may play a role in melanoma development, although the weight of evidence favors mutations in *CDKN2A* as the most prevalent germline event in the development of familial melanoma in humans [79].

Early estimates suggested that the penetrance of melanoma among *CDKN2A* carriers was up to 90%; however, recent studies have reported considerably lower risk estimates. For example, a population-based study estimated melanoma penetrance among *CDKN2A* mutation carriers to be 14% at the age of 50 years, 24% at 70 years, and 28% at 80 years [81]. These estimates were derived by comparing the incidence of melanoma among relatives of *CDKN2A* mutation carriers with the incidence of melanoma among relatives of non-carrier probands in a large, multinational cohort of patients with multiple primary melanomas. But even these estimates may be higher than the "true" population penetrance, since they were derived from the experience of relatives of carriers who themselves have had melanoma.

A population-based study in Iceland reported the prevalence of disease-related variants of *CDKN2A* among "healthy" controls in the range 0.08–0.38%, underscoring the notion that penetrance is far from universal, even for "high-risk" genes [82]. There have been reports that the penetrance of melanoma among *CDKN2A* mutation carriers increases with proximity to the equator, suggesting a gene–environment interaction [83], although this conclusion has since been challenged [81]. This is an issue of fundamental importance and clearly warrants further investigation in carefully designed, population-based studies.

Outside of melanoma kindreds, the prevalence of germline *CDKN2A* mutations among patients with "sporadic" melanoma is low. A large, population-based study in Queensland, Australia, found no germline *CDKN2A* mutations among 201 cases of sporadic melanoma [84]. A Canadian study of 254 patients reported an overall prevalence of germline *CDKN2A* mutations of 3.2% [85], although this may be an overestimate because the patients in that study included those likely to have a genetic basis, including patients with a strong family history of melanoma, early-onset disease, multiple primaries, and atypical nevus syndrome. The best estimate to date probably comes from the Icelandic study, which reported frequencies of disease-related variants of around 0.7–1.0% among "sporadic" melanoma cases [81].

Several other genes have been associated with a high risk of melanoma as part of an overall cancer syndrome. Patients with XP have one of several very specific mutations which render them unable to repair UV-damaged DNA. These patients develop cutaneous melanoma at more than thousand times the rate of the normal population [46, 86]. Cowden disease is another autosomal dominant syndrome which is caused by mutation in the *PTEN* gene. Affected individuals develop breast and thyroid cancer predominantly, but also melanoma. There is no evidence that germline *PTEN* mutations account for cases of melanoma outside of this syndrome however [87].

1.2.3.3.2 Low-Risk Genes

Until the recent advent of high-throughput genome-wide scans, the search for "low-risk" melanoma genes had been through the candidate gene approach. Typically these candidates were genes associated with pigmentation, or which encode DNA repair enzymes.

Most interest has focused on the melanocortin-1-receptor gene (*MC1R*), first identified in 1992 as the gene encoding a receptor for the melanocyte-stimulating hormone (MSH) [88]. This complex mediates the production of melanin by melanocytes. Variant *MC1R* genotypes are associated with red hair color and freckling on the skin [89–91]. More than 77 variants of the human *MC1R* gene have been identified [92], of which 3 (Arg151Cys, Arg160Trp, and Asp294His) are designated as "red hair genes." The prevalence of *MC1R* variants is high (50%), even among southern European populations in whom red hair is uncommon [93].

Because *MC1R* genotypes are associated with both red hair and skin type, and because these characteristics are both associated with increased risks of melanoma, a logical extension was to test for an association between *MC1R* genotype and melanoma. Numerous studies have tested this hypothesis; a systematic review and meta-analysis of 11 studies reported risks for melanoma on the order of 1.5–2.5 for seven of the nine *MC1R* variants tested [94]. Highest risks were associated with the Asp294His variant (OR 2.40; 95% CI 1.50–3.84). Unfortunately, that meta-analysis could not assess the effects of *MC1R* independently of the effects of other pigmentation characteristics, and so the magnitude of the risk estimates must be interpreted with caution. One recent study did estimate the extra risk conferred by *MC1R* genotype, over and above the contribution of skin color [95], and found a very modest increment. This suggests that the association of *MC1R* with melanoma is mediated almost entirely through the effects of this gene on pigmentation and not through other pathways.

Other "low-risk" candidate genes that have been investigated for possible associations with melanoma include polymorphisms in various DNA repair genes (e.g., from the XP gene family, *XPC* [96–99], *XPD* [98–100], and *BrCa2* [102] among others). At least one study has reported on risks associated with polymorphisms of the Vitamin D receptor [103]. From an epidemiologic perspective, all published studies to date have been underpowered, and most of the reported associations have been modest. Moreover, any positive associations have generally been observed within subgroups of populations, increasing the likelihood of type 1 error. It is therefore impossible to draw firm conclusions about the role, if any, of the low-risk candidates tested. This is a rapidly moving area however, and it is likely that very soon genome-wide association studies will provide new layers of information. All identified associations (including those already in the literature) will require formal testing in properly designed validation studies with large sample sizes before they can be accepted.

1.2.4 Multiple Causal Pathways to Melanoma?

The preceding sections have described the overall patterns of occurrence and risk factors for melanoma as they have been presented historically. That is, studies have been designed and data have been analyzed under the implicit assumption that all cutaneous melanomas are a single homogeneous group. Parallel lines of inquiry across a range of disciplines have resulted in findings that challenge this assumption, consistent with the view that melanomas are heterogeneous and may arise through several different causal pathways. A brief overview of those earlier findings is presented here, leading to the recently described divergent pathway hypothesis for melanoma.

1.2.4.1 Variations in Site-Specific Incidence of Melanoma with Age

The proposition that melanomas on different body sites might differ in their etiology has been around for at least three decades [104] and was initially based on the observation that people with melanomas of the face were generally older than patients with melanomas at other body sites. Following those anecdotal observations, two descriptive studies independently explored this hypothesis using reliable cancer data in populations with very different underlying rates of melanoma, namely in Canada [33] and New Zealand [37]. Importantly, both studies used similar methodology by adjusting the incidence of melanoma at different body sites for the relative surface area of each site. Both studies found that the area-adjusted incidence of melanomas in young adults was considerably higher on the trunk than the head and neck. Thereafter, melanoma on the trunk continued to rise steadily in adulthood, peaked in late middle age, and then declined slightly in older age groups. In contrast, the area-adjusted incidence of head and neck melanoma was low among the young and middle-aged, but then rose very rapidly among older age groups to far exceed the rate of melanoma on the trunk. These concordant findings from disparate populations suggested that the age dependence of melanoma by anatomical site is a real effect, possibly reflecting different subsets of tumors.

1.2.4.2 Risk Factors for Melanoma at Different Anatomical Sites

Several analytic studies conducted during the 1980s and 1990s performed post hoc analyses in which risk factors for melanoma were examined according to the anatomical site of the tumor. While the studies were not specifically designed to assess site-specific differences in melanoma risk, they nevertheless consistently reported that melanomas on the trunk or legs were statistically associated with high nevus counts, whereas melanomas on the head and neck were not [105–108]. In a case–control study in New South Wales, Australia, Bataille et al. [109] observed that patients with melanomas of the head and neck had substantially fewer nevi and more solar keratoses than patients with melanomas of the trunk or legs.

At about the same time, an immunohistochemical analysis of melanoma was reported which hinted at quite distinct patterns of risk factors based on the presence or absence of p53 immunoexpression [110]. Melanomas over-expressing p53 protein were found to occur more frequently on the head and neck than melanomas without evidence of p53 expression, and were associated with older age and high counts of solar keratoses. Further, p53 immunonegative melanomas occurred more commonly on the trunk, and were associated with greater numbers of nevi. These data suggested that the molecular profile of melanomas, at least in relation to p53 expression, may reflect their causal origins and provided a novel basis by which melanomas might be classified beyond their histological appearances.

1.2.4.3 Nevus-Associated Melanomas Differ from Other Melanomas

At about the same time as the risk factor studies, dermatopathologists began to note that melanomas with evidence of neval remnants had different characteristics from melanomas without such remnants. Depending upon the series, around 25% of cutaneous melanomas have remnants of neval tissue upon histological examination [106, 111–114]. The co-occurrence of these two histological entities (melanoma and nevus) is substantially higher than expected assuming a random distribution of melanomas and nevi on the skin surface [115, 116], and is certainly higher than the co-occurrence of nevi with other tumors of the skin [116]. Green first proposed the concept that melanomas arising from nevi may reflect a distinct pathway for the origins of these cancers, and suggested that the propensity for malignant progression was determined, at least in part, by the anatomical site of the target cell [117]. An analysis of pathology reports provided support for this theory [42]. Several other groups also investigated the anatomical distribution of melanoma with contiguous neval remnants (hereafter "CN+ melanoma") compared with other melanomas without neval remnants (CN− melanoma). Each study found that CN+ melanomas occur more commonly on the trunk than on the head and neck [106, 114, 116]. Further, patients with CN+ melanomas were significantly more likely to have high nevus counts and to report episodes of severe sunburn than controls [115]. In contrast, CN− melanoma patients were significantly more likely than controls to have red or blond hair, but had similar histories of sunburn and only modestly higher nevus counts. These observations suggest that CN+ melanomas differ from CN− melanomas in their association with phenotypic and environmental risk factors, and provided new insights into the likely multiplicity of pathways through which melanomas can arise [117].

In a histological review of 943 melanoma specimens from three study sites in Ontario and British Columbia (Canada) and New South Wales (Australia), 36% had contiguous neval remnants [118]. Patients with CN+ melanomas were significantly more likely to have high nevus counts and their tumors were more likely to arise on the trunk. In contrast, CN− melanomas were more likely among older people, among LMM subtypes, among those with melanomas arising on the head and neck, and those with pronounced solar elastosis. Very similar patterns of association for CN+ and CN− melanomas were also reported in another independent study [119], thereby confirming earlier reports.

1.2.4.4 Population Heterogeneity in Nevus Burden

Because of the close epidemiologic and histologic association between nevi and melanoma, there has been much research into the origins of these benign melanocytic tumors. Studies in environments of low ambient sunlight [120–123] and high ambient sunlight [124–127] have reported that children exposed to high levels of sunlight, however measured, have greater numbers of nevi than those who report lower levels of exposure. Moreover, studies which have used common protocols to count nevi on children from similar ethnic backgrounds residing in areas of differing ambient UVR consistently report significantly higher nevus counts among those children residing in higher solar environments [128, 129].

A strong genetic contribution to nevus burden is also apparent, based on the findings of twin studies conducted in high- and low-solar environments [130, 131]. Because monozygotic (MZ, or identical) twin pairs share all of their genes, whereas dizygotic (DZ, or fraternal) twin pairs share only half of their genes on average, comparisons of the within-pair correlations of nevus counts for MZ and DZ twins permit inferences about heritability. The heritability estimates for nevus counts among twins residing in Australia and the UK were strikingly similar (MZ twins $r \sim 0.94$; DZ twins $r \sim 0.60$), despite the very large differences in insolation between Australia and the UK, and the systematically higher nevus counts among Australian twins.

Taken together, these studies demonstrate the importance of both sunlight and genes as determinants of nevi. They show that within fair-skinned populations, there exist some people with a high propensity to develop nevi, while others have a low propensity, and that this propensity is genetically determined. The degree of expression of the phenotype ("nevus burden") is then determined by the ambient solar radiation of the environment in which an individual resides and modified by their outdoor exposure.

1.2.4.5 The Hypothesis of Divergent Causal Pathways to Melanoma

By the close of the 1990s, the collected findings from studies across the epidemiologic spectrum suggested that cutaneous melanomas were not a single homogeneous entity. Moreover, the nevus heritability studies indicated that a person's tendency for nevus development (a putative proxy for melanocytic proliferative capacity, and hence melanoma susceptibility) was under strong genetic control. These observations led to the "divergent pathway hypothesis" for melanoma, which proposes that people with an inherently low propensity for melanocyte proliferation (identified by low nevus counts) develop melanoma through chronic exposure to sunlight [110, 132]. In contrast, among people having an inherently high propensity for melanocyte proliferation (identified by high nevus counts), the hypothesis predicts that sun exposure is required only to initiate melanoma development, after which inherited host factors supervene to drive progression of the tumor. Among this latter group, melanomas are expected to develop on body sites with unstable melanocyte populations such as the trunk, and will do so at younger ages. In the relatively brief interval since the hypothesis was first proposed, there have been numerous studies that tested melanomas using a variety of approaches.

1.2.4.5.1 Ecological Studies

A number of studies have tested the divergent pathway model by comparing the age-specific incidence of melanoma by anatomic site. Lachiewicz et al. [31] compared the age-specific incidence curve for melanomas arising on the trunk with those arising on the head and neck for 48,673 melanoma patients notified to the US SEER registries between 2000 and 2004. Strikingly different curves were observed by body site, with the age distribution of melanomas of the trunk peaking 10 years before those of the face and ear (64 vs. 74 years).

A Swiss study compared the relative melanoma density (RMD) by anatomical site and age group [133] (the RMD is the ratio of the "observed" to the "expected" number of melanomas at any given anatomical site, and where the "expected" number is that which would be anticipated at that site assuming an even distribution of tumors over the whole body surface). Among those aged less than 50 years, melanomas occurred most densely on the trunk in both males and females whereas in those aged more than 65 years, RMD was highest on the face and lowest on the thighs and buttocks. Similar analyses with ostensibly the same findings have since been reported from Sweden [35], Scotland, and Australia [54]. Overall, these studies provide strong evidence that melanomas tend to arise on the trunk at younger ages and on the face and head at older ages, and that this phenomenon occurs in all populations.

1.2.4.5.2 Risk Factor Studies

Several studies have directly tested the divergent pathway hypothesis for melanoma by comparing the prevalence of risk factors within subgroups of melanoma patients. Using data from 178,153 eligible participants followed up within three large, prospective studies, Cho et al. assessed risk factors for melanoma across anatomical sites [134]. Significant differences in melanoma risk across anatomical sites were seen, especially for associations with nevi (test for heterogeneity $p = 0.04$). High nevus counts were more strongly associated with melanomas of the trunk (OR 4.67) than the head (OR 3.45) or upper (OR 2.50) or lower limbs (OR 2.00).

Two publications arising from a large, hospital-based case–control study in Italy concluded that they did not find evidence of differences in risk factors by anatomical site. The first publication estimated the relative risks associated with various measures of past sun exposure (numbers of sunburns etc.) and phenotype (hair color, eye color, numbers of nevi) for melanomas at different anatomical sites [135]. Some modest variations in the magnitude of association were noted for some exposures, but overall, there was no statistically significant evidence of heterogeneity by body site. The second publication assessed the risks of site-specific melanomas associated with nevus counts at specific anatomical sites [136] and reported that people with higher nevus counts had higher risks of melanomas of the trunk than other sites. So, while the authors concluded that their data did not support differences in melanoma risk by site, their data confirm the findings of earlier studies that people with large numbers of nevi are more likely to develop melanomas on the trunk than on the head and neck.

1.2.4.5.3 Somatic Mutation Studies

Much work has been undertaken to document the molecular phenotypes of melanoma since the original observations of Maldonado [66] that *BRAF* mutations are more strongly associated with melanomas from non-sun-exposed sites than from sun-exposed sites. Those original findings have been confirmed in subsequent studies [137, 138] and it is now clear that *BRAF* mutant melanomas are associated with particular phenotypic and sun-exposure attributes, including high nevus counts, truncal location, and young age [139, 140]. Interestingly, both studies have also reported that *BRAF* mutant melanomas have stronger associations with early life sun exposure than wild-type melanoma, consistent with a role for sunlight in initiating these tumors in early life. Such a pathway is supported by the finding that *BRAF* mutations are also more likely in melanomas with histological evidence of contiguous neval remnants [141, 142]. The supposition that *BRAF* mutations in nevocytes are acquired following sun exposure in early life has been given indirect support from an intricate study comparing *BRAF* mutations in two types of "congenital" nevi. The investigators reported that none of 32 nevi that were present at birth were found to harbor BRAF mutations [143]. In contrast, 20 of 28 (71%) of the melanocytic nevi with a "congenital pattern" but that were known to have arisen in childhood showed the common BRAF V600E mutation.

Recently, interest has focused on identifying possible genetic modifiers of *BRAF* mutation, with some evidence that constitutional *MC1R* variants confer a substantially increased risk of such mutations among people with only limited amounts of sun exposure [144]. Such findings await confirmation in large, population-based studies however, since the numbers of participants examined to date have been small and the resultant risk estimates have been imprecise. With the advent of high-throughput technologies, molecular studies of this type are being reported with increasing frequency, and it is inevitable that these gene–gene and gene–environment associations will be clarified in due course. For the moment, the emerging picture appears largely congruent with the concept that distinct subsets of melanomas can be defined on the basis of their molecular phenotype, and that these phenotypes are associated with different risk factors.

1.2.5 Conclusions

Melanomas are epidermal cancers arising predominantly in fair-skinned people. The incidence of melanoma has risen rapidly in many populations during recent decades, and rates continue to rise in most populations. Encouraging trends in Australia and the USA suggest that melanoma rates may have stabilized among younger people, and these trends will be closely monitored. Such trends might be anticipated in northern and western Europe; continued surveillance in these areas is required.

The principal environmental determinant of cutaneous melanoma is sunlight, with incidence rates varying more than tenfold between ethnically similar populations residing in environments with different levels of ambient sunlight. Epidemiological studies have identified a number of phenotypic risk factors for melanoma, many of which appear to be genetically determined. Recent studies suggest that epidermal melanocytes develop into malignant tumors through more than one pathway, as evidenced by differing molecular profiles, anatomical distributions, and risk factor profiles for subgroups of melanomas. This field is moving rapidly, and it is likely that in the near future, a clearer understanding of the molecular origins of melanomas will be delivered. It is hoped that such knowledge will be of value in designing interventions to control this cancer.

References

1. Ries, L.A.G., Eisner, M.P., Kosary, C.L., Hankey, B.F., Miller, B.A., Clegg, L., et al.: SEER Cancer Statistics Review, 1973–1997. National Cancer Institute, Bethesda (2000)
2. Fraumeni Jr., J.F.: Genes and the Environment in Cancer Causation. National Cancer Institute, Washington (2007)
3. Lancaster, H.O.: Some geographical aspects of the mortality from melanoma in Europeans. Med. J. Aust. **1**, 1082–1087 (1956)
4. Lancaster, H.O., Nelson, J.: Sunlight as a cause of melanoma: a clinical survey. Med. J. Aust. **1**, 452–456 (1957)
5. Deapen, D., Bernstein, L., Liu, L., Kerford, D., Balcius, P., Morrell, D., et al.: Cancer incidence in Los Angeles county. In: Curado, M.P., Edwards, B., Shin, H.R., Storm, H., Ferlay, J., Heanue, M. (eds.) Cancer Incidence in Five Continents, vol. IX. IARC Scientific, Lyon (2007)
6. Ministry of Health: Cancer in New Zealand: Trends and Projections. Ministry of Health, Wellington (2002)
7. Australian Institute of Health and Welfare (AIHW). ACIM (Australian Cancer Incidence and Mortality) Books. AIHW. Canberra (2010)
8. Crombie, I.K.: Variation of melanoma incidence with latitude in North America and Europe. Br. J. Cancer **40**, 774–781 (1979)
9. Bulliard, J.L., Cox, B., Elwood, J.M.: Latitude gradients in melanoma incidence and mortality in the non-Maori population of New Zealand. Cancer Causes Control **5**, 234–240 (1994)
10. Magnus, K.: Incidence of malignant melanoma of the skin in Norway, 1955–1970: Variations in time and space and solar radiation. Cancer **32**, 1275–1286 (1973)
11. Armstrong, B.K.: Epidemiology of malignant melanoma: intermittent or total accumulated exposure to the sun. J. Dermatol. Surg. Oncol. **14**, 835–849 (1988)
12. Coory, M., Baade, P., Aitken, J., Smithers, M., McLeod, G.R., Ring, I.: Trends for in situ and invasive melanoma in Queensland, Australia, 1982–2002. Cancer Causes Control **17**(1), 21–27 (2006)
13. Marrett, L.D., Nguyen, H.L., Armstrong, B.K.: Trends in the incidence of cutaneous malignant melanoma in New South Wales, 1983–1996. Int. J. Cancer **92**(3), 457–462 (2001)
14. Jemal, A., devesa, S.S., Fears, T.R., Hartge, P., Tucker, M.A.: Recent trends in cutaneous melanoma incidence among whites in the United States. J. Natl. Cancer Inst. **93**, 678–683 (2001)
15. Ulmer, M.J., Tonita, J.M., Hull, P.R.: Trends in invasive cutaneous melanoma in Saskatchewan 1970–1999. J. Cutan. Med. Surg. **7**(6), 433–442 (2003)
16. MacKie, R.M., Bray, C.A., Hole, D.J.: Incidence and survival from malignant melanoma in Scotland. Lancet **360**, 587–591 (2002)
17. Lasithiotakis, K.G., Leiter, U., Gorkievicz, R., Eigentler, T., Breuninger, H., Metzler, G., et al.: The incidence and mortality of cutaneous melanoma in Southern Germany: trends by anatomic site and pathologic characteristics, 1976 to 2003. Cancer **107**(6), 1331–1339 (2006)
18. Stang, A., Pukkala, E., Sankila, R., Soderman, B., Hakulinen, T.: Time trend analysis of the skin melanoma incidence of Finland from 1953 through 2003 including 16,414 cases. Int. J. Cancer **119**(2), 380–384 (2006)
19. Lipsker, D., Engel, F., Cribier, B., Velten, M., Hedelin, G.: Trends in melanoma epidemiology suggest three different types of melanoma. Br. J. Dermatol. **157**(2), 338–343 (2007)
20. de Vries, E., Bray, F.I., Coebergh, J.W., Parkin, D.M.: Changing epidemiology of malignant cutaneous melanoma in Europe 1953–1997: rising trends in incidence and mortality but recent stabilizations in western Europe and decreases in Scandinavia. Int. J. Cancer **107**(1), 119–126 (2003)
21. Whiteman, D.C., Bray, C.A., Siskind, V., Green, A.C., Hole, D.J., Mackie, R.M.: Changes in the incidence of cutaneous melanoma in the west of Scotland and Queensland, Australia: hope for health promotion? Eur. J. Cancer Prev. **17**(3), 243–250 (2008)
22. Garbe, C., McLeod, G.R., Buettner, P.G.: Time trends of cutaneous melanoma in Queensland, Australia and Central Europe. Cancer **89**(6), 1269–1278 (2000)
23. Welch, H.G., Woloshin, S., Schwartz, L.M.: Skin biopsy rates and incidence of melanoma: population based ecological study. Br. Med. J. **331**(7515), 481 (2005)
24. Burton, R.C., Coates, M.S., Hersey, P., Roberts, G., Chetty, M.P., Chen, S., et al.: An analysis of a melanoma epidemic. Int. J. Cancer **55**, 765–776 (1993)
25. Burton, R.C., Armstrong, B.K.: Recent incidence trends imply a nonmetastasizing form of invasive melanoma. Melanoma Res. **4**(2), 107–113 (1994)

26. Jemal, A., Devesa, S.S., Fears, T.R., Hartge, P.: Cancer surveillance series: changing patterns of cutaneous malignant melanoma mortality rates among whites in the United States. J. Natl. Cancer Inst. **92**(10), 811–818 (2000)

27. de Vries, E., Bray, F.I., Eggermont, A.M., Coebergh, J.W.: Monitoring stage-specific trends in melanoma incidence across Europe reveals the need for more complete information on diagnostic characteristics. Eur. J. Cancer Prev. **13**(5), 387–395 (2004)

28. de Vries, E., Coebergh, J.W.: Cutaneous malignant melanoma in Europe. Eur. J. Cancer **40**(16), 2355–2366 (2004)

29. Giles, G.G., Armstrong, B.K., Burton, R.C., Staples, M.J., Thursfield, V.J.: Has mortality from melanoma stopped rising in Australia? Analysis of trends between 1931 and 1994. Br. Med. J. **312**, 1121–1125 (1996)

30. Baade, P., Coory, M.: Trends in melanoma mortality in Australia: 1950–2002 and their implications for melanoma control. Aust. N. Z. J. Public Health **29**(4), 383–386 (2005)

31. Lachiewicz, A.M., Berwick, M., Wiggins, C.L., Thomas, N.E.: Epidemiologic support for melanoma heterogeneity using the surveillance, epidemiology, and end results program. J. Invest. Dermatol. **128**(5), 1340–1342 (2008)

32. Stang, A., Stabenow, R., Eisinger, B., Jockel, K.H.: Site- and gender-specific time trend analyses of the incidence of skin melanomas in the former German Democratic Republic (GDR) including 19351 cases. Eur. J. Cancer **39**(11), 1610–1618 (2003)

33. Elwood, J.M., Gallagher, R.P.: Body site distribution of cutaneous malignant melanoma in relationship to patterns of sun exposure. Int. J. Cancer **78**, 276–280 (1998)

34. Bulliard, J.-L.: Site-specific risk of cutaneous malignant melanoma and pattern of sun exposure in New Zealand. Int. J. Cancer **85**, 627–632 (2000)

35. Perez-Gomez, B., Aragones, N., Gustavsson, P., Lope, V., Lopez-Abente, G., Pollan, M.: Do sex and site matter? Different age distribution in melanoma of the trunk among Swedish men and women. Br. J. Dermatol. **158**(4), 766–772 (2008)

36. MacKie, R., Hunter, J.A., Aitchison, T.C., Hole, D., McLaren, K., Rankin, R.: Cutaneous malignant melanoma, Scotland, 1979–89. The Scottish Melanoma Group. Lancet **339**, 971–975 (1992)

37. Bulliard, J.L., Cox, B.: Cutaneous malignant melanoma in New Zealand: trends by anatomical site, 1969–1993. Int. J. Epidemiol. **29**(3), 416–423 (2000)

38. Osterlind, A., Hou-Jensen, K., Moller-Jensen, O.: Incidence of cutaneous malignant melanoma in Denmark 1978–1982. Anatomic site distribution, histologic types and comparison with non-melanoma skin cancer. Br. J. Cancer **58**, 385–391 (1988)

39. Magnus, K.: Habits of sun exposure and risk of malignant melanoma: an analysis of incidence rates in Norway 1955–1977 by cohort, sex, age and primary tumor site. Cancer **48**, 2329–2335 (1981)

40. Popescu, N.A., Beard, C.M., Treacy, P.J., Winkelmann, R.K., O'Brien, P.C., Kurland, L.T.: Cutaneous malignant melanoma in Rochester, Minnesota: trends in incidence and survivorship, 1950 through 1985. Mayo Clin. Proc. **65**, 1293–1302 (1990)

41. Masback, A., Westerdahl, J., Ingvar, C., Olsson, H., Jonsson, N.: Cutaneous malignant melanoma in South Sweden 1965, 1975, and 1985. A histopathologic review. Cancer **73**, 1625–1630 (1994)

42. Green, A., MacLennan, R., Youl, P., Martin, N.: Site distribution of cutaneous melanoma in Queensland. Int. J. Cancer **53**, 232–236 (1993)

43. Chen, Y.T., Zheng, T., Holford, T.R., Berwick, M., Dubrow, R.: Malignant melanoma incidence in Connecticut (United States): time trends and age-period-cohort modeling by anatomic site. Cancer Causes Control **5**, 341–350 (1994)

44. Armstrong, B.K., Kricker, A.: How much melanoma is caused by sun exposure? Melanoma Res. **3**, 395–401 (1993)

45. Whiteman, D.C., Whiteman, C.A., Green, A.C.: Childhood sun exposure as a risk factor for melanoma: a systematic review of epidemiologic studies. Cancer Causes Control **12**, 69–82 (2001)

46. Kraemer, K.H., Lee, M.M., Andrews, A.D., Lambert, W.C.: The role of sunlight and DNA repair in melanoma and nonmelanoma skin cancer. The xeroderma pigmentosum paradigm. Arch. Dermatol. **130**, 1018–1021 (1994)

47. Green, A.C., O'Rourke, M.G.E.: Cutaneous malignant melanoma in association with other skin cancers. J. Natl. Cancer Inst. **74**, 977–980 (1985)

48. Levi, F., Randimbison, L., La-Vecchia, C., Erler, G., Te, V.C.: Incidence of invasive cancers following squamous cell skin cancer. Am. J. Epidemiol. **146**(9), 734–739 (1997)

49. Bliss, J.M., Ford, D., Swerdlow, A.J., Armstrong, B.K., Cristofolini, M., Elwood, J.M., et al.: Risk of cutaneous melanoma associated with pigmentation characteristics and freckling: systematic overview of 10 case-control studies. Int. J. Cancer **62**, 367–376 (1995)

50. Noonan FP, Recio JA, Takayama H, et al. Neonatal sunburn and melanoma in mice. Nature. Sep 20 2001;413(6853):271–272.

51. Tucker, M.A.: Is sunlight important to melanoma causation? Cancer Epidemiol. Biomarkers Prev. **17**(3), 467–468 (2008)

52. Shuster, S.: Is sun exposure a major cause of melanoma? No. Br. Med. J. **337**, a764 (2008)

53. Elwood, J.M., Jopson, J.: Melanoma and sun exposure: an overview of published studies. Int. J. Cancer **73**(2), 198–203 (1997)

54. Whiteman, D.C., Bray, C.A., Siskind, V., Hole, D., MacKie, R.M., Green, A.C.: A comparison of the anatomic distribution of cutaneous melanoma in two populations with different levels of sunlight: the west of Scotland and Queensland, Australia 1982–2001. Cancer Causes Control **18**(5), 485–491 (2007)

55. Cooke, K.R., Fraser, J.: Migration and death from malignant melanoma. Int. J. Cancer **36**(2), 175–178 (1985)

56. Khlat, M., Vail, A., Parkin, M., Green, A.: Mortality from melanoma immigrants to Australia: variation by age at arrival and duration of stay. Am. J. Epidemiol. **135**, 1103–1113 (1992)

57. Wynder, E.L., Stellman, S.D.: The "over-exposed" control group. Am. J. Epidemiol. **135**, 459–461 (1992)

58. Autier, P., Dore, J.F.: Influence of sun exposures during childhood and during adulthood on melanoma risk. EPIMEL and EORTC Melanoma Cooperative Group. European Organisation for Research and Treatment of Cancer. Int. J. Cancer **77**(4), 533–537 (1998)

59. Dobson, A.J., Leeder, S.R.: Mortality from malignant melanoma in Australia: effects due to country of birth. Int. J. Epidemiol. **11**(3), 207–211 (1982)

60. Elwood, J.M., Gallagher, R.P., Hill, G.B., Pearson, J.C.: Cutaneous melanoma in relation to intermittent and constant sun exposure–the Western Canada Melanoma Study. Int. J. Cancer **35**, 427–433 (1985)

61. Osterlind, A., Tucker, M.A., Stone, B.J., Jensen, O.M.: The Danish case-control study of cutaneous malignant melanoma. II. Importance of UV-light exposure. Int. J. Cancer **42**, 319–324 (1988)

62. Nelemans, P.J., Rampen, F.H.J., Ruiter, D.J., Verbeek, A.L.M.: An addition to the controversy on sunlight exposure and melanoma risk: a meta-analytical approach. J. Clin. Epidemiol. **48**, 1331–1342 (1995)

63. Gandini, S., Sera, F., Cattaruzza, M.S., Pasquini, P., Picconi, O., Boyle, P., et al.: Meta-analysis of risk factors for cutaneous melanoma: II. Sun exposure. Eur. J. Cancer **41**(1), 45–60 (2005)

64. Whiteman, D.C., Stickley, M., Watt, P., Hughes, M.C., Davis, M.B., Green, A.C.: Anatomic site, sun exposure, and risk of cutaneous melanoma. J. Clin. Oncol. **24**(19), 3172–3177 (2006)

65. Rivers, J.K.: Is there more than one road to melanoma? Lancet **363**(9410), 728–730 (2004)

66. Maldonado, J.L., Fridlyand, J., Patel, H., Jain, A.N., Busam, K., Kageshita, T., et al.: Determinants of BRAF mutations in primary melanomas. J. Natl. Cancer Inst. **95**(24), 1878–1890 (2003)

67. Curtin, J.A., Fridlyand, J., Kageshita, T., Patel, H.N., Busam, K.J., Kutzner, H., et al.: Distinct sets of genetic alterations in melanoma. N. Engl. J. Med. **353**(20), 2135–2147 (2005)

68. Gallagher, R.: Sunbeds–do they increase risk of melanoma or not? Eur. J. Cancer **41**(14), 2038–2039 (2005)

69. Gallagher, R.P., Spinelli, J.J., Lee, T.K.: Tanning beds, sunlamps, and risk of cutaneous malignant melanoma. Cancer Epidemiol. Biomarkers Prev. **14**(3), 562–566 (2005)

70. IARC Working Group on Risk of Skin Cancer and Exposure to Artificial Ultraviolet Light: Exposure to Artificial UV Radiation and Skin Cancer. International Agency for Research on Cancer, Lyon (2005)

71. Gandini, S., Sera, F., Cattaruzza, M.S., Pasquini, P., Abeni, D., Boyle, P., et al.: Meta-analysis of risk factors for cutaneous melanoma: I. Common and atypical naevi. Eur. J. Cancer **41**(1), 28–44 (2005)

72. Ford, D., Bliss, J.M., Swerdlow, A.J., et al.: Risk of cutaneous melanoma associated with a family history of the disease. Int. J. Cancer **62**, 377–381 (1995)

73. Petty, E.M., Gibson, L.H., Fountain, J.W., Bologna, J.L., Yang-Feng, T.L., Housman, D.E., et al.: Molecular definition of a chromosome 9p21 germ-line deletion in a woman with multiple melanomas and a plexiform neurofibroma: implications for 9p tumor-suppressor gene(s). Am. J. Hum. Genet. **53**(1), 96–104 (1993)

74. Cannon-Albright, L.A., Goldgar, D.E., Meyer, L.J., et al.: Assignment of a locus for familial melanoma,MLM, to chromosome 9p13-p22. Science **258**, 1148–1152 (1992)

75. Nancarrow, D.J., Mann, G.J., Holland, E.A., et al.: Confirmation of chromosome 9p linkage in familial melanoma. Am. J. Hum. Genet. **53**, 936–942 (1993)

76. Gruis, N.A., van der Velden, P.A., Sandkuijl, L.A., et al.: Homozygotes for CDKN2 (p16) germline mutation in Dutch familial melanoma kindreds. Nat. Genet. **10**, 351–353 (1995)

77. Harland, M., Meloni, R., Gruis, N., Pinney, E., Brookes, S., Spurr, N.K., et al.: Germline mutations of the CDKN2 gene in UK melanoma families. Hum. Mol. Genet. **6**(12), 2061–2067 (1997)

78. Hussussian, C., Struewing, J.P., Goldstein, A.M., et al.: Germline p16 mutations in familial melanoma. Nat. Genet. **8**, 15–21 (1994)

79. Peters, G.: Tumor suppression for ARFicionados: the relative contributions of p16INK4a and p14ARF in melanoma. J. Natl. Cancer Inst. **100**(11), 757–759 (2008)

80. Zuo, L., Weger, J., Yang, Q., Goldstein, A.M., Tucker, M.A., Walker, G.J., et al.: Germline mutations in the p16INK4a binding domain of CDK4 in familial melanoma. Nat. Genet. **12**(1), 97–99 (1996)

81. Begg, C.B., Orlow, I., Hummer, A.J., Armstrong, B.K., Kricker, A., Marrett, L.D., et al.: Lifetime risk of melanoma in CDKN2A mutation carriers in a population-based sample. J. Natl. Cancer Inst. **97**(20), 1507–1515 (2005)

82. Goldstein, A.M., Stacey, S.N., Olafsson, J.H., Jonsson, G.F., Helgason, A., Sulem, P., et al.: CDKN2A mutations and melanoma risk in the Icelandic population. J. Med. Genet. **45**(5), 284–289 (2008)

83. Bishop, D.T., Demenais, F., Goldstein, A.M., Bergman, W., Bishop, J.N., Paillerets Bressac-de, B., et al.: Geographical variation in the penetrance of CDKN2A mutations for melanoma. J. Natl. Cancer Inst. **94**(12), 894–903 (2002)

84. Aitken, J., Welch, J., Duffy, D., Milligan, A., Green, A., Martin, N., et al.: CDKN2A variants in a population-based sample of Queensland families with melanoma. J. Natl. Cancer Inst. **91**(5), 446–452 (1999)

85. Ung-Juurlink, C.: American Academy of Dermatology 1999 Awards for Young Investigators in Dermatology. The prevalence of CDKN2A in patients with atypical nevi and malignant melanoma. J. Am. Acad. Dermatol. **41**(3), 461–462 (1999)

86. Kraemer, K.H.: Sunlight and skin cancer: another link revealed. Proc. Natl. Acad. Sci. U S A **94**(1), 11–14 (1997)

87. Boni, R., Vortmeyer, A.O., Burg, G., Hofbauer, G., Zhuang, Z.: The PTEN tumour suppressor gene and malignant melanoma. Melanoma Res. **8**(4), 300–302 (1998)

88. Chhajlani, V., Wikberg, J.E.: Molecular cloning and expression of the human melanocyte stimulating hormone receptor cDNA. FEBS Lett. **309**(3), 417–420 (1992)

89. Valverde, P., Healy, E., Jackson, I., Rees, J.L., Thody, A.J.: Variants of the melanocyte-stimulating hormone receptor gene are associated with red hair and fair skin in humans. Nat. Genet. **11**, 328–330 (1995)

90. Smith, R., Healy, E., Siddiqui, S., Flanagan, N., Steijlen, P.M., Rosdahl, I., et al.: Melanocortin 1 receptor variants in an Irish population. J. Invest. Dermatol. **111**(1), 119–122 (1998)

91. Box, N.F., Wyeth, J.R., O'Gorman, L.E., Martin, N.G., Sturm, R.A.: Characterization of melanocyte stimulating hormone receptor variant alleles in twins with red hair. Hum. Mol. Genet. **6**(11), 1891–1897 (1997)

92. Wong, T.H., Rees, J.L.: The relation between melanocortin 1 receptor (MC1R) variation and the generation of phenotypic diversity in the cutaneous response to ultraviolet radiation. Peptides **26**(10), 1965–1971 (2005)

93. Stratigos, A.J., Dimisianos, G., Nikolaou, V., Poulou, M., Sypsa, V., Stefanaki, I., et al.: Melanocortin receptor-1 gene polymorphisms and the risk of cutaneous melanoma in a low-risk southern European population. J. Invest. Dermatol. **126**(8), 1842–1849 (2006)

94. Raimondi, S., Sera, F., Gandini, S., Iodice, S., Caini, S., Maisonneuve, P., et al.: MC1R variants, melanoma and red hair color phenotype: a meta-analysis. Int. J. Cancer **122**(12), 2753–2760 (2008)

95. Dwyer, T., Stankovich, J.M., Blizzard, L., FitzGerald, L.M., Dickinson, J.L., Reilly, A., et al.: Does the addition of information on genotype improve prediction of the risk of melanoma and non-melanoma skin cancer beyond that obtained from skin phenotype? Am. J. Epidemiol. **159**(9), 826–833 (2004)

96. Zhang, D., Chen, C., Fu, X., Gu, S., Mao, Y., Xie, Y., et al.: A meta-analysis of DNA repair gene XPC polymorphisms and cancer risk. J. Hum. Genet. **53**(1), 18–33 (2008)

97. Blankenburg, S., Konig, I.R., Moessner, R., Laspe, P., Thoms, K.M., Krueger, U., et al.: Assessment of 3 xeroderma pigmentosum group C gene polymorphisms and risk of cutaneous melanoma: a case-control study. Carcinogenesis **26**(6), 1085–1090 (2005)

98. Blankenburg, S., Konig, I.R., Moessner, R., Laspe, P., Thoms, K.M., Krueger, U., et al.: No association between three xeroderma pigmentosum group C and one group G gene polymorphisms and risk of cutaneous melanoma. Eur. J. Hum. Genet. **13**(2), 253–255 (2005)

99. Millikan, R.C., Hummer, A., Begg, C., Player, J., de Cotret, A.R., Winkel, S., et al.: Polymorphisms in nucleotide excision repair genes and risk of multiple primary melanoma: the Genes Environment and Melanoma Study. Carcinogenesis **27**(3), 610–618 (2006)

100. Han, J., Colditz, G.A., Liu, J.S., Hunter, D.J.: Genetic variation in XPD, sun exposure, and risk of skin cancer. Cancer Epidemiol. Biomarkers Prev. **14**(6), 1539–1544 (2005)

101. Baccarelli, A., Calista, D., Minghetti, P., Marinelli, B., Albetti, B., Tseng, T., et al.: XPD gene polymorphism and host characteristics in the association with cutaneous malignant melanoma risk. Br. J. Cancer **90**(2), 497–502 (2004)

102. Debniak, T., Scott, R.J., Gorski, B., Cybulski, C., van de Wetering, T., Serrano-Fernandez, P., et al.: Common variants of DNA repair genes and malignant melanoma. Eur. J. Cancer **44**(1), 110–114 (2008)

103. Li, C., Liu, Z., Wang, L.E., Gershenwald, J.E., Lee, J.E., Prieto, V.G., et al.: Haplotype and genotypes of the VDR gene and cutaneous

melanoma risk in non-Hispanic whites in Texas: a case-control study. Int. J. Cancer **122**(9), 2077–2084 (2008)

104. Houghton, A., Flannery, J., Viola, M.V.: Malignant melanoma in Connecticut and Denmark. Int. J. Cancer **25**(1), 95–104 (1980)

105. Weinstock, M.A., Colditz, G.A., Willett, W.C., Stampfer, M.J., Bronstein, B.R., Mihm, M.C., et al.: Moles and site-specific cutaneous malignant melanoma in women. J. Natl. Cancer Inst. **81**, 948–952 (1989)

106. Kruger, S., Garbe, C., Buttner, P., Stadler, R., Guggenmoos-Holzmann, I., Orfanos, C.E.: Epidemiologic evidence for the role of melanocytic nevi as risk markers and direct precursors of cutaneous malignant melanoma. J. Am. Acad. Dermatol. **26**, 920–926 (1992)

107. Rieger, E., Soyer, H.P., Garbe, C., et al.: Overall and site-specific risk of malignant melanoma associated with nevus counts at different body sites: a multicenter case-control study of the German central malignant-melanoma registry. Int. J. Cancer **62**, 393–397 (1995)

108. Chen, Y.T., Dubrow, R., Holford, T.R., Zheng, T., Barnhill, R.L., Fine, J., et al.: Malignant melanoma risk factors by anatomic site: a case-control study and polychotomous logistic regression analysis. Int. J. Cancer **67**(5), 636–643 (1996)

109. Bataille, V., Sasieni, P., Grulich, A., Swerdlow, A., McCarthy, W., Hersey, P., et al.: Solar keratoses: A risk factor for melanoma but negative association with melanocytic naevi. Int. J. Cancer **78**, 8–12 (1998)

110. Whiteman, D.C., Green, A., Parson, P.G.: p53 Expression and risk factors for cutaneous melanoma: a case-control study. Int. J. Cancer **77**, 843–848 (1998)

111. Urso, C., Giannotti, V., Reali, U.M., Giannotti, B., Bondi, R.: Spatial association of melanocytic naevus and melanoma. Melanoma Res. **1**(4), 245–249 (1991)

112. Marks, R., Dorevitch, A.P., Mason, G.: Do all melanomas come from "moles"? A study of the histological association between melanocytic naevi and melanoma. Australas. J. Dermatol. **31**(2), 77–80 (1990)

113. Kaddu, S., Smolle, J., Zenahlik, P., Hofmann-Wellenhof, R., Kerl, H.: Melanoma with benign melanocytic naevus components: reappraisal of clinicopathological features and prognosis. Melanoma Res. **12**(3), 271–278 (2002)

114. Carli, P., Massi, D., Santucci, M., Biggeri, A., Gianotti, B.: Cutaneous melanoma histologically associated with a nevus and melanoma de novo have a different profile of risk: results from a case-control study. J. Am. Acad. Dermatol. **40**, 549–557 (1999)

115. Carli, P., Massi, D., Santucci, M., Biggeri, A., Giannotti, B.: Cutaneous melanoma histologically associated with a nevus and melanoma de novo have a different profile of risk: results from a case-control study. J. Am. Acad. Dermatol. **40**(4), 549–557 (1999)

116. Skender-Kalnenas, T.M., English, D.R., Heenan, P.J.: Benign melanocytic lesions: risk markers or precursors of cutaneous melanoma? J. Am. Acad. Dermatol. **33**, 1000–1007 (1995)

117. Green, A.: A theory of site distribution of melanomas: Queensland, Australia. Cancer Causes Control **3**, 513–516 (1992)

118. Purdue, M.P., From, L., Armstrong, B.K., Kricker, A., Gallagher, R.P., McLaughlin, J.R., et al.: Etiologic and other factors predicting nevus-associated cutaneous malignant melanoma. Cancer Epidemiol. Biomarkers Prev. **14**(8), 2015–2022 (2005)

119. Winnepenninckx, V., van den Oord, J.J.: p16INK4A expression in malignant melanomas with or without a contiguous naevus remnant: a clue to their divergent pathogenesis? Melanoma Res. **14**, 321–322 (2004)

120. Autier, P., Dore, J.F., Cattaruzza, M.S., Renard, F., Luther, H., Gentiloni-Silverj, F., et al.: Sunscreen use, wearing clothes, and number of nevi in 6- to 7-year-old European children. J. Natl. Cancer Inst. **90**, 1873–1880 (1998)

121. Gallagher, R.P., McLean, D.I., Yang, C.P., et al.: Suntan, sunburn and pigmentation factors and the frequency of acquired melanocytic nevi in children. Arch. Dermatol. **126**, 770–776 (1990)

122. Wiecker, T.S., Luther, H., Buettner, P., Bauer, J., Garbe, C.: Moderate sun exposure and nevus counts in parents are associated with development of melanocytic nevi in childhood: a risk factor study in 1,812 kindergarten children. Cancer **97**(3), 628–638 (2003)

123. Wachsmuth, R.C., Turner, F., Barrett, J.H., Gaut, R., Randerson-Moor, J.A., Bishop, D.T., et al.: The effect of sun exposure in determining nevus density in UK adolescent twins. J. Invest. Dermatol. **124**(1), 56–62 (2005)

124. Green, A., Sorohan, T., Pope, D., et al.: Moles in Australian and British schoolchildren. Lancet **2**, 1497 (1988)

125. English, D.R., Armstrong, B.K.: Melanocytic nevi in children. I. Anatomic sites and demographic and host factors. Am. J. Epidemiol. **139**, 390–401 (1994)

126. Harrison, S.L., MacLennan, R., Speare, R., Wronski, I.: Sun exposure and melanocytic naevi in young Australian children. Lancet **344**, 1529–1532 (1994)

127. Whiteman, D.C., Brown, R.M., Purdie, D.M., Hughes, M.C.: Melanocytic nevi in very young children: the role of phenotype, sun exposure, and sun protection. J. Am. Acad. Dermatol. **52**(1), 40–47 (2005)

128. Fritschi, L., McHenry, P., Green, A., MacKie, R., Green, L., Siskind, V.: Naevi in schoolchildren in Scotland and Australia. Br. J. Dermatol. **130**, 599–603 (1994)

129. Kelly, J.W., Rivers, J.K., MacLennan, R., Harrison, S., Lewis, A.E., Tate, B.J.: Sunlight: A major factor associated with the development of melanocytic nevi in Australian schoolchildren. J. Am. Acad. Dermatol. **30**, 40–48 (1994)

130. Zhu, G., Duffy, D.L., Eldridge, A., Grace, M., Mayne, C., O'Gorman, L., et al.: A major quantitative-trait locus for mole density is linked to the familial melanoma gene CDKN2A: a maximum-likelihood combined linkage and association analysis in twins and their sibs. Am. J. Hum. Genet. **65**(2), 483–492 (1999)

131. Wachsmuth, R.C., Gaut, R.M., Barrett, J.H., Saunders, C.L., Randerson-Moor, J.A., Eldridge, A., et al.: Heritability and gene-environment interactions for melanocytic nevus density examined in a U.K. adolescent twin study. J. Invest. Dermatol. **117**(2), 348–352 (2001)

132. Whiteman, D.C., Watt, P., Purdie, D.M., Hughes, M.C., Hayward, N.K., Green, A.C.: Melanocytic nevi, solar keratoses, and divergent pathways to cutaneous melanoma. J. Natl. Cancer Inst. **95**(11), 806–812 (2003)

133. Bulliard, J.L., De Weck, D., Fisch, T., Bordoni, A., Levi, F.: Detailed site distribution of melanoma and sunlight exposure: aetiological patterns from a Swiss series. Ann. Oncol. **18**(4), 789–794 (2007)

134. Cho, E., Rosner, B.A., Colditz, G.A.: Risk factors for melanoma by body site. Cancer Epidemiol. Biomarkers Prev. **14**(5), 1241–1244 (2005)

135. Naldi, L., Altieri, A., Imberti, G.L., Gallus, S., Bosetti, C., La Vecchia, C.: Sun exposure, phenotypic characteristics, and cutaneous malignant melanoma. An analysis according to different clinico-pathological variants and anatomic locations (Italy). Cancer Causes Control **16**(8), 893–899 (2005)

136. Randi, G., Naldi, L., Gallus, S., Di Landro, A., La Vecchia, C.: Number of nevi at a specific anatomical site and its relation to cutaneous malignant melanoma. J. Invest. Dermatol. **126**(9), 2106–2110 (2006)

137. Thomas, N.E.: BRAF somatic mutations in malignant melanoma and melanocytic naevi. Melanoma Res. **16**(2), 97–103 (2006)

138. Lang, J., MacKie, R.M.: Prevalence of exon 15 BRAF mutations in primary melanoma of the superficial spreading, nodular, acral,

and lentigo maligna subtypes. J. Invest. Dermatol. **125**(3), 575–579 (2005)

139. Thomas, N.E., Edmiston, S.N., Alexander, A., Millikan, R.C., Groben, P.A., Hao, H., et al.: Number of nevi and early-life ambient UV exposure are associated with BRAF-mutant melanoma. Cancer Epidemiol. Biomarkers Prev. **16**(5), 991–997 (2007)

140. Liu, W., Kelly, J.W., Trivett, M., Murray, W.K., Dowling, J.P., Wolfe, R., et al.: Distinct clinical and pathological features are associated with the BRAF(T1799A(V600E)) mutation in primary melanoma. J. Invest. Dermatol. **127**(4), 900–905 (2007)

141. Poynter, J.N., Elder, J.T., Fullen, D.R., Nair, R.P., Soengas, M.S., Johnson, T.M., et al.: BRAF and NRAS mutations in melanoma and melanocytic nevi. Melanoma Res. **16**(4), 267–273 (2006)

142. Edlundh-Rose, E., Egyhazi, S., Omholt, K., Mansson-Brahme, E., Platz, A., Hansson, J., et al.: NRAS and BRAF mutations in melanoma tumours in relation to clinical characteristics: a study based on mutation screening by pyrosequencing. Melanoma Res. **16**(6), 471–478 (2006)

143. Bauer, J., Curtin, J.A., Pinkel, D., Bastian, B.C.: Congenital melanocytic nevi frequently harbor NRAS mutations but no BRAF mutations. J. Invest. Dermatol. **127**(1), 179–182 (2007)

144. Landi, M.T., Bauer, J., Pfeiffer, R.M., Elder, D.E., Hulley, B., Minghetti, P., et al.: MC1R germline variants confer risk for BRAF-mutant melanoma. Science **313**(5786), 521–522 (2006)

Epidemiology of Cutaneous Lymphomas

Mirjana Urosevic-Maiwald

Primary cutaneous lymphomas represent the second most frequent type of extranodal non-Hodgkin lymphomas (NHLs) after gastrointestinal lymphomas [9]. The worldwide annual incidence of primary cutaneous lymphomas is estimated to be 1:100,000 [1, 6, 9]. Despite the existence of several large, often clinic-based registries dealing with cutaneous lymphomas (Netherlands Lymphoma Registry, Lymphoma Registry Graz/Austria, Lymphoma Registry Stanford/USA, German Registry for Cutaneous Lymphomas, National Cancer Institute's Surveillance, Epidemiology, and End Results Program (NCI SEER)) there is a paucity of comparable population-based data concerning this group of diseases. Until 2005, one of the main obstacles for the correct reporting was the lack of appropriate classification to cover all clinicopathological entities, when the new WHO-EORTC was introduced [23]. The comparison of age distribution in different lymphoma registries shows that primary cutaneous lymphomas most commonly arise in older adults, with a median onset time after 60 years of age [1]. One exception to this distribution is lymphomatoid papulosis, which often develops in young adults and can even manifest in childhood [2]. Males seem to be more affected than females, with a male/female ratio reaching up to 4:1 [7, 11, 27].

With respect to the cell of origin, roughly three-fourths of primary cutaneous lymphomas are of T-cell origin (cutaneous T-cell lymphomas, CTCL), whereas one-fourth encompasses cutaneous B-cell lymphomas (CBCL) and other rare forms. Depending on the source of the data, CTCL represent between 75% (data from the registry of the Dutch and Austrian Cutaneous Lymphoma Group [23], and from SEER [6]) and 85% of primary cutaneous lymphomas (data from the German Registry for Cutaneous Lymphomas ZRKL [1]), while CBCL account for 25% [6, 23] to 15% [1]

of the remaining cases. The incidence of CTCL has risen dramatically and consistently since 1973. Recent evaluation of the data obtained through SEER program in the USA for the period from 1973 to 2002 showed an overall annual age-adjusted incidence of CTCL of 0.64 per 100,000 persons [5]. Furthermore, annual incidence increased by 0.29:100,000 per decade over the study period. Changes in classification schemes may have contributed to the rise in incidence, as may improvement in detection or an increase in the underlying etiologic agent(s). Demographic correlates from this study show that incidence was strongly correlated with the density of physicians [5]. Therefore, the observed rise in incidence may be due, at least in part, to the increased efficiency of diagnosis and detection of CTCL due to improvement in medical care in the past few decades. The CTCL incidence was higher among men than among women (men/women ratio 1.9:1). These sex differences tended to increase with age and to decrease over time. Inconsistent classification of the lymphomas included in the NCI SEER database has led to their improper categorization (mostly as "not other specified") and disabled the possibility to directly evaluate changes in incidence trends of different lymphoma subtypes.

Even though an uncommon lymphoma, mycosis fungoides (MF) represents the most common primary lymphoma of the skin. According to the data of nine cancer population-based registries in the USA for the period from 1973 to 1984, the incidence of MF was initially reported to be 0.29:100,000 per year [22]. During the period of the study, a dramatic increase in the incidence of MF of 3.2-fold was noted. The factors responsible for this increase are same as the ones described above. The prevalence of MF seems to show differences between countries and ranges between 35% (in Japan [27]) to 69% (in Austria [7]). The prevalence rate around 45% is encountered in the Netherlands [24], USA [15], and Korea [6]. Register-to-register differences in relative frequencies of different cutaneous lymphoma subtypes are shown in Table 1.3.1. These regional differences most likely reflect the underlying pathogenesis of the given

M. Urosevic-Maiwald
Department of Dermatology, University Hospital Zurich,
Gloriastrasse 31, 8091 Zurich, Switzerland
e-mail: mirjana.urosevic@usz.ch

R. Dummer et al. (eds.), *Skin Cancer – A World-Wide Perspective*,
DOI: 10.1007/978-3-642-05072-5_1.3, © Springer-Verlag Berlin Heidelberg 2011

Table 1.3.1 Relative frequencies of primary cutaneous lymphomas in different countries

Entity (according to WHO-EORTC)	Dutch [24] 1986–1994 (%)	Austrian [7] 1960–1999 (%)	German [1] 1999–2004 (%)	Dutch-Austrian [23] 1986–2002 (%)	USA [6] 1992–2002 (%)	Japan [27] (Hokkaido) 1994–2004 (%)	Japan [17] (Osaka) 1988–1999 (%)	Korea [15] 1998–2000 (%)
Primary cutaneous T-cell lymphomas								
Indolent clinical behavior								
Mycosis fungoides	44	69	59	44	45	35	31	43
Folliculotropic MF (MF-associated follicular mucinosis)	4	6	2	4				
Pagetoid reticulosis	<1	<1	1	<1				
Granulomatous slack skin	<1	0	<1	<1				
Primary cutaneous anaplastic large cell lymphoma	9	4	7	8	5	3	10	19
Lymphomatoid papulosis	11	11	7	12		13	10	
Subcutaneous panniculitis-like T-cell lymphoma	3	<1	5	1	<1	3		11
Primary cutaneous CD4+ small/medium pleomorphic T-cell lymphoma	3	2		2			4	
(EORTC: primary cutaneous CD30- large T-cell lymphoma)	*(5)*	*(<1)*	*(1)*					
(WHO: peripheral T-cell lymphoma)						*(13)*	*(10)*	*(8)*
Aggressive clinical behavior								
Sézary syndrome	2	5	2	3	1	6	2	
Primary cutaneous NK/T-cell lymphoma, nasal-type	<1	<1	<1	<1	<1	6	8	15
Primary cutaneous aggressive CD8+ T-cell lymphoma	1	1	1	<1				
Primary cutaneous γ/δ T-cell lymphoma				<1				
Primary cutaneous peripheral T-cell lymphoma, unspecified				2	26			
Primary cutaneous B-cell lymphomas								
Indolent clinical behavior								
Primary cutaneous marginal zone B-cell lymphoma	2	15	4	7	5	3		1
Primary cutaneous follicle center lymphoma	13	15	7	11	5	0	15	3
Intermediate clinical behavior								
Primary cutaneous diffuse large B-cell lymphoma, leg type	3	6	2	4	2		2	
Primary cutaneous diffuse large B-cell lymphoma, other				<1	9	13		
Primary cutaneous intravascular large B-cell lymphoma	<1			<1		3		
Classification used	EORTC	EORTC	EORTC	WHO-EORTC	WHO-EORTC	WHO	EORTC	WHO

lymphoma subtype. Extranodal NK/T-cell lymphoma of the nasal type is more frequently observed in Asia (Japan, Korea) than in other countries included in this comparison. Indeed, these patients show a peculiar geographic distribution, as they are mainly reported in Far Eastern (Hong Kong, Japan, and Korea) and in Central American (Mexico, Guatemala) countries, while they are uncommon in North America and Europe [4, 18]. Similarly, adult T-cell leukemia/lymphoma (ATLL), which is caused by human T-cell lymphotropic virus-1 (HTLV-1), is endemic in southwest Japan, the Caribbean islands, South America, and parts of Central Africa [23]. ATLL accounts for 20–30% of T-cell lymphomas in Japan [11, 27], which is proportional to general occurrence of HTLV-1 in Japanese population [19]. The dominance of HTLV-1-associated ATLL could, therefore, explain a relatively lower frequency of MF in Japanese vs. other Western populations. Interestingly, CD30+ lymphoproliferative disorders, such as anaplastic large-cell lymphoma and lymphomatoid papulosis, also show somewhat higher occurrence in Japan [11, 17, 27]. The causal relationship, however, could be excluded, since HTLV-1 genome could not be detected by PCR in anaplastic large-cell lymphoma and lymphomatoid papulosis lesions obtained from diverse geographical locations including USA (Ohio, California), Switzerland, and Japan [26].

On the other hand, the frequency of patients with follicle center and in particular of marginal zone B-cell lymphomas is highest in Austria, as compared to other countries [7]. Analogous to gastric marginal zone lymphomas, which arise as in the setting of chronic antigenic stimulation due to microbacterial antigens (i.e., *Helicobacter pylori*), an association with *Borrelia burgdorferi* infection (Lyme disease) has been suggested for a significant minority of European cases [3, 8], but not in Asian cases [16] or cases from USA [25]. Diagnostic pitfalls may also contribute to an artificial increase in the relative frequency of a lymphoma subtype. The discrimination between the follicle center B-cell lymphomas of classical follicular type from the marginal zone lymphomas may represent a histological challenge, particularly when the latter display reactive follicle centers. Furthermore, differentiating a follicle center B-cell lymphoma of diffuse type from the diffuse large B-cell lymphoma of leg type can pose a difficulty, despite available immunohistochemical markers [23].

Most of the CTCL have an indolent clinical behavior with the disease-specific 5-year survival between 80% and 100%. Pleomorphic T-cell lymphoma seems to have a slightly worse outcome than the other indolent lymphoma types (5-year survival rate from 50% to 80%). Register-to-register differences

in 5-year survival of different cutaneous lymphoma subtypes are shown in Table 1.3.2. Aggressive entities like Sézary syndrome (SS) or cytotoxic CD8- or NK-cells lymphoma have a significantly reduced 5-year survival rate ranging from 11% to 42%, depending on the country. On the other hand, follicle center and marginal B-cell lymphomas also show indolent clinical course with a 5-year survival rate between 92% and 100%. In contrast, large-cell B-cell lymphomas, irrespective of the type, are with the worse outcome and have a 5-year survival rate 50–65%.

A recent study by Huang et al. evaluating data from nine population-based cancer registries in the USA as well as from the Stanford University referral center cohort of patients with cutaneous lymphoma revealed that patients with MF and SS have an overall increased risk for development of secondary malignancies, especially lymphomas [10]. This study constitutes the largest cohort of patients with MF and SS that have been followed up for second cancers to date. In the SEER-9 cohort, significantly elevated risk was observed for Hodgkin disease and NHLs as well as an elevated risk to develop melanoma and urinary cancer. In the Stanford University Cohort, elevated risk was also observed for Hodgkin disease as well as billiary cancer. This study confirms the reports of at least two previous studies, showing increased risk for NHL, lung and colon cancer [12, 21]. It is conceivable that these second cancers are due to impaired immune response either primary or secondary induced by MF/SS therapy [14, 20]. Together with disturbed cellular interactions between B- and T-cells, as often encountered in older individuals [13], these immunologic alterations may predispose these patients to develop second malignancies, particularly Hodgkin disease and NHLs. Alternatively, these patients may have a common underlying environmental/etiologic factor or inherent predisposition to develop particular malignant neoplasms.

With an increasing incidence of MF (including SS) and probably of other lymphomas, more studies are needed on larger population cohorts. Regrettably, the estimation of incidence trends in other countries (cohorts) is not possible on the basis of the existing data, thus making this need an imperative. The data from population-based epidemiological studies not only help in evaluating the demographics but may also be useful in planning public health strategies, indentifying risk factors, and understanding the etiology of these group of diseases so that effective prevention strategies can be developed. The introduction of the new clinically as well as pathologically oriented WHO-EORTC classification system will surely help to achieve this goal.

Table 1.3.2 Five-year survival related to primary cutaneous lymphomas in different countries

Entity (according to WHO-EORTC)	Dutch [24] 1986–1994 (%)	Austrian [7] 1960–1999 (%)	Dutch-Austrian [23] 1986–2002 (%)	USA [6] 1992–2002 (%)	Japan [17] (Osaka) 1988–1999 (%)
Primary cutaneous T-cell lymphomas					
Indolent clinical behavior					
Mycosis fungoides	87	89	88	92	70
Folliculotropic MF (MF-associated follicular mucinosis)	70	93	80		
Pagetoid reticulosis	100	100	100		
Granulomatous slack skin	–[a]		100		
Primary cutaneous anaplastic large cell lymphoma	90	100	95	83	100
Lymphomatoid papulosis	100	100	100		100
Subcutaneous panniculitis-like T-cell lymphoma		100	82	–	
Primary cutaneous CD4+ small/medium pleomorphic T-cell lymphoma	62	80	75		50
(EORTC: primary cutaneous CD30- large T-cell lymphoma)	*(15)*	*(100)*			*(0)*
(WHO: peripheral T-cell lymphoma)					
Aggressive clinical behavior					
Sézary syndrome	11	33	24	42	–
Primary cutaneous NK/T-cell lymphoma, nasal-type		0	–	–	0
Primary cutaneous aggressive CD8+ T-cell lymphoma		0	18		
Primary cutaneous γ/δ T-cell lymphoma			–		
Primary cutaneous peripheral T-cell lymphoma, unspecified			16	83	
Primary cutaneous B-cell lymphomas					
Indolent clinical behavior					
Primary cutaneous marginal zone B-cell lymphoma	100	98	99	95	
Primary cutaneous follicle center lymphoma	97	94	95	92	100
Intermediate clinical behavior					
Primary cutaneous diffuse large B-cell lymphoma, leg type	58	58	55	65	–
Primary cutaneous diffuse large B-cell lymphoma, other			50	85	
Primary cutaneous intravascular large B-cell lymphoma	50		65		
Classification used	EORTC	EORTC	WHO-EORTC	WHO-EORTC	EORTC

[a]Case number for evaluation not reached; empty cells – data not available

References

1. Assaf, C., Gellrich, S., Steinhoff, M., et al.: Cutaneous lymphomas in Germany: an analysis of the Central Cutaneous Lymphoma Registry of the German Society of Dermatology (DDG). J. Dtsch. Dermatol. Ges. **5**, 662–668 (2007)
2. Bekkenk, M.W., Geelen, F.A., van Voorst Vader, P.C., et al.: Primary and secondary cutaneous CD30(+) lymphoproliferative disorders: a report from the Dutch Cutaneous Lymphoma Group on the long-term follow-up data of 219 patients and guidelines for diagnosis and treatment. Blood **95**, 3653–3661 (2000)
3. Cerroni, L., Zöchling, N., Pütz, B., et al.: Infection by Borrelia burgdorferi and cutaneous B-cell lymphoma. J. Cutan. Pathol. **24**, 457–461 (1997)
4. Chim, C., Ma, S., Au, W., et al.: Primary nasal natural killer cell lymphoma: long-term treatment outcome and relationship with the International Prognostic Index. Blood **103**, 216–221 (2004)
5. Criscione, V.D., Weinstock, M.A.: Incidence of cutaneous T-cell lymphoma in the United States, 1973–2002. Arch. Dermatol. **143**, 854–859 (2007)
6. Dores, G.M., Anderson, W.F., Devesa, S.S.: Cutaneous lymphomas reported to the National Cancer Institute's surveillance, epidemiology, and end results program: applying the new WHO-European Organisation for Research and Treatment of Cancer classification system. J. Clin. Oncol. **23**, 7246–7248 (2005)
7. Fink-Puches, R., Zenahlik, P., Bäck, B., et al.: Primary cutaneous lymphomas: applicability of current classification schemes (European Organization for Research and Treatment of Cancer, World Health Organization) based on clinicopathologic features observed in a large group of patients. Blood **99**, 800–805 (2002)
8. Goodlad, J.R., Davidson, M.M., Hollowood, K., et al.: Primary cutaneous B-cell lymphoma and Borrelia burgdorferi infection in patients from the Highlands of Scotland. Am. J. Surg. Pathol. **24**, 1279–1285 (2000)
9. Groves, F.D., Linet, M.S., Travis, L.B., et al.: Cancer surveillance series: non-Hodgkin's lymphoma incidence by histologic subtype in the United States from 1978 through 1995. J. Natl Cancer Inst. **92**, 1240–1251 (2000)
10. Huang, K.P., Weinstock, M.A., Clarke, C.A., et al.: Second lymphomas and other malignant neoplasms in patients with mycosis fungoides and Sezary syndrome: evidence from population-based and clinical cohorts. Arch. Dermatol. **143**, 45–50 (2007)
11. Ishiji, T., Takagi, Y., Niimura, M.: Cutaneous lymphomas in Tokyo: analysis of 62 cases in a dermatology clinic. Int. J. Dermatol. **40**, 37–40 (2001)
12. Kantor, A.F., Curtis, R.E., Vonderheid, E.C., et al.: Risk of second malignancy after cutaneous T-cell lymphoma. Cancer **63**, 1612–1615 (1989)
13. Lazuardi, L., Jenewein, B., Wolf, A.M., et al.: Age-related loss of naïve T cells and dysregulation of T-cell/B-cell interactions in human lymph nodes. Immunology **114**, 37–43 (2005)
14. Lee, B.N., Duvic, M., Tang, C.K., et al.: Dysregulated synthesis of intracellular type 1 and type 2 cytokines by T cells of patients with cutaneous T-cell lymphoma. Clin. Diagn. Lab. Immunol. **6**, 79–84 (1999)
15. Lee, M.: Characteristics of cutaneous lymphomas in Korea. Clin. Exp. Dermatol. **28**, 639–646 (2003)
16. Li, C., Inagaki, H., Kuo, T., et al.: Primary cutaneous marginal zone B-cell lymphoma: a molecular and clinicopathologic study of 24 asian cases. Am. J. Surg. Pathol. **27**, 1061–1069 (2003)
17. Nagasawa, T., Miwa, H., Nakatsuka, S., et al.: Characteristics of cutaneous lymphomas in Osaka, Japan (1988–1999) based on the European Organization for Research and Treatment of Cancer classification. Am. J. Dermatopathol. **22**, 510–514 (2000)
18. Pagano, L., Gallamini, A., Trape, G., et al.: NK/T-cell lymphomas 'nasal type': an Italian multicentric retrospective survey. Ann. Oncol. **17**, 794–800 (2006)
19. Tajima, K.: Malignant lymphomas in Japan: epidemiological analysis of adult T-cell leukemia/lymphoma (ATL). Cancer Metastasis Rev. **7**, 223–241 (1988)
20. Urosevic, M., Fujii, K., Calmels, B., et al.: Type I IFN innate immune response to adenovirus-mediated IFN-gamma gene transfer contributes to the regression of cutaneous lymphomas. J. Clin. Invest. **117**, 2834–2846 (2007)
21. Väkevä, L., Pukkala, E., Ranki, A.: Increased risk of secondary cancers in patients with primary cutaneous T cell lymphoma. J. Invest. Dermatol. **115**, 62–65 (2000)
22. Weinstock, M.A., Horm, J.W.: Mycosis fungoides in the United States. Increasing incidence and descriptive epidemiology. JAMA **260**, 42–46 (1988)
23. Willemze, R., Jaffe, E.S., Burg, G., et al.: WHO-EORTC classification for cutaneous lymphomas. Blood **105**, 3768–3785 (2005)
24. Willemze, R., Kerl, H., Sterry, W., et al.: EORTC classification for primary cutaneous lymphomas: a proposal from the Cutaneous Lymphoma Study Group of the European Organization for Research and Treatment of Cancer. Blood **90**, 354–371 (1997)
25. Wood, G.S., Kamath, N.V., Guitart, J., et al.: Absence of Borrelia burgdorferi DNA in cutaneous B-cell lymphomas from the United States. J. Cutan. Pathol. **28**, 502–507 (2001)
26. Wood, G.S., Schaffer, J.M., Boni, R., et al.: No evidence of HTLV-I proviral integration in lymphoproliferative disorders associated with cutaneous T-cell lymphoma. Am. J. Pathol. **150**, 667–673 (1997)
27. Yasukawa, K., Kato, N., Kodama, K., et al.: The spectrum of cutaneous lymphomas in Japan: a study of 62 cases based on the World Health Organization Classification. J. Cutan. Pathol. **33**, 487–491 (2006)

Epidemiology of Histocytoses

1.4

Marie C. Zipser and Reinhard Dummer

1.4.1 Langerhans Cell Histiocytosis

Langerhans cell histiocytisis (LCH) is the most common of the histiocytic disorders [39]. It represents a spectrum of several clinical entities chracterized by a disorder of antigen-presenting dendritic cells of the immune system. Its epidemiology is poorly understood and based mainly on a few international and regional studies of defined populations [34]. The overall incidence rate varies from 2.6 to 8.9 children per million per year [1, 19, 34, 36]. Children of any age can be affected, however the peak age of presentation, in children, is between the ages of one and three [34]. LCH is also diagnosed in adults [37] but only a few reports are available describing LCH patients with onset during adulthood [3]. Some studies reveal a greater prevalence of LCH among male children [19]. On the other hand, in adults, a preponderance of females is documented with onset as late as the ninth decade of life [26]. Dissemitaned LCH is described to present most frequently in the first year of life [19]. Congenital self-healing LCH is an uncommon form of LCH, which is usually present at birth or in the neonatal period [23].

1.4.2 Indeterminate Cell Histiocytosis

Indeterminate cell histiocytosis is a rare disease that shows both histological and phenotypic features of LCH and non-Langerhans cell histiocytosis (NLCH). There are approximately 40 cases reported in the literature [32]. The disease usually occurs during adulthood. However there are cases reported in teenagers as well as children [17, 24, 27, 28, 33].

1.4.3 Sinus Histiocytosis with Massive Lymphadenopathy (Rosai–Dorfman Disease)

Sinus histiocytosis is a rare, proliferateve, histiocytic disorder seen primarily in children and young adult males [18]. The purely cutaneous form is particularly seen in older females [7].

1.4.4 Juvenile Xanthogranuloma

Juvenile xanthogranuloma (JXG) is the most common of the NLCH. It is primarily seen in the first two decades of life, especially within the first year of life [14]. However, a number of adult cases have been reported [35]. A male preponderance is observed [14].

1.4.5 Reticulohistiocytosis

In adults, the most frequent form is the multicentric reticulohistiocytosis with systemic involvement (MR). Approximately 100 cases have been reported in the literature between 1977 and 2001 [25]. The mean age of onset of MR is in the fourth decade of life. However it ranges from childhood [22] to old age [16]. A female predominance has been reported [4, 25].

M.C. Zipser
University Hospital of Zürich, Department of Dermatology F2,
Gloriastrasse 31, 8091 Zürich,
Switzerland
e-mail: marie.zipser@usz.ch

R. Dummer (✉)
Department of Dermatology, University Hospital of Zürich,
Gloriastrasse 31, 8091 Zürich,
Switzerland
e-mail: reinhard.dummer@usz.ch

R. Dummer et al. (eds.), *Skin Cancer – A World-Wide Perspective*,
DOI: 10.1007/978-3-642-05072-5_1.4, © Springer-Verlag Berlin Heidelberg 2011

References

1. Alston, R.D., Tatevossian, R.G., et al.: Incidence and survival of childhood Langerhans cell histiocytosis in Northwest England from 1954 to 1998. Pediatr Blood Cancer **48**(5), 555–560 (2007)

2. Annels, N.E., Da Costa, C.E., et al.: Aberrant chemokine receptor expression and chemokine production by Langerhans cells underlies the pathogenesis of Langerhans cell histiocytosis. J Exp Med **197**(10), 1385–1390 (2003)

3. Arico, M.: Langerhans cell histiocytosis in adults: more questions than answers? Eur J Cancer **40**(10), 1467–1473 (2004)

4. Barrow, M.V., Holubar, K.: Multicentric reticulohistiocytosis. A review of 33 patients. Medicine (Baltimore) **48**(4), 287–305 (1969)

5. Bergman, R., Aviram, M., et al.: Enhanced low-density lipoprotein degradation and cholesterol synthesis in monocyte-derived macrophages of patients with adult xanthogranulomatosis. J Invest Dermatol **101**(6), 880–882 (1993)

6. Beverley, P.C., Egeler, R.M., et al.: The Nikolas Symposia and histiocytosis. Nat Rev Cancer **5**(6), 488–494 (2005)

7. Brenn, T., Calonje, E., et al.: Cutaneous Rosai–Dorfman disease is a distinct clinical entity. Am J Dermatopathol **24**(5), 385–391 (2002)

8. Campbell, D.A., Edwards, N.L.: Multicentric reticulohistiocytosis: systemic macrophage disorder. Baillieres Clin Rheumatol **5**(2), 301–319 (1991)

9. Caputo, R., Alessi, E., et al.: Collagen phagocytosis in multicentric reticulohistiocytosis. J Invest Dermatol **76**(5), 342–346 (1981)

10. Catterall, M.D., White, J.E.: Multicentric reticulohistiocytosis and malignant disease. Br J Dermatol **98**(2), 221–224 (1978)

11. Caux, C., Dezutter-Dambuyant, C., et al.: GM-CSF and TNF-alpha cooperate in the generation of dendritic Langerhans cells. Nature **360**(6401), 258–261 (1992)

12. da Costa, C.E., Annels, N.E., et al.: Presence of osteoclast-like multinucleated giant cells in the bone and nonostotic lesions of Langerhans cell histiocytosis. J Exp Med **201**(5), 687–693 (2005)

13. da Costa, C.E., Egeler, R.M., et al.: Differences in telomerase expression by the CD1a+ cells in Langerhans cell histiocytosis reflect the diverse clinical presentation of the disease. J Pathol **212**(2), 188–197 (2007)

14. Dehner, L.P.: Juvenile xanthogranulomas in the first two decades of life: a clinicopathologic study of 174 cases with cutaneous and extracutaneous manifestations. Am J Surg Pathol **27**(5), 579–593 (2003)

15. Egeler, R.M., Favara, B.E., et al.: Differential In situ cytokine profiles of Langerhans-like cells and T cells in Langerhans cell histiocytosis: abundant expression of cytokines relevant to disease and treatment. Blood **94**(12), 4195–4201 (1999)

16. Fedler, R., Frantzmann, Y., et al.: Multicenter reticulohistiocytosis. Therapy with azathioprine and prednisolone. Hautarzt **46**(2), 118–120 (1995)

17. Ferran, M., Toll, A., et al.: Acquired mucosal indeterminate cell histiocytoma. Pediatr Dermatol **24**(3), 253–256 (2007)

18. Gaitonde, S.: Multifocal, extranodal sinus histiocytosis with massive lymphadenopathy: an overview. Arch Pathol Lab Med **131**(7), 1117–1121 (2007)

19. Guyot-Goubin, A., Donadieu, J., et al.: Descriptive epidemiology of childhood Langerhans cell histiocytosis in France, 2000–2004. Pediatr Blood Cancer **51**(1), 71–75 (2008)

20. Janssen, D., Folster-Holst, R., et al.: Clonality in juvenile xanthogranuloma. Am J Surg Pathol **31**(5), 812–813 (2007)

21. Kolde, G., Brocker, E.B.: Multiple skin tumors of indeterminate cells in an adult. J Am Acad Dermatol **15**(4 pt. 1), 591–597 (1986)

22. Kuramoto, Y., Iizawa, O., et al.: Multicentric reticulohistiocytosis in a child with sclerosing lesion of the leg. Immunohistopathologic studies and therapeutic trial with systemic cyclosporine. J Am Acad Dermatol **20**(2 Pt 2), 329–335 (1989)

23. Larralde, M., Rositto, A., et al.: Congenital self-healing Langerhans cell histiocytosis: the need for a long term follow up. Int J Dermatol **42**(3), 245–246 (2003)

24. Levisohn, D., Seidel, D., et al.: Solitary congenital indeterminate cell histiocytoma. Arch Dermatol **129**(1), 81–85 (1993)

25. Luz, F.B., Gaspar, T.A.P., et al.: Multicentric reticulohistiocytosis. J Eur Acad Dermatol Venereol **15**(6), 524–531 (2001)

26. Malpas, J.S., Norton, A.J.: Langerhans cell histiocytosis in the adult. Med Pediatr Oncol **27**(6), 540–546 (1996)

27. Flores-Stadler, M., Gonzalez-Crussi, E.F., et al.: Indeterminate-cell histiocytosis: immunophenotypic and cytogenetic findings in an infant. Med Pediatr Oncol **32**(4), 250–254 (1999)

28. Miracco, C., Raffaelli, M., et al.: Solitary cutaneous reticulum cell tumor. Enzyme-immunohistochemical and electron-microscopic analogies with IDRC sarcoma. Am J Dermatopathol **10**(1), 47–53 (1988)

29. Murakami, I., Gogusev, J., et al.: Detection of molecular cytogenetic aberrations in Langerhans cell histiocytosis of bone. Hum Pathol **33**(5), 555–560 (2002)

30. Nunnink, J.C., Krusinski, P.A., et al.: Multicentric reticulohistiocytosis and cancer: a case report and review of the literature. Med Pediatr Oncol **13**(5), 273–279 (1985)

31. Oliver, G.F., Umbert, I., et al.: Reticulohistiocytoma cutis – review of 15 cases and an association with systemic vasculitis in two cases. Clin Exp Dermatol **15**(1), 1–6 (1990)

32. Ratzinger, G., Burgdorf, W.H., et al.: Indeterminate cell histiocytosis: fact or fiction? J Cutan Pathol **32**(8), 552–560 (2005)

33. Saijo, S., Hara, M., et al.: Generalized eruptive histiocytoma: a report of a variant case showing the presence of dermal indeterminate cells. J Cutan Pathol **18**(2), 134–136 (1991)

34. Salotti, J.A., Nanduri, V., et al.: Incidence and clinical features of Langerhans cell histiocytosis in the UK and Ireland. Arch Dis Child **94**(5), 376–380 (2008)

35. Shoo, B.A., Shinkai, K., et al.: Xanthogranulomas associated with hematologic malignancy in adulthood. J Am Acad Dermatol **59**(3), 488–493 (2008)

36. Stalemark, H., Laurencikas, E., et al.: Incidence of Langerhans cell histiocytosis in children: a population-based study. Pediatr Blood Cancer **51**(1), 76–81 (2008)

37. Tatevossian, R., Nanduri, V., et al.: Adults with LCH – orphans with an orphan disease. Clin Med **6**(4), 404–408 (2006)

38. Vener, C., Soligo, D., et al.: Indeterminate cell histiocytosis in association with later occurrence of acute myeloblastic leukaemia. Br J Dermatol **156**(6), 1357–1361 (2007)

39. Weitzman, S., Egeler, R.M.: Langerhans cell histiocytosis: update for the pediatrician. Curr Opin Pediatr **20**(1), 23–29 (2008)

Epidemiology of Kaposi Sarcoma

1.5

Nagwa M. Elwan

Kaposi sarcoma (KS) is a spindle-cell tumor derived from endothelial cells, first described by a Hungarian dermatologist, Mortiz Kaposi [22]. KS is a very heterogeneous group of neoplasms that is usually divided with regard to its clinical and epidemiologic characteristics into four types [37]. Its classic or Mediterranean form tends to be benign. In transplant recipients it may be less so. As part of the AIDS pandemic, it may be life-threatening [35].

Classic KS: It is also known as chronic, European, or sporadic (Fig. 1.5.1). It is an uncommon disease among middle-aged and elderly men of Mediterranean or Jewish lineage [20, 28, 37]. It mainly affects males over 60 years old, with a male-to-female ratio 10:1 or 15:1 [23]. KS incidence in the Mediterranean had been up to tenfold higher than in the rest of Europe and the USA [16], with a particularly high incidence in Italy, Greece, Turkey, and Israel [20]. The incidence of classic KS in Italy has been estimated to be 1.0 for men and 0.4 for women per 100,000 population per year, while in southern Italy, the incidence in men has been estimated at 3.01/100,000 [11, 12], which is about 2–3 times higher than in the USA and 10–20 times higher than in England [15, 20]. The incidence of classic KS in the USA has been estimated to be 0.34 for men and 0.08 for women per 100,000 population per year [9]. Possible risk factors for classic KS are evident in Italy. Hot spots are in the Po River Valley, Sardinia, and southern Italy, all of which have not only silicaceous volcanic soil but also abundant blood-sucking insects [7]. Age too is an important risk factor. Subjects more than 50 years of age had a higher HHV-8 seroprevalence as compared to younger individuals. A strong direct correlation between HHV-8 prevalence and classic KS incidence was documented. Other risk factors for classic KS have been postulated, including patients receiving quinine to treat malaria and subjects farming cereals [10, 32].

Classic KS in Greece exhibits some special characteristics, including an older age of onset, a lower male-to-female

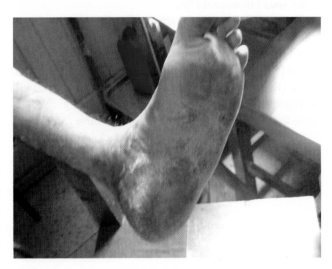

Fig. 1.5.1 Bluish erythematous nodules and plaques of classic KS in the foot of an elderly Egyptian patient

ratio, endemic clustering, disseminated skin disease at diagnosis, often accompanied by lymphedema and a more common visceral or lymph node involvement and a more frequent association with second malignancies [36]. KS may be as common among Arabians as among the Mediterranean population [2]. Classic KS in South America showed low seroprevalence of HHV-8, whereas high seroprevalence rates were seen in Amerindian population [27].

1.5.1 Endemic African KS

In the 1950s, KS was recognized as being common in portions of Africa [3]. Endemic African KS has accounted for 10% of cancers in central Africa, with a male-to-female ratio near unity in childhood KS cases but often rising in puberty to 15:1 [4, 5, 17, 24]. In those under 15 years of age, the median age was 4 years, with male-to-female ratio being 1.7:1 and 78% testing positive for HIV [41].

Endemic KS is divided into two subtypes. In the first one, skin involvement is usually observed with only local

N.M. Elwan
Department of Medicine, Tanta University, Tanta-Egypt
e-mail: elwan2egy@yahoo.com

R. Dummer et al. (eds.), *Skin Cancer – A World-Wide Perspective*,
DOI: 10.1007/978-3-642-05072-5_1.5, © Springer-Verlag Berlin Heidelberg 2011

aggressiveness and sometimes massive edema. The affected populations are middle-aged adults (25–50 years old) residing in several sub-Saharan countries such as Uganda, Sudan, Congo, Rowanda, and Burundi as well as Malawi, eastern Zaire, and the coast of Cameroon [21, 38]. The Kampala Cancer Registry has shown a significant alteration in the incidence of KS in the area of AIDs [39]. In Uganda, KS is responsible for almost one half (48.6%) of the cases of cancer in men and 17.9% in women. The incidence in men (30.1 cases/100,000 people) represents a more than tenfold increase since the 1950s, and is approximately three times the incidence found in women [39].

The second subtype of endemic KS affects mainly Bantu children under 10 years of age. It is characterized by generalized lymphadenopathy, more pronounced in the cervical region [21]. In Uganda, lymphadenopathic KS affected 12% of total cases; 42% of childhood cases were of this type [39]. In Zambia, the disorder was aggressive among children, more than 80% of whom were HIV seropositive (5). KS was found to represent as much as 25% of childhood cancers. Although lymphadenopathic KS is very rare in Egypt, a case of a 3-year-old boy with cutaneous and lymphangiopathic KS was reported [19].

1.5.2 Epidemic or AIDS Associated KS

KS is the most frequent neoplasm in homosexual and bisexual men with AIDS [13, 14]. The incidence of KS varies among groups of patients with AIDS; 21–40% of homosexuals with AIDS develop KS [8]. A decline in new HIV infection reduced KS frequency in AIDS patients in the mid-1990s to about 15–25% [31]. Also, the incidence has been declining with the use of highly active antiretroviral therapy (HAART) for HIV disease [34]. The AIDS epidemic has altered KS epidemiology worldwide [35]. There is a high incidence of AIDS in Brazil [40]. In Zambia, KS in infants and young children was found to occur more commonly since the advent of the HIV epidemic [5].

1.5.3 Immunosuppression: Associated or Iatrogenic KS

The incidence of KS in transplant recipients is 400–500 times greater than that in the general population [41]. KS may develop within months after starting the immunosuppressive therapy; particularly with calcineurin inhibitors [25]. Also, differences in immunosuppressive therapy may favor HHV-8 reactivation in transplant recipients [26]. KS

may develop after using prednisone [1], or other immunosuppressive including cyclosporine, which may reactivate HHV-8 from latency to lytic replication in tissue culture [18]. Iatrogenic KS occurs in only about 0.4% of transplant patients in the USA and Western Europe [29], but in about 4.0–5.3% of renal transplant patients in Saudi Arabia [30].

1.5.4 Epidemiology of KS Associated Herpes Virus (KSHV)

The epidemiology of KSHV points strongly to a critical role for this infection in KS pathogenesis [33]. In societies where classical KS is common, seroprevalence of KSHV is high (20–25%) in the population in the Mediterranean and up to 60% in parts of Africa [33]. Moreover, among male homosexuals in the USA, there is clear evidence of sexual transmission of KSHV, in accord with the epidemiologic predictions [8]. An increased prevalence of HHV-8 among injection drug users has been noted. In the USA, relative risks for KS associated with injection drug use were 1.3/100 person years [6].

References

1. Agbaht, K., Pepedil, F., Kirkpantur, A., et al.: A case of Kaposi's sarcoma following treatment of membranoproliferative glomerulonephritis and a review of the literature. Ren. Fail. 29, 107–110 (2007)
2. Alzahrani, A.J., El-Harith el, H.A., Milzer, J., et al.: Increased seroprevalence of human herpes virus-8 in renal transplant recipients in Saudi Arabia. Nephrol. Dial. Transplant. 20, 2532–2536 (2005)
3. Antman, K., Chang, Y.: Kaposi's sarcoma. N. Engl. J. Med. 342, 1027–1038 (2000)
4. Antón, E.: Kaposi's sarcoma in an immunocompetent patient following corticosteroid therapy. Eur. J. Intern. Med. 19, 226 (2008)
5. Athale, U.H., Patil, P.S., Chintu, C., et al.: Influence of HIV epidemic on the incidence of Kaposi's sarcoma in Zambian children. J. Acquir. Immune Defic. Syndr. Hum. Retrovirol. 8, 96–100 (1995)
6. Atkinson, J.O., Biggar, R.J., Goedert, J.J., et al.: The incidence of Kaposi sarcoma among injection drug users with AIDS in the United States. J. Acquir. Immune Defic. Syndr. 37, 1282–1287 (2004)
7. Ascoli, V., Zambon, P., Manno, D., et al.: Variability in the incidence of classic Kaposi's sarcoma in the Veneto region, Northern Italy. Tumori 89, 122–124 (2003)
8. Beral, V., Peterman, T.A., Berkelman, R.L., et al.: Kaposi's sarcoma among persons with AIDS: a sexually transmitted infection? Lancet 335, 123–128 (1990)
9. Cook, P.M., Whitby, D., Calabro, M.L., et al.: Variability and evolution of Kaposi's sarcoma-associated herpesvirus in Europe and Africa. International Collaborative Group. AIDS 13, 1165–1176 (1999)
10. Cottoni, F., Masala, M.V., Budroni, M., et al.: The role of occupation and a past history of malaria in the etiology of classic Kaposi's sarcoma: a case-control study in north-east Sardinia. Br. J. Cancer. 76, 1518–1520 (1997)

11. Crispo, A., Tamburini, M., De Marco, M.R., et al.: HHV-8 prevalence, immunosuppression and Kaposi's sarcoma in South Italy. Int. J. Mol. Med. **7**, 535–538 (2001)

12. Dal Maso, L., Polesel, J., Ascoli, V., et al.: Cancer and AIDS Registry Linkage Study. Classic Kaposi's sarcoma in Italy, 1985–1998. Br. J. Cancer **92**, 188–193 (2005)

13. Dourmishev, L.A., Dourmishev, A.L., Palmeri, D., et al.: Molecular genetics of Kaposi's sarcoma-associated herpesvirus (human herpesvirus-8) epidemiology and pathogenesis. Microbiol. Mol. Biol. Rev. **67**, 175–212 (2003)

14. Goedert, J.J.: The epidemiology of acquired immunodeficiency syndrome malignancies. Semin. Oncol. **27**, 390–401 (2000)

15. Grabar, S., Lanoy, E., Allavena, C., et al.: Clinical Epidemiology Group of the French Hospital Database on HIV. Causes of the first AIDS-defining illness and subsequent survival before and after the advent of combined antiretroviral therapy. HIV Med. **9**, 246–256 (2008)

16. Grulich, A.E., Beral, V., Swerdlow, A.J.: Kaposi's sarcoma in England and Wales before the AIDS epidemic. Br. J. Cancer **66**, 1135–1137 (1992)

17. Hengge, U.R., Ruzicka, T., Tyring, S.K., et al.: Update on Kaposi's sarcoma and other HHV8 associated diseases. Part 1: epidemiology, environmental predispositions, clinical manifestations, and therapy. Lancet Infect. Dis. **2**, 281–292 (2002)

18. Hudnall, S.D., Rady, P.L., Tyring, S.K., et al.: Hydrocortisone activation of human herpesvirus 8 viral DNA replication and gene expression in vitro. Transplantation **67**, 648–652 (1999)

19. Hussein, M.R.: Cutaneous and lymphadenopathic Kaposi's sarcoma: a case report and review of literature. J. Cutan. Pathol. **35**, 575–578 (2008)

20. Iscovich, J., Boffetta, P., Franceschi, S., et al.: Classic kaposi sarcoma: epidemiology and risk factors. Cancer **88**, 500–517 (2000)

21. James, W., Berger, T., Eston, D.: Andrew's diseases of the skin. Clinical dermatology, 10th edn. Saunders Elsevier, Philadelphia (2006)

22. Kaposi, M.: Idiopathisches multiples pigments arkom der haut. Arch. Dermatol. Syph. **4**, 265–272 (1872)

23. Laor, Y., Schwartz, R.A.: Epidemiologic aspects of American Kaposi's sarcoma. J. Surg. Oncol. **12**, 299–303 (1979)

24. Meditz, A.L., Borok, M., MaWhinney, S., et al.: Gender differences in AIDS-associated Kaposi sarcoma in Harare, Zimbabwe. J. Acquire. Immune Defic. Syndr. **44**, 306–308 (2007)

25. Mendez, J.C., Paya, C.V.: Kaposi's Sarcoma and Transplantation. Herpes **7**, 18–23 (2000)

26. Micali, G., Gasparri, O., Nasca, M.R., et al.: Kaposi's sarcoma occurring de novo in the surgical scar in a heart transplant recipient. J. Am. Acad. Dermatol. **27**, 273–274 (1992)

27. Mohanna, S., Maco, V., Bravo, F., et al.: Epidemiology and clinical characteristics of classic Kaposi's sarcoma, seroprevalence, and variants of human herpesvirus 8 in South America: a critical review of an old disease. Int. J. Infect. Dis. **9**, 239–250 (2005)

28. Morand, J.J., Lightburn, E., Simon, F., et al.: Update on Kaposi's sarcoma. Med. Trop. (Mars) **67**, 123–130 (2007)

29. Penn, I.: Cancers following cyclosporine therapy. Transplant. Proc. **19**, 2211–2213 (1987)

30. Qunibi, W., Al-Furayh, O., Almeshari, K., et al.: Serologic association of human herpesvirus eight with posttransplant Kaposi's sarcoma in Saudi Arabia. Transplantation **65**, 583–585 (1998)

31. Renwick, N., Halaby, T., Weverling, G.J., et al.: Seroconversion for human herpesvirus 8 during HIV infection is highly predictive of Kaposi's sarcoma. AIDS **12**, 2481–2488 (1998)

32. Ruocco, V., Schwartz, R.A., Ruocco, E.: Lymphedema: an immunologically vulnerable site for development of neoplasms. J. Am. Acad. Dermatol. **47**, 124–127 (2002)

33. Schulz, T.F.: Epidemiology of Kaposi's sarcoma-associated herpesvirus/human herpesvirus 8. Adv. Cancer Res. **76**, 121–160 (1999)

34. Schwartz, R.A.: Kaposi's sarcoma: advances and perspectives. J. Am. Acad. Dermatol. **34**, 804–814 (1996)

35. Schwartz, R.A., Micali, G., Nasca, M.R., et al.: Kaposi sarcoma: a continuing conundrum. J. Am. Acad. Dermatol. **59**, 179–206 (2008)

36. Stratigos, J.D., Katoulis, A.C., Stavrianeas, N.G.: An overview of classic Kaposi's sarcoma in Greece. Adv. Exp. Med. Biol. **455**, 503–506 (1999)

37. Szajerka, T., Jablecki, J.: Kaposi's sarcoma revisited. AIDS Rev. **9**, 230–236 (2007)

38. Taylor, J.F., Smith, P.G., Bull, D., et al.: Kaposi's sarcoma in Uganda: geographic and ethnic distribution. Br. J. Cancer **26**, 483–497 (1973)

39. Wabinga, H.R., Parkin, D.M., Wabwire-Mangen, F., et al.: Cancer in Kampala, Uganda, in 1989–91: changes in incidence in the era of AIDS. Int. J. Cancer **54**, 26–36 (1993)

40. Yoshioka, M.C., Alchorne, M.M., Porro, A.M., et al.: Epidemiology of Kaposi's sarcoma in patients with acquired immunodeficiency syndrome in São Paulo, Brazil. Int. J. Dermatol. **43**, 643–647 (2004)

41. Zavos, G., Bokos, J., Papaconstantinou, I., et al.: Clinicopathological aspects of 18 Kaposi's sarcoma among 1055 Greek renal transplant recipients. Artif. Organs. **28**, 595–599 (2004)

Epidemiology of Dermatofibrosarcoma Protuberans

1.6

Selma Ugurel and Lauren Lockwood

Dermatofibrosarcoma protuberans (DFSP) is a fibroblastic skin tumor [6]. According to the WHO classification of mesenchymal tumors, DFSP belongs to the *Intermediate Malignancy Group*, characterized by locally aggressive, rarely metastasizing tumors. DFSP is one of the rarest skin cancers (less than 1 case per 100,000 people annually) [3]. However, it is the most common cutaneous sarcoma. The tumor generally presents in middle age, with an average age of onset at 40 years. Tumors presenting at birth or in childhood have, however, been reported [1]. Males and females are equally affected; the mortality rate accompanying low metastatic rate is very low.

DFSP exhibits a storiform growth pattern, is subject to local recurrence, and rarely, metastatic spread (in less than 5% of cases) [2, 3].

Fibrosarcomatous DFSP, a progressive variant of DFSP, exhibits an increased metastatic rate and is currently classified as a G-2 tumor. Another unique variant is pigmented DFSP, the so-called *Bednar-tumor*. Unlike typical DFSP, pigmented DFSP displays an excess of melanin-containing dendritic cells upon histological evaluation. Giant cell fibroblastoma, despite differences in morphology, reveals similar genetic alterations to DFSP and, thus, is characterized as a variant of DFSP [4, 5]. Furthermore, there are certain tumors that show characteristics of both DFSP and giant cell fibroblastoma.

References

1. Checketts, S.R., Hamilton, T.K., et al.: Congenital and childhood dermatofibrosarcoma protuberans: a case report and review of the literature. J. Am. Acad. Dermatol. **42**, 907–913 (2000)
2. Fish, F.S.: Soft tissue sarcomas in dermatology. Dermatol. Surg. **22**, 268–273 (1996)
3. Gloster Jr., H.M.: Dermatofibrosarcoma protuberans. J. Am. Acad. Dermatol. **35**, 355–374 (1996)
4. O'Brien, K.P., Seroussi, F., et al.: Various regions within the alpha-helical domain of the COL1A1 gene are fused to the second exon of the PDGFB gene in dermatofibrosarcomas and giant-cell fibroblastomas. Genes Chromosomes Cancer **23**, 187–193 (1998)
5. Simon, M.P., Pedeutour, F., et al.: Deregulation of the platelet-derived growth factor B-chain gene via fusion with collagen gene COL1A1 in dermatofibrosarcoma protuberans and giant-cell fibroblastoma. Nat. Genet. **15**, 95–98 (1997)
6. Weiss, S.W., Goldblum, J.R. (eds.): Fibrohistiocytic tumors of intermediate malignancy. In: Enzinger and Weiss's Soft Tissue Tumors, pp. 491–506. Mosby, St. Louis (2001)

S. Ugurel (✉)
Klinik und Poliklinik für Dermatologie, Venerologie und Allergologie der Universität Würzburg, Josef-Schneider-Strasse 2, 97080 Würzburg, Germany
e-mail: ugurel_s@klinik.uni-wuerzburg.de

L. Lockwood
Department of Dermatology, University Hospital of Zürich, Zürich, Switzerland

R. Dummer et al. (eds.), *Skin Cancer – A World-Wide Perspective*,
DOI: 10.1007/978-3-642-05072-5_1.6, © Springer-Verlag Berlin Heidelberg 2011

Epidemiology of Merkel Cell Carcinoma

Jean Kanitakis and Wen Lyn Ho

1.7.1 Definition

Merkel cell carcinoma (MCC), also known as primary neuroendocrine or trabecular carcinoma of the skin, is an aggressive primary cutaneous carcinoma first described by Toker in 1972 [21]. MCC cells share ultrastructural and immunohistochemical neuroendocrine features with epidermal Merkel cells, but their precise histogenetic origin remains uncertain.

1.7.2 Incidence

MCC is regarded as a rare tumor, and detailed descriptive epidemiological data are lacking. Referring to data from the US Surveillance, Epidemiology, and End Results (SEER) Program, it has been estimated that the annual incidence of MCC in the USA is 0.23 per 100,000 people in the white population [16]. Worth noting is a later analysis of SEER data that included 1,124 MCC cases; the incidence of MCC was found to have tripled between 1986 and 2001, i.e., from 0.15 to 0.44 per 100,000, especially among men [9]. Possible explanations for the 8% annual increase include improved detection (attributed to the advent of reliable ancillary diagnostic techniques such as immunohistochemistry) and reporting, increasing rates of ultraviolet light (UV) exposure, and higher risk for immunosuppression in the general population.

Some other estimates of MCC incidence rates have been reported for residents of South East Scotland, Minnesota, Finland, and Connecticut [4, 11, 17, 18], but these are difficult to interpret since the data are often not population-based/or age-adjusted. Nowadays, there are approximately 1,500 MCC cases per year in the USA, i.e., more cases than cutaneous T-cell lymphoma [13]. Overall, MCC is 65–100-fold rarer than melanoma [12, 16].

1.7.3 Sex

Despite some variations in the published series, most MCC series have shown a slight predilection for men (male: female ratio 1.4–2:1 in whites and blacks, and 1.5:1 in other ethnic groups) [1, 2, 15, 16].

1.7.4 Age

MCC has been described in a wide range of ages (8–101 years) but occurs predominantly in elderly people with a mean age of 70–74 years [1–3, 14, 17]. The 85+ age group has the highest age-specific incidence, at 4.3 per 100,000 [9]. More than two-thirds of MCC cases occur in people 65 years or older, and patients over 75 years of age account for almost 50% of all cases; men seem to be affected at a younger age than women [1].

1.7.5 Ethnic Groups

As above MCC has been reported in several ethnic groups (including white, black, and Asian people) [7], but it clearly prevails in Caucasian patients who account for well over 90% of cases [1, 7]. The incidence of MCC in black populations (0.01 cases per 100,000) is one twentieth the corresponding figure in whites [16]. According to another study [1], the incidence rate in whites is 11.3 times higher than in blacks and 2.2 times higher than other ethnic groups.

J. Kanitakis (✉)
Department of Dermatology, Ed. Herriot Hospital, 69437 Lyon, France
e-mail: jean.kanitakis@univ-lyon1.fr

W.L. Ho
Department of Dermatology, Beaumont Hospital, Dublin, Ireland

R. Dummer et al. (eds.), *Skin Cancer – A World-Wide Perspective*,
DOI: 10.1007/978-3-642-05072-5_1.7, © Springer-Verlag Berlin Heidelberg 2011

1.7.6 Anatomic Site

MCC usually occurs on sun-exposed skin, occasionally in association with other UV-induced skin cancers such as Bowen's disease and squamous cell carcinomas [10]. According to various series, 40–50% of cases occur on the head and neck, 11–23% on the trunk, and 33–40% on the upper and lower extremities [1, 2, 15, 18]. There are some variations depending on age at diagnosis; for instance, with advancing age, the head becomes a progressively more prevailing site, whereas patients (especially males) younger than 65 years of age have a greater proportion of tumors developing on the limbs and trunk [1]. MCC occurs exceptionally (4.5% of cases) on mucosal surfaces such as the nasal cavity, mouth, pharynx, larynx, and vagina [1].

1.7.7 Risk Factors

The etiopathogenesis of MCC has long remained a mystery. Very recently, a new polyoma virus, named Merkel cell polyoma virus (MCPyV or MCPV), was detected in a majority of MCC cases [5]. This virus is integrated into the genome of tumor cells before their clonal expansion, and it thus appears to be involved in the development of the tumor.

Possible risk factors that could favor the development of MCC include:

(a) UV radiation. This is suggested by the predominance of MCC on sun-exposed sites and its possible association with basal cell and squamous cell carcinomas (known to be triggered by UV), the development of MCC following PUVA treatment, and the increased incidence within the same ethnic group in geographic areas of higher sun exposure [9]. The detection of some genetic abnormalities shared with squamous cell carcinomas, such as UVB-induced mutations on *p53* and *H-ras* genes [20], also speaks in favor of UV radiation as a risk factor.

(b) Immunosuppression is suggested as a risk factor by the fact that the incidence of MCC seems to be increased among immunosuppressed patients including those with HIV infection, lymphomas/leukemias, and organ transplants [10] and by occasional observations of tumor regression upon cessation of immunosuppressive treatment [6]. Immunosuppressed patients are significantly younger than non-immunosuppressed patients at the mean age of presentation (e.g., 47 years in those with organ grafts) [10], and around 29% of MCC cases in immunosuppressed patients present before the age of 50 years [19]. The role of immunosuppression is consistent with the involvement of the above-mentioned newly discovered virus, MCPV, in MCC development.

(c) Exposure to arsenic has been suggested as favoring the development of MCC, but relevant epidemiological evidence remains sparse [8].

References

1. Agelli, M., Clegg, L.: Epidemiology of primary Merkel cell carcinoma in the United States. J. Am. Acad. Dermatol. **49**, 832–841 (2003)
2. Akhtar, S., Oza, K., Wright, J.: Merkel cell carcinoma: report of 10 cases and review of the literature. J. Am. Acad. Dermatol. **43**, 755–767 (2000)
3. Brennner, B., Katz, A., Rakowski, E., et al.: Merkel cell carcinoma in Israel. Isr. J. Med. Sci. **32**, 1235–1238 (1996)
4. Chuang, T., Su, W., Muller, S.: Incidence of T cell lymphoma and other rare skin cancers in a defined population. J. Am. Acad. Dermatol. **23**(2 pt 1), 254–256 (1990)
5. Feng, H., Shuda, M., Chang, Y., Moore, P.: Clonal integration of a polyomavirus in human Merkel cell carcinoma. Science **319**, 1096–1100 (2008)
6. Friedlaender, M., Rubinger, D., Rosenbaum, E., Amir, G., Siguencia, E.: Temporary regression of Merkel cell carcinoma metastases after cessation of cyclosporine. Transplantation **73**, 1849–1850 (2002)
7. Heath, M., Jaimes, N., Lemos, B., et al.: Clinical characteristics of Merkel cell carcinoma at diagnosis in 195 patients: the AEIOU features. J. Am. Acad. Dermatol. **58**, 375–381 (2008)
8. Ho, S.Y., Tsai, Y.C., Lee, M.C., Guo, H.R.: Merkel cell carcinoma in patients with long-term ingestion of arsenic. J. Occup. Health. **47**, 188–192 (2005)
9. Hodgson, N.: Merkel cell carcinoma: changing incidence trends. J. Surg. Oncol. **89**, 1–4 (2005)
10. Kanitakis, J., Euvrard, S., Chouvet, B., et al.: Merkel cell carcinoma in renal transplant recipients. Report of two new cases with unusual histological features and literature review. J. Cutan. Pathol. **33**, 686–694 (2006)
11. Koljonen, V., Bohling, T., Granhroth, G., Tukiainen, E.: Merkel cell carcinoma: a clinicopathologic study of 34 patients. Eur. J. Surg. Oncol. **29**, 607–610 (2003)
12. Landis, S., Murray, T., Bolden, S., Wingo, P.: Cancer statistics, 1998. CA Cancer J. Clin. **48**, 6–29 (1998)
13. Lemos, B., Nghiem, P.: Merkel cell carcinoma: more deaths but still no pathway to blame. J. Invest. Dermatol. **12**, 2100–2103 (2007)
14. Liapakis, I., Korkolis, D., Koutsoumbi, A., et al.: Merkel cell carcinoma: clinicopathological aspects of an unusual neoplasm. J. BUON **12**, 173–179 (2007)
15. Medina-Franco, H., Urist, M., Fiveash, J., et al.: Multimodality treatment of Merkel cell carcinoma: case series and literature review of 1024 cases. Ann. Surg. Oncol. **8**, 204–208 (2001)
16. Miller, R., Rabkin, C.: Merkel cell carcinoma and melanoma: etiological similarities and differences. Cancer Epidemiol. Biomarkers Prev. **8**, 153–158 (1999)
17. Mills, L., Durrani, A., Watson, J.: Merkel cell carcinoma in South East Scotland, 1993–2003. Surgeon **4**, 133–138 (2006)
18. Pan, D., Naryan, D., Ariyan, S.: Merkel cell carcinoma: five case reports using sentinel lymph node biopsy and review of 110 new cases. Plast. Reconstr. Surg. **110**, 1259–1265 (2002)
19. Penn, I., First, M.R.: Merkel's cell carcinoma in organ recipients: report of 41 cases. Transplantation **68**, 1717–1721 (1999)
20. Popp, S., Waltering, S., Herbst, C., Moll, I., Boukamp, P.: UV-B-type mutations and chromosomal imbalances indicate common pathways for the development of Merkel and skin squamous cell carcinomas. Int. J. Cancer **99**, 352–360 (2002)
21. Toker, C.: Trabecular carcinoma of the skin. Arch. Dermatol. **105**, 107–110 (1972)

Pathogenesis of Nonmelanoma Skin Cancer

2.1

Petra Boukamp

Nonmelanoma skin cancers (NMSC), that is, basal cell carcinomas (BCC) and squamous cell carcinomas (SCC), are the most common cancers, and their incidence continues to increase worldwide [32]. Immunosuppression in organ transplant patients strongly contributes to this increased incidence. While BCCs are more frequent than SCCs in the general population, with a ratio of 4–1, this proportion reverses in organ transplant patients, with a ratio of 3.8:1 SCCs to BCCs. This makes skin cancer, particularly SCCs, 65–250 times more frequent in immune-suppressed organ transplant patients than in the general population. Often these patients suffer from second and third lesions. SCCs in these patients also appear to be more aggressive. They tend to grow rapidly, show a higher rate of local recurrences, and metastasize in 5–8% of patients (reviewed in [35]). This may suggest that "dormant" SCC precursor cells/lesions are present at a high frequency but are well controlled by the immune system. BCCs may be less dependent on immune surveillance, thereby highlighting their different etiology.

2.1.1 BCC Pathology

It is suggested that BCCs develop de novo from the basal germinative cells and are initiated by one or few major sunburns early in life. The generally slow-growing BCCs are differentiated into nodular, superficial, morpheaform, and ulcerating subtypes [2, 84]. Typically, the nodular form of BCCs appears on sun-exposed skin and is often characterized by smooth and intensive telangiectasia and inner ulceration [88]. Despite the fact that BCCs frequently develop on the face, about 30% develop in sun-protected locations, indicating that in addition to UV radiation, UV-independent

mechanisms contribute to BCC development. BCCs rarely metastasize (<0.1%); however, they are highly invasive and locally destructive and, therefore, a burden for patients.

2.1.2 SCC Pathology

SCC development, on the other hand, is viewed as a multistep process with cumulative lifetime exposure to UV radiation (especially UVB) thought to be a causative factor. As an early and potentially primary event, mutations in the p53 tumor suppressor gene have been found in otherwise unsuspicious epidermis [53, 62, 69]. They are detectable by immunohistochemistry in individual cells and also in patches of cells. Indeed, 70% of these p53 patches had an underlying mutation in the p53 gene [53, 82]. It was reasoned that these patches are early precancerous lesions and, therefore, may serve as risk markers for SCC development. However, a retrospective study of 250 cases did not establish statistically significant differences between skin from patients with solitary and multiple skin carcinomas. Instead, this study highlighted an increased frequency of p53 patches with age [60].

Actinic keratosis (AK), on the other hand, is a well-established precancerous skin lesion, and it is suggested that about 10% will develop into skin SCCs [52]. In fact, p53 mutations and, in particular, UV-type mutations are frequently found in AK, further substantiating that they may develop through p53-positive patches. Bowen's disease (BD), also known as carcinoma in situ (CIS), is a further advanced preinvasive stage. AK and CIS can occur at multiple sites as well as in vicinity of SCCs, supporting the hypothesis of field cancerization, already suggested by the immunopositive p53 distribution [55]. Although still controversially discussed, keratoacanthomas (KAs) may also be potential precursor lesions [15]. KAs are benign, cutaneous, squamous tumors arising preferentially on sun-exposed skin. They are characterized by a rapid growth phase for the first 4–8 weeks and a possible, spontaneous, self-induced regression after 3–6 months. Due to their initial growth rate and morphology, which are very similar to well-differentiated SCCs [6], it is

P. Boukamp
Division of Genetics of Skin Carcinogenesis, German Cancer
Research Center, Im Neuenheimer Feld 280, 69120 Heidelberg,
Germany
e-mail: p.boukamp@DKFZ-Heidelberg.de

R. Dummer et al. (eds.), *Skin Cancer – A World-Wide Perspective*,
DOI: 10.1007/978-3-642-05072-5_2.1, © Springer-Verlag Berlin Heidelberg 2011

still debated whether KAs are a specific type of SCC or an independent tumor entity [46]. This said, in many cases, a defined clinical classification is difficult, allowing for KA-like SCCs or SCCs with KA-like characteristics. We recently demonstrated that at least some KAs are genetically incomplete SCCs [15]. This may well argue for a fluent transition and, depending on the combination of aberrations present, KAs may either still be able to spontaneously regress or may have already lost this ability.

2.1.3 Genetic Aberrations

2.1.3.1 p53 and Skin Cancer

As mentioned above, UV radiation is a major contributor to skin cancer development and progression. UV exposure induces specific types of aberrations, one of which – mutation in the p53 tumor suppressor gene – is particularly well characterized. It is now well established that more than 50% of all SCCs and BCCs show p53 mutations, and this frequency rises to 90% in tumors of patients with xeroderma pigmentosum, that is, patients who suffer from a defect in nucleotide excision repair that is responsible for hyperphotosensitivity and a high incidence of skin cancer (reviewed in [37]. Many p53 mutations show a very specific pattern, that is, C to T transitions with a high frequency of CC to TT double base changes. Since these mutations are exclusive to skin tumors and since it was shown that UVB radiation can induce such changes [95], these types of mutations are now accepted as UVB signatures. Furthermore, the authors found that repair is slow at these sites suggesting that repair inefficiency may strongly contribute to the mutation spectrum. Pfeifer and colleagues also showed that the presence of photodimers, the most common UV-dependent lesions, strongly inhibited binding of several important cell cycle regulatory and DNA damage-responsive transcription factors [94], thereby, providing a potential explanation for the fact that promoter regions are repaired inefficiently.

As a second characteristic, skin carcinomas differ from, for example, colon cancer because the second p53 allele is not lost during tumor progression but frequently mutated. Since the two mutations occur at different sites, this strongly supports the mutational power of UVB radiation [12, 76]. Additionally, the mutations do not appear to occur at random but accumulate in hot spots [104]. These hot spots differ from those of internal malignancies, and it is actually proposed that the mutation in codon 177 is specific for BCCs, while mutations in codon 278, though occasionally seen in certain internal cancers, are specific for SCCs [37]. Such specificity argues for a selective advantage in these mutations, not only causing inactivation of the protein but providing some gain of

function [57]. Since such mutations can precede visible tumors, it is suggested that p53 mutations are early if not initial events. Actually, with p53 being the guardian of the genome [59], it is tempting to suggest that these mutations allow for a first pulse of genomic instability, a mechanism required for additional genetic changes to occur.

2.1.3.2 BCCs are Characterized by a Defective SONIC Hedgehog Pathway

While mutations in the p53 gene are common in BCCs and SCCs, most other known genetic aberrations are rather exclusive for one skin tumor type or the other. The best defined aberration in BCCs is their aberrant sonic hedgehog-patched-smoothened pathway. The finding that patients with nevoid basal cell carcinoma (NBCC) syndrome – who develop multiple BCCs at an early age – showed frequent loss of chromosome 9q has allowed for the identification of the putative tumor suppressor gene from 9q22 to q32, the *PTCH* gene. *PTCH* is the cell surface receptor of the secreted signaling molecule, sonic hedgehog (*SHH*) (for review, see [93]). In the absence of *SHH*, patched1, the protein product of *PTCH*, inhibits smoothened (*SMO*), a G-protein-coupled-like receptor. *SMO* is released upon binding of *SHH* to patched1 and can initiate a signal transduction cascade that causes activation of the transcription factor Gli. Thus, deregulation of this pathway, by either loss of *PTCH* or forced expression of *SMO*, results in elevated levels of Gli1 and, as a consequence, induces hair follicle tumors. Most importantly, loss-of-function mutations in *PTCH* have been found in a number of sporadic BCCs, and most of them showed the UVB signature, arguing that UV is responsible for abrogating the *SHH* pathway in sporadic BCCs [44]. Similarly, mutations activating *SMO* and Gli have been found in sporadic human BCCs and even more often in BCC from xeroderma pigmentosum patients, as well as mutations in *SHH* [23, 81]. Furthermore, studies with a BCC mouse model have shown that the function of Gli2 is to prevent apoptosis and promote microvascularization. This model implicates that preventing Gli2 function may also inhibit BCC formation [48]. Thus, it is now widely accepted that abrogation of the SHH pathway is the major cause of BCC development. Furthermore, since the *SHH* pathway is known to be essential for hair follicle development [19], it is strongly believed that BCCs originate from hair follicle precursor cells.

Recently, there has been evidence that the TGF-β/Smad pathway plays a role in BCC pathogenesis [36]. The authors found significant mRNA overexpression of TGF-β1 and Smad pathway constituents, Smad 3 and Smad 7, in the center of BCCs as compared to adjacent healthy skin sites [36]. However, functional studies are still missing.

2.1.3.3   Other Genetic Aberrations in BCCs

14-3-3sigma: Many tumors are characterized by defined changes in cell cycle regulators. While 16^{INK4} and cyclin D1 play important roles in skin SCCs (see later), abrogation of 14-3-3sigma, a member of a protein family that regulates cellular activity by binding and sequestering, for example, cyclin B1 and cdc2, seems to be responsible for an aberrant growth control in BCCs. 14-3-3-sigma, which is controlled by p53, promotes premitotic cell cycle arrest following DNA damage and thereby prevents "mitotic catastrophe" [20]. Indeed, expression of 14-3-3sigma was found to be, partially or completely lost in BCCs, mainly due to CpG-hypermethylation [63]. Since it is generally believed that p16^{INK4} remains wildtype in BCCs and, accordingly, no methylation was found, 14-3-3sigma may substitute for p16^{INK4} in BCCs, and its silencing may thus contribute to evasion of senescence in BCC [63].

Cytogenetic changes: Most BCCs are characterized by a relatively "simple" genotype with only one to three aberrations per tumor [51]. More surprising was the finding of extensive, intratumoral heterogeneity. From the 44 BCCs analyzed, 21 contained genetically independent subclones, while only ten tumors contained genetically related subclones. The most frequent aberrations the authors identified were gains of chromosomes 18, X, 7, and 9 and losses of the terminal parts of chromosomes 6q, 13q, 4q, 1q, 8q, and 9p. While no clear-cut association existed between the karyotypic patterns and histological subtypes or sites of the tumor, the frequency of cytogenetically unrelated clones was significantly higher in recurrent BCCs than in primary lesions, suggesting that the aggressiveness of BCCs may be determined by the presence of genetically unrelated tumor cell clones, which may allow for better adaptation to environmental changes and thus provide a selective growth advantage.

2.1.3.4   SCCs are Characterized by Multiple Genetic Aberrations

2.1.3.4.1   Potential Involvement of Aberrant Signal Transduction Pathways

Wnt/β-catenin pathway activation: Unlike BCCs, where *SHH* pathway abrogation is the most prominent genetic change, the search for pathway alterations in SCCs is ongoing. Recently, Doglioni et al. found mutated β-catenin and suggested the involvement of the TCF-1/MITF-mediated pathway [29]. In line with these observations, Hülsken and coworkers reported a high number of SCCs containing nuclear β-catenin, arguing for an activated Wnt/β-catenin pathway in skin SCCs [64]. From their experimental mouse studies, the authors proposed that cutaneous cancer stem cell maintenance is dependent on β-catenin signaling. On the other hand, Brasanac et al. [11] could detect nuclear β-catenin in AKs but only in a few SCCs. Our own studies demonstrate β-catenin-positive nuclei in KAs and SCCs (Wischermann and Boukamp, unpublished results). While it is well established that an activated Wnt pathway is essential for hair follicle development (reviewed in [73]), and constitutive SH signaling was shown to induce Wnt/β-catenin signaling in BCCs (reviewed in [85]), its role in the interfollicular epidermis and skin SCC is still unclear. Accordingly, the functional consequences of an activated Wnt pathway in human HaCaT keratinocytes are underway.

On the other hand, evidence is emerging that TGFβ and its canonical Smad pathway are involved in skin carcinogenesis. This said, an active *TGFβ/Smad pathway* is essential for normal keratinocyte growth and differentiation (Buschke et al., submitted). In human SCCs, two distribution patterns of TGFβ were found either (1) predominantly in suprabasal layers or (2) throughout the tumor epithelia, including the basal proliferative cells [61]. Several keratinocyte-specific, transgenic mouse models were generated with TGFβ-1 being overexpressed, either predominantly in the suprabasal epidermis or in the basal layer of the epidermis and hair follicles. Suprabasal TGFβ-1 inhibited keratinocyte proliferation and suppressed chemically induced skin carcinogenesis in early stages, but promoted tumor invasion at later stages. In contrast, TGFβ-1 overexpressed in the basal layer of the epidermis and hair follicles caused severe inflammation and epidermal hyperproliferation, thus highlighting the dual action of TGFβ, acting as a tumor suppressor in early stages but promoting carcinogenesis during tumor progression.

NF-kapaB signaling pathway: A most unexpected result was reported by Gottipati et al. [39]. The authors demonstrated that passive smoking hindered UVB-dependent skin carcinogenesis in SKH-1 hairless mice. They suggested that passive smoking inhibited activation of the NF-kappaB signaling pathway and thereby hindered tumorigenesis.

2.1.3.5   Other Genetic Aberrations in SCCs

The ras oncogene: As discussed above, in the primary lesion in skin cancer development, mutational inactivation of the p53 tumor suppressor gene occurs, allowing for survival in spite of subsequent damage, which then manifests and thus causes a certain degree of genomic instability. Another aberration discussed as being essential for SCC development is mutational activation of the ras oncogene. From the three *ras* genes, *Harvey- (Ha)*, *Kirsten- (Ki)*, and *N-ras*, mutations in

Ha-ras predominate in the general population, and interestingly, the characteristic mutations in codons 12, 13, and 61 are all opposite UV-sensitive CC sites. This led to the conclusion that in skin SCCs, *ras* mutations are also caused by UVB radiation. Early (early 1990s) studies suggested that it was the *ras* oncogene that significantly contributed to skin cancer development, but finally, a mutation frequency of only 10–20% was established (reviewed in [8]). However, a high mutation frequency and prevalence of *N-ras* mutations were reported in xeroderma pigmentosum patients, being in good agreement with the more important role of UV radiation in SCC development and different mutation profile in the tumors of these patients [25].

The role of *ras* mutations in skin carcinogenesis is best demonstrated in mouse models using skin carcinogenesis initiation – promotion protocol with one treatment of the carcinogen di-methyl-benzanthracene (DMBA) followed by biweekly application of phorbol ester (TPA). This model causes *ras*-dependent formation of papillomas, which in part progress to SCCs (reviewed in [28]). Although these mouse tumors show remarkable phenotypic similarities to human skin carcinomas, it remains unknown how far molecular findings, based on chemical carcinogenesis, that is, "*ras*-dependent" skin carcinogenesis, can be extrapolated to human SCCs and will help to unravel the still poorly understood genetic pathway of human UV-induced skin carcinogenesis. This said, the SKH1 hairless mouse model may be more relevant (for review, see [97]). Reproducible and quantitative data were established for dose, time, and wavelength of UV radiation required for SCC development [27]. In this model, a high frequency of p53 mutations was found, while only 1 out of 32 tumors carried a *ras* mutation [98]. The majority of the p53 mutations were located in a codon matching a hotspot for p53 mutations in human skin carcinomas, thus largely mimicking human UV-induced skin cancer. Nevertheless, also these data must be taken with caution. Differences between mouse and human physiology exist in, for example, the composition of melanin and, with that, the level of protection against UV radiation. Depending on skin type, various compositions of pheomelanin and eumelanin, another form of melanin, are observed. Increased pheomelanin photosensitizes DNA and thus induces DNA damage, while eumelanin predominates in mouse melanocytes [71].

In line with some functional consequences of the *ras* oncogene in SCC development, a novel keratinocyte-specific chemokine, CCL27, was recently proposed to play a critical role in the organization of skin-associated immune responses, by regulating T cell homing under homeostatic and inflammatory conditions. CCL27 mRNA and protein expression were progressively lost in AKs, BCCs, and SCCs. Since it was suggested that downregulation of CCL27 occurs through activation of the Ras-MAPK-signaling pathways, and because precancerous skin lesions as well as cutaneous carcinomas show significantly elevated levels of phosphorylated ERK when compared to normal skin, oncogenic ras may be involved in a skin tumor mechanism used to evade host antitumor immune responses [75].

The role of cell cycle inhibitors: Deregulation of cell cycle regulators plays an important role in epithelial transformation, the most extensively analyzed being the cyclin-dependent kinase inhibitor p16INK4. p16INK4 specifically inhibits progression through the G1 phase of the cell cycle by blocking the cyclin-dependent kinase 4 from phosphorylating the retinoblastoma protein [87]. p16INK4 mutations were detected, although at a low frequency, in SCC from the general population as well as in patients suffering from xeroderma pigmentosum [58, 89, 90]. It was discussed that p16INK4 mutations may be late events in skin cancer development and, therefore, may have been missed in studies evaluating precancerous lesions or small tumors, that is, microinvasive SCCs [90]. On the other hand, loss of heterozygosity (LOH) as well as loss of parts of or the entire short term of chromosome 9 – p16INK4 maps to 9p21 – was frequently observed in SCCs [76, 79]. We recently showed that p16INK4, which is largely undetectable in normal skin, was highly expressed in KAs but absent in most of the SCCs. Although some of these SCCs had lost a copy of 9p, we did not find a strong correlation, suggesting that besides chromosomal loss, loss of heterogeneity (small microdeletions), point mutations, or epigenetic mechanisms, such as promoter methylation, as previously detected [13], were causal. We, however, also found SCCs that expressed high levels of p16INK4. Interestingly, none of those showed loss of 9p and all were undifferentiated. SCCs, while the p16INK4-negative tumors were well-to-highly differentiated ones. As suggested from cervical carcinomas, human papilloma virus (HPV) can induce expression of p16INK4 [24], and it is tempting to suggest that p16INK4 is wild-type in this subgroup of SCCs and that HPV may have been responsible for the p16INK4 immune-reactivity. In agreement with our results, Salama et al. [86] also showed little immunostaining for AK, a high frequency of positive BDs, and no staining for SCC. In a third study, not only the BDs but also all AKs were positive [45]. This may allow for two interpretations. First, p16INK4 expression is required for premalignant lesions to control their growth and thus allow for tumor regression. Second, for invasive growth, the function of this cell cycle inhibitor needs to be abrogated. The differential expression of p16INK4 in well vs. poorly differentiated SCCs, however, may highlight two different developmental pathways, that is, UV-related vs. HPV-related.

While abrogation of p16INK4 function seems to be a late event, upregulation of the cell cycle activator cyclin D1 was similarly detected in premalignant KAs and SCCs [16, 96]. Protein overexpression occurred as a consequence of chromosome duplication and gene locus amplification, as well as by a still unknown translational mechanism. While increased cyclin D1 expression suggested improved proliferation, this was not confirmed by our experimental data using the HaCaT model [10]. Instead, tissues generated by these cells were characterized by disorganized proliferation and differentiation, that is, proliferating and differentiating cells throughout the entire epithelium, suggesting that overexpression of cyclin D1 seriously disturbed tissue homeostatsis [16]. Transplantation studies also demonstrated an unexpected interaction with the stroma. Unlike control cells, the cyclin D1 overexpressing HaCaT cells caused a massive inflammatory response [15]. Nevertheless, the cells remained nontumorigenic. Only cells that, in addition, had upregulated the cyclin-dependent kinase Cdk4 formed KA-like tumors [16]. This clearly demonstrates the need for changes exceeding p53 mutation and cyclin D1 upregulation to obtain fully malignant SCCs.

Glutathione peroxidase: Another potential early aberration was suggested by Walshe et al. [99]. They reported that perturbation in glutathione peroxidase activity (GPX) leads to an elevated peroxide burden and thus an increased risk of skin damage [99]. Indeed, they observed that reduced GPX in vivo could be reversed by agents that reduce the burden of oxidatives/peroxidatives and concluded that the disruption of peroxide and reactive oxygen species' (ROS) metabolism directly contributes to UV-induced skin SCC.

The angiogenic switch: One of the essential changes allowing for malignant growth is the so-called angiogenic switch. In order to acquire an invasive phenotype, blood vessels need to infiltrate the tumor [68]. We recently showed that the angiogenic inhibitor thrombospondin 1 (TSP-1) is able to halt tumor vascularization and thereby to suppress invasive growth [7]. We recently added that TSP-1, a component of the provisional matrix during wound healing, was strongly expressed by KAs but absent or minimal in SCCs [15]. Interestingly, a lack of TSP-1 in SCCs correlated with the expression of the matrix degradation enzyme, matrix metalloprotease 13 (MMP13), in either the tumor cells or surrounding stroma; however, MMP13 expression was largely absent in KAs (Burnworth and Boukamp, unpublished). Similarly, MMP2 and MMP9 expression were found to be more extensive in the stroma of SCCs than BDs [72]. These data suggest that TSP-1 inhibition, correlated with MMP upregulation, is a late event in tumor progression and is responsible for malignant progression. The data also suggest that premalignant KAs interact with their environment like continuous wounds; a tumor is a wound that never heals, as originally stated by Cairns, but a change is necessary for progression to SCC. A potential mechanism for TSP-1 inhibition is the loss of copies of chromosome 15 [15]; however, other mechanisms are also likely to contribute.

Requirements for metastasis: The genetic changes that allow cells to metastasize are still poorly understood. For a specific sequence of tumors, we could show that the metastasis genetically developed directly from the primary tumor, while two independent recurrences had a different genetic makeup and had developed from a common precursor lesion, in parallel to the primary tumor [76]. Whether this is a general rule, metastases always establishing detectable new aberrations (when compared to primary tumors), is still unclear. Using single nucleotide polymorphism (SNP) microarray analyses [78], Purdie et al. identified the protein-tyrosin-phosphatase-receptor type D (PTPRD) locus as a tumor suppressor gene candidate in SCCs, with a potential association with metastasis. Functional proof, however, is still awaited. Similarly open is the functional consequence of chemokine receptor changes. It was recently reported that downregulation of CCR6, in concert with upregulation of CCR7 and CXCR4, was correlated with metastasis-competent SCCs but not AKs or BCCs, and it was proposed – as for metastatic melanoma and SCC of the head and neck – that chemokine receptors may influence biological behavior and thereby add to metastasis [5].

Molecular and cytogenetic changes: In 1994, Rees and coworkers reported on LOH in 9q in as many as 77% of BCCs but only 12% of SCCs. In contrast, LOH in 9p markers was frequent in SCC [79]. Recently, a gene was identified, the Brahma gene (BRM), an ATPase subunit of the SWI/SNF chromatin remodeling complex. It plays important roles in transcription, splicing, replication, and DNA repair [41] and may account for aberrations occurring due to lack of 9p [67]. In addition to chromosome 9p, a number of other chromosomes were shown to carry LOH in SCCs, such as 3p, 13p, 17p, and 17q [80]. Comparison with AKs and KAs revealed that AKs shared many of the same loci as SCCs, while the frequency of LOH in KAs was low with only isolated losses at 9p, 9q, and 10q [80, 100]. Cytogenetic analysis and comparative genomic hybridization, the latter allowing a genome-wide screen for gains and losses of chromosomal parts [54], revealed great karyotypic complexity and cytogenetic heterogeneity in SCCs [49, 50, 76, 77]. Jin et al. found that many structural aberrations affected centromeric regions, particularly those of chromosomes 3q, 8q, 9q, and 5p. These caused whole-arm translocations and duplication of one chromosome arm, thereby generating iso-chromosomes [49]. They additionally observed genetically unrelated clones within the same tumor, suggesting that, as described for BCCs, a multifocal development is also frequent in SCCs. AKs, on the other hand, only revealed few numerical changes, for example, gain of chromosomes 7, 9, and 18, while recurrent iso-chromosomes were not seen [49]. In line with these findings, our CGH studies also suggest a much simpler aberration profile for KAs than SCCs. Unexpectedly, gains and losses of the same chromosomes (in particular loss of 3p, 9p and gain of 11q) were involved in both tumor types. However, the important difference was that the individual KA only carried one or two of these aberrations, while in SCCs, several different aberrations were commonly present together (Popp et al., unpublished). This further strengthened the hypothesis that KAs are genetically incomplete SCCs. Finally, multiplex fluorescence in situ hybridization (M-FISH), which identifies all chromosomes of a metaphase simultaneously [91], highlighted complex translocations in the SCC-derived cell lines [77], substantiating the important role of ongoing genomic instability in skin SCC development.

2.1.4 UVA May be Causal for Structural Chromosomal Aberrations

UVB radiation is thought to be the major risk factor for human skin carcinogenesis because its energy is sufficient to enter the nuclei of epidermal cells. It directly damages DNA by inducing cyclobutane pyrimidine dimers (CPDs) and pyrimidine (6–4) pyrimidine photoproducts at dipyrimidine sites, thereby giving rise to very specific mutation patterns (summarized in [9]). Recently, more interest in UVA radiation's role in aberrations has been expressed. Although the photon energy may be insufficient to damage DNA directly, UVA radiation is able to penetrate into the epidermis down to the proliferative basal cells and, even further, to the dermal compartment, where it contributes to photoaging (for review, see [38]). Using albino hairless mice, de Gruijl et al. provided evidence that UVA may also be relevant for skin cancer development (for review, see [26]). Accordingly, the immortal human HaCaT keratinocytes became tumorigenic when irradiated with UVA, and we showed that as little as 20 J/cm^2 UVA for 5 weeks was sufficient to induce first tumor growth [43, 102].

The action of UVA is thought to be indirect. By activating cellular chromophores and inducing photo-oxidative cellular stress [103], ROS can modify guanine to 8-oxo-7,8-dihydro-7'-deoxyguanosine (8-oxo-guanine) resulting in transversion mutations, changing guanine to thymine during replication [17]. Most importantly, ROS is also involved in generating DNA single strand (ss) breaks [56]. If ss breaks are not repaired during the G1 phase of the cell cycle, they generate double strand (ds) breaks during S-phase, which then can result in chromosomal aberrations such as amplifications, deletions, or translocations. In agreement with this scenario, we recently showed that UVA can induce a dose-dependent and long lasting induction of DNA strand breaks in HaCaT cells and normal keratinocytes as well as a significant induction and maintenance of micronuclei (MN) with more acentric fragments (indicative of ds breaks) than entire chromosomes. Finally, all tumors recultivated from the UVA-treated HaCaT cells were characterized by new chromosomal changes, that is, loss of chromosomes or exchange of chromosomal material, that is, translocation chromosomes [102]. Although not yet firmly proven, this strongly suggests that UVA radiation has enough energy to cause these types of chromosomal aberrations, which are both hallmarks of human SCCs [76, 77].

2.1.4.1 The Role of Human Papillomavirus (HPV)

Similar to mutations, p53 function can be abrogated in human skin carcinomas by the action of human papillomaviruses (HPV) (reviewed in [33]). More than 100 subtypes have been identified, but only a subgroup of so-called high-risk mucosotropic HPV types, including HPV-16, 18, 31, 33, 35, and 58, are believed to be causative agents in the development of cancer, that is, cervical cancer. The E6 gene of these high-risk HPV types is able to induce rapid proteasomal degradation of p53, thereby abolishing the induction of cell cycle arrest or apoptosis. As in cervical carcinomas, a high prevalence of HPV infection is characteristic of immune-competent (47%) and even more so of immune-suppressed patients (75%). However, more than 40 different HPV types were identified [70], and the typical high-risk HPV types (e.g., HPV 16 and 18) were not yet found (reviewed in [40]). Therefore, it was suggested that mechanisms different from those of HPV oncoproteins in genital cancer may be involved in skin neoplastic transformation [18]. Only in epidermodysplasia verruciformis patients, known for their clinically apparent infections with HP viruses, HPV-5 and -8 are believed to have carcinogenic potential (reviewed in [33]). Furthermore, in forehead skin swab samples from 50 healthy males who were frequently exposed to the sun and 50 healthy males who were not, HPV prevalence was higher in the first group. Most interestingly, however, HPV-76 was only detected in the latter group, suggesting that UV radiation may lead to a difference in prevalence of cutaneous HPV types [21].

One HPV type that recently gained interest is HPV-38. HPV-38 was detected in about 50% of skin SCCs but in only 10% of healthy skin [65]. An Australian study additionally revealed HPV-38 DNA in 43% of solar keratoses, as well as 13% and 16% of SCCs and BCCs, respectively [1]. Furthermore, HPV-38 was shown to actively support longevity/immortalization of cultured human skin keratinocytes [65]. Additionally, HPV-38's early genes E6 and E7 affected the interferon-reduced upregulation of major histocompatibility (MHC) class 1, indicating that HPV-38 may contribute to the evasion of host immune surveillance [22]. HPV-8, on the other hand, is thought to be involved in the rare inherited disorder, epidermodysplasia verruciformis, which is characterized by life-long occurrence of multiple flat warts and macular lesions. HPV-8 was expressed in the epidermis of mice (Keratin 14 promoter), and these transgenic mice spontaneously developed single or multiple benign skin tumors [47]. In contrast and unexpectedly, HPV-16 transgenic mice – carrying the high-risk HPV for cervical cancer – only developed hyperplasia, associated with hyperkeratosis [66]. Also, other HPV types, including 12, 14, 15, 24, 36, and 49, proved to have significant transforming potential when introduced into primary baby rat kidney cells [65].

Nevertheless, some uncertainties remain about the role of HPV in skin carcinogenesis. A broad spectrum of HPV types and multiple infections are generally found in immune-suppressed patients (reviewed in [74]). Furthermore, it was recently reported that HPV DNA was frequently detected in swab samples collected from the superficial layers of skin tumors, while only little HPV DNA was found in biopsies of the same tumors [34]. Last but not least, HP viruses not only occur in tumors but infect skin cells as a common flora. Already 1 month after birth, Antonsson et al. found HPV DNA in 37% of the samples of forehead skin swabs and, after 1 year, 50% were positive [3]. Thus, the role of HPV in skin SCCs is still far from being understood, and further studies are needed to support the relevance of the "high-risk" cutaneous HPV types for NMSC.

If HPV is involved, it clearly can serve several functions. First, it is well established that high-risk HPV abrogates p53 as well as Rb (reviewed in [33]). Second, HPV-induced genomic instability is documented with HPV-16 E6 causing structural chromosomal changes [101], while E7 is correlated with numerical chromosomal abnormalities [42, 101]. Duensing et al. further showed that E6 and E7 cooperate to induce genomic instability by uncoupling centrosome duplication from cell division [31] and that E7 is responsible for abnormal centrosome synthesis [30]. Thus, it remains to be seen whether the HPV types associated with skin SCCs can function in a similar way as cervical HPV types and, besides interfering with p53 and Rb function, cause centrosome abnormalities and, with that, numerical chromosomal changes, that is, aneuploidy.

Recently, the presence of polyomavirus has been detected in 80% of Merkel cell carcinomas (MCCs), a very rare but highly aggressive skin tumor (reviewed in [14]). A follow-up study investigated polyomavirus DNA in 85 SCCs, 37 KAs, 28 BDs, and 6 AK from organ transplant recipients. With the exception of 1 KA, no polyomavirus DNA was detected [83]. This may suggest that, different from MCCs, polyomaviruses are not of importance for NMSC.

2.1.5   Conclusions and Further Perspective

Comparison of the two NMSCs, BCC and SCC, clearly demonstrates that most of their oncogenes, tumor suppressor genes, and signal transduction pathways responsible for genesis are quite different and, particularly in respect to SCCs, our knowledge about the role of a number of the genetic changes required for malignant tumor growth are still poorly understood. On the one hand, BCC exhibits a relatively simple genotype, with only few aberrations and a high degree of independence of the immune system. With the identification of an aberrant SH pathway, a major cause of BCC development was identified. Correspondingly, the plant-derived teratogen cyclopamine has been shown to reverse the effects of oncogenic mutations in *SMO* and *PTCH* [92]. Its efficacy in BCC treatment in humans remains to be seen and thus its application as a successful therapy to eliminate this common, highly destructive tumor.

On the other hand, skin SCCs develop, at least in part, from precursor lesions and accumulate a highly complex genotype. While relatively few causal genes for tumor development and progression are known, a lot remains to be learned – for example, involvement of specific signal transduction pathways and the role of the environments/immune system. As demonstrated by the reversion rate of BCC to SCCs in immune-suppressed transplant patients, the immune system is particularly important for SCC development while largely negligible for BCC development. Whether it is the aberrant SH pathway that accounts for BCCs' loss of sensitivity remains to be seen. The most intriguing feature of SCCs, at present, is their large number of chromosomal aberrations and the recurrent involvement of specific chromosomes in gains, losses, and translocations. With increasing evidence that certain chromosomal aberrations and, in particular, certain combinations of aberrations are required for a fully malignant SCC, it is now important not only to understand their resulting functional changes but also to unravel the mechanisms underlying the induction of these genetic alterations. Recent studies have shown that the ends of the chromosomes, the telomeres, are more and more related to genomic instability and that telomeres are targets of oxidative damage (for review, see [4, 9]). Since UVA in addition to UVB is more extensively discussed for its contributions to skin carcinogenesis (reviewed in [71]) and since UVA is supposed to cause chromosomal aberrations via oxidative damage [102], which in turn may act on telomeres, it will now be of interest to investigate the role of UV-dependent telomere erosion, as a potential risk factor for chromosomal aberrations and thus development of skin cancer. Understanding and fighting genomic instability may be a promising future approach, particularly for tumors such as skin SCCs that suffer from numerous and highly complex aberrations.

Acknowledgments   The author wishes to thank Angelika Lampe for her help in editing the manuscript. This work was in part supported by the, European Union (LSHC-CT-2004-502943), the Deutsche Krebshilfe eV, Tumorzentrum Heidelberg-Mannheim, Baden-Württemberg Stiftung, and the Bmbf (UVA-03NUK003A).

References

1. Accardi, R., Dong, W., Smet, A., Cui, R., Hautefeuille, A., Gabet, A.S., Sylla, B.S., Gissmann, L., Hainaut, P., Tommasino, M.: Skin human papillomavirus type 38 alters p53 functions by accumulation of deltaNp73. EMBO Rep. **7**, 334–340 (2006)

2. Ackerman, A.B., Kerl, H., Sanchez, J.: Clinical Atlas of 101 Common Skin Diseases with Histopathologic Correlation. Ardor Scribendi, New York (2000)

3. Antonsson, A., Karanfilovska, S., Lindqvist, P.G., Hansson, B.G.: General acquisition of human papillomavirus infections of skin occurs in early infancy. J. Clin. Microbiol. **41**, 2509–2514 (2003)

4. Ayouaz, A., Raynaud, C., Heride, C., Revaud, D., Sabatier, L.: Telomeres: hallmarks of radiosensitivity. Biochimie **90**, 60–72 (2008)

5. Basile, J., Thiers, B., Maize Sr., J., Lathers, D.M.: Chemokine receptor expression in non-melanoma skin cancer. J. Cutan. Pathol. **35**, 623–629 (2008)

6. Billingsley, E.M., Davis, N., Helm, K.F.: Rapidly growing squamous cell carcinoma. J. Cutan. Med. Surg. **3**, 193–197 (1999)

7. Bleuel, K., Popp, S., Fusenig, N.E., Stanbridge, E.J., Boukamp, P.: Tumor suppression in human skin carcinoma cells by chromosome 15 transfer or thrombospondin-1 overexpression through halted tumor vascularization. Proc. Natl. Acad. Sci. U. S. A. **96**, 2065–2070 (1999)

8. Boukamp, P.: Non-melanoma skin cancer: what drives tumor development and progression? Carcinogenesis **26**, 1657–1667 (2005)

9. Boukamp, P.: UV-induced skin cancer: similarities – variations. J. Dtsch. Dermatol. Ges. **3**, 493–503 (2005)

10. Boukamp, P., Petrussevska, R.T., Breitkreutz, D., Hornung, J., Markham, A., Fusenig, N.E.: Normal keratinization in a spontaneously immortalized aneuploid human keratinocyte cell line. J. Cell Biol. **106**, 761–771 (1988)

11. Brasanac, D., Boricic, I., Todorovic, V., Tomanovic, N., Radojevic, S.: Cyclin A and beta-catenin expression in actinic keratosis, Bowen's disease and invasive squamous cell carcinoma of the skin. Br. J. Dermatol. **153**, 1166–1175 (2005)

12. Brash, D.E., Ziegler, A., Jonason, A.S., Simon, J.A., Kunala, S., Leffell, D.J.: Sunlight and sunburn in human skin cancer: p53, apoptosis, and tumor promotion. J. Investig. Dermatol. Symp. Proc. **1**, 136–142 (1996)

13. Brown, V.L., Harwood, C.A., Crook, T., Cronin, J.G., Kelsell, D.P., Proby, C.M.: p16INK4a and p14ARF tumor suppressor genes are commonly inactivated in cutaneous squamous cell carcinoma. J. Invest. Dermatol. **122**, 1284–1292 (2004)

14. Buck, C.B., Lowy, D.R.: Getting stronger: the relationship between a newly identified virus and merkel cell carcinoma. J. Invest. Dermatol. **129**, 9–11 (2009)

15. Burnworth, B., Arendt, S., Muffler, S., Steinkraus, V., Brocker, E.B., Birek, C., Hartschuh, W., Jauch, A., Boukamp, P.: The multi-step process of human skin carcinogenesis: a role for p53, cyclin D1, hTERT, p16, and TSP-1. Eur. J. Cell Biol. **86**, 763–780 (2007)

16. Burnworth, B., Popp, S., Stark, H.J., Steinkraus, V., Brocker, E.B., Hartschuh, W., Birek, C., Boukamp, P.: Gain of 11q/cyclin D1 overexpression is an essential early step in skin cancer development and causes abnormal tissue organization and differentiation. Oncogene **25**, 4399–4412 (2006)

17. Cadet, J., Sage, E., Douki, T.: Ultraviolet radiation-mediated damage to cellular DNA. Mutat. Res. **571**, 3–17 (2005)

18. Caldeira, S., Zehbe, I., Accardi, R., Malanchi, I., Dong, W., Giarre, M., de Villiers, E.M., Filotico, R., Boukamp, P., Tommasino, M.: The E6 and E7 proteins of the cutaneous human papillomavirus type 38 display transforming properties. J. Virol. **77**, 2195–2206 (2003)

19. Callahan, C.A., Oro, A.E.: Monstrous attempts at adnexogenesis: regulating hair follicle progenitors through Sonic hedgehog signaling. Curr. Opin. Genet. Dev. **11**, 541–546 (2001)

20. Chan, T.A., Hermeking, H., Lengauer, C., Kinzler, K.W., Vogelstein, B.: 14-3-3Sigma is required to prevent mitotic catastrophe after DNA damage. Nature **401**, 616–620 (1999)

21. Chen, A.C., McMillan, N.A., Antonsson, A.: Human papillomavirus type spectrum in normal skin of individuals with or without a history of frequent sun exposure. J. Gen. Virol. **89**, 2891–2897 (2008)

22. Cordano, P., Gillan, V., Bratlie, S., Bouvard, V., Banks, L., Tommasino, M., Campo, M.S.: The E6E7 oncoproteins of cutaneous human papillomavirus type 38 interfere with the interferon pathway. Virology **377**, 408–418 (2008)

23. Couve-Privat, S., Le Bret, M., Traiffort, E., Queille, S., Coulombe, J., Bouadjar, B., Avril, M.F., Ruat, M., Sarasin, A., Daya-Grosjean, L.: Functional analysis of novel sonic hedgehog gene mutations identified in basal cell carcinomas from xeroderma pigmentosum patients. Cancer Res. **64**, 3559–3565 (2004)

24. Dallenbach-Hellweg, G., Trunk, M.J., von Knebel, D.M.: Traditional and new molecular methods for early detection of cervical cancer. Arkh. Patol. **66**, 35–39 (2004)

25. Daya-Grosjean, L., Robert, C., Drougard, C., Suarez, H., Sarasin, A.: High mutation frequency in ras genes of skin tumors isolated from DNA repair deficient xeroderma pigmentosum patients. Cancer Res. **53**, 1625–1629 (1993)

26. de Gruijl, F.R.: Photocarcinogenesis: UVA vs. UVB radiation. Skin Pharmacol. Appl. Skin Physiol. **15**, 316–320 (2002)

27. de Gruijl, F.R., Forbes, P.D.: UV-induced skin cancer in a hairless mouse model. Bioessays **17**, 651–660 (1995)

28. Dlugosz, A., Merlino, G., Yuspa, S.H.: Progress in cutaneous cancer research. J. Investig. Dermatol. Symp. Proc. **7**, 17–26 (2002)

29. Doglioni, C., Piccinin, S., Demontis, S., Cangi, M.G., Pecciarini, L., Chiarelli, C., Armellin, M., Vukosavljevic, T., Boiocchi, M., Maestro, R.: Alterations of beta-catenin pathway in non-melanoma skin tumors: loss of alpha-ABC nuclear reactivity correlates with the presence of beta-catenin gene mutation. Am. J. Pathol. **163**, 2277–2287 (2003)

30. Duensing, S., Duensing, A., Crum, C.P., Munger, K.: Human papillomavirus type 16 E7 oncoprotein-induced abnormal centrosome synthesis is an early event in the evolving malignant phenotype. Cancer Res. **61**, 2356–2360 (2001)

31. Duensing, S., Lee, L.Y., Duensing, A., Basile, J., Piboonniyom, S., Gonzalez, S., Crum, C.P., Munger, K.: The human papillomavirus type 16 E6 and E7 oncoproteins cooperate to induce mitotic defects and genomic instability by uncoupling centrosome duplication from the cell division cycle. Proc. Natl. Acad. Sci. U. S. A. **97**, 10002–10007 (2000)

32. Euvrard, S., Kanitakis, J., Claudy, A.: Skin cancers after organ transplantation. N. Engl. J. Med. **348**, 1681–1691 (2003)

33. Feltkamp, M.C., de Koning, M.N., Bavinck, J.N., Ter, S.J.: Betapapillomaviruses: Innocent bystanders or causes of skin cancer. J. Clin. Virol. **43**, 353–360 (2008)

34. Forslund, O., Lindelof, B., Hradil, E., Nordin, P., Stenquist, B., Kirnbauer, R., Slupetzky, K., Dillner, J.: High prevalence of cutaneous human papillomavirus DNA on the top of skin tumors but not in "stripped" biopsies from the same tumors. J. Invest. Dermatol. **123**, 388–394 (2004)

35. Freedberg, I., Eisen, A., Wolff, K., Austen, K.F., Goldspith, L., Katz, S., Fitzpatrick, T.: Fitzpatrick's Dermatology in General Medicine. McGraw-Hill Health Professional Division, New York (1999)

36. Gambichler, T., Skrygan, M., Kaczmarczyk, J.M., Hyun, J., Tomi, N.S., Sommer, A., Bechara, F.G., Boms, S., Brockmeyer, N.H., Altmeyer, P., Kreuter, A.: Increased expression of TGF-beta/Smad proteins in basal cell carcinoma. Eur. J. Med. Res. **12**, 509–514 (2007)

37. Giglia-Mari, G., Sarasin, A.: TP53 mutations in human skin cancers. Hum. Mutat. **21**, 217–228 (2003)

38. Gilchrest, B.A., Krutmann, J.: Photoaging. Springer, New York (2006)
39. Gottipati, K.R., Poulsen, H., Starcher, B.: Passive cigarette smoke exposure inhibits ultraviolet light B-induced skin tumors in SKH-1 hairless mice by blocking the nuclear factor kappa B signalling pathway. Exp. Dermatol. **17**, 780–787 (2008)
40. Hall, L., Struijk, L., Neale, R.E., Feltkamp, M.C.: Re: Human papillomavirus infection and incidence of squamous cell and basal cell carcinomas of the skin. J. Natl. Cancer Inst. **98**, 1425–1426 (2006)
41. Halliday, G.M., Bock, V.L., Moloney, F.J., Lyons, J.G.: SWI/SNF: a chromatin-remodelling complex with a role in carcinogenesis. Int. J. Biochem. Cell. Biol. **41**, 725–728 (2009)
42. Hashida, T., Yasumoto, S.: Induction of chromosome abnormalities in mouse and human epidermal keratinocytes by the human papillomavirus type 16 E7 oncogene. J. Gen. Virol. **72**(pt 7), 1569–1577 (1991)
43. He, Y.Y., Pi, J., Huang, J.L., Diwan, B.A., Waalkes, M.P., Chignell, C.F.: Chronic UVA irradiation of human HaCaT keratinocytes induces malignant transformation associated with acquired apoptotic resistance. Oncogene **25**, 3680–3688 (2006)
44. Heitzer, E., Lassacher, A., Quehenberger, F., Kerl, H., Wolf, P.: UV fingerprints predominate in the PTCH mutation spectra of basal cell carcinomas independent of clinical phenotype. J. Invest. Dermatol. **127**, 2872–2881 (2007)
45. Hodges, A., Smoller, B.R.: Immunohistochemical comparison of p16 expression in actinic keratoses and squamous cell carcinomas of the skin. Mod. Pathol. **15**, 1121–1125 (2002)
46. Hurt, M.A.: Keratoacanthoma vs. squamous cell carcinoma in contrast with keratoacanthoma is squamous cell carcinoma. J. Cutan. Pathol. **31**, 291–292 (2004)
47. Ibiebele, T.I., van der Pols, J.C., Hughes, M.C., Marks, G.C., Williams, G.M., Green, A.C.: Dietary pattern in association with squamous cell carcinoma of the skin: a prospective study. Am. J. Clin. Nutr. **85**, 1401–1408 (2007)
48. Ji, J., Kump, E., Wernli, M., Erb, P.: Gene silencing of transcription factor Gli2 inhibits basal cell carcinomalike tumor growth in vivo. Int. J. Cancer **122**, 50–56 (2008)
49. Jin, Y., Jin, C., Salemark, L., Wennerberg, J., Persson, B., Jonsson, N.: Clonal chromosome abnormalities in premalignant lesions of the skin. Cancer Genet. Cytogenet. **136**, 48–52 (2002)
50. Jin, Y., Martins, C., Jin, C., Salemark, L., Jonsson, N., Persson, B., Roque, L., Fonseca, I., Wennerberg, J.: Nonrandom karyotypic features in squamous cell carcinomas of the skin. Genes Chromosomes Cancer **26**, 295–303 (1999)
51. Jin, Y., Martins, C., Salemark, L., Persson, B., Jin, C., Miranda, J., Fonseca, I., Jonsson, N.: Nonrandom karyotypic features in basal cell carcinomas of the skin. Cancer Genet. Cytogenet. **131**, 109–119 (2001)
52. Johnson, T.M., Rowe, D.E., Nelson, B.R., Swanson, N.A.: Squamous cell carcinoma of the skin (excluding lip and oral mucosa). J. Am. Acad. Dermatol. **26**, 467–484 (1992)
53. Jonason, A.S., Kunala, S., Price, G.J., Restifo, R.J., Spinelli, H.M., Persing, J.A., Leffell, D.J., Tarone, R.E., Brash, D.E.: Frequent clones of p53-mutated keratinocytes in normal human skin. Proc. Natl. Acad. Sci. U. S. A. **93**, 14025–14029 (1996)
54. Kallioniemi, A., Kallioniemi, O.P., Sudar, D., Rutovitz, D., Gray, J.W., Waldman, F., Pinkel, D.: Comparative genomic hybridization for molecular cytogenetic analysis of solid tumors. Science **258**, 818–821 (1992)
55. Kanjilal, S., Strom, S.S., Clayman, G.L., Weber, R.S., el Naggar, A.K., Kapur, V., Cummings, K.K., Hill, L.A., Spitz, M.R., Kripke, M.L.: p53 mutations in nonmelanoma skin cancer of the head and neck: molecular evidence for field cancerization. Cancer Res. **55**, 3604–3609 (1995)
56. Kielbassa, C., Roza, L., Epe, B.: Wavelength dependence of oxidative DNA damage induced by UV and visible light. Carcinogenesis **18**, 811–816 (1997)
57. Kim, E., Deppert, W.: Transcriptional activities of mutant p53: when mutations are more than a loss. J. Cell Biochem. **93**, 878–886 (2004)
58. Kubo, Y., Urano, Y., Matsumoto, K., Ahsan, K., Arase, S.: Mutations of the INK4a locus in squamous cell carcinomas of human skin. Biochem. Biophys. Res. Commun. **232**, 38–41 (1997)
59. Lane, D.P.: Cancer. p53, guardian of the genome. Nature **358**, 15–16 (1992)
60. Le Pelletier, F., Soufir, N., de la, S.P., Janin, A., Basset-Seguin, N.: p53 Patches are not increased in patients with multiple nonmelanoma skin cancers. J. Invest. Dermatol. **117**, 1324–1325 (2001)
61. Li, A.G., Lu, S.L., Han, G., Hoot, K.E., Wang, X.J.: Role of TGFbeta in skin inflammation and carcinogenesis. Mol. Carcinog. **45**, 389–396 (2006)
62. Ling, G., Persson, A., Berne, B., Uhlen, M., Lundeberg, J., Ponten, F.: Persistent p53 mutations in single cells from normal human skin. Am. J. Pathol. **159**, 1247–1253 (2001)
63. Lodygin, D., Yazdi, A.S., Sander, C.A., Herzinger, T., Hermeking, H.: Analysis of 14-3-3sigma expression in hyperproliferative skin diseases reveals selective loss associated with CpG-methylation in basal cell carcinoma. Oncogene **22**, 5519–5524 (2003)
64. Malanchi, I., Peinado, H., Kassen, D., Hussenet, T., Metzger, D., Chambon, P., Huber, M., Hohl, D., Cano, A., Birchmeier, W., Huelsken, J.: Cutaneous cancer stem cell maintenance is dependent on beta-catenin signalling. Nature **452**, 650–653 (2008)
65. Massimi, P., Thomas, M., Bouvard, V., Ruberto, I., Campo, M.S., Tommasino, M., Banks, L.: Comparative transforming potential of different human papillomaviruses associated with non-melanoma skin cancer. Virology **371**, 374–379 (2008)
66. McNaughton, S.A., Marks, G.C., Green, A.C.: Role of dietary factors in the development of basal cell cancer and squamous cell cancer of the skin. Cancer Epidemiol. Biomarkers Prev. **14**, 1596–1607 (2005)
67. Moloney, F.J., Lyons, J.G., Bock, V.L., Huang, X.X., Bugeja, M.J., Halliday, G.M.: Hotspot mutation of brahma in non-melanoma skin cancer. J. Invest. Dermatol. **129**, 1012–1015 (2009)
68. Mueller, M.M., Fusenig, N.E.: Tumor-stroma interactions directing phenotype and progression of epithelial skin tumor cells. Differentiation **70**, 486–497 (2002)
69. Nakazawa, H., English, D., Randell, P.L., Nakazawa, K., Martel, N., Armstrong, B.K., Yamasaki, H.: UV and skin cancer: specific p53 gene mutation in normal skin as a biologically relevant exposure measurement. Proc. Natl. Acad. Sci. U. S. A. **91**, 360–364 (1994)
70. Nindl, I., Gottschling, M., Stockfleth, E.: Human papillomaviruses and non-melanoma skin cancer: basic virology and clinical manifestations. Dis. Markers **23**, 247–259 (2007)
71. Nishigori, C., Hattori, Y., Toyokuni, S.: Role of reactive oxygen species in skin carcinogenesis. Antioxid. Redox Signal. **6**, 561–570 (2004)
72. O'Grady, A., Dunne, C., O'Kelly, P., Murphy, G.M., Leader, M., Kay, E.: Differential expression of matrix metalloproteinase (MMP)-2, MMP-9 and tissue inhibitor of metalloproteinase (TIMP)-1 and TIMP-2 in non-melanoma skin cancer: implications for tumour progression. Histopathology **51**, 793–804 (2007)
73. Perez-Moreno, M., Fuchs, E.: Catenins: keeping cells from getting their signals crossed. Dev. Cell **11**, 601–612 (2006)
74. Pfister, H.: HPV and skin neoplasia. Hautarzt **59**, 26–30 (2008)
75. Pivarcsi, A., Muller, A., Hippe, A., Rieker, J., Steinhoff, M., Seeliger, S., Kubitza, R., Pippirs, U., Meller, S., Gerber, P.A., Liersch, R., Buenemann, E., Sonkoly, E., Wiesner, U., Hoffmann, T.K., Schneider, L., Piekorz, R., Enderlein, E., Reifenberger, J., Rohr, U.P., Haas, R., Boukamp, P., Haase, I., Nurnberg, B., Ruzicka, T., Zlotnik, A., Homey, B.: Tumor immune escape by the loss of homeostatic chemokine expression. Proc. Natl. Acad. Sci. U. S. A. **104**, 19055–19060 (2007)

76. Popp, S., Waltering, S., Herbst, C., Moll, I., Boukamp, P.: UV-B-type mutations and chromosomal imbalances indicate common pathways for the development of Merkel and skin squamous cell carcinomas. Int. J. Cancer **99**, 352–360 (2002)

77. Popp, S., Waltering, S., Holtgreve-Grez, H., Jauch, A., Proby, C., Leigh, I.M., Boukamp, P.: Genetic characterization of a human skin carcinoma progression model: from primary tumor to metastasis. J. Invest. Dermatol. **115**, 1095–1103 (2000)

78. Purdie, K.J., Lambert, S.R., Teh, M.T., Chaplin, T., Molloy, G., Raghavan, M., Kelsell, D.P., Leigh, I.M., Harwood, C.A., Proby, C.M., Young, B.D.: Allelic imbalances and microdeletions affecting the PTPRD gene in cutaneous squamous cell carcinomas detected using single nucleotide polymorphism microarray analysis. Genes Chromosomes Cancer **46**, 661–669 (2007)

79. Quinn, A.G., Sikkink, S., Rees, J.L.: Basal cell carcinomas and squamous cell carcinomas of human skin show distinct patterns of chromosome loss. Cancer Res. **54**, 4756–4759 (1994)

80. Rehman, I., Takata, M., Wu, Y.Y., Rees, J.L.: Genetic change in actinic keratoses. Oncogene **12**, 2483–2490 (1996)

81. Reifenberger, J., Wolter, M., Knobbe, C.B., Kohler, B., Schonicke, A., Scharwachter, C., Kumar, K., Blaschke, B., Ruzicka, T., Reifenberger, G.: Somatic mutations in the PTCH, SMOH, SUFUH and TP53 genes in sporadic basal cell carcinomas. Br. J. Dermatol. **152**, 43–51 (2005)

82. Ren, Z.P., Hedrum, A., Ponten, F., Nister, M., Ahmadian, A., Lundeberg, J., Uhlen, M., Ponten, J.: Human epidermal cancer and accompanying precursors have identical p53 mutations different from p53 mutations in adjacent areas of clonally expanded non-neoplastic keratinocytes. Oncogene **12**, 765–773 (1996)

83. Ridd, K., Yu, S., Bastian, B.C.: The presence of polyomavirus in non-melanoma skin cancer in organ transplant recipients is rare. J. Invest. Dermatol. **129**, 250–252 (2009)

84. Rook, A., Wilkinson, D.S., Ebling, F.J.G.: Textbook of Dermatology. Blackwell Scientific, Oxford (1992)

85. Roop, D., Toftgard, R.: Hedgehog in wnterland. Nat. Genet. **40**, 1040–1041 (2008)

86. Salama, M.E., Mahmood, M.N., Qureshi, H.S., Ma, C., Zarbo, R.J., Ormsby, A.H.: p16INK4a expression in actinic keratosis and Bowen's disease. Br. J. Dermatol. **149**, 1006–1012 (2003)

87. Serrano, M., Hannon, G.J., Beach, D.: A new regulatory motif in cell-cycle control causing specific inhibition of cyclin D/CDK4. Nature **366**, 704–707 (1993)

88. Shvartzman, L.: Non-Melanoma Cancer of the Skin. Northeast Florida Medicine **58**, 37–39 (2007), http://www.dcmsonline.org

89. Soufir, N., Daya-Grosjean, L., de la, S.P., Moles, J.P., Dubertret, L., Sarasin, A., Basset-Seguin, N.: Association between INK4a-ARF and p53 mutations in skin carcinomas of xeroderma pigmentosum patients. J. Natl. Cancer Inst. **92**, 1841–1847 (2000)

90. Soufir, N., Ribojad, M., Magnaldo, T., Thibaudeau, O., Delestaing, G., Daya-Grosjean, L., Rivet, J., Sarasin, A., Basset-Seguin, N.: Germline and somatic mutations of the INK4a-ARF gene in a xeroderma pigmentosum group C patient. J. Invest. Dermatol. **119**, 1355–1360 (2002)

91. Speicher, M.R., Gwyn, B.S., Ward, D.C.: Karyotyping human chromosomes by combinatorial multi-fluor FISH. Nat. Genet. **12**, 368–375 (1996)

92. Taipale, J., Chen, J.K., Cooper, M.K., Wang, B., Mann, R.K., Milenkovic, L., Scott, M.P., Beachy, P.A.: Effects of oncogenic mutations in Smoothened and Patched can be reversed by cyclopamine. Nature **406**, 1005–1009 (2000)

93. Toftgard, R.: Hedgehog signalling in cancer. Cell Mol. Life Sci. **57**, 1720–1731 (2000)

94. Tommasi, S., Swiderski, P.M., Tu, Y., Kaplan, B.E., Pfeifer, G.P.: Inhibition of transcription factor binding by ultraviolet-induced pyrimidine dimers. Biochemistry **35**, 15693–15703 (1996)

95. Tornaletti, S., Pfeifer, G.P.: Slow repair of pyrimidine dimers at p53 mutation hotspots in skin cancer. Science **263**, 1436–1438 (1994)

96. Utikal, J., Udart, M., Leiter, U., Kaskel, P., Peter, R.U., Krähn, G.: Numerical abnormalities of the cyclin D1 gene locus on chromosome 11q13 in non-melanoma skin cancer. Cancer Lett. **219**, 197–204 (2005)

97. van Kranen, H.J., de Gruijl, F.R.: Mutations in cancer genes of UV-induced skin tumors of hairless mice. J. Epidemiol. **9**, S58–S65 (1999)

98. van Kranen, H.J., de Gruijl, F.R., de Vries, A., Sontag, Y., Wester, P.W., Senden, H.C., Rozemuller, E., van Kreijl, C.F.: Frequent p53 alterations but low incidence of ras mutations in UV-B-induced skin tumors of hairless mice. Carcinogenesis **16**, 1141–1147 (1995)

99. Walshe, J., Serewko-Auret, M.M., Teakle, N., Cameron, S., Minto, K., Smith, L., Burcham, P.C., Russell, T., Strutton, G., Griffin, A., Chu, F.F., Esworthy, S., Reeve, V., Saunders, N.A.: Inactivation of glutathione peroxidase activity contributes to UV-induced squamous cell carcinoma formation. Cancer Res. **67**, 4751–4758 (2007)

100. Waring, A.J., Takata, M., Rehman, I., Rees, J.L.: Loss of heterozygosity analysis of keratoacanthoma reveals multiple differences from cutaneous squamous cell carcinoma. Br. J. Cancer **73**, 649–653 (1996)

101. White, A.E., Livanos, E.M., Tlsty, T.D.: Differential disruption of genomic integrity and cell cycle regulation in normal human fibroblasts by the HPV oncoproteins. Genes Dev. **8**, 666–677 (1994)

102. Wischermann, K., Popp, S., Moshir, S., Scharfetter-Kochanek, K., Wlaschek, M., de, G.F., Hartschuh, W., Greinert, R., Volkmer, B., Faust, A., Rapp, A., Schmezer, P., Boukamp, P.: UVA radiation causes DNA strand breaks, chromosomal aberrations and tumorigenic transformation in HaCaT skin keratinocytes. Oncogene **27**, 4269–4280 (2008)

103. Wondrak, G.T., Jacobson, M.K., Jacobson, E.L.: Endogenous UVA-photosensitizers: mediators of skin photodamage and novel targets for skin photoprotection. Photochem. Photobiol. Sci. **5**, 215–237 (2006)

104. Ziegler, A., Leffell, D.J., Kunala, S., Sharma, H.W., Gailani, M., Simon, J.A., Halperin, A.J., Baden, H.P., Shapiro, P.E., Bale, A.E.: Mutation hotspots due to sunlight in the p53 gene of nonmelanoma skin cancers. Proc. Natl. Acad. Sci. U. S. A. **90**, 4216–4220 (1993)

Keith S. Hoek

2.2.1 Transformation I: Genetic Mutation

It has long been known that cancer arises most frequently from cells in tissues which undergo constant renewal [12]. For example, epithelial tissues of the skin and intestine are composed of cells which are renewed throughout life and are also often the source of adult malignancies [4, 64]. Although the process is periodic rather than constant, melanocytes also undergo frequent renewal and thus increase the risk of malignant transformation. In the hair follicle bulge region melanocyte stem cells produce daughter cells for each hair cycle and are themselves considered a possible source for melanoma [31, 88]. By contrast, epidermal melanocyte proliferation is stimulated by UV radiation [43, 77]. Sun exposure is believed to be involved in the malignant transformation of cutaneous melanocytes, as epidemiological studies point to increased incidence rates among fair-skinned peoples living at lower (and sunnier) latitudes [62]. Excessive and cumulative exposure to UV radiation results in increasing levels of DNA damage to proliferating melanocytes, which eventually overcome the capacity for DNA repair mechanisms to compensate [74]. Usually this evokes mechanisms which precipitate apoptotic cell death [48], but occasionally a cell undergoes malignant transformation and nucleates a melanoma. No one genetic aberration has been identified as the sole cause for malignant transformation, rather it is thought that melanoma is initiated by aggregated genetic changes within different loci. Genes that are frequently changed in melanoma include those which code for p16, B-raf, N-ras, PTEN, p53, Mitf, c-Kit, and Mc1r. Consequently, these genes are high on the list of suspects whose mutation, deletion, or amplification are thought to contribute to melanocytic transformation.

Cyclin-dependent kinase inhibitor 2A (p16) is a cell cycle regulator which binds cyclin-dependent kinase 4 (Cdk4) and inhibits that enzyme's phosphorylation of the retinoblastoma (Rb) protein [81]. Rb phosphorylation by Cdk4 releases E2F-transcription factors and activates genes responsible for S-phase progression [1]. Therefore, by sequestering Cdk4 from the Rb-phosphorylation complex in an appropriately timely fashion, p16 acts as a critical regulator for cell-cycle G1-S transition. In melanoma, the gene encoding p16 is deleted or mutated in approximately 69% of cases and its promoter is inactivated by DNA methylation in a further 9% [6]. Familial melanomas, defined as being from a cluster of at least two immediate family members with the disease, represent less than 10% of all melanoma cases. For these only p16 and Cdk4 have been identified as high-risk genes and, while only six families present with a germline mutation in Cdk4 which abrogates p16 binding, approximately one-third of all other familial melanomas correlate with an inherited p16-inactivating deletion or mutation [35, 63, 70, 89, 108]. The inactivation of p16 and subsequent loss of regulation at the G1-S transition is likely to be a major contributor to the loss of proliferative control in most cases of melanocytic transformation.

The v-raf murine sarcoma viral oncogene homolog B1 (B-raf) is a serine/threonine protein kinase which functions as a part of the mitogen-activated protein (MAP) kinase pathway in the transmission of mitogenic signals from surface receptors to the nucleus. In melanoma the MAP kinase pathway is reported to be usually activated, as measured by high constitutive ERK activity, and this is assumed to drive proliferation [85]. In at least half of all melanomas the *B-raf* gene carries a narrowly specific mutation (B-raf[V600E]) which constitutively activates its kinase function [21]. Although it is not typical of UV-mediated DNA damage, exposure to UV is still thought to be sufficient for generating this mutation [8], and B-raf[V600E] has not been detected in mucosal melanomas [18]. However, while other sites yield primary melanomas that frequently carry the mutation, it is less common (<10%) in melanomas originating from chronically UV-exposed skin [75]. The high frequency of its mutation in melanoma has led to the general belief that active MAP kinase signaling is critical for melanoma development. For example, it has been shown that transformation of melan-a

K.S. Hoek
Department of Dermatology, University Hospital Zurich,
Gloriastrasse 31, 8091 Zurich, Switzerland
e-mail: keith.hoek@usz.ch

R. Dummer et al. (eds.), *Skin Cancer – A World-Wide Perspective*,
DOI: 10.1007/978-3-642-05072-5_2.2, © Springer-Verlag Berlin Heidelberg 2011

cells, a line of immortalized mouse melanocytes [7], to express B-raf^{V600E} allows them to proliferate without mitogenic stimulation and form tumors when injected subcutaneously into immunocompromised mice [102]. Importantly, melan-a cells lack functional p16 [95] and this is very probably a contributing factor. B-raf^{V600E} coexists with p16 mutants in 60% of melanomas and it has been shown that simultaneous B-raf knockdown and p16 overexpression results in significant growth inhibition of melanoma cells in vitro [104]. For many melanomas, therefore, synergism between p16 inactivation (which abrogates cell cycle control) and B-raf activation (which drives cell proliferation) contributes to the transformation process. Interestingly, whether or not the B-raf mutation is detrimental to patient survival remains to be firmly established. While it has been calculated that patients with B-raf^{V600E} primary lesions have a significantly worse prognosis than those with wild-type B-raf [45], other researchers have found that B-raf^{V600E} appears to be a marker for longer disease-free survival [50, 101].

The neuroblastoma RAS viral oncogene homolog (N-ras) is another member of the MAP kinase pathway. Like *B-raf*, the *N-ras* gene is also subject to activating mutations in melanoma and occurs in 21% of cases [6]. In MAP kinase signaling, N-ras is upstream of B-raf, which suggests that its oncogenic mechanism is identical. Indeed there is evidence that its activation similarly promotes cell proliferation [3, 30, 67]. However, activating N-ras^{Q61R} or N-ras^{Q61K} mutations, which are almost always mutually exclusive of B-raf^{V600E}, have no significant association with patient survival [45]. Recently it was determined that while N-ras is upstream of B-raf it is also upstream of the v-raf-1 murine leukemia viral oncogene homolog (c-Raf). In melanocytes, c-Raf signaling is suppressed by cAMP activation of protein kinase A, so MAP kinase signaling follows the N-ras/B-raf axis. In melanoma, activating N-ras mutations suppress cAMP metabolism and thus switch MAP kinase signaling to the N-ras/c-Raf axis [28]. There is no clear evidence for a link to N-ras mutation and patient survival.

Phosphoinositide 3-kinase (PI3K) function drives activation of the V-akt murine thymoma viral oncogene homolog (Akt), which inhibits the activity of cell cycle regulators p27^{Kip1} and p27^{Cip1}. Additionally, activated Akt blocks glycogen synthase kinase 3β (GSK3β) from degrading cyclin D1, augmenting its interaction with Cdk4 and Cdk6 to promote cell cycle G1/S transition. Furthermore, PI3K/Akt signaling is reported to inactivate proapoptotic factors including Bcl2-binding protein, caspase 9, and forkhead family transcription factors [11, 13, 20, 25, 51, 105]. Therefore, activation of the PI3K pathway is often associated with cancer progression and several groups have looked for pathway-specific mutations to account for this. The phosphatase and tensin homolog (PTEN) is a phosphatase with broad specificity involved in regulating the cell cycle and apoptosis. Like p53, PTEN

aberrations are frequently found in cancer and it is deleted or mutated in 28% of melanomas [6]. As the normal function of PTEN is to block PI3K activation of Akt it is considered to be a tumor suppressor [24, 84, 91]. PTEN's tumor suppressor role is supported by studies in which its reexpression was seen to inhibit tumorigenecity and metastasis [40]. Interestingly, there is a high correlation in melanoma between the BRAF-activating mutations and PTEN-disabling mutations/deletions [97], which suggests that they may act synergistically in selecting for cells with a proliferative advantage. A recent immunohistochemical analysis of primary lesions showed a significant association between ulceration (a strong predictor for nodal involvement) and reduced PTEN expression, but it has no significant connection to either disease-free survival or overall survival [59]. This lack of a significant association was confirmed in another report. Interestingly, this different study did find that decreased phospho-Akt *was* significantly associated with reduced disease-free survival, which indicates that the role of PI3K/Akt pathway activation in melanoma is not yet fully understood [84].

The p53 tumor suppressor (p53) is a potent stress response factor which can regulate target genes to induce cell cycle arrest, DNA repair, senescence or apoptotic cell death and while active it represents a significant barrier for tumorigenesis [15]. Inactivating mutations or deletions in p53 are a generally frequent phenomenon in cancer and occur in about half of all cases [90]. However, in melanoma it has been found to have a frequency of only 9% [69]. Interestingly, the hypomorphic Arg72Pro allele of p53 is associated with melanoma, where the Pro/Pro geneotype has an incidence of approximately 5–10% and carries a significantly increased risk of melanoma over the Arg/Arg genotype [93].

The microphthalmia-associated transcription factor (Mitf) is a master regulator of melanocytic cell development and survival [94]. Various isoforms of Mitf are also important for the development and function of other cell types including retinal pigment epithelia, osteoclasts, and mast cells [47, 65, 71]. In mature melanocytes, Mitf functions to halt the cell cycle by upregulating cyclin-dependent kinase inhibitors to drive cell cycle exit [53]. Conversely, Mitf is reported to be a critical factor in promoting melanoma cell proliferation [14, 38]. Furthermore, its gene is subject to occasional amplification. The frequency of Mitf amplification is approximately 15%, although less than a third of these represent focal amplifications which exceed one or two extra copies [44, 92]. Nevertheless, Mitf amplification has been shown to correlate with reduced patient survival and is held to be an example of "oncogene addiction" similar to that described for BCR-ABL in chronic myeloid leukemia [27, 32, 98].

The v-kit Hardy-Zuckerman 4 feline sarcoma viral oncogene homolog (c-Kit) is a receptor tyrosine kinase whose normal function is important for melanocyte development. When bound by its ligand, cytokine stem cell factor, c-Kit dimerizes and serves as a docking site for signal transducers which in turn activate PI3K signaling [9]. In melanoma, the *c-Kit* gene is reported to be amplified in about 14% of cases [17]. While mutations in this gene are reported to be most common in acral (23%) and mucosal (16%) melanomas, and rare in cutaneous forms [5], there is little information regarding the consequences of most of these. However, the L576P mutation is an activator (abrogating a negative-feedback mechanism) but its incidence is rare [5, 6]. Nevertheless, by whatever means, activation of the c-Kit/PI3K axis is likely to contribute to the loss of proliferative control and melanocytic transformation.

The last gene to be specifically discussed here in the context of melanocytic transformation has no direct role in proliferative control. Rather it is a factor which is critical for protection against UV-mediated DNA damage. The melanocyte-stimulating hormone receptor (Mc1r) is a G protein-coupled receptor which has an important role in eumelanin synthesis. Eumelanins, dark brown/black pigments, are the principal photoprotective agents made by melanocytes. Accordingly, Mc1r mutants unable to make eumelanin are associated with red hair, freckles, and an increased sensitivity to sun exposure. Mc1r variants, including those which do not necessarily interrupt its function, are present in more than half of fair-skinned people [68]. While it is reasonably evident why Mc1r loss-of-function can contribute to melanocytic transformation, its impact on melanoma incidence has most relevance in the context of other melanoma-related mutations. For example, the presence of any of three active Mc1r alleles (R151C, R160W, N294H) significantly increases the penetrance of p16 mutation [10]. There are other, less common genomic aberrations not discussed here which have also been described for melanoma [6]. While there is some indication of how these and those discussed above may cooperate to drive melanoma initiation the overall picture remains unclear. However, it seems certain that melanoma initiation may result from several different combinations of genomic aberration.

Another aspect of structural DNA alteration which correlates with melanoma is the pattern of common gross chromosomal copy number changes. High throughput methods of genomic analysis have recently allowed us to examine, with increasing detail, the changes in copy number (including deletions and amplifications) that occur on each chromosome (Table 2.2.1).

Table 2.2.1 Chromosomal copy number gains and losses reported for melanoma

Gains	Losses	Reference
6p, 7, 8q, 17q, and 20	6q, 9p, 10, and 21q	[18]
1q, 6p, 7, 8q, 17q, and 20	4, 6q, 9p, 10, and 11q	[44]
2p, 6p, 7, 19q, 20, and 22q	9, 10, and 17	[92]
1q, 6p, 7, 8q, 15q, 17q, 20, and 22	4, 6q, 9, 10, and 11q	[52]

Comparative hybridization studies show that the reported genomic differences between melanoma primary lesion subtypes are also related to where on the body they occur. For example, BRAF mutation is most frequent in melanoma types arising in sites of intermittent sun exposure [54]. While most SSM lesions have their origins in sites of intermittent sun exposure, the association between BRAF mutation and location is stronger than between BRAF mutation and subtype [18].

2.2.2 Transformation II: Gene Expression Changes

Clinical observations of melanoma gene expression have principally rested on factors whose expression is *maintained* during transformation, because pigment gene expression is tightly restricted to melanocytic cell types and this is helpful in identifying melanoma cells. Experimental analyses, on the other hand, have typically looked for genes whose expression has *changed* in order to understand the process of malignant transformation of melanocytes. Before DNA microarrays permitted large-scale screening for de novo factors, many laboratories concentrated on monitoring gene expression changes in genes already linked through mutation studies or borrowed from other cancers. For example, p16 expression is decreased from benign nevi to primary melanoma without metastasis to primary melanoma with metastasis [58]. For p53, which in melanoma has a relatively low mutation or deletion rate, its expression was reported to be rarely altered by melanocytic transformation [78]. However, more recent studies show that expression of the *p53* gene can be blocked by promoter methylation, which is found in up to 25% of tested melanomas [19], or by a repressor complex of MAGE proteins with Tripartate motif-containing protein 28 [103]. Furthermore, p53 function may also be inhibited by overexpression of MDM2, a major E3 ubiquitin ligase which binds and ubiquitinates p53 for degradation [41]. Therefore, while the mutation rate for p53 is low in melanoma, there are additional mechanisms adopted by melanoma cells to abrogate its tumor-suppressive function. The expression of v-Myc myelocytomatosis viral oncogene homolog (cMyc) is increased in more than half of human cancers [2, 66]. Its overexpression in melanoma is thought to contribute to the suppression of oncogene-induced senescence and participate in proliferation [56, 106].

Many researchers, looking to identify novel practical clinical markers or comprehend the role of transcriptional change in neoplastic transformation, have used gene expression arrays to document the up- and downregulation of genes in melanoma when compared with healthy cells and tissue. The initial studies used small arrays to identify by fold-change filtering a small number of genes with expression differences between healthy and malignant samples [22, 26, 61, 82, 107]. The combined results of these small studies are that there is almost no agreement between them. The reasons for this are very likely due to their use of small platforms, few replicates, and insufficient statistical stringency. There have been three studies using larger array formats to compare melanoma against normal cells or tissues and each identified putative molecular markers [34, 36, 96]. Systematic analysis of their respective gene lists shows that only two genes (melanocyte-specific gene 1 and placental cadherin) were identified by all groups as being differentially expressed. For programs interrogating the greater fraction of expressed genes, this is a diminishingly small yield. However, the comparison is probably not a particularly fair one for several reasons. One is that two studies looked at biopsy materials while the third used cell lines. Another is that the cell line study used only two control samples.

A recent meta-analysis compared data obtained from different sources, including five separate melanoma cell line sets and two separate melanocyte culture sets. It was found that the comparison recapitulated a large number of factors well known to melanoma research. These include the downregulation of epithelial cadherin, pipeptidyl peptidase IV, and c-Kit and the upregulation of known melanoma antigens, neuronal cadherin, and osteopontin. Additional genes confirm earlier reports such as the upregulation of Notch-2. Less familiar factors include a downregulated putative tumor suppressor (WFDC1) and upregulated tumor protein D52, neither of which has been specifically associated with melanoma before. Overall, the results confirm the overexpression in melanoma cells of several growth factors and receptors reported to confer growth advantage and metastasis. Furthermore, novel pathways and patterns of associated expression were identified. These included activation of the Notch pathway, changed expression of transcriptional regulators involved in embryonic development and epidermal/mesenchymal transition, activation of cancer/testis antigens, and downregulation of membrane trafficking factors and growth suppressors [36, 37].

2.2.3 Molecular Biology of Progression

From a clinical perspective, the progression from a primary melanoma lesion to distal metastases is a well-characterized phenomenon. The Clark model of melanoma progression describes a clear series of histologic changes including melanocytic proliferation, dysplasia, hyperplasia, invasion, and metastasis [16]. How melanoma achieves each of these steps, the last of which is itself a highly complex multistep process, is not understood. There are three general hypotheses:

melanoma stem cells (MSCs), clonal selection, and phenotype switching.

Despite several decades of concentrated effort, no therapy has been shown to significantly affect melanoma patient survival. It had been suggested that this was because the therapies tested had failed to target a putative population of cells which are solely responsible for progression of the disease, MSCs [31]. The melanoma stem cell hypothesis, invoking the stem cell property of asymmetric division, also supplied an attractive explanation for the observed heterogeneity of melanoma cells within lesions. Schatton et al. demonstrated that only a tiny population of melanoma cells, less than one in a million, expressing ABCB5 (a chemoresistance mediator) could propagate tumor growth when injected subcutaneously into an immunocompromised (NOD/SCID) mouse model [79]. However, another group using a more acutely immunocompromised (NOD/SCID $Il2rg^{-/-}$) mouse model showed that the proportion of cells with tumorigenic qualities is as much as one in four. Most powerfully, these authors could repeatedly demonstrate xenograft tumor growth upon the injection of a *single* melanoma cell. Finally, they demonstrated through fractionation studies that whatever known stem cell factors or putative melanoma stem cell markers were expressed was of no consequence [72]. This strongly indicates that melanoma does *not* follow a cancer stem cell model.

Despite the continuing controversy over putative MSCs, there is widespread agreement that melanoma progression nevertheless involves accumulation of gene expression changes which lead to increased metastatic potential. Currently, melanoma progression is generally accepted to involve a downregulation of factors including melanocytic markers (e.g., HMB45, S100, Melan-A), melastatin, and epithelial cadherin, and concomitant upregulation of other cadherins, integrins, and matrix metalloproteinases [60]. This is an essentially linear model, in which early-stage melanoma should be clearly differentiable from late-stage metastases by changes in gene expression (Fig. 2.2.1).

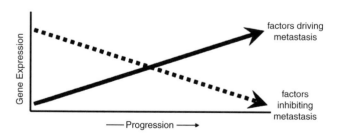

Fig. 2.2.1 Accumulation of molecular change drives melanoma progression. The current accepted model stipulates that gene expression changes in a unidirectional fashion during malignant progression of melanoma. Genes whose expression drives metastatic progression are upregulated and genes whose expression inhibits metastasis are downregulated [60]. The model rests on the assumption that early-stage melanoma has less metastatic potential than late-stage melanoma

Several groups have pursued this using high-throughput techniques to survey the whole genome for gene expression changes during melanoma progression. Haqq et al. profiled gene expression in skin, nevi, primary melanoma lesions, and metastases. For one primary lesion they compared the gene expression profile of the radial growth component against that obtained from cells extracted from the vertical growth phase, finding a number of genes that were down-regulated in the vertical growth phase. Despite the weakness of this single-sample analysis, frequent vertical phase down-regulation of matrix metallopeptidase 10 and placental cadherin was confirmed by immunohistochemical examination of additional samples [34]. These workers also compared primary melanoma lesions against nevus tissue and metastatic lesions, identifying a discriminator set of more than 2,000 genes. Unfortunately, the authors' interpretation of the nevi/primary/metastasis discriminator gene set was restricted to a diagnostic context and little about the molecular biology of progression was discussed. Another study used class discovery analysis to first cluster samples without reference to their clinical stage. The purpose of this was to see if unbiased data analysis could appropriately cluster stage-specific samples. Two distinct groups of samples emerged, respectively, comprising early-stage (skin, nevi and in situ melanoma) and advanced-stage lesions (vertical growth phase, lymph node metastases, and distal metastases). This suggested that the most significant change in gene expression during melanoma progression takes place between in situ and vertical growth phase. Multiple testing-corrected ANOVA analyses were used to pick out genes with significant differences between early- and late-stage groups. These authors identified changes in many factors involved in mitotic cell cycle regulation and cell proliferation [86]. Others made superficial use of DNA microarrays to specifically assess pro-apoptotic gene expression. This showed that many of these genes are downregulated at the transition between thin and thick primary melanoma lesions [42]. The conclusion to be drawn from these studies is that vertical growth phase melanoma lesions have in many respects already adopted the stage-specific expression complement of late-stage metastases (Fig. 2.2.2).

One of the inferred benefits of sourcing tissue samples for DNA microarray-based studies, rather than cell cultures or lines, is their greater biological relevance. However, it must therefore be assumed that any given lesion will be sufficiently homogeneous for its contribution to statistically meaningful findings. This is critical because the piece of tissue sampled from a lesion for analysis is often small and taken without detailed foreknowledge of its cellular or molecular complement. That cell cultures and cell lines are usually established from small fragments of whole lesions is because as much of the original lesion as possible must be preserved for diagnostic purposes. The issue is that we are forced to assume that the fraction taken is sufficiently representative of the whole,

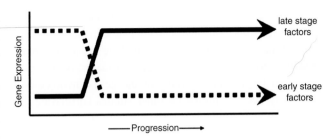

Fig. 2.2.2 Gene expression changes at the RGP/VGP transition. Gene expression studies of tissue samples taken from different stages indicate that the most significant shift in gene expression takes place during transition to the vertical growth phase of a primary melanoma lesion [86]

but this may not be the case. The laboratory of Meenhard Herlyn was among the first to establish cell lines from lesions and metastases which had been thoroughly staged and characterized with the express purpose of looking for stage-specific molecular markers. This group participated in a genome-wide DNA microarray analysis of gene expression in melanoma cultures and melanoma lines, where three separate laboratories supplied libraries of cultures or lines for analysis. What was striking about this study is that a search for internal structure in the DNA microarray data obtained from Herlyn's group (called the Philadelphia data set) helped to identify clustering patterns for their cell lines, which had *no relationship* with the stages from which they were derived [39]. This contrasts strongly with the study done with biopsy material by Smith et al., where a similar search for internal structure in the data revealed a clear division between early- and late-stage tissues [86].

It is tempting to dismiss the cell line studies because in vitro culturing removes cells from tissue environments which may be crucial for maintaining stage-specific patterns of gene expression. However, hundreds of the genes with expression patterns that determined the subclustering pattern of Herlyn's library of cell lines were also found determining an identical clustering pattern in the cell culture libraries of two other laboratories. Again, it could be reasonable to suppose that the common culturing conditions in use contributed to this pattern identity. Although it fails to explain why there *are* different subtypes of otherwise identically cultured melanoma cells, what significance this apparent taxonomy of cell types has for melanoma biology is not yet fully understood, but there is strong evidence that it is related to metastatic potential.

Principally, there are two major in vitro cell types and they are most immediately differentiated by the expression pattern of a large number of melanocytic genes. One (melanocytic) cell type expresses genes encoding the microphthalmia-associated transcription factor (Mitf) and many of its known targets, including tyrosinase, melan-A, gp100, and tyrosinase-related protein 2. The other (nonmelanocytic) cell type suppresses the expression of these genes and instead expresses many genes associated with modifying the extracellular environment. These include basic fibroblast growth factor, connective tissue growth factor, type V collagen and lysyl oxidase. Many of the genes involved had previously been identified by other studies correlating the expression of individual factors with melanoma metastatic potential. For example, both gelatinase A and the urokinase plasminogen activator were each identified by multiple groups as being upregulated in melanomas with increased metastatic potential [55, 80, 99]. Similarly, genes like melastatin, the AP2 transcription factor, and the type B endothelin receptor were previously reported as being upregulated in melanomas with *decreased* metastatic potential [29, 46, 87]. These and others are among a total of at least 134 genes whose expression was correlated with metastatic potential [39]. Of these there were 20 (including the five just mentioned) whose expression differences correlated with variation in melanoma metastatic potential and were among the 223 whose expression patterns define the new melanoma cell taxonomy. Such an overlap occurring by chance is extremely unlikely ($p < 10^{-26}$) and strongly argues that the cell types delineated by gene expression are reflections of differences in metastatic potential [39].

Several experiments were conducted on the gene expression delineated cell types to determine if there were correlating in vitro characteristics. For example, a characteristic attributed to early phase or poorly metastatic melanoma cells is their susceptibility to growth inhibition by the cytokine TGF-β [49, 57, 76]. It was found that the melanocytic cell type was significantly more susceptible to growth inhibition by TGF-β than the nonmelanocytic cell type. This suggested that the melanocytic type represented early phase or poorly metastatic cells, while nonmelanocytic cells represented later phase or more metastatic cells. Furthermore, it was found that melanocytic cells were far less motile than nonmelanocytic cells, which again correlates with the notion that motility is a trait acquired with increasing metastatic potential. Therefore, melanocytic cells had the appearance of early phase, poorly metastatic cells while the nonmelanocytic cells appeared to be later phase, highly metastatic cells. However, as demonstrated by the Philadelphia data set derived from Meenhard Herlyn's carefully characterized cell lines, whether a cell was melanocytic or nonmelanocytic was no reflection of whether it was derived from a radial growth phase, vertical growth phase, or metastatic lesion. Furthermore, melanocytic cells are significantly more proliferative, both in vitro and in vivo, than nonmelanocytic cells [38] – which runs counter to the notion that later phase, highly metastatic cells should gain rather than lose proliferative capacity. These findings do not fit with the existing molecular model of melanoma progression, in which genes are upregulated or downregulated according to stage of progression. Finally, the immunohistochemical record provides many instances of late-stage melanoma lesion cells expressing genes for whom the existing model of melanoma pathology predicts are specific for early-stage lesions. The reverse, in which genes expected to be expressed in late-stage tumors are instead absent, is also frequently observed. Together, these in vitro and in situ studies point out a significant shortcoming of the existing model's molecular context – that it does not sufficiently describe observed biologies.

An alternative model for melanoma progression is one which takes into account both the melanocytic and nonmelanocytic cell types characterized by gene expression profiling and other in vitro tests, and also accounts for apparent discrepancies uncovered by the immunohistochemical record. This new model begins by evoking an interpretation of metastatic potential as being split between separate programs of invasion and proliferation, and that disease progression is achieved not by the steady intensification of both (as inferred by the current model) but by repeated switching between them. This necessarily entails that lesions are frequently heterogeneous composites of both melanocytic and nonmelanocytic melanoma cells. That melanocytic cells can give rise to nonmelanocytic cells and vice versa has been demonstrated in vivo. Each cell type was separately injected subcutaneously into the flanks of immunocompromised nude mice and the resulting tumors were analyzed immunohistochemically for cell-type-specific markers. It was found that no matter what cell type was used, the resulting tumors were always a composite of the two [38]. This particular observation was later duplicated by another study which isolated melanoma cells from biopsy material into marker-positive and marker-negative fractions. It was similarly found that whether a cell population was negative or positive for a given marker, the resulting xenograft was *always* a composite of marker-negative and marker-positive cells [72]. It is thus likely that in the earliest stages after melanocytic transformation, thin primary melanomas are composed entirely of proliferative but poorly invasive melanocytic cell type. Later, due to the possible influence of increasing hypoxia within the growing lesion, some of these switch to the invasive but poorly proliferative nonmelanocytic cell type. Some or even many of these cells escape to distal environments where they switch back to the melanocytic type and reinitiate the proliferative program, possibly to begin the cycle of type-switching anew (Fig. 2.2.3). Other evidence in support of this includes gene expression profiling of spontaneously regressing melanoma lesions in a miniature pig model [73]. In this model the genes being expressed by growing lesions are the same as those expressed by proliferative melanocytic cell types, while the cells in regressing lesions express genes which are expressed by invasive nonmelanocytic cell types. Colin Goding's laboratory has performed several studies investigating cellular heterogeneity in melanoma metastases,

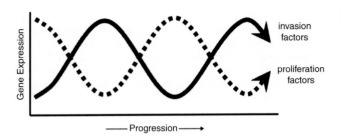

Fig. 2.2.3 Phenotype switching model for melanoma progression. An alternative model describing gene expression change during malignant progression of melanoma. Melanoma cells switch between genetic programs of invasion and proliferation [38]. This hypothesis accounts for in vivo immunohistochemical heterogeneity of lesions and the observation that in vitro cultures present with different molecular and phenotypic characteristics of metastatic potential

showing distinct populations of melanocytic (Mitf-expressing) and nonmelanocytic cells and pointing out that neither population reaches clonal dominance within a tumor [14, 33]. That this is true for primary lesions was shown by the different expression profiles obtained by Haqq et al. from RGP and VGP regions of the same primary lesion [34].

How are we to reconcile the differences encountered between in vivo and in vitro gene-expression profiling studies in melanoma? Why do studies of melanoma biopsy samples yield stage-specific results while similar studies of melanoma lines do not? Gene expression of cells in tissue is certainly affected by the environment in which the cells reside. Until a primary lesion thickens, most melanoma cells remain in proximity to keratinocytes, which are known to maintain normal melanocyte differentiation [100] and their influence is known to affect early-stage expression patterns [83]. As the lesion thickens keratinocyte influence is presumably lost in an increasing number of melanoma cells. The inference is that stage is dominated more by microenvironmental context than anything intrinsic to the melanoma cell itself. A case in point would be the ability for melanoma cells removed from a thin primary lesion to nevertheless form a subcutaneous xenograft lesion, an environment arguably more familiar to cutaneous melanoma metastases [23].

The molecular biology of melanoma progression is dominated by melanoma cell response to changing microenvironments. At the same time, accumulating changes within the cell nucleus seems less likely to contribute to the process of metastatic progression and anyway fails to explain the molecular heterogeneity of metastatic lesions. Therefore, it is important that researchers work toward an understanding of the mechanisms of microenvironmentally controlled phenotype switching. Furthermore, it is critical that clinicians understand that they are faced with *two* very different types of melanoma cells in the lesions of melanoma patients, both with the capacity to promote disease progression.

References

1. Adams, P.D.: Regulation of the retinoblastoma tumor suppressor protein by cyclin/cdks. Biochim. Biophys. Acta **1471**, M123–M133 (2001)
2. Adhikary, S., Eilers, M.: Transcriptional regulation and transformation by Myc proteins. Nat. Rev. Mol. Cell Biol. **6**, 635–645 (2005)
3. Albino, A.P., Nanus, D.M., Mentle, I.R., Cordon-Cardo, C., McNutt, N.S., Bressler, J., Andreeff, M.: Analysis of ras oncogenes in malignant melanoma and precursor lesions: correlation of point mutations with differentiation phenotype. Oncogene **4**, 1363–1374 (1989)
4. Bach, S.P., Renehan, A.G., Potten, C.S.: Stem cells: the intestinal stem cell as a paradigm. Carcinogenesis **21**, 469–476 (2000)
5. Beadling, C., Jacobson-Dunlop, E., Hodi, F.S., Le, C., Warrick, A., Patterson, J., Town, A., Harlow, A., Cruz III, F., Azar, S., et al.: KIT gene mutations and copy number in melanoma subtypes. Clin. Cancer Res. **14**, 6821–6828 (2008)
6. Bennett, D.C.: How to make a melanoma: what do we know of the primary clonal events? Pigment Cell Melanoma Res. **21**, 27–38 (2008)
7. Bennett, D.C., Cooper, P.J., Hart, I.R.: A line of non-tumorigenic mouse melanocytes, syngeneic with the B16 melanoma and requiring a tumour promoter for growth. Int. J. Cancer **39**, 414–418 (1987)
8. Besaratinia, A., Pfeifer, G.P.: Sunlight ultraviolet irradiation and BRAF V600 mutagenesis in human melanoma. Hum. Mutat. **29**, 983–991 (2008)
9. Blume-Jensen, P., Janknecht, R., Hunter, T.: The kit receptor promotes cell survival via activation of PI 3-kinase and subsequent Akt-mediated phosphorylation of Bad on Ser136. Curr. Biol. **8**, 779–782 (1998)
10. Box, N.F., Duffy, D.L., Chen, W., Stark, M., Martin, N.G., Sturm, R.A., Hayward, N.K.: MC1R genotype modifies risk of melanoma in families segregating CDKN2A mutations. Am. J. Hum. Genet. **69**, 765–773 (2001)
11. Brunet, A., Bonni, A., Zigmond, M.J., Lin, M.Z., Juo, P., Hu, L.S., Anderson, M.J., Arden, K.C., Blenis, J., Greenberg, M.E.: Akt promotes cell survival by phosphorylating and inhibiting a Forkhead transcription factor. Cell **96**, 857–868 (1999)
12. Cairns, J.: Mutation selection and the natural history of cancer. Nature **255**, 197–200 (1975)
13. Cardone, M.H., Roy, N., Stennicke, H.R., Salvesen, G.S., Franke, T.F., Stanbridge, E., Frisch, S., Reed, J.C.: Regulation of cell death protease caspase-9 by phosphorylation. Science **282**, 1318–1321 (1998)
14. Carreira, S., Goodall, J., Denat, L., Rodriguez, M., Nuciforo, P., Hoek, K.S., Testori, A., Larue, L., Goding, C.R.: Mitf regulation of dia1 controls melanoma proliferation and invasiveness. Genes Dev. **20**, 3426–3439 (2006)
15. Chumakov, P.M.: Versatile functions of p53 protein in multicellular organisms. Biochemistry (Mosc) **72**, 1399–1421 (2007)
16. Clark Jr., W.H., Elder, D.E., Guerry, Dt, Epstein, M.N., Greene, M.H., Van Horn, M.: A study of tumor progression: the precursor lesions of superficial spreading and nodular melanoma. Hum. Pathol. **15**, 1147–1165 (1984)
17. Curtin, J.A., Busam, K., Pinkel, D., Bastian, B.C.: Somatic activation of KIT in distinct subtypes of melanoma. J. Clin. Oncol. **24**, 4340–4346 (2006)
18. Curtin, J.A., Fridlyand, J., Kageshita, T., Patel, H.N., Busam, K.J., Kutzner, H., Cho, K.H., Aiba, S., Brocker, E.B., LeBoit, P.E., et al.: Distinct sets of genetic alterations in melanoma. N. Engl. J. Med. **353**, 2135–2147 (2005)
19. Dahl, C., Guldberg, P.: The genome and epigenome of malignant melanoma. APMIS **115**, 1161–1176 (2007)

20. Datta, S.R., Dudek, H., Tao, X., Masters, S., Fu, H., Gotoh, Y., Greenberg, M.E.: Akt phosphorylation of BAD couples survival signals to the cell-intrinsic death machinery. Cell **91**, 231–241 (1997)

21. Davies, H., Bignell, G.R., Cox, C., Stephens, P., Edkins, S., Clegg, S., Teague, J., Woffendin, H., Garnett, M.J., Bottomley, W., et al.: Mutations of the BRAF gene in human cancer. Nature **417**, 949–954 (2002)

22. de Wit, N.J., Rijntjes, J., Diepstra, J.H., van Kuppevelt, T.H., Weidle, U.H., Ruiter, D.J., van Muijen, G.N.: Analysis of differential gene expression in human melanocytic tumour lesions by custom made oligonucleotide arrays. Br. J. Cancer **92**, 2249–2261 (2005)

23. Degen, W.G., Agterbos, M.A., Muyrers, J.P., Bloemers, H.P., Swart, G.W.: memA/DRS, a putative mediator of multiprotein complexes, is overexpressed in the metastasizing human melanoma cell lines BLM and MV3. Biochim. Biophys. Acta **1444**, 384–394 (1999)

24. Di Cristofano, A., Pandolfi, P.P.: The multiple roles of PTEN in tumor suppression. Cell **100**, 387–390 (2000)

25. Diehl, J.A., Cheng, M., Roussel, M.F., Sherr, C.J.: Glycogen synthase kinase-3beta regulates cyclin D1 proteolysis and subcellular localization. Genes Dev. **12**, 3499–3511 (1998)

26. Dooley, T.P., Curto, E.V., Davis, R.L., Grammatico, P., Robinson, E.S., Wilborn, T.W.: DNA microarrays and likelihood ratio bioinformatic methods: discovery of human melanocyte biomarkers. Pigment Cell Res. **16**, 245–253 (2003)

27. Druker, B.J., Talpaz, M., Resta, D.J., Peng, B., Buchdunger, E., Ford, J.M., Lydon, N.B., Kantarjian, H., Capdeville, R., Ohno-Jones, S., et al.: Efficacy and safety of a specific inhibitor of the BCR-ABL tyrosine kinase in chronic myeloid leukemia. N. Engl. J. Med. **344**, 1031–1037 (2001)

28. Dumaz, N., Hayward, R., Martin, J., Ogilvie, L., Hedley, D., Curtin, J.A., Bastian, B.C., Springer, C., Marais, R.: In melanoma, RAS mutations are accompanied by switching signaling from BRAF to CRAF and disrupted cyclic AMP signaling. Cancer Res. **66**, 9483–9491 (2006)

29. Duncan, L.M., Deeds, J., Cronin, F.E., Donovan, M., Sober, A.J., Kauffman, M., McCarthy, J.J.: Melastatin expression and prognosis in cutaneous malignant melanoma. J. Clin. Oncol. **19**, 568–576 (2001)

30. Eskandarpour, M., Hashemi, J., Kanter, L., Ringborg, U., Platz, A., Hansson, J.: Frequency of UV-inducible NRAS mutations in melanomas of patients with germline CDKN2A mutations. J. Natl Cancer Inst. **95**, 790–798 (2003)

31. Fang, D., Nguyen, T.K., Leishear, K., Finko, R., Kulp, A.N., Hotz, S., Van Belle, P.A., Xu, X., Elder, D.E., Herlyn, M.: A tumorigenic subpopulation with stem cell properties in melanomas. Cancer Res. **65**, 9328–9337 (2005)

32. Garraway, L.A., Widlund, H.R., Rubin, M.A., Getz, G., Berger, A.J., Ramaswamy, S., Beroukhim, R., Milner, D.A., Granter, S.R., Du, J., et al.: Integrative genomic analyses identify MITF as a lineage survival oncogene amplified in malignant melanoma. Nature **436**, 117–122 (2005)

33. Goodall, J., Carreira, S., Denat, L., Kobi, D., Davidson, I., Nuciforo, P., Sturm, R.A., Larue, L., Goding, C.R.: Brn-2 represses microphthalmia-associated transcription factor expression and marks a distinct subpopulation of microphthalmia-associated transcription factor-negative melanoma cells. Cancer Res. **68**, 7788–7794 (2008)

34. Haqq, C., Nosrati, M., Sudilovsky, D., Crothers, J., Khodabakhsh, D., Pulliam, B.L., Federman, S., Miller 3rd, J.R., Allen, R.E., Singer, M.I., et al.: The gene expression signatures of melanoma progression. Proc. Natl. Acad. Sci. USA **102**, 6092–6097 (2005)

35. Hayward, N.K.: Genetics of melanoma predisposition. Oncogene **22**, 3053–3062 (2003)

36. Hoek, K., Rimm, D.L., Williams, K.R., Zhao, H., Ariyan, S., Lin, A., Kluger, H.M., Berger, A.J., Cheng, E., Trombetta, E.S., et al.: Expression profiling reveals novel pathways in the transformation of melanocytes to melanomas. Cancer Res. **64**, 5270–5282 (2004)

37. Hoek, K.S.: DNA microarray analyses of melanoma gene expression: a decade in the mines. Pigment Cell Res. **20**, 466–484 (2007)

38. Hoek, K.S., Eichhoff, O.M., Schlegel, N.C., Doebbeling, U., Schaerer, L., Hemmi, S., Dummer, R.: In vivo switching of human melanoma cells between proliferative and invasive states. Cancer Res. **68**, 650–656 (2008)

39. Hoek, K.S., Schlegel, N.C., Brafford, P., Sucker, A., Ugurel, S., Kumar, R., Weber, B.L., Nathanson, K.L., Phillips, D.J., Herlyn, M., et al.: Metastatic potential of melanomas defined by specific gene expression profiles with no BRAF signature. Pigment Cell Res. **19**, 290–302 (2006)

40. Hwang, P.H., Yi, H.K., Kim, D.S., Nam, S.Y., Kim, J.S., Lee, D.Y.: Suppression of tumorigenicity and metastasis in B16F10 cells by PTEN/MMAC1/TEP1 gene. Cancer Lett. **172**, 83–91 (2001)

41. Iwakuma, T., Lozano, G.: Crippling p53 activities via knock-in mutations in mouse models. Oncogene **26**, 2177–2184 (2007)

42. Jensen, E.H., Lewis, J.M., McLoughlin, J.M., Alvarado, M.D., Daud, A., Messina, J., Enkemann, S., Yeatman, T.J., Sondak, V.K., Riker, A.I.: Down-regulation of pro-apoptotic genes is an early event in the progression of malignant melanoma. Ann. Surg. Oncol. **14**, 1416–1423 (2007)

43. Jimbow, K., Uesugi, T.: New melanogenesis and photobiological processes in activation and proliferation of precursor melanocytes after UV-exposure: ultrastructural differentiation of precursor melanocytes from Langerhans cells. J. Invest. Dermatol. **78**, 108–115 (1982)

44. Jonsson, G., Dahl, C., Staaf, J., Sandberg, T., Bendahl, P.O., Ringner, M., Guldberg, P., Borg, A.: Genomic profiling of malignant melanoma using tiling-resolution arrayCGH. Oncogene **26**, 4738–4748 (2007)

45. Jovanovic, B., Krockel, D., Linden, D., Nilsson, B., Egyhazi, S., Hansson, J.: Lack of cytoplasmic ERK activation is an independent adverse prognostic factor in primary cutaneous melanoma. J. Invest. Dermatol. **128**, 2696–2704 (2008)

46. Karjalainen, J.M., Kellokoski, J.K., Mannermaa, A.J., Kujala, H.E., Moisio, K.I., Mitchell, P.J., Eskelinen, M.J., Alhava, E.M., Kosma, V.M.: Failure in post-transcriptional processing is a possible inactivation mechanism of AP-2alpha in cutaneous melanoma. Br. J. Cancer **82**, 2015–2021 (2000)

47. Kawaguchi, N., Noda, M.: Mitf is expressed in osteoclast progenitors in vitro. Exp. Cell Res. **260**, 284–291 (2000)

48. Kim, Y.G., Kim, H.J., Kim, D.S., Kim, S.D., Han, W.S., Kim, K.H., Chung, J.H., Park, K.C.: Up-Regulation and redistribution of Bax in ultraviolet B-irradiated melanocytes. Pigment Cell Res. **13**, 352–357 (2000)

49. Krasagakis, K., Kruger-Krasagakes, S., Fimmel, S., Eberle, J., Tholke, D., von der Ohe, M., Mansmann, U., Orfanos, C.E.: Desensitization of melanoma cells to autocrine TGF-beta isoforms. J. Cell. Physiol. **178**, 179–187 (1999)

50. Kumar, R., Angelini, S., Czene, K., Sauroja, I., Hahka-Kemppinen, M., Pyrhonen, S., Hemminki, K.: BRAF mutations in metastatic melanoma: a possible association with clinical outcome. Clin. Cancer Res. **9**, 3362–3368 (2003)

51. Liang, J., Zubovitz, J., Petrocelli, T., Kotchetkov, R., Connor, M.K., Han, K., Lee, J.H., Ciarallo, S., Catzavelos, C., Beniston, R., et al.: PKB/Akt phosphorylates p27, impairs nuclear import of p27 and opposes p27-mediated G1 arrest. Nat. Med. **8**, 1153–1160 (2002)

52. Lin, W.M., Baker, A.C., Beroukhim, R., Winckler, W., Feng, W., Marmion, J.M., Laine, E., Greulich, H., Tseng, H., Gates, C., et al.: Modeling genomic diversity and tumor dependency in malignant melanoma. Cancer Res. **68**, 664–673 (2008)

53. Loercher, A.E., Tank, E.M., Delston, R.B., Harbour, J.W.: MITF links differentiation with cell cycle arrest in melanocytes by transcriptional activation of INK4A. J. Cell Biol. **168**, 35–40 (2005)

54. Maldonado, J.L., Fridlyand, J., Patel, H., Jain, A.N., Busam, K., Kageshita, T., Ono, T., Albertson, D.G., Pinkel, D., Bastian, B.C.: Determinants of BRAF mutations in primary melanomas. J. Natl. Cancer Inst. **95**, 1878–1890 (2003)

55. Maniotis, A.J., Folberg, R., Hess, A., Seftor, E.A., Gardner, L.M., Pe'er, J., Trent, J.M., Meltzer, P.S., Hendrix, M.J.: Vascular channel formation by human melanoma cells in vivo and in vitro: vasculogenic mimicry. Am. J. Pathol. **155**, 739–752 (1999)

56. Mannava, S., Grachtchouk, V., Wheeler, L.J., Im, M., Zhuang, D., Slavina, E.G., Mathews, C.K., Shewach, D.S., Nikiforov, M.A.: Direct role of nucleotide metabolism in C-MYC-dependent proliferation of melanoma cells. Cell Cycle **7**, 2392–2400 (2008)

57. Medrano, E.E.: Repression of TGF-beta signaling by the oncogenic protein SKI in human melanomas: consequences for proliferation, survival, and metastasis. Oncogene **22**, 3123–3129 (2003)

58. Mihic-Probst, D., Mnich, C.D., Oberholzer, P.A., Seifert, B., Sasse, B., Moch, H., Dummer, R.: p16 expression in primary malignant melanoma is associated with prognosis and lymph node status. Int. J. Cancer **118**, 2262–2268 (2006)

59. Mikhail, M., Velazquez, E., Shapiro, R., Berman, R., Pavlick, A., Sorhaindo, L., Spira, J., Mir, C., Panageas, K.S., Polsky, D., et al.: PTEN expression in melanoma: relationship with patient survival, Bcl-2 expression, and proliferation. Clin. Cancer Res. **11**, 5153–5157 (2005)

60. Miller, A.J., Mihm Jr., M.C.: Melanoma. N. Engl. J. Med. **355**, 51–65 (2006)

61. Mirmohammadsadegh, A., Baer, A., Nambiar, S., Bardenheuer, W., Hengge, U.R.: Rapid identification of dysregulated genes in cutaneous malignant melanoma metastases using cDNA technology. Cells Tissues Organs **177**, 119–123 (2004)

62. Moan, J., Porojnicu, A.C., Dahlback, A.: Ultraviolet radiation and malignant melanoma. Adv. Exp. Med. Biol. **624**, 104–116 (2008)

63. Molven, A., Grimstvedt, M.B., Steine, S.J., Harland, M., Avril, M.F., Hayward, N.K., Akslen, L.A.: A large Norwegian family with inherited malignant melanoma, multiple atypical nevi, and CDK4 mutation. Genes Chromosomes Cancer **44**, 10–18 (2005)

64. Morris, R.J.: A perspective on keratinocyte stem cells as targets for skin carcinogenesis. Differentiation **72**, 381–386 (2004)

65. Nechushtan, H., Zhang, Z., Razin, E.: Microphthalmia (mi) in murine mast cells: regulation of its stimuli-mediated expression on the translational level. Blood **89**, 2999–3008 (1997)

66. Nesbit, C.E., Tersak, J.M., Prochownik, E.V.: MYC oncogenes and human neoplastic disease. Oncogene **18**, 3004–3016 (1999)

67. Omholt, K., Karsberg, S., Platz, A., Kanter, L., Ringborg, U., Hansson, J.: Screening of N-ras codon 61 mutations in paired primary and metastatic cutaneous melanomas: mutations occur early and persist throughout tumor progression. Clin. Cancer Res. **8**, 3468–3474 (2002)

68. Palmer, J.S., Duffy, D.L., Box, N.F., Aitken, J.F., O'Gorman, L.E., Green, A.C., Hayward, N.K., Martin, N.G., Sturm, R.A.: Melanocortin-1 receptor polymorphisms and risk of melanoma: is the association explained solely by pigmentation phenotype? Am. J. Hum. Genet. **66**, 176–186 (2000)

69. Petitjean, A., Mathe, E., Kato, S., Ishioka, C., Tavtigian, S.V., Hainaut, P., Olivier, M.: Impact of mutant p53 functional properties on TP53 mutation patterns and tumor phenotype: lessons from recent developments in the IARC TP53 database. Hum. Mutat. **28**, 622–629 (2007)

70. Piepkorn, M.: Melanoma genetics: an update with focus on the CDKN2A(p16)/ARF tumor suppressors. J. Am. Acad. Dermatol. **42**, 705–722 (2000). quiz 723–6

71. Planque, N., Raposo, G., Leconte, L., Anezo, O., Martin, P., Saule, S.: Microphthalmia transcription factor induces both retinal pigmented

epithelium and neural crest melanocytes from neuroretina cells. J. Biol. Chem. **279**, 41911–41917 (2004)

72. Quintana, E., Shackleton, M., Sabel, M.S., Fullen, D.R., Johnson, T.M., Morrison, S.J.: Efficient tumour formation by single human melanoma cells. Nature **456**, 593–598 (2008)

73. Rambow, F., Malek, O., Geffrotin, C., Leplat, J.J., Bouet, S., Piton, G., Hugot, K., Bevilacqua, C., Horak, V., Vincent-Naulleau, S.: Identification of differentially expressed genes in spontaneously regressing melanoma using the MeLiM swine model. Pigment Cell Melanoma Res. **21**, 147–161 (2008)

74. Rass, K., Reichrath, J.: UV damage and DNA repair in malignant melanoma and nonmelanoma skin cancer. Adv. Exp. Med. Biol. **624**, 162–178 (2008)

75. Rivers, J.K.: Is there more than one road to melanoma? Lancet **363**, 728–730 (2004)

76. Rodeck, U., Bossler, A., Graeven, U., Fox, F.E., Nowell, P.C., Knabbe, C., Kari, C.: Transforming growth factor beta production and responsiveness in normal human melanocytes and melanoma cells. Cancer Res. **54**, 575–581 (1994)

77. Rosen, C.F., Seki, Y., Farinelli, W., Stern, R.S., Fitzpatrick, T.B., Pathak, M.A., Gange, R.W.: A comparison of the melanocyte response to narrow band UVA and UVB exposure in vivo. J. Invest. Dermatol. **88**, 774–779 (1987)

78. Saenz-Santamaria, M.C., McNutt, N.S., Bogdany, J.K., Shea, C.R.: p53 expression is rare in cutaneous melanomas. Am. J. Dermatopathol. **17**, 344–349 (1995)

79. Schatton, T., Murphy, G.F., Frank, N.Y., Yamaura, K., Waaga-Gasser, A.M., Gasser, M., Zhan, Q., Jordan, S., Duncan, L.M., Weishaupt, C., et al.: Identification of cells initiating human melanomas. Nature **451**, 345–349 (2008)

80. Seftor, E.A., Meltzer, P.S., Kirschmann, D.A., Pe'er, J., Maniotis, A.J., Trent, J.M., Folberg, R., Hendrix, M.J.: Molecular determinants of human uveal melanoma invasion and metastasis. Clin. Exp. Metastasis **19**, 233–246 (2002)

81. Serrano, M., Lee, H., Chin, L., Cordon-Cardo, C., Beach, D., DePinho, R.A.: Role of the INK4a locus in tumor suppression and cell mortality. Cell **85**, 27–37 (1996)

82. Seykora, J.T., Jih, D., Elenitsas, R., Horng, W.H., Elder, D.E.: Gene expression profiling of melanocytic lesions. Am. J. Dermatopathol. **25**, 6–11 (2003)

83. Shih, I.M., Elder, D.E., Hsu, M.Y., Herlyn, M.: Regulation of Mel-CAM/MUC18 expression on melanocytes of different stages of tumor progression by normal keratinocytes. Am. J. Pathol. **145**, 837–845 (1994)

84. Slipicevic, A., Holm, R., Nguyen, M.T., Bohler, P.J., Davidson, B., Florenes, V.A.: Expression of activated Akt and PTEN in malignant melanomas: relationship with clinical outcome. Am. J. Clin. Pathol. **124**, 528–536 (2005)

85. Smalley, K.S.: A pivotal role for ERK in the oncogenic behaviour of malignant melanoma? Int. J. Cancer **104**, 527–532 (2003)

86. Smith, A.P., Hoek, K., Becker, D.: Whole-genome expression profiling of the melanoma progression pathway reveals marked molecular differences between nevi/melanoma in situ and advanced-stage melanomas. Cancer Biol. Ther. **4**, 1018–1029 (2005)

87. Smith, S.L., Damato, B.E., Scholes, A.G., Nunn, J., Field, J.K., Heighway, J.: Decreased endothelin receptor B expression in large primary uveal melanomas is associated with early clinical metastasis and short survival. Br. J. Cancer **87**, 1308–1313 (2002)

88. Sommer, L.: Checkpoints of melanocyte stem cell development. Sci. STKE **2005**, pe42 (2005)

89. Soufir, N., Avril, M.F., Chompret, A., Demenais, F., Bombled, J., Spatz, A., Stoppa-Lyonnet, D., Benard, J., Bressac-de Paillerets, B.: Prevalence of p16 and CDK4 germline mutations in 48 melanoma-prone families in France. The French Familial Melanoma Study Group. Hum. Mol. Genet. **7**, 209–216 (1998)

90. Soussi, T., Beroud, C.: Assessing TP53 status in human tumours to evaluate clinical outcome. Nat. Rev. Cancer **1**, 233–240 (2001)

91. Stambolic, V., Suzuki, A., de la Pompa, J.L., Brothers, G.M., Mirtsos, C., Sasaki, T., Ruland, J., Penninger, J.M., Siderovski, D.P., Mak, T.W.: Negative regulation of PKB/Akt-dependent cell survival by the tumor suppressor PTEN. Cell **95**, 29–39 (1998)

92. Stark, M., Hayward, N.: Genome-wide loss of heterozygosity and copy number analysis in melanoma using high-density single-nucleotide polymorphism arrays. Cancer Res. **67**, 2632–2642 (2007)

93. Stefanaki, I., Stratigos, A.J., Dimisianos, G., Nikolaou, V., Papadopoulos, O., Polydorou, D., Gogas, H., Tsoutsos, D., Panagiotou, P., Kanavakis, E., et al.: p53 codon 72 Pro homozygosity increases the risk of cutaneous melanoma in individuals with dark skin complexion and among noncarriers of melanocortin 1 receptor red hair variants. Br. J. Dermatol. **156**, 357–362 (2007)

94. Steingrimsson, E., Copeland, N.G., Jenkins, N.A.: Melanocytes and the microphthalmia transcription factor network. Annu. Rev. Genet. **38**, 365–411 (2004)

95. Sviderskaya, E.V., Hill, S.P., Evans-Whipp, T.J., Chin, L., Orlow, S.J., Easty, D.J., Cheong, S.C., Beach, D., DePinho, R.A., Bennett, D.C.: p16(Ink4a) in melanocyte senescence and differentiation. J. Natl. Cancer Inst. **94**, 446–454 (2002)

96. Talantov, D., Mazumder, A., Yu, J.X., Briggs, T., Jiang, Y., Backus, J., Atkins, D., Wang, Y.: Novel genes associated with malignant melanoma but not benign melanocytic lesions. Clin. Cancer Res. **11**, 7234–7242 (2005)

97. Tsao, H., Goel, V., Wu, H., Yang, G., Haluska, F.G.: Genetic interaction between NRAS and BRAF mutations and PTEN/MMAC1 inactivation in melanoma. J. Invest. Dermatol. **122**, 337–341 (2004)

98. Ugurel, S., Houben, R., Schrama, D., Voigt, H., Zapatka, M., Schadendorf, D., Brocker, E.B., Becker, J.C.: Microphthalmia-associated transcription factor gene amplification in metastatic melanoma is a prognostic marker for patient survival, but not a predictive marker for chemosensitivity and chemotherapy response. Clin. Cancer Res. **13**, 6344–6350 (2007)

99. Vaisanen, A., Tuominen, H., Kallioinen, M., Turpeenniemi-Hujanen, T.: Matrix metalloproteinase-2 (72 kD type IV collagenase) expression occurs in the early stage of human melanocytic tumour progression and may have prognostic value. J. Pathol. **180**, 283–289 (1996)

100. Valyi-Nagy, I.T., Hirka, G., Jensen, P.J., Shih, I.M., Juhasz, I., Herlyn, M.: Undifferentiated keratinocytes control growth, morphology, and antigen expression of normal melanocytes through cell-cell contact. Lab. Invest. **69**, 152–159 (1993)

101. Viros, A., Fridlyand, J., Bauer, J., Lasithiotakis, K., Garbe, C., Pinkel, D., Bastian, B.C.: Improving melanoma classification by integrating genetic and morphologic features. PLoS Med. **5**, e120 (2008)

102. Wellbrock, C., Ogilvie, L., Hedley, D., Karasarides, M., Martin, J., Niculescu-Duvaz, D., Springer, C.J., Marais, R.: V599EB-RAF is an oncogene in melanocytes. Cancer Res. **64**, 2338–2342 (2004)

103. Yang, B., O'Herrin, S.M., Wu, J., Reagan-Shaw, S., Ma, Y., Bhat, K.M., Gravekamp, C., Setaluri, V., Peters, N., Hoffmann, F.M., et al.: MAGE-A, mMage-b, and MAGE-C proteins form complexes with KAP1 and suppress p53-dependent apoptosis in MAGE-positive cell lines. Cancer Res. **67**, 9954–9962 (2007)

104. Zhao, Y., Zhang, Y., Yang, Z., Li, A., Dong, J.: Simultaneous knockdown of BRAF and expression of INK4A in melanoma cells leads to potent growth inhibition and apoptosis. Biochem. Biophys. Res. Commun. **370**, 509–513 (2008)

105. Zhou, B.P., Liao, Y., Xia, W., Spohn, B., Lee, M.H., Hung, M.C.: Cytoplasmic localization of p21Cip1/WAF1 by Akt-induced phosphorylation in HER-2/neu-overexpressing cells. Nat. Cell Biol. **3**, 245–252 (2001)

106. Zhuang, D., Mannava, S., Grachtchouk, V., Tang, W.H., Patil, S., Wawrzyniak, J.A., Berman, A.E., Giordano, T.J., Prochownik, E.V., Soengas, M.S., et al.: C-MYC overexpression is required for continuous suppression of oncogene-induced senescence in melanoma cells. Oncogene **27**, 6623–6634 (2008)

107. Zuidervaart, W., van der Velden, P.A., Hurks, M.H., van Nieuwpoort, F.A., Out-Luiting, C.J., Singh, A.D., Frants, R.R., Jager, M.J., Gruis, N.A.: Gene expression profiling identifies tumour markers potentially playing a role in uveal melanoma development. Br. J. Cancer **89**, 1914–1919 (2003)

108. Zuo, L., Weger, J., Yang, Q., Goldstein, A.M., Tucker, M.A., Walker, G.J., Hayward, N., Dracopoli, N.C.: Germline mutations in the p16INK4a binding domain of CDK4 in familial melanoma. Nat. Genet. **12**, 97–99 (1996)

Pathogenesis of Primary Cutaneous Lymphomas

2.3

Sean Whittaker

Primary cutaneous lymphomas are now defined in the WHO EORTC classification on the basis of specific clinico-pathologic features [1], but the underlying pathogenesis of these extranodal lymphomas has yet to be fully characterised. Primary cutaneous T-cell lymphomas do not show disease-specific translocations and are distinct from nodal lymphomas with a similar pathology. In contrast, primary cutaneous B-cell lymphomas appear to be much closer pathogenetically to their nodal or extranodal counterparts and can share specific chromosomal translocations.

2.3.1 Primary Cutaneous T-Cell Lymphomas

The underlying molecular pathogenesis of mycosis fungoides (MF) and Sezary syndrome (SS) has not yet been fully characterised. No disease-specific translocations have been identified [2], but studies have shown consistent abnormalities of cell cycle, DNA repair and apoptotic pathways, which contribute to both genomic instability and a failure of activation-induced cell death leading to dysregulation of T-cell homeostasis.

2.3.1.1 Cytogenetic Studies

Extensive studies have shown complex recurrent numerical and structural chromosomal abnormalities in all stages of disease [2–10]. In SS, an abnormal karotype is a poor prognostic factor [11]. These studies, using conventional cytogenetics, allelotyping, metaphase and array CGH techniques, have shown consistent patterns of chromosomal losses (1p, 13, 19, 17p and 10q) and gains (4, 8q and 17q), as well as loss of heterozygosity (9p, 10q and 17p) in both MF and SS suggesting a shared pathogenesis. In contrast, array CGH studies in primary cutaneous CD30+ anaplastic large-cell lymphoma (pcCD30+ALCL) and subcutaneous panniculitis-like T-cell lymphomas have shown different chromosomal imbalances with gains of chromosomes 1p and 5 and amplification of several different oncogenes [12, 13]. In MF/SS minimal regions of deletion have been detected on 10q suggesting a number of potential candidate genes [14, 15]. High-resolution array CGH studies have confirmed these findings in SS and suggest a high frequency (40–75% of cases) of candidate gene abnormalities including gains of *CMYC* and *STAT3/5* and loss of *CMYC* antagonists including *MXI1* and *MNT* and *p53* [16]. Gains of *HER 2/NEU* gene copy number at 17q have also been detected using FISH in a small series of SS patients [17]. High-resolution array CGH studies in early stages of MF have also shown recurrent losses (7p, 7q, 9q, 12q, 16q and 19) with gains (8q and 21q) and specific deletions of tumor suppressor genes *BCL7A*, *SMAC/DIABLO* and *RHOF* [18].

Specific chromosomal abnormalities have been detected in early stages of MF suggesting that chromosomal instability occurs at an early stage of disease [19]. Microsatellite instability (MSI) has been detected and attributed to hypermethylation of the mismatch repair enzyme gene promoter, *MLH1*, in some studies [20]. Telomerase activity is increased in MF/SS [21] which is essential to prevent tumor cell senescence but also potentially contributes to genomic instability.

A balanced t(12;18)(q21;21.2) translocation described in a patient with SS subsequently led to the identification of a *NAV3* gene deletion on chromosome 12q21–22 using interphase FISH in a majority of MF and SS patients [22]. However, subsequent studies have not detected specific *NAV3* deletions in a separate series of MF and SS patients; 12q losses were detected in a few cases but in only two cases did the 12q deletions include *NAV3* [23]. In pcCD30+ALCL the t(2;5) chromosomal translocation, producing the fusion protein NPM-ALK, seen in a high proportion of nodal CD30+ anaplastic lymphomas is not detected [24].

S. Whittaker
St John's Institute of Dermatology, King's College,
London, WC2R 2LS, UK
e-mail: sean.whittaker@kcl.ac.uk

R. Dummer et al. (eds.), *Skin Cancer – A World-Wide Perspective*,
DOI: 10.1007/978-3-642-05072-5_2.3, © Springer-Verlag Berlin Heidelberg 2011

2.3.1.2 Genomic and Epigenetic Abnormalities (Fig. 2.3.1)

Specific gene abnormalities in MF/SS include over-expression and mutation of *p53* in advanced stages of disease [25–28]. In one study, UVB-type *p53* mutations were found [27]. Additional 17p copy number losses also contribute to loss of *p53* function in MF/SS [7]. *p53* abnormalities are not found in early stages of disease, suggesting that inactivation of *p53* is related to disease progression, similar to findings in other nodal and extranodal lymphomas. At present, it is unclear if *p53* abnormalities are associated with treatment resistance and a poor prognosis as seen in other non-Hodgkin's lymphomas but loss of p53 would contribute to both apoptotic defects and genomic instability. Inactivation of *p14*, *p15* and *p16* genes has also been detected in MF [29–31]. This is a consequence of 9p deletions involving the *CDKN2A/2B* locus and epigenetic abnormalities due to hypermethylation of gene-promoter sequences rather than mutation. It is still unclear whether this is restricted to late-stage disease and transformation. Allelic losses at 9p21–22 have also been shown in pcCD30+ALCL, although the frequency of p16 loss/inactivation has yet to be determined [32]. Other genes shown to be inactivated in MF/SS through epigenetic mechanisms involving promoter hypermethylation include tumor suppressor genes, *BCL7A, PTPRG* and *p73* [33]. Deletions of *BCL7A* have also been demonstrated in early stages of MF [18]. The tumor suppressor gene on 10q, *PTEN*, has been shown to be homozygously deleted in a proportion of patients suggesting that the pro-apoptotic AKT signalling pathway is dysregulated [14]. Recent studies have identified infrequent mutations of the *Fas* gene on 10q in early stages of MF and

loss of *Fas* expression in advanced disease, providing a further mechanism by which tumor cells may escape apoptosis [34, 35]. Fas-mediated apoptosis may also be inhibited in tumor cells by over-expression of cFLIP, which inhibits the extrinsic apoptotic pathway [36]. Dysregulation of the intrinsic apoptotic pathway has also been detected in MF/SS [37]. Gains of oncogenes including *RAF1* and *CTSB* have been detected in a small series of MF/SS cases [38]. In addition, gains of *JUNB* on chromosome 19p have been detected in a large series of MF/SS patients and pcCD30+ALCL [39, 40]. This appears to be due to chromosomal amplification in some cases with over-expression in tumor cells identified in tumor samples as well [39]. JunB is a member of the AP1 transcription factor family involved in controlling cell proliferation and differentiation. JunB is also essential for expression of a Th2 cytokine profile and so over-expression in MF/SS may explain the characteristic Th2 cytokine expression by MF/SS [41] (Fig. 2.3.1).

2.3.1.3 Gene Expression Profiling

Gene expression studies in MF have shown abnormalities of TNF signalling pathways and gene expression signatures which reportedly distinguish inflammatory dermatoses from MF [42]. A further array cDNA study of MF has identified three signature profiles using consensus clustering which distinguishes (1) those patients with early-stage disease (IA–IIA) who respond to therapy, (2) an intermediate group (stage IB/III) who show a degree of resistance to therapy and (3) a poor prognostic group (predominantly stage IIB) [43]. These findings have yet to be validated and may explain

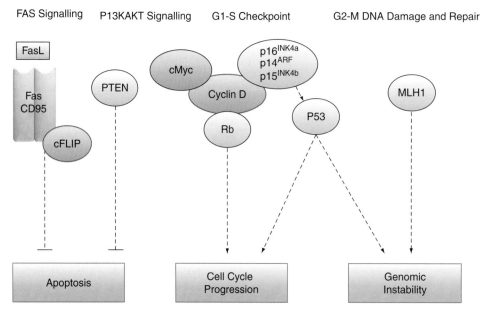

Fig. 2.3.1 Molecular features of MF/SS: *Grey* – loss of function; *Red* – gain of function

more about the host immune response than the actual tumor gene expression profile.

In SS cDNA array studies have identified a gene signature which is reported to be associated with a poor prognosis in SS and a diagnostic gene signature which can be used to distinguish inflammatory dermatoses from SS has also been described [44, 45]. A further study using a different array platform showed expression of a tyrosine kinase receptor, EphA4 and a transcription factor, Twist [46]. The functional relevance and validation of these findings require further study. Several studies have now confirmed overexpression of T-plastin in SS. This is an actin bundling protein and the T-plastin isoform is normally only expressed in epithelial tissues and could prove to be an important biomarker [44, 47].

2.3.1.4 Conclusion

Fundamental questions remaining include the cause(s) of the genomic instability which defines MF/SS even at early stages as well as a need to define the specific genomic abnormalities which distinguish SS from MF. However, it is apparent that critical abnormalities of apoptosis are prevalent in both MF and SS and almost certainly this affects T-cell homeostasis. Such defects are probably essential, allowing tumor cells in MF/SS to adopt a malignant phenotype. Defective activation-induced cell death in MF/SS is further exemplified by other key findings (Fig. 2.3.2); constitutive expression of STAT3 protein which is integral to cytokine-mediated T-cell activation and inhibition of IL-2-mediated expression of STAT5 have been clearly defined in advanced stages of disease such as SS [48–50]. In addition constitutive expression of NFκB has also been shown in both MF and SS [51, 52]. The consequent dysregulation of multiple signalling pathways controlled by STAT and NFκB

will contribute to prevention of tumor cell apoptosis in MF/SS and these pathways may also be potential therapeutic targets.

2.3.2 Primary Cutaneous B-Cell Lymphomas

The pathogenetic relationship between primary cutaneous B-cell lymphomas and their nodal counterparts remains unclear. Specific translocations characteristic of marginal-zone (MALT, mucosa-associated lymphoid tissue) lymphomas of nodal and extranodal origin have been detected in a proportion of primary cutaneous marginal zone lymphomas (pcMZL), and genomic abnormalities detected in nodal diffuse large B-cell lymphomas have also been identified in primary cutaneous large B-cell lymphoma (pcLBCL) suggesting a similar pathogenesis [53]. However, primary cutaneous follicle centre lymphomas (pcFCL) appear to be pathogenetically distinct from nodal follicular lymphomas [53].

Studies in nodal DLBCL using array technology have confirmed that these tumors are heterogeneous in origin with the detection of three distinct gene expression profiles with prognostic significance: one characteristic of germinal centre cells; one with an expression profile consistent with activated peripheral blood B-cells and one with an indeterminate profile [54, 55]. In primary cutaneous B-cell lymphomas, studies have shown that pcLBCL has an origin from activated B-cells, while pcFCL shows a germinal centre B-cell gene expression profile [56] and pcMZL, as would be expected, shows a plasma cell cDNA signature in a subset of cases [57].

2.3.3 Primary Cutaneous Marginal Zone Lymphoma

pcMZL is part of the spectrum of extranodal marginal zone B-cell lymphomas which were first described in the stomach, so-called MALT lymphoma, and have since been described in the thyroid, salivary gland, orbit and lung as well as the skin.

Development of immunocytomas has been reported in patients with acrodermatitis chronica atrophicans and has led to speculation about the role of *Borrelia burgdorferi* producing chronic antigen stimulation leading to neoplastic transformation. The detection of *Borrelia* DNA in some cutaneous lesions of pcMZL using PCR has provided support for this role, but the frequency of positivity varies considerably in different geographical regions with positive results in central

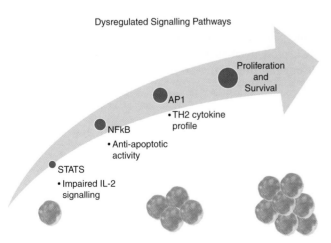

Fig. 2.3.2 Dysregulated T-cell signalling pathways in MF/SS

Europe and Scotland [58, 59] but no evidence of an association in the USA [60, 61]. To date, most cases of pcMZL associated with *Borrelia*, have been λ-chain-positive.

2.3.3.1 Cytogenetics

Recent studies have clearly demonstrated that approximately a third of pcMZL have identical translocations to those found in other extra-nodal MALT lymphomas including the t(14;18) involving the *IgH* gene locus and the *MALT1* gene, which is mostly found in monocytoid variants [62–64]. The t(14;18) involving *BCl2* has not been detected consistently in pcMZL [64, 65] but some studies have reported the presence of this translocation in a minority of cases [62, 66]. The t(11;18) which produces a fusion protein involving the *AP12* gene and the *MALT1* gene has been detected in some [67, 68], but not all studies of pcMZL [64, 69, 70]. Other translocations found in extra-nodal marginal zone B-cell lymphomas, such as the t(1;14) involving the *BCl-10* gene on 1q have not yet been identified in pcMZL [64, 67, 69, 70]. Trisomy 3 and 18 have been detected in up to 25% of cases [64, 67]. CGH techniques have also shown 18q gains in rare cases [71].

2.3.3.2 Genomic and Epigenetic Abnormalities

FAS mutations have rarely been described [69], but generally there is a lack of studies identifying specific gene mutations in pcMZL.

2.3.4 Primary Cutaneous Follicle Centre Lymphoma

The relationship between pcFCL and nodal systemic follicular and diffuse large B-cell lymphomas remains unclear. While there are morphological similarities, pcFCL follows an indolent clinical course and the immunophenotypic features, are distinct.

2.3.4.1 Cytogenetic Studies

While the t(14;18), characteristic of nodal systemic follicular lymphoma and a significant proportion of DLBCLs, has not been consistently detected in most studies of pcFCL [63, 65, 72, 73], some studies have detected the t(14;18) in a proportion of CD10+ and Bcl-2 positive pcFCL with a follicular growth pattern [74, 75], suggesting that there might be an unexplained geographical or histologic subset distinction

despite a lack of obvious prognostic differences. A recent study using a FISH-based technique has detected the t(14;18) translocation involving *BCl2* in 41% of 27 cases in which a PCR-based technique had failed to identify any *BCl2* rearrangement [76]. However, this study restricted the cases of pcFCL to those with a follicular growth pattern only. In contrast, in one study using microdissection of tumor cells, no evidence of the t(14;18) translocation was found [77].

FISH studies have not identified chromosomal breakpoints involving the *IGH*, *MYC* or *BCL-6* loci [78], although one study did show a t(3;14) in 2 of 27 cases involving Bcl6 and *IGH* in pcFCL and *BCl6* rearrangements/mutations have also been detected [76]. CGH studies have also identified patterns of chromosomal gains and losses associated with specific oncogene abnormalities in pcFCL including *cREL* amplification but a consistent pattern has not yet emerged [71, 79].

2.3.4.2 Genomic and Epigenetic Abnormalities

Inactivation of both the cyclin-dependent kinase inhibitors, namely the *p15* and *p16* genes, by promoter hypermethylation has been detected in a proportion of cases but the clinical significance is not yet clear [80]. A recent study has identified aberrant somatic hypermutation affecting certain oncogenes in pcFCL including *BCL6*, *PAX5*, *MYC* and *RHOH/TTF* similar to findings in nodal and primary cutaneous LBCL [81].

2.3.5 Primary Cutaneous Large B-Cell Lymphoma

Although pcLBCL by definition arises de novo in the skin, some tumors might result from high-grade transformation of a low-grade primary cutaneous B-cell lymphoma such as pcFCL. At present it is unclear whether pcLBCL has the same pathogenesis as primary nodal DLBCL. When pcL-BCL presents at sites other than the leg, it is important to distinguish from diffuse forms of pcFCL, because the latter has an excellent prognosis.

2.3.5.1 Cytogenetics

No disease-specific cytogenetic abnormalities have been identified. The t(14;18) translocation has not been identified in Bcl-2 positive pcLBCL [65, 78, 82, 83], except in rare cases from one series [84], In contrast, the t(14;18) is a common feature of nodal DLBCL reflecting a likely transformation from nodal follicular lymphoma and this translocation is also found in nodal DLBCL with secondary cutaneous

Table 2.3.1 Incidence of cytogenetic abnormalities in primary cutaneous B-cell lymphoma subtypes

Cytogenetic abnormality	pcMZL	pcFCL	pcLBCL	References
t(14;18) IgH:MALT1	22% (21/95)	0% (0/6)	0% (0/14)	[62–64]
t(14;18) IgH:BCL2	11% (9/80)	17% (24/143)	7% (4/54)	[62–66, 72–78, 82, 83]
t(11;18) AP12:MALT1	4% (4/96)	0% (0/1)	0% (0/6)	[64, 67–70]
t(1;14) BCL10:IgH	0% (0/63)	ND	ND	[64, 67, 69, 70]
t(8;14) MYC:IgH	0% (0/9)	0% (0/6)	36% (5/14)	[78, 84]
t(3;14) BCL6:IgH	0% (0/9)	6% (2/33)	14% (2/14)	[76]
Trisomy 3	17% (11/63)	ND	ND	[64, 67]
Trisomy 18	6% (4/63)	ND	ND	[64, 67]
BCL2/MALT1 amplification	0% (0/11)	8% (2/25)	60% (12/20)	[65, 78, 82, 83]
BCL10 mutation	3% (1/33)	50% (2/4)	ND	[69]
BCL6 mutation	0% (0/9)	37% (7/19)	47% (15/32)	[81, 84]
cMYC amplification	0% (0/9)	0% (0/6)	17% (3/18)	[81]
cREL amplification	ND	25% (3/12)	63% (12/19)	[71, 79]
9p21.3 (p16/p14ARF) deletion	ND	0% (0/19)	62% (43/64)	[80, 85]

Multiple techniques used including PCR, FISH and CGH
ND not done

involvement [82]. Unlike pcFCL and pcMZL, 6q losses and 2p, 12 and 18q gains are characteristic findings in pcLBCL, while chromosomal amplification of the *BCL2* gene on 18q is reported frequently and is associated with bcl-2 over-expression in pcLBCL [71, 79, 84]. Studies have also shown the t(8;14) translocation involving *CMYC* and *IGH* in a significant proportion of pcLBCL, which is likely to have clinical relevance as this translocation is associated with a poor prognosis in nodal DLBCL [78, 84].

2.3.5.2 Genomic and Epigenetic Abnormalities

Specific oncogene abnormalities including *cREL* and *MALT1* gene amplification have been reported in a high proportion of patients [71, 79]. In addition, inactivation of *p15* and *p16* genes by promoter hypermethylation and deletion of the 9p21.3 locus containing the *P16/14ARF* genes have been detected [79, 80]. Recent studies suggest that *P16/p14ARF* loss may have critical prognostic significance with 62% showing deletions of this locus [85]. *BCL6* rearrangements have only rarely been detected in pcLBCL but mutations of the *BCL6* gene have been reported which provides an alternative explanation for over-expression of Bcl6 [84].

2.3.5.3 Conclusion

The current findings suggest that pcMZL are pathogenetically similar to other extranodal MZL and that these low grade lymphomas may arise from chronic antigenic stimulation. The small studies reported to date also suggest that pcLBCL is related to nodal DLBCL although recent evidence that *P16/P14ARF* deletions may have prognostic significance is a novel finding. In contrast, a detailed characterization of the molecular abnormalities in pcFCL is still required to clarify the pathogenetic relationship between pcFCL and both nodal follicular and diffuse large B-cell lymphomas. The discrepancy in some of the published cytogenetic studies in pcFCL may relate to different methodologies and approaches to classification, which emphasises the importance of multi-centre collaborative studies (Table 2.3.1).

References

Pathogenesis of Primary Cutaneous Lymphomas

1. Willemze, R., Jaffe, E., Burg, G., et al.: WHO-EORTC classification for cutaneous lymphomas. Blood **105**, 3768–3785 (2005)

Primary Cutaneous T-Cell Lymphomas

2. Thangavelu, M., Finn, W., Yelavarthi, K., et al.: Recurring structural chromosomal abnormalities in peripheral blood lymphocytes of patients with mycosis fungoides/Sézary syndrome. Blood **89**, 3371 (1997)
3. Karenko, L., Kahkonen, M., Hyytinen, E., et al.: Notable losses at specific regions of chromosome 10q and 13q in the Sézary syndrome detected by comparative genomic hybridization. J. Invest. Dermatol. **112**, 392 (1999)

4. Mao, X., Lillington, D., Scarisbrick, J., et al.: Molecular cytogenetic analysis of cutaneous T-cell lymphomas: identification of common genetic alterations in Sézary syndrome and mycosis fungoides. Br. J. Dermatol. **147**, 464–475 (2002)

5. Karenko, L., Sarna, S., Kahkonen, M., Ranki, A.: Chromosomal abnormalities in relation to clinical disease in patients with cutaneous T-cell lymphoma: a 5 year follow-up study. Br. J. Dermatol. **148**, 55–64 (2003)

6. Scarisbrick, J.J., Woolford, A.J., Russell-Jones, R., Whittaker, S.J.: Allelotyping in mycosis fungoides and Sézary syndrome: common regions of allelic loss identified on 9p, 10q, and 17p. J. Invest. Dermatol. **117**, 663–670 (2001)

7. Mao, X., Lillington, D., Czepulkowski, B., et al.: Molecular cytogenetic characterization of Sézary syndrome. Genes Chromosomes Cancer **36**, 250–260 (2003)

8. Batista, D., Vonderheid, E., Hawkins, A., Morsberger, L., Long, P., Murphy, K., Griffin, C.: Multicolor fluoresecence in situ hybridization (SKY) in mycosis fungoides and Sezary syndrome: search for recurrent chromosome abnormalities. Genes Chromosomes Cancer **45**, 383–391 (2006)

9. Padilla-Nash, H., Wu, K., Just, H., Ried, T., Thestrup-Pedersen, K.: Spectral karyotyping demonstrates genetically unstable skin homing T lymphocytes in cutaneous T-cell lymphoma. Exp. Dermatol. **16**, 98–103 (2006)

10. Prochazkova, M., Chevret, E., Mainhaguiet, G., et al.: Common chromosomal abnormalities in mycosis fungoides transformation. Genes Chromosomes Cancer **46**, 828–838 (2007)

11. Whang-Peng, J., Bunn, P., Knutsen, T., et al.: Clinical implications of cytogenetic studies in cutaneous T-cell lymphoma (CTCL). Cancer **50**, 1539–1553 (1982)

12. Mao, X., Orchard, G., Lillington, D., et al.: Genetic alterations in primary cutaneous CD30+ anaplastic large cell lymphoma. Genes Chromosomes Cancer **37**, 176–185 (2003)

13. Hahtola, S., Burghart, E., Jeskanen, L., et al.: Clinicopathological characterisation and genomic aberrations in subcutaneous panniculitis-like T-cell lymphoma. J. Invest. Dermatol. **128**, 2304–2309 (2008)

14. Scarisbrick, J., Woolford, A., Russell-Jones, R., et al.: Loss of heterozygosity on 10q and microsatellite instability in advanced stages of primary cutaneous T-cell lymphoma and possible association with homozygous deletion of *PTEN*. Blood **95**, 2937–2942 (2000)

15. Wain, M., Mitchell, T., Russell Jones, R., Whittaker, S.: Fine mapping of chromosome 10q deletions in mycosis fungoides and Sezary syndrome: identification of two discrete regions of deletion at 10q23.33-24.1 and 10q24.33-25.1. Genes Chromosomes Cancer **42**, 184–192 (2005)

16. Vermeer, M., van Doorn, R., Dijkman, R., et al.: Novel and highly recurrent chromosomal alterations in Sezary syndrome. Cancer Res. **68**, 268–298 (2008)

17. Utikal, J., Poenitz, N., Gratchev, A., et al.: Additional Her 2/*neu* gene copies in patients with Sezary syndrome. Leuk. Res. **30**, 755–760 (2006)

18. Carbone, A., Bernardini, L., Valenzano, F., et al.: Array-based comparative genomic hybridization in early-stage mycosis fungoides: recurrent deletion of tumor suppressor genes *BCL7A, SMAC/DIABLO* and *RHOF*. Genes Chromosomes Cancer **47**(12), 1067–1075 (2008)

19. Barab, G., Matteucci, C., Girolomoni, G., et al.: Comparative genomic hybridization identifies 17q11.2-q12 duplication as an early event in cutaneous T-cell lymphomas. Cancer Genet. Cytogenet. **184**, 48–51 (2008)

20. Scarisbrick, J., Mitchell, T., Calonje, E., et al.: Microsatellite instability is associated with hypermethylation of the hMLH1 gene and reduced expression in mycosis fungoides. J. Invest. Dermatol. **121**, 894–901 (2003)

21. Wu, K., Lund, M., Bang, K., Thestrup-Pedersen, K.: Telomerase activity and telomere length in lymphocytes from patients with cutaneous T-cell lymphoma. Cancer **86**, 1056–1063 (1999)

22. Karenko, L., Hahtola, S., Paivinen, S., et al.: Primary cutaneous T-cell lymphomas show a deletion or translocation affecting *NAV3*, the human *UNC-53* homologue. Cancer Res. **65**, 8101–8110 (2005)

23. Marty, M., Prochazkova, M., Lahranne, E., et al.: Primary cutaneous T-cell lymphomas do not show specific *NAV3* gene deletion or translocation. J. Invest. Dermatol. **128**, 2458–2466 (2008)

24. DeCoteau, J., Butmarc, J., Kinney, M., Kadin, M.: The t(2;5) chromosomal translocation is not a common feature of primary cutaneous CD30+ lymphoproliferative disorders: comparison with anaplastic large cell lymphoma of nodal origin. Blood **87**, 3437–3441 (1996)

25. Lauritzen, A., Vejlsgaard, G., Hou-Jensen, K., et al.: P53 protein expression in cutaneous T-cell lymphomas. Br. J. Dermatol. **133**, 32–36 (1995)

26. MacGregor, J., Dublin, E., Levison, D., et al.: P53 immunoreactivity is uncommon in primary cutaneous lymphoma. Br. J. Dermatol. **132**, 353 (1995)

27. MacGregor, J., Crook, T., Fraser-Andrews, E., et al.: Spectrum of *p53* gene mutations suggests a possible role for ultraviolet radiation in the pathogenesis of advanced cutaneous lymphomas. J. Invest. Dermatol. **112**, 317–321 (1999)

28. Marrogi, A., Khan, M., Vonderheid, E., Wood, G., McBurney, E.: *P53* tumor suppressor gene mutations in transformed cutaneous T-cell lymphoma: a study of 12 cases. J. Cutan. Pathol. **26**, 369–378 (1999)

29. Peris, K., Stanta, G., Fargnoli, C., et al.: Reduced expression of CDKN2a/p16 in mycosis fungoides. Arch. Dermatol. Res. **291**, 207–211 (1999)

30. Navas, I., Oritz-Romero, P., Villuendas, R., et al.: *P16* gene alterations are frequent in lesions of mycosis fungoides. Am. J. Pathol. **156**, 1565–1572 (2000)

31. Scarisbrick, J.J., Woolford, A.J., Calonje, E., et al.: Frequent abnormalities of the *p15* and *p16* genes in mycosis fungoides and Sézary syndrome. J. Invest. Dermatol. **118**, 493–499 (2002)

32. Boni, R., Xin, H., Kamarashev, J., et al.: Allelic deletion at 9p21-22 in primary cutaneous CD30+ large cell lymphoma. J. Invest. Dermatol. **115**, 1104–1107 (2000)

33. van Doorn, R., Zoutman, W., Dijkman, R., et al.: Epigenetic profiling of cutaneous T-cell lymphoma: promoter hypermethylation of multiple tumor suppressor genes including *BCL7a, PTPRG* and *p73*. J. Clin. Oncol. **23**, 3886–3896 (2005)

34. Dereure, O., Levi, E., Vonderhied, E., Kadin, M.: Infrequent Fas mutations but no BAX or p53 mutations in early mycosis fungoides: a possible mechanism for the accumulation of malignant T lymphocytes in the skin. J. Invest. Dermatol. **118**, 949–956 (2002)

35. Zoi-Toli, O., Vermmer, M., De Vries, E., et al.: Expression of Fas and Fas-ligand in primary cutaneous T-cell lymphoma (CTCL): association between lack of Fas expression and aggressive types of CTCL. Br. J. Dermatol. **143**, 313–319 (2000)

36. Contassot, E., Kerl, K., Roques, S., et al.: Resistance to FasL and tumor necrosis factor-related apoptosis-inducing ligand-mediated apoptosis in Sezary syndrome T-cells associated with impaired death receptor and FLICE-inhibitory protein expression. Blood **111**, 4780–4787 (2006)

37. Zhang, C.-L., Kamarashev, J., Qin, J.-Z., et al.: Expression of apoptosis regulators in cutaneous T-cell lymphoma (CTCL) cells. J. Pathol. **200**, 249–254 (2003)

38. Mao, X., Orchard, G., Lillington, D., et al.: Amplification and overexpression of *JUNB* is associated with primary cutaneous T-cell lymphomas. Blood **101**, 1513–1519 (2003)

39. Mao, X., Orchard, G., Mitchell, T., et al.: A genomic and expression study of AP-1 in primary cutaneous T-cell lymphoma: evidence for dysregulated expression of JUNB and JUND in MF and SS. J. Cutan. Pathol. **35**(10), 899–910 (2008)

40. Mao, X., Orchard, G., Russell Jones, R., Whittaker, S.: Abnormal activator 1 protein expression in primary cutaneous CD30 positive large cell lymphomas. Br. J. Dermatol. **157**, 914–921 (2007)

41. Hahtola, S., Tuomela, S., Elo, L., et al.: Th1 response and cytotoxicity genes are down-regulated in cutaneous T-cell lymphoma. Clin. Cancer Res. **12**, 4812–4821 (2006)

42. Tracey, L., Villuendas, R., Dotor, A., et al.: Mycosis fungoides shows concurrent deregulation of multiple genes involved in the TNF signaling pathway: an expression profile study. Blood **102**, 1042–1050 (2003)

43. Shin, J., Monti, S., Aires, D., et al.: Lesional gene expression profiling in cutaneous T cell lymphoma reveals natural clusters associated with disease outcome. Blood **110**(8), 3015–3027 (2007)

44. Kari, L., Loboda, A., Nebozhyn, M., et al.: Classification and prediction of survival in patients with the leukemic phase of cutaneous T cell lymphoma. J. Exp. Med. **197**, 1477–1488 (2003)

45. Nebozhyn, M., Loboda, A., Kari, L., et al.: Quantitative PCR on 5 genes reliably identifies CTCL patients with 5% to 99% circulating tumor cells with 90% accuracy. Blood **107**, 3189–3196 (2006)

46. van Doorn, R., Dijkman, R., Vermeer, M., et al.: Aberrant expression of the tyrosine kinase receptor EphA4 and the transcription factor Twist in Sezary syndrome identified by gene expression analysis. Cancer Res. **64**, 5578–5586 (2004)

47. Su, M., Dorocicz, I., Dragowska, W., et al.: Aberrant expression of T-plastin in Sezary cells. Cancer Res. **63**, 7122–7127 (2003)

48. Zhang, Q., Nowak, I., Vonderheid, E., et al.: Activation of Jak/STAT proteins involved in signal transduction pathway mediated by receptor for interleukin 2 in malignant T lymphocytes derived from cutaneous anaplastic large T-cell lymphoma and Sezary syndrome. Proc. Natl. Acad. Sci. U.S.A. **93**, 9148–9153 (1996)

49. Qin, J.-Z., Kamarashev, J., Zhang, C.-L., Dummer, R., Burg, G., Dobbeling, U.: Constitutive and interleukin-7 and interleukin-15 stimulated DNA binding of STAT and novel factors in cutaneous T cell lymphoma cells. J. Invest. Dermatol. **117**, 583–589 (2001)

50. Mitchell, T., Whittaker, S., John, S.: Dysregulated expression of COOH-terminally truncated Stat5 and loss of IL2-inducible Stat5-dependent gene expression in Sezary syndrome. Cancer Res. **63**, 9048–9054 (2003)

51. Izban, K., Ergin, M., Qin, J.-Z., et al.: Constitutive expression of NF-kB is a characteristic feature of mycosis fungoides: implications for apoptosis resistance and pathogenesis. Hum. Pathol. **31**, 1482–1490 (2000)

52. Sors, A., Jean-Loius, F., Pellet, C., et al.: Down-regulating constitutive activation of the NFkB canonical pathway overcomes the resistance of cutaneous T-cell lymphoma to apoptosis. Blood **107**, 2354–2363 (2006)

Primary Cutaneous B-Cell Lymphomas NB

53. Willemze, R., Jaffe, E., Burg, G., et al.: WHO-EORTC classification for cutaneous lymphomas. Blood **105**, 3768–3785 (2005)

54. Rosenwald, A., Wright, G., Chan, W., et al.: The use of molecular profiling to predict survival after chemotherapy for diffuse large B-cell lymphoma. N. Engl. J. Med. **346**, 1937–1947 (2002)

55. Alizadeh, A., Eisen, M., Davis, R., et al.: Distinct types of diffuse large B-cell lymphoma identified by gene expression profiling. Nature **403**, 503–511 (2000)

56. Hoefnagel, J., Dijkman, R., Basso, K., et al.: Distinct types of primary cutaneous large B-cell lymphoma identified by gene expression profiling. Blood **105**, 3671–3678 (2005)

57. Storz, M., van de Rijn, M., Kim, Y., et al.: Gene expression profiles of cutaneous B-cell lymphoma. J. Invest. Dermatol. **120**, 865–870 (2003)

Primary Cutaneous Marginal B-Cell Lymphoma

58. Cerroni, L., Zochling, N., Putz, B., et al.: Infection by *Borrelia burgdorferi* and cutaneous B-cell lymphoma. J. Cutan. Pathol. **24**, 457–461 (1997)

59. Goodlad, J., Davidson, M., Hollowood, K., et al.: Primary cutaneous B-cell lymphoma and *Borrelia burgdorferi* infection in patients from the highlands of Scotland. Am. J. Surg. Pathol. **245**, 1279–1285 (2000)

60. Wood, G., Kamath, N., Guitart, J., et al.: Absence of *Borrelia burgdorferi* DNA in cutaneous B-cell lymphomas from the United States. J. Cutan. Pathol. **28**, 502–507 (2001)

61. Dillon, W., Saed, G., Fivenson, D.: *Borrelia burgdorferi* DNA is undetectable by polymerase chain reaction in skin lesions of morphoea, scleroderma or lichen sclerosis et atrophicus of patients from North America. J. Am. Acad. Dermatol. **33**, 617–620 (1995)

62. Palmedo, G., Hautschke, M., Rutten, A., et al.: Primary cutaneous marginal zone B-cell lymphoma may exhibit both the t(14;18) (q32;21) IGH/BCL2 and the t(14;18)(q32;21) IGH/MALT1 translocation: an indicator for clonal transformation towards higher grade B-cell lymphoma. Am. J. Dermatopathol. **29**, 231–236 (2007)

63. Streubel, B., Lamprecht, A., Dierlamm, J., et al.: T(14;18)(q32;q21) involving IGH and MALT1 is a frequent chromosomal aberration in MALT lymphoma. Blood **101**, 2335–2339 (2003)

64. Schreuder, M., Hoefnagel, J., Jansen, P., Krieken, J., Willemze, R., Hebeda, K.: FISH analysis of MALT lymphoma-specific translocations and aneuploidy in primary cutaneous marginal zone lymphoma. J. Pathol. **205**, 302–310 (2005)

65. Child, F., Russell Jones, R., Woolford, A., et al.: Absence of the t(14;18) translocation in primary cutaneous B-cell lymphomas. Br. J. Dermatol. **144**, 735–744 (2001)

66. Servitje, O., Gallardo, F., Estrach, T., et al.: Prirmary cutaneous marginal zone B-cell lymphoma: a clinical, histopathological, immunophenotypic and molecular genetic study of 22 cases. Br. J. Dermatol. **147**, 1147–1158 (2002)

67. Streubel, B., Simonitsch-Klupp, I., Mullauer, L., et al.: Variable frequency of MALT lymphoma-associated genetic aberrations in MALT lymphomas of different sites. Leukemia **18**, 1722–1726 (2004)

68. Remstein, E., James, C., Kurtin, P.: Incidence and subtype specificity of AP12 MALT1 fusion translocations in extranodal, nodal and splenic marginal zone lymphomas. Am. J. Pathol. **156**, 1183–1188 (2000)

69. Gronbaek, K., Ralfkiaer, E., Kalla, J., Skovgard, G., Guldberg, P.: Infrequent somatic FAS mutations but no evidence of Bcl10 mutations or t(11;18) in primary cutaneous MALTtype lymphoma. J. Pathol. **201**, 134–140 (2003)

70. Li, C., Inagaki, H., Kuo, T., Hu, S., Okabe, M., Eimoto, T.: Primary cutaneous marginal zone B-cell lymphoma: a molecular and clinicopathologic study of 24 asian cases. Am. J. Surg. Pathol. **27**, 1061–1069 (2003)

71. Mao, X., Lillington, D., Child, F., et al.: Comparative genomic hybridization analysis of primary cutaneous B-cell lymphoma: identification of common genetic alterations in disease pathogenesis. Genes Chromosomes Cancer **35**, 144–155 (2002)

Primary Cutaneous Follicle Centre Lymphoma

72. Goodlad, J., Krajewski, A., Batstone, P., et al.: Primary cutaneous follicular lymphoma; a clinicopathologic and molecular study of 16 cases in support of a distinct entity. Am. J. Surg. Pathol. **26**, 733–741 (2002)
73. Mirza, I., Macpherson, N., Paproski, R., et al.: Primary cutaneous follicular lymphoma: an assessment of clinical, histopathologic, immunophenotypic, and molecular features. J. Clin. Oncol. **20**, 647–655 (2002)
74. Bergman, R., Kurtin, P., Gibson, L., et al.: Clinicopathologic, immunophenotypic and molecular characterization of primary cutaneous B-cell lymphoma. Arch. Dermatol. **137**, 432–439 (2001)
75. Yang, B., Tubbs, R., Finn, W., et al.: Clinicopathologic reassessment of primary cutaneous B-cell lymphomas with immunophenotypic and molecular genetic characterization. Am. J. Surg. Pathol. **24**, 694–702 (2000)
76. Streubel, B., Scheucher, B., Valencak, J., et al.: Molecular cytogenetic evidence of t(14;18)(IGH;BCL2) in a substantial proportion of primary cutaneous follicle center lymphomas. Am. J. Surg. Pathol. **30**, 529–536 (2006)
77. Gellrich, S., Rutz, S., Golembowski, S., et al.: Primary cutaneous follicle center cell lymphomas and large B-cell lymphomas of the leg descend from germinal center cells: a single cell polymerase chain reaction analysis. J. Invest. Dermatol. **117**, 1512–1520 (2001)
78. Hallerman, C., Kaune, K., Gesk, S., et al.: Molecular cytogenetic analysis of chromosomal breakpoints in the IGH, MYC, BCL6 and MALT1 gene loci in primary cutaneous B-cell lymphomas. J. Invest. Dermatol. **123**, 213–219 (2004)
79. Dijkman, R., Tensen, C., Jordanova, E., et al.: Array based comparative hybridization analysis reveals recurrent chromosomal alterations and prognostic parameters in primary cutaneous large B-cell lymphomas. J. Clin. Oncol. **24**, 296–305 (2006)
80. Child, F., Scarisbrick, J., Calonje, E., et al.: Inactivation of tumor suppressor genes *p15* (INK4b) and *p16* (INK4a) in primary cutaneous B cell lymphoma. J. Invest. Dermatol. **118**, 941–948 (2002)
81. Dijkman, R., Tensen, C., Buettner, M., et al.: Primary cutaneous follicle center lymphoma and primary cutaneous large B-cell lymphoma, leg type, are both targeted by aberrant somatic hypermutation but demonstrate differential expression of AID. Blood **107**, 4926–4929 (2006)

Primary Cutaneous Large B-Cell Lymphoma

82. Kim, B., Surti, U., Pandya, A., Swerdlow, S.: Primary and secondary cutaneous diffuse large B-cell lymphomas. Am. J. Surg. Pathol. **27**, 356–364 (2003)
83. Hallerman, C., Kaune, K., Siebert, R., et al.: Chromosomal aberration patterns differ in subtypes of primary cutaneous B-cell lymphomas. J. Invest. Dermatol. **122**, 1495–1502 (2004)
84. Wiesner, T., Streubel, B., Huber, D., Kerl, H., Chott, A., Cerroni, L.: Genetic aberrations in primary cutaneous large B-cell lymphoma. Am. J. Surg. Pathol. **29**, 666–673 (2005)
85. Senff, N.J., Zoutman, W.H., Vermeer, M.H., et al.: An EORTC study: Fine-mapping chromosomal loss at 9p21: correlation with prognosis in primary cutaneous diffuse large B-cell lymphoma, leg type. J. Invest. Dermatol. **129**(5), 1149–1155 (2009)

Pathogenesis of Histiocytoses

2.4

Marie C. Zipser and Reinhard Dummer

2.4.1 Langerhans Cell Histiocytosis

Langerhans cell histiocytosis (LCH) is a disease of unknown etiology showing clonal proliferation of Langerhans-like cells or their precursors [1, 16]. Pathologic LCH cells appear to be in an immature state of activation and/or differentiation [1]. They accumulate in peripheral tissue and express inflammatory cytokines resulting in their own recruitment and retention [21]. Moreover, activated CD40 ligand expressing T helper cells are found to be the predominant source of cytokines and growth factors in LCH lesions [3]. The "cytokine storm" seems to be further enhanced by the interaction of CD40 expressing LCH cells and CD40 ligand expressing T-cells [3]. High levels of granulocyte-macrophage colony-stimulating factor, tumor-necrosis factor alpha, interleukin-3, and other cytokines are potential chemoattractants for recruiting eosinophils, neutrophils, marcrophages, and CD34+ Langerhans cell precursors into the LCH lesion [3, 7]. These cytokines are known to contribute directly to the development of fibrosis, necrosis, and osteolysis [11]. They are also supposed to play a role in the presence of several other myeloid cell types; the multinucleated giant cell (MGC), amongst others, was found in LCH lesions [8]. MGCs are believed to play a major role in tissue destruction, as they are express osteoclast markers [8]. Remarkably, though various inflammatory cytokines are present in LCH lesions, LCH cells remain immature and do not maturate [3]. Lesional microenvironment seems to play a role in the maintenance of the phenotype of LCH cells [3].

The clonality of LCH cells is suggestive of a neoplastic process. Moreover, there is an increase in the incidence of related second neoplasms, and up to 1% of probands have another first- or second-degree relative with the disease [3]. The molecular basis indeed includes aberrant expression of several adhesion molecules and elevated expression of oncogene products such as p53, c-myc, and H-ras [16]. Loss of heterozygosity has been reported on chromosomes 1, 4, 6, 7, 9, 16, 17, and 22 [16].

Recent studies identified differences in telomesase expression and telomere shortening by LCH cells, also supporting this being a neoplastic disorder [9]. Arguments supporting a reactive disease, resulting from environmental or infectious triggers, include the granulomatous character of LCH lesions and frequent cases of spontaneous regression [9]. A clear risk factor for pulmonary LCH in adults is smoking [21]. The relationship between this sometimes polyclonal lung disease and monoclonal LCH remains to be elucidated [21].

2.4.2 Indeterminate Cell Histiocytosis

Various hypotheses exist regarding the relationship between Langerhans cells and indeterminate cells [19]. Indeterminate cells may be immature precursors of Langerhans cells arrested during the process of migration and maturation [14] or members of the epidermal/dermal dendritic cell system, which migrate from skin to regional lymph nodes [20]. Indeterminate cell histiocytosis, therefore, might be a disorder caused by locally arrested dermal indeterminate cells that proliferate before the departure for the lymph nodes [20]. Neoplastic cells express S-100, CD1a, and CD68; they are CD207 (Langerin) negative and Birbeck granules are absent [15, 20].

M.C. Zipser
University Hospital of Zürich, Department of Dermatology F2,
Gloriastrasse 31, 8091 Zürich,
Switzerland
e-mail: marie.zipser@usz.ch

R. Dummer (✉)
Department of Dermatology, University Hospital of Zürich,
Gloriastrasse 31, 8091 Zürich,
Switzerland
e-mail: reinhard.dummer@usz.ch

R. Dummer et al. (eds.), *Skin Cancer – A World-Wide Perspective*,
DOI: 10.1007/978-3-642-05072-5_2.4, © Springer-Verlag Berlin Heidelberg 2011

2.4.3 Sinus Histiocytosis with Massive Lymphadenopathy (Rosai–Dorfman Disease)

The pathogenesis is unknown. Sinus histiocytosis lesions consist of a nonmalignant proliferating subset of distinctive histiocytes [12]. These histiocytes characteristically present in their cytoplasm a variable number of lymphoctes, a phenomenon called lymphophagocytosis or emperipolesis [12].

2.4.4 Juvenile Xanthogranuloma

The etiology of juvenile xanthogranuloma (JXG) is unknown. Recently JXG was found to represent a clonal proliferation of histiocytic/dendritic cells [13]. Typical histopathological presentation of JXG is infiltration of Touton giant cells staining positive for CD68 and negative for CD1a and S-100 protein [10].

In adult xanthograulomatosis, dermal macrophages accumulate cholesterol intracellularly, despite normal plasma cholesterol [2].

2.4.5 Reticulohistiocytosis

The etiopathogenesis of multicentric reticulohistiocytosis is unknown. It may reflect a reactive inflammatory response to an undetermined stimulus [4]. An association with internal malignancy has been reported in about a third of patients [6, 17]. Solitary cutaneous forms may be associated with local trauma such as insect bites, folliculitis, or ruptured infundibular cysts [5]. Cutaneous reticulohistiocytosis could also be associated with autoimmune diseases such as vasculitis [18].

References

1. Annels, N.E., Da Costa, C.E., et al.: Aberrant chemokine receptor expression and chemokine production by Langerhans cells underlies the pathogenesis of Langerhans cell histiocytosis. J. Exp. Med. **197**(10), 1385–1390 (2003)
2. Bergman, R., Aviram, M., et al.: Enhanced low-density lipoprotein degradation and cholesterol synthesis in monocyte-derived mac- rophages of patients with adult xanthogranulomatosis. J. Invest. Dermatol. **101**(6), 880–882 (1993)
3. Beverley, P.C., Egeler, R.M., et al.: The Nikolas Symposia and his- tiocytosis. Nat. Rev. Cancer **5**(6), 488–494 (2005)
4. Campbell, D.A., Edwards, N.L.: Multicentric reticulohistiocytosis: systemic macrophage disorder. Baillières Clin. Rheumatol. **5**(2), 301–319 (1991)
5. Caputo, R., Alessi, E., et al.: Collagen phagocytosis in multi- centric reticulohistiocytosis. J. Invest. Dermatol. **76**(5), 342–346 (1981)
6. Catterall, M.D., White, J.E.: Multicentric reticulohistiocytosis and malignant disease. Br. J. Dermatol. **98**(2), 221–224 (1978)
7. Caux, C., Dezutter-Dambuyant, C., et al.: GM-CSF and TNF-alpha cooperate in the generation of dendritic Langerhans cells. Nature **360**(6401), 258–261 (1992)
8. da Costa, C.E., Annels, N.E., et al.: Presence of osteoclast-like multinucleated giant cells in the bone and nonostotic lesions of Langerhans cell histiocytosis. J. Exp. Med. **201**(5), 687–693 (2005)
9. da Costa, C.E., Egeler, R.M., et al.: Differences in telomerase expression by the CD1a+ cells in Langerhans cell histiocytosis reflect the diverse clinical presentation of the disease. J. Pathol. **212**(2), 188–197 (2007)
10. Dehner, L.P.: Juvenile xanthogranulomas in the first two decades of life: a clinicopathologic study of 174 cases with cutaneous and extracutaneous manifestations. Am. J. Surg. Pathol. **27**(5), 579–593 (2003)
11. Egeler, R.M., Favara, B.E., et al.: Differential In situ cytokine pro- files of Langerhans-like cells and T cells in Langerhans cell histio- cytosis: abundant expression of cytokines relevant to disease and treatment. Blood **94**(12), 4195–4201 (1999)
12. Gaitonde, S.: Multifocal, extranodal sinus histiocytosis with mas- sive lymphadenopathy: an overview. Arch. Pathol. Lab. Med. **131**(7), 1117–1121 (2007)
13. Janssen, D., Folster-Holst, R., et al.: Clonality in juvenile xan- thogranuloma. Am. J. Surg. Pathol. **31**(5), 812–813 (2007)
14. Kolde, G., Brocker, E.B.: Multiple skin tumors of indeterminate cells in an adult. J. Am. Acad. Dermatol. **15**(4 Pt 1), 591–597 (1986)
15. Martin Flores-Stadler, E., Gonzalez-Crussi, F., et al.: Indeterminate- cell histiocytosis: immunophenotypic and cytogenetic findings in an infant. Med. Pediatr. Oncol. **32**(4), 250–254 (1999)
16. Murakami, I., Gogusev, J., et al.: Detection of molecular cytoge- netic aberrations in langerhans cell histiocytosis of bone. Hum. Pathol. **33**(5), 555–560 (2002)
17. Nunnink, J.C., Krusinski, P.A., et al.: Multicentric reticulohistiocy- tosis and cancer: a case report and review of the literature. Med. Pediatr. Oncol. **13**(5), 273–279 (1985)
18. Oliver, G.F., Umbert, I., et al.: Reticulohistiocytoma cutis–review of 15 cases and an association with systemic vasculitis in two cases. Clin. Exp. Dermatol. **15**(1), 1–6 (1990)
19. Ratzinger, G., Burgdorf, W.H., et al.: Indeterminate cell histiocyto- sis: fact or fiction? J. Cutan. Pathol. **32**(8), 552–560 (2005)
20. Vener, C., Soligo, D., et al.: Indeterminate cell histiocytosis in asso- ciation with later occurrence of acute myeloblastic leukaemia. Br. J. Dermatol. **156**(6), 1357–1361 (2007)
21. Weitzman, S., Egeler, R.M.: Langerhans cell histiocytosis: update for the pediatrician. Curr. Opin. Pediatr. **20**(1), 23–29 (2008)

Nagwa M. Elwan

The pathogenesis of Kaposi sarcoma is still confusing. Multifactorial theory has been implicated including mainly human immunodeficiency virus (HIV), herpes virus 8 (HHV-8), and abnormal cytokine profile associated with these viral infections.

2.5.1 HIV and Kaposi Sarcoma

In 1983, a retrovirus named HIV was cultured from T-cells of a homosexual man with lymphadenopathy [16], the majority of scientists believed at that time that HIV can stimulate mesenchymal tissue to undergo a metaplasia and form sarcoma. In, 1984, it became apparent that HIV was absent in the KS cells, and hence, it was unlikely to cause the lesions directly [24]. On the other hand, the HIV type-1 (HIV-1) *tat* gene was found to induce nodules resembling KS in 33 of 37 male transgenic mice, but in none of 15 females [26]. These findings suggested that HIV might directly cause KS (Fig. 2.5.1). Another important finding was a result of efforts to grow KS cells in culture, requiring a long-term growth factor. Media containing T-cells infected with human T-cell leukemia virus type II favored the growth and long-term culture of KS cell derived from KS-AIDS tissue, whereas that with T-cells infected with HIV-1 or human T-cell leukemia virus type I did not [26].

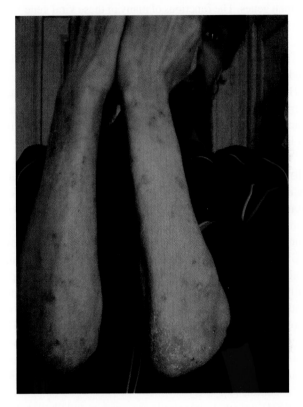

Fig. 2.5.1 Multiple disseminated erythematous plaques and nodules of AIDS-KS Egyptian patient

2.5.2 Cytokines and Kaposi Sarcoma

In 1992, the growth factor required for growth of KS cells in culture was proved to be a cytokine previously termed oncostatin M [20]. Another cytokine, scatter factor, was evident in large quantities in this medium, inducing endothelial cells to demonstrate a KS tumor cell-like phenotype [19]. The significance of oncostatin M and scatter factor has been shown in the pathogenesis of KS, often working synergistically with HIV (*tat*) gene product [23].

Other cytokines may work synergistically with HIV *tat* gene product, including interleukin 1 (IL-1), tumor necrosis factor, IL-6 and basic fibroblastic growth factor (bFGF) [7]. Therefore, KS seemed to be a cytokine-induced neoplasm. However, neither the HIV *tat* gene nor the cytokine interactions fully explained KS; a third and defining infections element was missing [23].

N.M. Elwan
Department of Medicine, Tanta University, Tanta-Egypt
e-mail: elwan2egy@yahoo.com

R. Dummer et al. (eds.), *Skin Cancer – A World-Wide Perspective*,
DOI: 10.1007/978-3-642-05072-5_2.5, © Springer-Verlag Berlin Heidelberg 2011

2.5.3 Herpes Virus and Kaposi Sarcoma

Herpes-type viruses have been associated with KS for more than 30 years [10]. A major landmark occurred in 1994 when Chang et al. showed short DNA sequences of a unique human herpes virus in KS tissues of a patient with AIDS [4]. This herpes virus, now termed HHV-8, appears to interact with the HIV *tat* protein, excess levels of basic fibroblast growth factor, scatter factor, and IL-6 [12]. The discovery of HHV-8 was followed by elucidation of its complete sequence denoting that the virus had co-opted a wide armamentarium of human genes. The functions of many of these viral gene variants in cell growth control, signaling apoptosis, angiogenesis, and immunomodulation have been characterized [21], perhaps explaining the long latent period between infection and KS [3]. The immune evasion strategies employed by HHV-8 in targeting tumor suppressor pathways, activated during immune system signaling may produce counterproductive cell proliferation and tumorigenesis in susceptible individuals [14].

Kaposi sarcoma herpes virus (KSHV) DNA is present in all KS tumors, irrespective of clinical type. Viral infection selectively targets spindle cells [11], with little or no infection of other cell types [2]. Like all herpes viruses, KSHV can adopt either of two replicative programs, which are known as latency and lytic replication. In most de novo KSHV infections of cultured cells, latency is the default pathway. In contrast, lytic replication involves the temporally regulated expression of virtually the entire viral genome, with viral DNA replication and production of infectious progeny, in the course of which the host cell dies [25]. The high prevalence of latent infection in the spindle-cell compartment and its escalating density as KS progresses, clearly point to an important role for latent gene expression in KS pathogenesis [9].

KSHV-infected tumor cells can express endothelial (EC) marker and viral genes like V-cyclin, which is a homolog of cellular D-type cyclins. V-cyclin induces replicative stress in ECs, which leads to activation of the DNA damage response. It was found that antiproliferative checkpoints are activated upon KSHV infection of ECs, and in early-stage but not late-stage lesions of clinical Kaposi sarcoma. This suggested that DNA damage checkpoint response also functions as an anticancer barrier in virally induced cancers [13].

2.5.4 Is Kaposi Sarcoma a True Neoplasm or a Reactive Hyperplasia? [18, 21]

It remains unclear whether KS is a true neoplasm, a reactive proliferation or both. Early KS seems to be a reactive process which might remain so, or progress to become a true sarcoma

[5, 8]. HHV-8 is the most frequent cause of malignancy in patients with AIDS, producing not only KS but, less commonly, others as non-Hogkin's lymphoma [6, 17]. Viral oncogene induced DNA damage response is activated in KS tumorigenesis[13]. Also, the role of HHV-8 oncogene kaposin and lytic reaction of HHV-8 are points of interest in KS pathogenesis [8, 21]. It was observed in vitro that human herpes virus 6 (HHV-6) may have a role in KS pathogenesis by promoting HHV-8 replication and increasing HHV-8 viral load [15].

On the other hand, some reports suggested that KS cell biology affirms that KS is not a typical cancer. Classically, one criterion for malignant transformation in cell culture is the reduced dependence upon exogenous growth factors; however, cultured KS spindle cells, unlike classical tumor cells, remain highly dependent upon exogenous growth factors [9]. Ensoli and colleagues were the first to grow KS spindle cells in culture and found them to be strongly dependent upon a cytokine-rich medium derived from supernatants of activated T-cell cultures [8].

Another hallmark of traditional cancers is displaying genetic instability. KS spindle cells are generally diploid and no characteristic chromosomal rearrangements are shared by multiple tumors. Classical KS lesions do not display microsatellite instability, although some advanced AIDS-KS do [1]. Cultured KS spindle cells also lack other markers of transformation; they do not form foci, nor grow in soft agar, nor form tumors in nude mice [22]. Although they do not generate a tumor, they do survive for a brief interval, during which slit-like new vessels of murine origin appear in the surrounding tissue. This suggests a KS model in which spindle cells require growth factors from their microenvironment for their survival and proliferation, but also produce angiogenic and proinflammatory substances to develop the other components of the lesions [9].

Most clinical and experimental observations about KS suggest that the differences between this disorder and classical cancers are at least as numerous as their similarities. Perhaps, the viral contributions to KS pathogenesis may be more variegated than those of other tumor viruses to more traditional cancers [9]. Nonetheless, whether KS is a hyperplasia or a true neoplasm is a question that is not fully answered up until now.

References

1. Bedi, G.C., Westra, W.H., Farzadegan, H., et al.: Microsatellite instability in primary neoplasms from HIV + patients. Nat. Med. **1**, 65–68 (1995)
2. Blasig, C., Zietz, C., Haar, B., et al.: Monocytes in Kaposi's sarcoma lesions are productively infected by human herpesvirus 8. J. Virol. **71**, 7963–7968 (1997)

3. Cerimele, D., Cottoni, F., Masala, M.V.: Long latency of human herpesvirus type 8 infection and the appearance of classic Kaposi's sarcoma. J. Am. Acad. Dermatol. **43**, 731–732 (2000)

4. Chang, Y., Cesarman, E., Pessin, M.S., Lee, F., et al.: Identification of herpesvirus-like DNA sequences in AIDS-associated Kaposi's sarcoma. Science **266**, 1865–1869 (1994)

5. Duprez, R., Lacoste, V., Brière, J., et al.: Evidence for a multiclonal origin of multicentric advanced lesions of Kaposi sarcoma. J. Natl. Cancer Inst. **99**, 1086–1094 (2007)

6. Engels, E.A., Rosenberg, P.S., Frisch, M., et al.: Cancers associated with Kaposi's sarcoma (KS) in AIDS: a link between KS herpesvirus and immunoblastic lymphoma. Br. J. Cancer **85**, 1298–1303 (2001)

7. Ensoli, B., Gendelman, R., Markham, P., et al.: Synergy between basic fibroblast growth factor and HIV-1 Tat protein in induction of Kaposi's sarcoma. Nature **371**, 674–680 (1994)

8. Ensoli, B., Sgadari, C., Barillari, G., et al.: Biology of Kaposi's sarcoma. Eur. J. Cancer **37**, 1251–1269 (2001)

9. Ganem, D.: KSHV infection and the pathogenesis of Kaposi's sarcoma. Annu. Rev. Pathol. **1**, 273–296 (2006)

10. Giraldo, G., Beth, E., Haguenau, F.: Herpes-type virus particles in tissue culture of Kaposi's sarcoma from different geographic regions. J. Natl. Cancer Inst. **49**, 1509–1526 (1972)

11. Herndier, B., Ganem, D.: The biology of Kaposi's sarcoma. Cancer Treat. Res. **104**, 89–126 (2001)

12. Huang, L.M., Chao, M.F., Chen, M.Y., Hm, S., et al.: Reciprocal regulatory interaction between human herpesvirus 8 and human immunodeficiency virus type 1. J. Biol. Chem. **276**, 13427–13432 (2001)

13. Koopal, S., Furuhjelm, J.H., Järviluoma, A., et al.: Viral oncogene-induced DNA damage response is activated in Kaposi sarcoma tumorigenesis. PLoS Pathog. **3**, 1348–1360 (2007)

14. Lee, B.S., Alvarez, X., Ishido, S., et al.: Inhibition of intracellular transport of B cell antigen receptor complexes by Kaposi's sarcoma-associated herpesvirus K1. J. Exp. Med. **192**, 11–21 (2000)

15. Lu, C., Zeng, Y., Huang, Z., et al.: Human herpesvirus 6 activates lytic cycle replication of Kaposi's sarcoma-associated herpesvirus. Am. J. Pathol. **166**, 173–183 (2005)

16. Montagnier, L., Barré-Sinoussi, F., Chermann, J.C., et al.: Isolation of a T-lymphotropic retrovirus from a patient at risk for (AIDS). Science **220**, 868–871 (1983)

17. Moore, P.S., Chang, Y.: Kaposi's sarcoma-associated herpesvirus immunoevasion and tumorigenesis: two sides of the same coin? Annu. Rev. Microbiol. **57**, 609–639 (2003)

18. Muralidhar, S., Pumfery, A.M., Hassani, M., et al.: Identification of kaposin (open reading frame K12) as a human herpesvirus 8 (Kaposi's sarcoma-associated herpesvirus) transforming gene. J. Virol. **72**, 4980–4988 (1998)

19. Naidu, Y.M., Rosen, E.M., Zitnick, R., et al.: Role of scatter factor in the pathogenesis of AIDS-related Kaposi sarcoma. Proc. Natl. Acad. Sci. U. S. A. **91**, 5281–5285 (1994)

20. Nair, B.C., DeVico, A.L., Nakamura, S., et al.: Identification of a major growth factor for AIDS-Kaposi's sarcoma cells as oncostatin M. Science **255**, 1430–1432 (1992)

21. Palmeri, D., Spadavecchia, S., Carroll, K.D., et al.: Promoter- and cell-specific transcriptional transactivation by the Kaposi's sarcoma-associated herpesvirus ORF57/Mta protein. J. Virol. **81**, 13299–13314 (2007)

22. Salahuddin, S.Z., Nakamura, S., Biberfeld, P., et al.: Angiogenic properties of Kaposi's sarcoma-derived cells after long-term culture in vitro. Science **242**, 430–433 (1988)

23. Schwartz, R.A., Micali, G., Nasca, M.R., et al.: Kaposi sarcoma: a continuing conundrum. J. Am. Acad. Dermatol. **59**, 179–206 (2008)

24. Shaw, G.M., Hahn, B.H., Arya, S.K., et al.: Molecular characterization of human T-cell leukemia (lymphotropic) virus type III in the acquired immune deficiency syndrome. Science **226**, 1165–1171 (1984)

25. Sun, R., Lin, S.F., Gradoville, L., et al.: A viral gene that activates lytic cycle expression of Kaposi's sarcoma-associated herpesvirus. Proc. Natl. Acad. Sci. U. S. A. **95**, 10866–10871 (1998)

26. Vogel, J., Hinrichs, S.H., Reynolds, R.K., et al.: The HIV tat gene induces dermal lesions resembling Kaposi's sarcoma in transgenic mice. Nature **335**, 606–611 (1988)

Pathogenesis of Dermatofibrosarcoma Protuberans

2.6

Selma Ugurel and Lauren Lockwood

Nongenetic risk factors for DFSP remain unknown; there are also no details on genetic influences in terms of prevalence within families. New molecular research evidences frequent presentation of *chromosomal translocations* in DFSP tumor cells, finding a translocation between chromosomes 17 and 22 in over 90% of cases (17q22; 22q13) [4]. This translocation occurs mostly through fusion of collagen encoding gene *(COL1A1) to cell-mediated growth factor platelet-derived growth factor beta* (PDGFβ) *encoding gene,* frequently, though not always, forming a ring chromosome [1, 3]. The gene product of this fusion, a COL1A1-PDGFβ-Fusionsprotein, acts on a DFSP-cell binding site constitutively expressing PDGF-receptor as a continuous autocrine, developmental stimulus for the tumor cells [2] (see Fig. 2.6.1). The acknowledgment of these *solitary, autocrine stimulation pathways* will allow for the development of a favorable, etiopathogenetically based, molecularly directed therapy for DFSP.

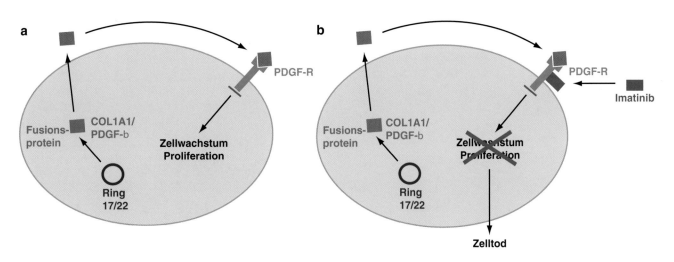

Fig. 2.6.1 Schematic view of the autocrine developmental stimulation of the PDGFβ signaling pathway in dermatofibrosarcoma cells (**a**), and its interruption with tyrosinkinase-inhibitor Imatinib (**b**)

S. Ugurel (✉)
Klinik und Poliklinik für Dermatologie,
Venerologie und Allergologie der Universität, Würzburg,
Germany
e-mail: ugurel_s@klinik.uni-wuerzburg.de

L. Lockwood
Department of Dermatology, University Hospital of Zürich,
Zürich, Switzerland

R. Dummer et al. (eds.), *Skin Cancer – A World-Wide Perspective,*
DOI: 10.1007/978-3-642-05072-5_2.6, © Springer-Verlag Berlin Heidelberg 2011

References

1. O'Brien, K.P., Seroussi, F., et al.: Various regions within the alpha-helical domain of the COL1A1 gene are fused to the second exon of the PDGFB gene in dermatofibrosarcomas and giant-cell fibroblastomas. Genes Chromosomes Cancer **23**, 187–193 (1998)
2. Shimizu, A., O'Brien, K.P., et al.: The dermatofibrosarcoma protuberans-associated collagen type Ialpha1/platelet-derived growth factor (PDGF) B-chain fusion gene generates a transforming protein that is processed to functional PDGF-BB. Cancer Res. **59**, 3719–3723 (1999)
3. Simon, M.P., Pedeutour, F., et al.: Deregulation of the platelet-derived growth factor B-chain gene via fusion with collagen gene COL1A1 in dermatofibrosarcoma protuberans and giant-cell fibroblastoma. Nat. Genet. **15**, 95–98 (1997)
4. Sirvent, N., Maire, G., et al.: Genetics of dermatofibrosarcoma protuberans family of tumors: from ring chromosomes to tyrosine kinase inhibitor treatment. Genes Chromosomes Cancer **37**, 1–19 (2003)

Pathogenesis of Merkel Cell Carcinoma

2.7

Jürgen C. Becker and Roland Houben

Despite a substantial research effort, the understanding of the molecular basis of MCC is still limited. Overexpression of the anti-apoptotic molecule bcl-2 was observed in three-fourths of MCC tumors in two independent studies [10, 21]. Inhibition of bcl-2 expression in vivo by antisense oligonucleotides in a SCID mouse/human tumor xenograft model resulted in tumor shrinkage [31]. The expression of this anti-apoptosis protein is a common finding in many cancers and suggests one of its mechanisms to avoid cell death; however, the same antisense oligonucleotides when tested in a phase II trial, demonstrated only a very limited, if any, efficacy in patients with MCC [32]. Moreover, bcl-2 overexpression does not illuminate the promitotic pathways that drive MCC.

Secreted Wingless type (Wnt) ligands have been shown to activate signal transduction pathways and trigger changes in gene expression, cell behavior, adhesion, and polarity [8]. The role of Wnt signaling in cancer was first suggested 20 years ago with the discovery of Wnt-1 as an integration site for mouse mammary tumor virus in mouse mammary carcinoma. Over time, a wealth of evidence has implicated Wnt signaling in tumor development and progression. The Wnt pathway and its role in MCC have been evaluated by determination of nuclear accumulation of β-catenin and mutations in β-catenin and three other related genes. Liu et al. observed elevated β-catenin accumulation in only one out of 12 tumors and no mutations in any tumors; thus, they concluded that the Wnt pathway is not implicated in MCC [25].

The classical mitogen-activated protein (MAP) kinase signaling pathway plays a key role in many processes such as proliferation, suppression of apoptosis, migration, and differentiation [42]. The relevance of the Raf/MEK/ERK cascade for tumorigenesis has been evident for a long time, but was underlined in 2002 with the discovery that B-Raf, one of the three isoforms of Raf, is present in a mutated form in many tumor entities, particularly melanoma [9]. Thus, MAP kinase signaling, a common feature of many epithelial cancers, is the most studied oncogenic pathway in MCC. The impact of dysregulated c-Kit as oncogenic tyrosine kinase for autocrine stimulation MAP kinase signaling in MCC has been addressed in several studies which have detected c-Kit expression in tumor samples [4, 11, 26, 35]. Recently, Swick et al. determined that although eight of nine MCC tumors were positive for c-Kit by immunohistochemical staining, no activating mutations were present in the four exons commonly found to have mutations in this gene [36]. Similarly, the analysis of MCC samples for the presence of activating B-Raf mutation did not reveal any of these [16, 43]. Moreover, immunohistochemical studies revealed that despite high proliferation indices and existing expression of ERK, the ERK protein generally occurs in the non-phosphorylated form and is thus inactive [16]. The lack of ERK phosphorylation was always accompanied by a strong expression of the Raf kinase inhibitor protein (RKIP), a negative regulator of the MAPK cascade that binds to Raf and MEK and thus inhibits their interaction. These observations suggested that RKIP is responsible for turning off this signaling pathway. That this is not the case was demonstrated in experiments where silencing of RKIP did not lead to an induction of ERK phosphorylation [17].

The general inactivity of the "mitogenic" cascade distinguishes MCC from many other tumors such as melanoma and raises the question if active MAP kinase signaling is perhaps even a negative selection factor for MCC cells. To test this notion, we developed UISO cells that express a Raf construct in which the natural regulatory domain is replaced by an artificial hydroxy tamoxifen (OHT)-sensitive regulatory domain (Raf-ER) derived from the estrogen receptor [18]. OHT stimulation results in MEK and ERK activation in these cells. This activation of the MAPK pathway leads to a collapse of the cytoskeleton and subsequent death of the MCC cells. The induced cell death was by apoptosis and this OHT-induced apoptosis could be prevented by specific MEK inhibition indicating that apoptosis is indeed an effect mediated by the MAPK cascade.

The inactivity of the MAP kinase pathway together with the report that inhibition of Ras farnesylation by apoptosis

J.C. Becker (✉) and R. Houben
Department of General Dermatology, Medical University of Graz,
Auenbruggerplatz 8, A-8010 Graz, Austria
e-mail: juergen.becker@medunigraz.at

induction suppresses the growth of MCC xenografts in the naked mouse model suggest that another Ras-dependent signaling pathway may be of special relevance in MCC [19]. The most important Ras-regulating signal pathway next to the Raf/MEK/ERK cascade involves class 1 phosphoinositide 3 kinase (PI3K) and the Akt kinase [22]. PI3K phosphorylates phosphatidylinositol 4,5-biphphosphate (PIP2) to phosphatidylinositol 3,4,5-triphosphate (PIP3), an important second messenger lipid.

The antagonist of PI3K that dephosphorylates PIP3 is the phosphate and tensin homologue deleted in chromosome 10 (PTEN) that is frequently inactivated in human tumors. Accumulation of PIP3 after PI3K activation leads to a translocation of Akt to the plasma membrane where it is phosphorylated by two PIP3-dependent kinases and thus activated. Akt develops its anti-apoptotic and cell-cycle-regulating effects via a series of target molecules (over 30 have already been described) such as, e.g., the pro-apoptotic protein Bad, pro-caspase 9, forkhead transcription factors, or the mammalian target of rapamycin (mTOR) [30]. Surprisingly mTOR functions, on the one hand, in a rapamycin-sensitive complex with raptor as an effector of Akt; on the other hand, it belongs in a rapamycin-insensitive complex with rictor to the Akt-activating kinases. Interestingly, an Akt/mTOR-regulated suppression of p53 protein expression that functions via induction of the translation of the p53-specific ubiquitin ligase mdm2 has been described. Furthermore, Akt can directly activate mdm2 and thus induce p53 protein degradation [22]. As the apoptosis induced by Ras inhibition in the MCC xenografts is accompanied by p53 induction, an involvement of the PI3K/Akt signal pathway in this process as well as in the molecular pathogenesis appears very likely [19].

The frequent heterozygous loss of chromosome 10 or the long arm of chromosome10 in MCC suggests that the tumor-suppressor PTEN encoded there plays a relevant role [41]. However, only rarely has loss of heterozygosity (LOH) been accompanied by inactivation of the second allele by mutation or deletion, which leads the authors to conclude that additional tumor suppressors located on 10q might be "targets" of the loss [40]. On the other hand, a recent study using MCC tissue arrays to measure the expression of various proteins (especially matrix metalloproteinases) revealed that PTEN could hardly be identified in the samples examined, which could indicate inactivation of the second allele, e.g., by epigenetic mechanisms [13].

The epigenetic silencing of another tumor-suppressor gene in MCC had been recently reported [23]. Lassacher et al. observed that promoter hypermethylation of the INK4a-ARF locus is common in MCC. Their analysis revealed the presence of methylated DNA at the p14ARF promoter in 8 of 19 MCC samples; in contrast, the p16INK4a promoter was only methylated in one case. This observation sheds important light on the pathogenesis of MCC because DNA methylation in promoter regions helps to regulate the gene expression. In particular, hypermethylation of CpG islands located in the promoter regions of tumor-suppressor genes such as p16INK4a, BRCA1, and hMLH is now established as an important mechanism of gene inactivation in cancer [3]. The INK4a-ARF locus encodes the two protein products (p16INK4a and p14ARF) whose respective mRNAs are generated from separate promoters. p16INK4a and p14ARF are integral parts of the two cell-cycle control pathways targeted most frequently during tumorigenesis, i.e., the pRB and p53 pathway [15]. In the case of MCC, alterations in the p53 pathway appear to be most crucial, as suggested by the high frequency of p14ARF promoter methylation and low frequency of p16INK4a promoter methylation.

A multitude of functions have been described for the tumor-suppressor p53. Most importantly, as a transcription factor following DNA damage p53 regulates the expression of genes involved in the control of the cell cycle, the induction of apoptosis or senescence, and DNA repair [15]. The anti-proliferative activity of p53 plays a significant role in the avoidance of tumor development, but also requires effective mechanisms to control p53 in normal proliferating cells. Probably the most important mechanism involves the control of protein stability with ubiquitination by the p53-specific ubiquitin ligase mdm2 and subsequent proteasomal degradation playing a central role. Oncogenic stress results in the induction of the tumor-suppressor protein p14ARF. P14 binds to mdm2, inactivates it, and thus prevents degradation of p53 [34].

p53 is the protein that is most frequently present in a mutated form in tumors. It is found altered in about 50% of human tumors, and in tumors with wild-type p53, its activation is often disturbed. p53 mutations are occasionally found in MCC. In 3 of 15 tumors examined and in 2 of 6 MCC cell lines p53 mutations were present [29, 39]. On the other hand, the previously mentioned apoptosis induction associated with p53 depression in MCC xenografts suggests that the regulation of p53 expression or stability may be disturbed in MCC [19]. For another member of the p53 family, p63, it has been shown that its expression in tumor cells correlates to an exceptionally high degree with the aggressiveness of the disease [1]. p63 is a transcription factor essential for proliferation of stem cells and for stratification in epithelia, mutated in human hereditary syndromes characterized by ectodermal dysplasia.

The proteins whose expression is induced by p53 include p21. Together with p27 and the proteins of the Ink4 family p21 belongs to the inhibitors of the cyclin-dependent kinas (CDK). These CDK inhibitors, expressed upon various extra- and intracellular stimuli, can prevent the transition from the G1 to the Sphase of the cell cycle [28]. By binding to cyclin/CDK complexes these are inactivated and the phosphorylation of Rb1 (product of the retinoblastoma susceptibility gene) does not take place. Rb1 is a key molecule in gene expression promoting the G1/S transition. In its hypo-phosphorylated state this tumor-suppressor protein prevents entry into the Sphase by forming an inhibiting complex with transcription factors of the E2Ffamily and by mediating the binding of DNA-modifying enzymes [7]. After multiple phosphorylations of Rb1 by cyclinD/CDK4/6 and cyclinE/CDK2 complexes, Rb1 is released and degraded, the inhibition of E2F is suspended and the transcription of genes for the G1/S transition is initiated. The RB//E2F signaling pathway is of such central significance for the control of cell proliferation that it is assumed that its regulation is disturbed in practically all tumors. Gene loss or inactivating mutations of Rb1, viral Rb1-incativating oncoproteins (e.g., human papilloma virus E7), overexpression and activating mutations of CDK4/6, amplification and overexpression of CDK2, amplification or translocation of cyclinD genes, as well as inactivating mutations and loss of expression of p16Ink4a and p15Ink4b have been described. For MCC little data on the regulation of the cell cycle by Rb1 exists and studies on a possible loss of Rb1 are contradictory. Leonard and Hayard found LOH for the marker D13S233 (13q14.3), which is located close to the Rb1 gene, in 18 of 24 examined MCC samples [24]. Further, in all 9 MCC cell lines they analyzed, no Rb1 could be detected in the Western blot. In contrast, Popp et al. reported no loss of the 13q region in 10 MCCs analyzed by comparative genome hybridization [29].

The role of UV light in the development of MCC is rather immunosuppressive than mutagenic. Pathogenetically, in addition to disturbed antigen presentation, the induction of immunosuppressive cytokines such as IL-10 and TNF-α, the isomerization of *trans*-urocanic acid to *cis*-urocanic acid and the formation of reactive oxygen species are blamed [37, 38]. This notion goes in parallel with the striking epidemiologic association between immunosuppression and MCC [5]. The observation that MCC occurs more frequently than expected among immunosuppressed transplant and AIDS patients is very similar to Kaposi's sarcoma. This similarity to Kaposi's sarcoma, an immune-related tumor caused by Kaposi's sarcoma-associated herpes virus, raised the possibility that MCC may also have an infectious origin. Indeed, Feng and coworkers recently were able to provide evidence for a possible viral oncogenesis [12]. They studied MCC samples using digital transcriptome subtraction, a method with which the same working group has already identified Kaposi sarcoma-associated herpes virus type 8. These studies resulted in the discovery of a genome encompassing 5,387 base pairs of a new polyomavirus, the Merkel cell polyomavirus (MCPyV).

Since the discovery of the mouse polyomavirus by Gross in 1953, polyomaviruses have been suspected as possible causes of cancer in humans [33, 44]. Even though polyomaviruses can induce tumors in animal models, there has not yet been any definitive proof that they play a relevant role in human carcinogenesis. These small (40–50 nm in diameter) double-stranded DNA viruses code for several proteins, among them large T(umor) antigen, in their circular genome. Polyomaviruses express genes in two waves: early and late. The early-expressed genes, including large and small T antigens, bind to host proteins to force the cell into S phase (the cell-cycle phase when the DNA is replicated) and facilitate viral replication [6, 27]. The late genes encode components of the viral coat and enable lysis.

The large T antigen regulates the life cycle of the virus as well as the cell cycle of the host cell. The last occurs via interaction with the tumor-suppressor gene p53 and the members of the Rb gene family (Fig. 2.7.1). This viral stimulation of the cell cycle is the main driving force of the oncogenic potential of polyomaviruses [6, 27]. Importantly, the predicted MCPyV large T antigen contains many of the features common to oncogenic polyomaviruses, including an LxCxE motif that may directly bind pRb [12].

Polyomaviruses often induce latent infections without manifest disease, but can, for example, in an immunosuppressed host, induce tumors. In animal models tumor development is usually preceded by the integration of the polyomavirus DNA into the host genome [44]. In this respect, it is important to note that when screening ten MCC tumors for MCPyV, it is found that seven were strongly positive for MCPyV DNA by PCR and an additional tumor was weakly positive. The strength of the PCR signals suggested that the viral DNA was integrated in a clonal fashion (Fig. 2.7.2). To test this notion genomic DNA from MCC tumors was digested with two restriction enzymes and analyzed by Southern hybridization using an MCPyV DNA probe. The resulting banding pattern in five of the eight MCPyV-positive MCC tumors indicated a monoclonal integration of the virus; in one tumor a monoclonally integrated viral concatemer and the remaining two other tumors an indeterminate integration pattern were observed [12]. Moreover, for one tumor with a monoclonal integration pattern, both primary and metastatic tumor tissue was available, and both specimens showed an identical viral integration pattern, demonstrating that integration of MCPyV preceded metastasis formation. Furthermore, the distinct integration patterns between tumors imply that the virus integrated at different locations within the human genome in the different tumors.

The presence of MCPyV in the majority of MCC samples as been confirmed by three independent groups [2, 14, 20]. Interestingly, our own data suggest a poorer prognosis for MCC patients with the identification of MCV in tumor tissue. In all published MCPyV genome sequences premature stop codons are predicted within the second exon of the large T antigen. The predicted truncated proteins potentially preserve some of the cell-cycle progression activities of the

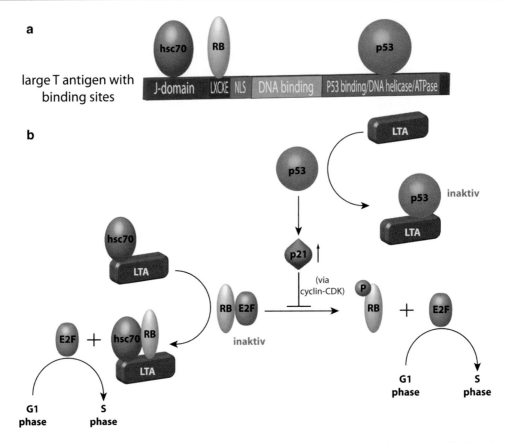

Fig. 2.7.1 Binding sites of the large T antigen for the tumor-suppressor gene *p53* and the members of the Rb gene family (**a**) and its impact on these pathways (**b**)

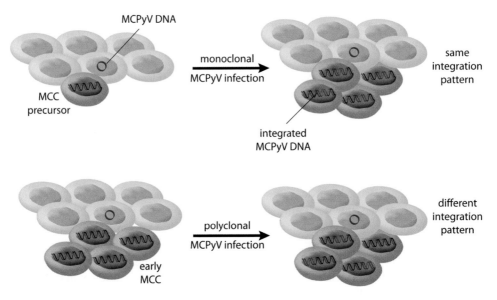

Fig. 2.7.2 Monoclonal vs. polyclonal MCPyV infection

amino terminus of large T but prevent cell-lethal genomic instability related to the replicative functions of the carboxyl terminus [6, 27]. If the large T antigen were intact, replication initiated at an integrated origin would lead to genomic instability and cell death. Indeed, in permissive cells transformed by SV40, the large T antigen is often mutated such that the viral replication functions are inactive but cell-cycle progression functions are preserved.

The presence of MCPyV DNA in Merkel tumors does not prove a causal involvement of this virus in Merkel carcinomas. The clonal pattern of integration in tumor tissue as well as in its metastasis, however, could favor this interpretation. The preferential occurrence of this cancer in immunosuppressed patients might also support a viral etiology. Merkel cell carcinoma seems to represent the first human malignancy with a relatively consistent presence of integrated sequences of a specific type of polyomavirus.

References

1. Asioli, S., Righi, A., Volante, M., Eusebi, V., Bussolati, G.: p63 expression as a new prognostic marker in Merkel cell carcinoma. Cancer 110, 640–647 (2007)
2. Becker, J.C., Houben, R., Ugurel, S., Trefzer, U., Pfohler, C., Schrama, D.: MC polyomavirus is frequently present in merkel cell carcinoma of European patients. J. Invest. Dermatol. 129, 248–250 (2009)
3. Becker, J.C., Ugurel, S., Brocker, E.B., Schrama, D., Houben, R.: New therapeutic approaches for solid tumors: histone deacetylase, methyltransferase and proteasome inhibitors. J. Dtsch. Dermatol. Ges. 4, 108–113 (2006)
4. Brunner, M., Thurnher, D., Pammer, J., Geleff, S., Heiduschka, G., Reinisch, C.M., Petzelbauer, P., Erovic, B.M.: Expression of VEGF-A/C, VEGF-R2, PDGF-alpha/beta, c-kit, EGFR, Her-2/Neu, Mcl-1 and Bmi-1 in Merkel cell carcinoma. Mod. Pathol. 21, 876–884 (2008)
5. Buell, J.F., Trofe, J., Hanaway, M.J., Beebe, T.M., Gross, T.G., Alloway, R.R., First, M.R., Woodle, E.S.: Immunosuppression and Merkel cell cancer. Transplant. Proc. 34, 1780–1781 (2002)
6. Caracciolo, V., Reiss, K., Khalili, K., De Falco, G., Giordano, A.: Role of the interaction between large T antigen and Rb family members in the oncogenicity of JC virus. Oncogene 25, 5294–5301 (2006)
7. Chau, B.N., Wang, J.Y.: Coordinated regulation of life and death by RB. Nat. Rev. Cancer 3, 130–138 (2003)
8. Chen, X., Yang, J., Evans, P.M., Liu, C.: Wnt signaling: the good and the bad. Acta Biochim. Biophys. Sin. (Shanghai) 40, 577–594 (2008)
9. Davies, H., Bignell, G.R., Cox, C., Stephens, P., Edkins, S., Clegg, S., Teague, J., Woffendin, H., Garnett, M.J., Bottomley, W., Davis, N., Dicks, E., Ewing, R., Floyd, Y., Gray, K., Hall, S., Hawes, R., Hughes, J., Kosmidou, V., Menzies, A., Mould, C., Parker, A., Stevens, C., Watt, S., Hooper, S., Wilson, R., Jayatilake, H., Gusterson, B.A., Cooper, C., Shipley, J., Hargrave, D., Pritchard-Jones, K., Maitland, N., Chenevix-Trench, G., Riggins, G.J., Bigner, D.D., Palmieri, G., Cossu, A., Flanagan, A., Nicholson, A., Ho, J.W., Leung, S.Y., Yuen, S.T., Weber, B.L., Seigler, H.F., Darrow, T.L., Paterson, H., Marais, R., Marshall, C.J., Wooster, R., Stratton, M.R., Futreal, P.A.: Mutations of the BRAF gene in human cancer. Nature 417, 949–954 (2002)
10. Feinmesser, M., Halpern, M., Fenig, E., Tsabari, C., Hodak, E., Sulkes, J., Brenner, B., Okon, E.: Expression of the apoptosis-related oncogenes bcl-2, bax, and p53 in Merkel cell carcinoma: can they predict treatment response and clinical outcome? Hum. Pathol. 30, 1367–1372 (1999)
11. Feinmesser, M., Halpern, M., Kaganovsky, E., Brenner, B., Fenig, E., Hodak, E., Sulkes, J., Okon, E.: c-kit Expression in primary and metastatic merkel cell carcinoma. Am. J. Dermatopathol. 26, 458–462 (2004)
12. Feng, H., Shuda, M., Chang, Y., Moore, P.S.: Clonal integration of a polyomavirus in human Merkel cell carcinoma. Science 319, 1096–1100 (2008)
13. Fernandez-Figueras, M.T., Puig, L., Musulen, E., Gilaberte, M., Lerma, E., Serrano, S., Ferrandiz, C., Ariza, A.: Expression profiles associated with aggressive behavior in Merkel cell carcinoma. Mod. Pathol. 20, 90–101 (2007)
14. Garneski, K.M., Warcola, A.H., Feng, Q., Kiviat, N.B., Leonard, J.H., Nghiem, P.: Merkel cell polyomavirus is more frequently present in North American than Australian Merkel cell carcinoma tumors. J. Invest. Dermatol. 129, 246–248 (2009)
15. Horn, H.F., Vousden, K.H.: Coping with stress: multiple ways to activate p53. Oncogene 26, 1306–1316 (2007)
16. Houben, R., Michel, B., Vetter-Kauczok, C.S., Pfohler, C., Laetsch, B., Wolter, M.D., Leonard, J.H., Trefzer, U., Ugurel, S., Schrama, D., Becker, J.C.: Absence of classical MAP kinase pathway signalling in Merkel cell carcinoma. J. Invest. Dermatol. 126, 1135–1142 (2006)
17. Houben, R., Ortmann, S., Becker, J.C.: RKIP does not contribute to MAP kinase pathway silencing in the Merkel Cell Carcinoma cell line UISO. J. Carcinog. 6, 16 (2007)
18. Houben, R., Ortmann, S., Schrama, D., Herold, M.J., Berberich, I., Reichardt, H.M., Becker, J.C.: Activation of the MAP kinase pathway induces apoptosis in the Merkel cell carcinoma cell line UISO. J. Invest. Dermatol. 127, 2116–2122 (2007)
19. Jansen, B., Heere-Ress, E., Schlagbauer-Wadl, H., Halaschek-Wiener, J., Waltering, S., Moll, I., Pehamberger, H., Marciano, D., Kloog, Y., Wolff, K.: Farnesylthiosalicylic acid inhibits the growth of human Merkel cell carcinoma in SCID mice. J. Mol. Med. 77, 792–797 (1999)
20. Kassem, A., Schopflin, A., Diaz, C., Weyers, W., Stickeler, E., Werner, M., Zur, H.A.: Frequent detection of Merkel cell polyomavirus in human Merkel cell carcinomas and identification of a unique deletion in the VP1 gene. Cancer Res. 68, 5009–5013 (2008)
21. Kennedy, M.M., Blessing, K., King, G., Kerr, K.M.: Expression of bcl-2 and p53 in Merkel cell carcinoma. An immunohistochemical study. Am. J. Dermatopathol. 18, 273–277 (1996)
22. Kim, D., Chung, J.: Akt: versatile mediator of cell survival and beyond. J. Biochem. Mol. Biol. 35, 106–115 (2002)
23. Lassacher, A., Heitzer, E., Kerl, H., Wolf, P.: p14ARF hypermethylation is common but INK4a-ARF locus or p53 mutations are rare in Merkel cell carcinoma. J. Invest. Dermatol. 128, 1788–1796 (2008)
24. Leonard, J.H., Hayard, N.: Loss of heterozygosity of chromosome 13 in Merkel cell carcinoma. Genes Chromosomes Cancer 20, 93–97 (1997)
25. Liu, S., Daa, T., Kashima, K., Kondoh, Y., Yokoyama, S.: The Wnt-signaling pathway is not implicated in tumorigenesis of Merkel cell carcinoma. J. Cutan. Pathol. 34, 22–26 (2007)
26. Llombart, B., Monteagudo, C., Lopez-Guerrero, J.A., Carda, C., Jorda, E., Sanmartin, O., Almenar, S., Molina, I., Martin, J.M., Llombart-Bosch, A.: Clinicopathological and immunohistochemical analysis of 20 cases of Merkel cell carcinoma in search of prognostic markers. Histopathology 46, 622–634 (2005)
27. Moens, U., Van Ghelue, M., Johannessen, M.: Oncogenic potentials of the human polyomavirus regulatory proteins. Cell Mol. Life Sci. 64, 1656–1678 (2007)
28. Ortega, S., Malumbres, M., Barbacid, M.: Cyclin D-dependent kinases, INK4 inhibitors and cancer. Biochim. Biophys. Acta 1602, 73–87 (2002)
29. Popp, S., Waltering, S., Herbst, C., Moll, I., Boukamp, P.: UV-B-type mutations and chromosomal imbalances indicate common pathways for the development of Merkel and skin squamous cell carcinomas. Int. J. Cancer 99, 352–360 (2002)
30. Sarbassov, D.D., Guertin, D.A., Ali, S.M., Sabatini, D.M.: Phosphorylation and regulation of Akt/PKB by the rictor-mTOR complex. Science 307, 1098–1101 (2005)
31. Schlagbauer-Wadl, H., Klosner, G., Heere-Ress, E., Waltering, S., Moll, I., Wolff, K., Pehamberger, H., Jansen, B.: Bcl-2 antisense oligonucleotides (G3139) inhibit Merkel cell carcinoma growth in SCID mice. J. Invest. Dermatol. 114, 725–730 (2000)

32. Shah, M.H., Varker, K.A., Collamore, M., Zwiebel J.A., Chung, K.Y., Coit, D., Kelsen, D.: Multicenter phase II trial of bcl-2 anti-sense therapy (Genasense®) in patients with advanced Merkel cell carcinoma. AACR (poster presentation) (2007)

33. Shah, K.V.: SV40 and human cancer: a review of recent data. Int. J. Cancer **120**, 215–223 (2007)

34. Sherr, C.J.: Divorcing ARF and p53: an unsettled case. Nat. Rev. Cancer **6**, 663–673 (2006)

35. Strong, S., Shalders, K., Carr, R., Snead, D.R.: KIT receptor (CD117) expression in Merkel cell carcinoma. Br. J. Dermatol. **150**, 384–385 (2004)

36. Swick, B.L., Ravdel, L., Fitzpatrick, J.E., Robinson, W.A.: Merkel cell carcinoma: evaluation of KIT (CD117) expression and failure to demonstrate activating mutations in the C-KIT proto-oncogene - implications for treatment with imatinib mesylate. J. Cutan. Pathol. **34**, 324–329 (2007)

37. Ullrich, S.E.: Mechanisms underlying UV-induced immune suppression. Mutat. Res. **571**, 185–205 (2005)

38. Ullrich, S.E.: Sunlight and skin cancer: lessons from the immune system. Mol. Carcinog. **46**, 629–633 (2007)

39. Van Gele, M., Kaghad, M., Leonard, J.H., Van Roy, N., Naeyaert, J.M., Geerts, M.L., Van Belle, S., Cocquyt, V., Bridge, J., Sciot, R., Wolf-Peeters, C., De Paepe, A., Caput, D., Speleman, F.: Mutation analysis of P73 and TP53 in Merkel cell carcinoma. Br. J. Cancer **82**, 823–826 (2000)

40. Van Gele, M., Leonard, J.H., Van Roy, N., Cook, A.L., De Paepe, A., Speleman, F.: Frequent allelic loss at 10q23 but low incidence of PTEN mutations in Merkel cell carcinoma. Int. J. Cancer **92**, 409–413 (2001)

41. Van Gele, M., Speleman, F., Vandesompele, J., Van Roy, N., Leonard, J.H.: Characteristic pattern of chromosomal gains and losses in Merkel cell carcinoma detected by comparative genomic hybridization. Cancer Res. **58**, 1503–1508 (1998)

42. Vogelstein, B., Kinzler, K.W.: Cancer genes and the pathways they control. Nat. Med. **10**, 789–799 (2004)

43. Worda, M., Sreevidya, C.S., Ananthaswamy, H.N., Cerroni, L., Kerl, H., Wolf, P.: T1796A BRAF mutation is absent in Merkel cell carcinoma. Br. J. Dermatol. **153**, 229–232 (2005)

44. zur Hausen H: Novel human polyomaviruses–re-emergence of a well known virus family as possible human carcinogens. Int. J. Cancer **123**, 247–250 (2008)

Michael B. Colgan, Mark A. Cappel, Mark R. Pittelkow,
Kazuyasu Fujii, Dorothea Terhorst, and Eggert Stockfleth

3.1.1 Basal Cell Carcinoma

**Michael B. Colgan, Mark A. Cappel,
and Mark R. Pittelkow**

3.1.1.1 Definition

Malignant cutaneous tumors characterized by bands, cords, nests, islands, or buds of basaloid cells.

3.1.1.2 ICD-O Code

8090/3

3.1.1.3 Synonyms

Recent terms – basal cell epithelioma, trophoblastic carcinoma.

M.B. Colgan (✉)
Department of Dermatology, Mayo Clinic College of Medicine,
Rochester, MN 55905, USA
e-mail: colgan.michael@mayo.edu

M.A. Cappel
Department of Dermatology, Mayo Clinic College of Medicine,
Jacksonville, FL, 32224, USA
e-mail: cappel.mark@mayo.edu

M.R. Pittelkow
Departments of Dermatology and Biochemistry and Molecular
Biology, Mayo Clinic College of Medicine, Mayo Medical School,
Rochester, MN 55905 USA
e-mail: pittelkow.mark@mayo.edu

K. Fujii
Department of Dermatology, Okayama University Graduate School of
Medicine, Dentistry, and Pharmaceutical Sciences, 2-5-1 Shikata-cho,
Okayama 700-8558, Japan
e-mail: kazfujii@cc.okayama-u.ac.jp

D. Terhorst and E. Stockfleth
Klinik für Dermatologie, Allergologie und Venerologie,
Charité – Universitätsmedizin,
Schumannstraße 20-21, 10117 Berlin, Deutschland
e-mail: dorothea.terhorst@charite.de

Previously used/other terms – chancroid ulcer, rodent ulcer, ulcus exedens, or basalioma [1].

3.1.1.4 History

The term basal cell carcinoma (BCC) is derived from the "basal" keratinocytes of the epidermis and the Greek words "carcinos" for crab-like and "oma" for swelling [2]. Hippocrates often described and made drawings of outwardly visible tumors on the skin, nose, and breasts, which may have represented the first descriptions or documentation of BCC; however, the first description in the medical literature is widely credited to Arthur Jacobs [2]. In 1827 Jacobs, an ophthalmologist described a "destructive ulceration of peculiar character which I have observed to attack the eyelids, and extend to the eyeball, orbit, and face. The characteristic features of the disease are the extraordinary slowness to progress; the peculiar condition at the edges and surface of the ulcer…." [3]. Jacobs did not name the tumor, but over the next century, this lesion would carry many names including chancroid ulcer, rodent ulcer, basal cell epithelioma, ulcus exedens, or basalioma [1]. Studies in the first half of the nineteenth century linked ionizing radiation and then ultraviolet (UV) B radiation to skin cancers in both mice, and subsequently, humans, initiating a path to the discovery that has led to our current understanding of this common malignancy.

3.1.1.5 BCC Epidemiology

Basal cell carcinoma (BCC) is the most common type of skin cancer as well as the most common malignancy among fair-skinned populations [4, 5]. It accounts for approximately 70–80% of all nonmelanoma skin cancer (NMSC), with NMSCs fully accounting for 90% of all skin cancers worldwide [5, 6]. In the U.S., 1 in 5 Americans will have a BCC in their lifetime, representing well over 2.5 million cases annually, and worldwide, these numbers approach four million diagnosed cancers annually [6–8]. Some estimate that the

R. Dummer et al. (eds.), *Skin Cancer – A World-Wide Perspective*,
DOI: 10.1007/978-3-642-05072-5_3.1, © Springer-Verlag Berlin Heidelberg 2011

incidence is increasing at a rate of 3–6% per year [9]. Due to its indolent course and ability to be treated in an outpatient setting, it is likely that a large portion of BCCs go unreported making the documented incidence an underestimation [10]. The true incidence may be as high as three-fold the current estimates.

BCC tends to involve the photodistributed areas including face, head, neck, arms, and the back of hands with particular concentration in the areas of ears, eyelids, nose, and lips [9, 11]. It is much more common in the elderly and twice as likely in men. Because BCC is slow growing, rarely metastasizes, and is usually visible, mortality associated with BCC is rare with estimates around 12 per 100,000 (age-adjusted) with increased mortality reported in men, Caucasians, and those with scrotal lesions [12]. Though mortality is low, there is a significant medical and societal burden. In the U.S. medicare population, it was estimated that in 2001 alone 426 million dollars was spent on BCC and SCC, making NMSC one of the most costly skin cancers to treat [13, 14]. With an aging population and increasing health care costs, these numbers are likely to continue to increase.

BCC has a direct link to UV radiation, therefore anything that predisposes a population to an increasing amount or intensity of UV exposure increases the incidence of BCC [9, 11, 15–18]. With the exception of uncommon genetic disorders, most people at risk fall into two broad categories. Individuals have an extrinsic increase in their exposure and/ or an intrinsic susceptibility to sunlight, with blistering sunburns conferring the greatest risk rather than lifetime cumulative exposure [9, 15, 19].

Those with intrinsic predisposition generally are Caucasians, often of Celtic, Scottish, or Welch descent, Fitzpatrick skin type I–II, with blue or green eyes, red or blond hair, inability to tan, and freckles [17, 18, 20, 21]. Darker pigmented individuals appear to be protected leading to the concept that melanin acts as a barrier to cancer causing UV mutations [19, 22]. Further supporting this hypothesis is the observation that Africans with albinism have an increased BCC risk, close to rates seen in regional Caucasian populations [23, 24]. Uncommon to rare genetic disorders mediate significant effects on the development of extreme numbers of BCCs such as basal cell nevus (Gorlin) syndrome and xeroderma pigmentosum [5]. The immune system also plays a critical role in the ability to suppress BCC and NMSC, with increased rates of BCC in patients with an organ transplant or HIV/AIDS [5].

Extrinsic factors associated with BCC incidence are numerous, but most have an association with UV exposure. Those living closer to the equator and those with jobs that increase exposure to sunlight are at increased risk, such as farmers, railway workers, masons, and quarrymen [18, 25, 26]. Latitude greatly impacts the rates of BCC both through UV exposure and lifestyle changes. As people move further from the latitudes of ancestral origin, rates of BCC and NMSC increase. U.S. citizens living near the equator in Hawaii have a four times greater risk than mainland US residents [5, 27]. Japanese living in Hawaii had a 45-fold increase compared to those living on mainland Japan, likely secondary to both UV intensity and cultural lifestyle variances [25]. Few studies have been done to link BCC association with altitude, but UV exposure is greatly increased in individuals who live, visit, or recreate at altitude [28, 29]. Therefore, populations living, working, or recreating at altitude likely have a greater risk of NMSC and BCC.

Evidence for non-UV-induced causes of BCC exists and continues to mount, but is less well studied. BCCs have been induced by exposures at sites of ionizing radiation contamination and have been found to be increased in Japanese atomic bomb survivors [26, 30]. Associations also have been established with diet, exposure to carcinogens, tobacco, coal-tar, asphalt, soot, crude paraffin, anthracene pitch, organic and inorganic solvents, mineral oil, burns, chronic ulcerations, chickenpox vaccination scars, venipuncture sites, leishmanial scars, and burn scars within tattoos [5, 19, 31–34].

Taking into account these intrinsic and extrinsic factors, it would be expected that Fitzpatrick skin type I–II populations living close to the equator with a lifestyle that increases sun exposure have the highest rates of BCC. This is, in fact, what epidemiologic studies have demonstrated, with the highest rates in the world in Australia and an incidence estimated at 1–2% per year [31]. In comparison, the lowest recorded rates (though very few large studies have been conducted) come from native populations in Africa where BCC makes up less than 2% of all skin cancer [23]. Lower incidences in those of African, Asians, or Mediterranean descent have all been well documented [5] (Table 3.1.1).

3.1.1.6 Pathogenesis

Basal cell carcinomas(BCCs) emerge from genetically altered keratinocytic precursor stem cells in the hair follicles, sebaceous glands, or possibly, interfollicular basal cells [43].

Table 3.1.1 Incidence rates of BCC in different geographic regions

BCC rates per 100,000
936 M and 497 F in Arizona 1985–1996 [35]
310 M and 166 F in New Hampshire 1993–1994 [36]
7,067 M and 3,379 in western Australia 1987–1992 [37]
2,074 M and 1,579 F Australia Nambour 1985–1992 [38]
69 M and 62 F in Switzerland 1991–1992 [39]
49 M and 45 F in Finland 1991–1995 [40]
19.7 M and 23.3 F in Jordan 1997–2001 [41]
87 M and 67 F in New Brunswick 1992–2001 [42]

These mutations frequently arise spontaneously, but are also associated with genetic predisposition as found in people with basal cell nevus (Gorlin) syndrome or xeroderma pigmentosum [43]. Sunlight, particularly within the UVB wavelength, is the most frequent mechanism inducing somatic mutations in these cells [5].

For BCC, the most well-characterized mutations are in the p53 and *patched* (PTCH1) genes, both of which play important roles in tumor suppression [43]. UVB induces a dipyrimidine-base substitution from C to T or CC to TT in the DNA of mutated keratinocytes [43]. This common substitution in photodamaged epidermis renders ineffective the tumor suppresser mechanism within the cell and leads to unchecked keratinocyte proliferation [43]. There is also evidence that the inflammatory response of the skin to UV sunburns in the form of prostaglandin E2 (PGE2), tumor necrosis factor (TNF)-a, interleukin (IL)-1, and other proinflammatory cytokines further creates an environment that promotes mutagenesis and tumor growth [44].

3.1.1.6.1 P53

P53 is the most commonly mutated gene that has thus far been identified in human cancers. As a tumor suppressor gene, it induces apoptosis in cells that have become damaged or stressed [45]. When p53 function is disrupted, damaged cells are more prone to survive and undergo unchecked proliferation. Mutations in p53 are more commonly associated with SCC, but have been identified in up to 56% of BCC in some studies. In the majority of these cases the UV-associated dipyrimidine substitution is identified [43].

3.1.1.6.2 PTCH1 and the SHH Pathway

The role of the PTCH1 gene (chromosome 9q22.3) as a tumor suppressor has been extensively studied since it was first discovered to be the cause of basal cell nevus or Gorlin syndrome [43]. PTCH1 is a critical component of the Hedgehog signaling pathway, which mediates development of a variety of structures including skeleton, limbs, craniofacial structures, neural tube, skin, and hair follicles. When functioning properly, the PTCH1 gene encodes for a protein that acts to suppress gene transcription and cell growth [43, 46]. The loss of PTCH1 function leads to continuous signaling from the smoothened (SMO) transmembrane signaling protein which, in turn, activates transcription of the GLI family of gene products [43, 47]. The GLI protein members upregulate a cascade of cyclins and other growth-promoting

proteins that ultimately lead to unchecked cell growth [43]. PTCH1 has been identified in 30–40% of sporadic tumors, with fully 30% of these demonstrating the dipyrimidine UV-associated mutation [43, 46]. In addition, SMO mutations have been identified in some 6–20% of sporadic BCCs, further implicating the Hedgehog pathway in BCC development [47]. In the basal cell nevus syndrome, patients have an inherited mutation in one copy of the PTCH gene and, following the classic two-hit hypothesis of heritable cancers, the loss of the other copy of PTCH1 leads to unregulated cell proliferation and eventually to frank tumor formation [43].

3.1.1.7 Clinico-Pathologic Features and Prognosis

3.1.1.7.1 Nodular

ICD-O

8097/3

Clinical

Nodular basal cell carcinoma is the most common subtype representing approximately 78% of all BCC that are biopsied. It frequently presents on the head and neck as a red or pink papule with a pearly or translucent appearance and prominent telangiectasias, rolled borders, central ulceration, with frequent bleeding or occasional symptoms such as pruritus [9, 48] (Fig. 3.1.1). It is generally more frequent in men and in the elderly with an average age at diagnosis of approximately 65.5 years [9].

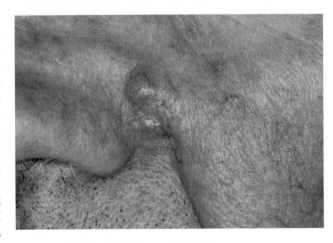

Fig. 3.1.1 Nodular BCC, left nasolabial fold

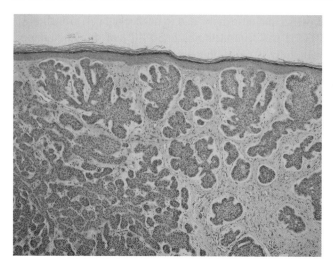

Fig. 3.1.2 Nodular and micronodular BCC (H&E) 100×

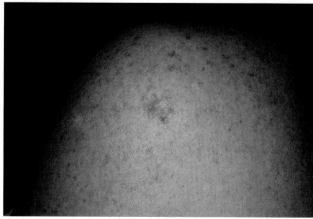

Fig. 3.1.3 Superficial BCC of the left posterior shoulder

Dermatopathology

The tumor shows well-defined smooth-bordered basophilic staining islands of neoplastic cells (Fig. 3.1.2). Peripheral palisading is often present, as well as retraction artifact due to stromal shrinkage during processing [48, 49].

On higher magnification individual cells are characterized by large uniform nuclei with scant cytoplasm and affinity for basophilic dye. A connection with the epidermis is often evident [50].

Inflammatory response is varied, but generally less frequent, and mitosis is rarely observed [51].

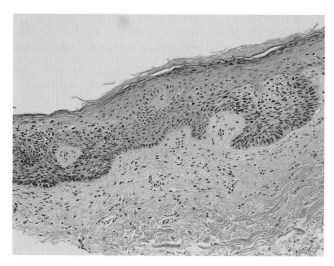

Fig. 3.1.4 Superficial BCC (H&E) 2×00

Prognosis

Most nodular BCCs have a slow growth rate with limited growth and have a fairly indolent course when treated promptly. However, they can be very locally destructive when left untreated, particularly on the more sensitive structures of the face such as the eyes and ears [50, 52].

3.1.1.7.2 Superficial BCC

ICD-O

8091/3

Clinical

Superficial BCCs are the second most common form of BCC representing approximately 15% of all biopsied BCC [48].

They are more frequently found on the trunk and extremities, but are also common on the head and neck [48]. They are found in a younger demographic than the nodular subtype, with an average age of 57.5 years [9, 48].

Clinically, they present as red/pink, scaly, thin plaques, or papules with occasionally rolled or raised borders (Fig. 3.1.3). They are often confused with inflammatory lesions, actinic keratosis, or squamous cell carcinoma in situ [53].

Dermatopathology

Multiple small superficially located buds of basaloid cells that do not extend beyond the papillary dermis are seen (Fig. 3.1.4). There are frequent "skip areas" along the epidermis, which has given rise to the synonym, superficial multifocal BCC; however, many believe that these are more a result of superficial three-dimensional finger-like projections being viewed in two dimensions [50].

Prognosis

Typically, these tumors progress to spread laterally, but can occasionally penetrate the deep dermis and cause increased morbidity. Overall, their prognosis is similar to that of nodular BCC, with local destruction of normal surrounding tissues as the most common associated complication [50]. They tend to have a higher rate of recurrence likely related to their "multifocal nature" with poorly defined margins.

3.1.1.7.3 Sclerosing (Morpheaform)

ICD-O

80921/3

Clinical

Sclerosing or morpheaform BCC is much less common than superficial and nodular BCCs accounting for approximately 6–12% of all BCCs diagnosed with variations across different population groups [48, 54, 55]. More than 90% of morpheaform BCCs are located on the face and scalp, with one third of these involving the nose [48]. By immunohistochemical staining, they are often associated with increased p53 and decreased Bcl-2 expression when compared to nodular and superficial subtypes [56, 57].

The clinical appearance of sclerosing BCC often resembles the plaque of morphea, which gives rise to one of its common terms, morpheaform. Typically, these lesions range from flat, atrophic lesions to whitish scar-like plaques with associated telangiectasias (Fig. 3.1.5a). Frequently the tumors are poorly demarcated and often have an actual size and extent of spread much greater than the apparent clinical lesion [50] (Fig. 3.1.5b).

Dermatopathology

Cords or strands of basaloid keratinocytes extend between collagen and fibrotic stroma of the dermis. Morpheaform nests are small, poorly demarcated, often lack peripheral palisading, and can penetrate deep into the dermis encompassing nerve bundles in the process [50] (Fig. 3.1.6a, b).

Prognosis

These tumors tend to be more aggressive and invade to a greater depth within the dermis, making them much more difficult to treat as compared to nodular and superficial BCC [58]. Their rate of recurrence has been documented to be as high as 60%, but more recent studies using Mohs surgery have shown rates around 14.8% [55, 59]. Similar to other types of BCC, their morbidity results from local destruction, but given that they are more challenging to detect, invade to

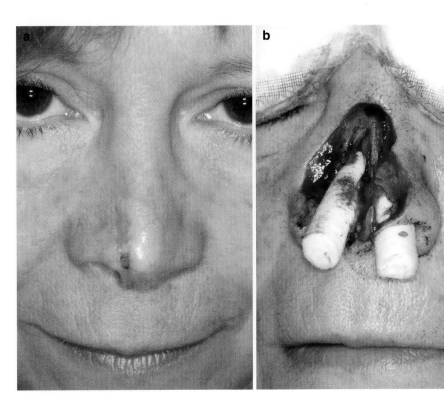

Fig. 3.1.5 (a) Morpheaform BCC, nasal tip, preoperative view. **(b)** Post-MOHS clearance of tumor

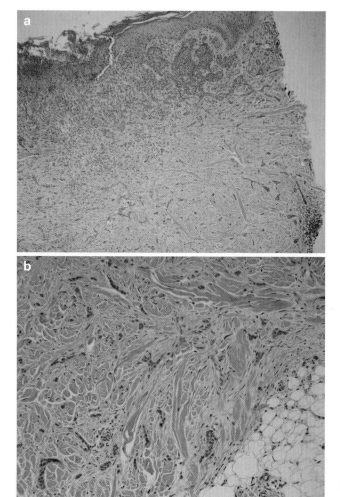

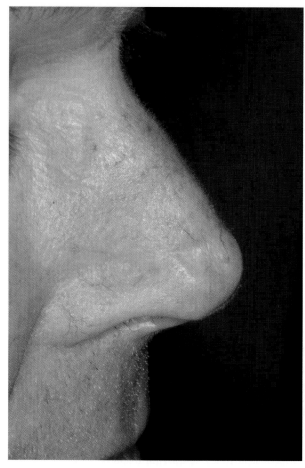

Fig. 3.1.7 Infiltrating BCC, right nasal tip

Fig. 3.1.6 (a) Morpheaform BCC (H&E) 100×. (b) Higher magnification of morpheaform BCC (H&E) 200×

a greater depth, and are more difficult to completely excise, morpheaform BCCs tend to have increased morbidity when compared to other subtypes.

3.1.1.7.4 Infiltrative

ICD-O

8092/3

Clinical

Infiltrative BCC is an important subtype to recognize as it has a similarly aggressive profile and is considered to be closely related to sclerosing BCC. Some studies have estimated that as much as 16% of BCC referred for MOHS surgery are infiltrative, though the true percentage is likely much lower due to a referral bias [60]. It typically presents as an opaque whitish to yellow poorly defined plaque that tends to blend with the surrounding skin (Fig. 3.1.7). When occurring along embryonic fusion lines, these tumors can be more infiltrative, and paresthesias in the surrounding tissue often signal perineural extension [60].

Dermatopathology

Infiltrative BCC presents with basophilic staining, elongated strands and islands. These islands generally have lost the round nest-like appearance seen in nodular BCC and no longer demonstrate peripheral palisading or retraction (Fig. 3.1.8). There is a great deal of variation from one island to the next and the tumors can extend quite deep into the dermis giving them there name. Generally, there is very little fibrosis identified which is the key differentiating factor when comparing these tumors to sclerosing BCC [60]. These tumors can also show a mixed histology with nodular or micronodular BCC centrally and the more infiltrative portions on the periphery of the biopsy [61]. It is important to make the proper diagnosis and not rely on a superficial biopsy as infiltrative BCCs can be much more challenging to treat [62].

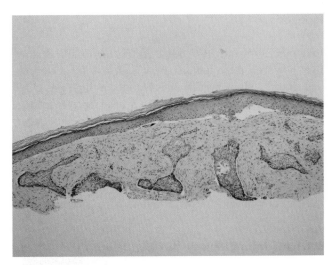

Fig. 3.1.8 Infiltrating BCC (H&E) 100×

Prognosis

These tumors are more aggressive and have a greater propensity to recur. Much like sclerosing BCC, these tumors can demonstrate a much greater subclinical spread and often have positive margins after traditional excisions. MOHS surgery is indicated for treatment of these lesions and long-term follow-up for recurrence is paramount [60, 62].

3.1.1.7.5 Micronodular

ICD-O

8090/3

Clinical

This histopathological variant is important to distinguish from typical nodular BCC as it has been shown to have a higher rate of recurrence and usually demonstrates greater depth of invasion on presentation [63]. In some studies micronodular BCC constitutes as much as 15% of BCC [63, 64]. Due to their infiltrative nature, micronodular BCC are generally considered, from a treatment standpoint, to be in the same class as morpheaform or sclerosing BCC [63].

Dermatopathology

Micronodular BCC is composed of multiple, approximately 0.15 mm diameter, small tumor islands. These islands typically demonstrate basaloid cells with peripheral palisading, but retraction artifact is not as common as in nodular BCC [50].

Prognosis

Because of their propensity for subclinical spread, and difficulty in obtaining margins due to multiple small nests, these tumors are generally more likely to recur. Though less information on rates of recurrence, metastatic potential, and morbidity is published on this subtype, it is accepted that these behave more like sclerosing or metatypical BCC. MOHS surgery is the treatment of choice [63].

3.1.1.7.6 Basosquamous (Metatypical)

ICD-O

8094/3

Clinical

Basosquamous carcinoma is thought to constitute between 0.4 and 12% of all BCCs with more recent reports placing its incidence at 1.2–2.7% [65–67]. The wide variance is likely due to the lack of concrete definitions used to categorize these tumors, and there is even continuing controversy as to whether this represents a true subtype or a combined lesion of SCC and BCC [67, 68]. Regardless, it is important to histopathologically differentiate this lesion from nodular or superficial spreading BCC as its course is more aggressive with more frequent metastases and recurrences warranting a more judicious clinical approach to treatment and follow-up [66, 67, 69].

Clinically, these occur most frequently on the face, neck, and ears. There appearance is similar to other more indolent forms of BCC presenting as red papules to ulcerative nodules [66, 69] (Fig. 3.1.9).

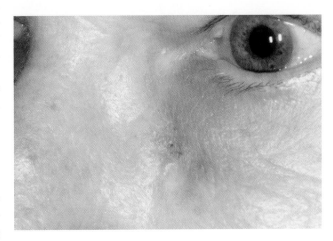

Fig. 3.1.9 Metatypical BCC

Dermatopathology

There are three major components that make up the histopathologic diagnostic criteria of basosquamous carcinoma. The first is a strongly basaloid component of dark staining, well-circumscribed cells that may demonstrate palisading and possible peripheral clefting. The second is a more squamous component with typical larger, lighter-staining cells with a tendency to consistently keratinize (Fig. 3.1.10). The third component is a well-differentiated transition zone or connection between the two populations of cells which essentially differentiates this single entity from the possibility of having two separate keratinocyte carcinomas in close proximity [70–72]. For comparison, a "collision" tumor of BCC and squamous cell carcinoma (SCC) is shown (Fig. 3.1.11).

Prognosis

Like other forms of BCC, these tumors are locally destructive; however, these tumors are at high risk for recurrence and spread with metastasis rates reported as high as 5–7.4% [66, 67, 69, 73]. Recurrence rates have been reported to range from 12 to 54% with traditional excision and approximately 4% with Mohs micrographic surgery [67]. From a clinical standpoint, they should be treated more like an aggressive SCC with wide excision or preferably MOHS and consideration of a sentinal lymph node biopsy if the tumor is large (>2 cm) or lymphatic or perineural invasion is identified.

3.1.1.7.7 Infundibulocystic BCC

ICD-O

Clinical

Infundibulocystic BCC has been recognized as its own entity with unique histopathology and more indolent course than other subtypes of BCC [74]. It presents as a very small, shiny flesh-colored papule with an acrochordon or "skin-tag" like appearance on the head, neck, extremities, and trunk.

Dermatopathology

Infundibulocystic BCC can have a unique combination of follicular differentiation including follicular germs and infundibula [74]. Overall, architecture demonstrates cords and strands of palisading basaloid cells with few scattered infundibular cysts [75] (Fig. 3.1.12).

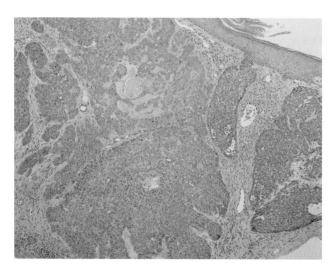

Fig. 3.1.10 Metatypical BCC (H&E) 100×

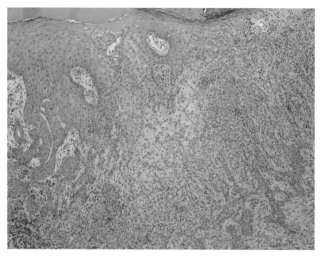

Fig. 3.1.11 Collision tumor of BCC and SCC (H&E) 100×

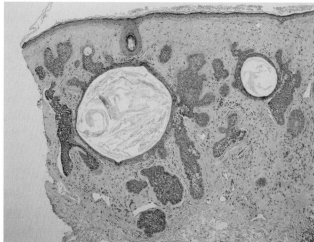

Fig. 3.1.12 Infundibulocystic BCC (H&E) 100×

Prognosis

This subtype tends to be very slow growing and therefore less destructive if treated in a reasonable time frame. They are typically treated in similar fashion to nodular BCC with local destruction, excision, or MOHS all representing viable treatment options.

3.1.1.7.8 Fibroepithelioma (Fibroepithelioma of Pinkus) or Fenestrated Trichoblastoma

ICD-O

8093/3

Clinical

Pinkus described "premalignant fibroepithelioma" as a proliferation that gave rise to many tiny basal cell carcinomas within each lesion [76]. Since its first description, many have argued over the proper classification of this tumor with some accepting it as a subtype of BCC and others calling for its classification as a subtype of trichoblastoma known as a fenestrated trichoblastoma [77]. Clinically, fibroepithelial BCCs appear as smooth, skin-colored to pink, polypoid, or papillomatous lesions with a marked predilection for occurrence on the trunk. Unlike other forms of BCC, they tend to be found more frequently in females [77].

Dermatopathology

Fibroepitheliomas show thin basaloid or squamous cell anastomosing strands with abundant surrounding stroma extending from the epidermis into the deep dermis (Fig. 3.1.13).

The strands can show follicular bulb and dermal papilla-like formations [77].

Prognosis

Very little information and studies have been done on the long-term prognosis and follow-up of fibroepithelial tumors. Regardless of their name and classification, they are generally thought to behave in a similar manner to other forms of BCC and therefore are treated in a similar fashion.

3.1.1.7.9 Basal Cell Carcinoma with Adnexal Differentiation (Sebaceous)

ICD-O

8098/3

Clinical

BCC with adnexal differentiation is more of a histopathological diagnosis as it has no distinguishing clinical features with a similar appearance to that of nodular BCC.

Dermatopathology

This form of BCC is distinguished by its adnexal differentiation including basaloid buds, ductal, sebaceous, and trichilemmal elements and, in some variants, eccrine or apocrine differentiation [78, 79] (Fig. 3.1.14a, b). Of greater importance than subclassifying this form of BCC is differentiating

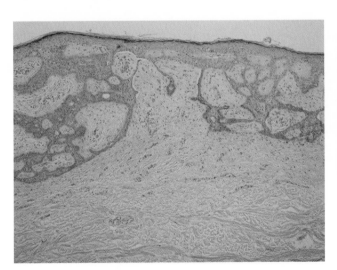

Fig. 3.1.13 Fibroepithelioma of Pinkus-type BCC (H&E) 100×

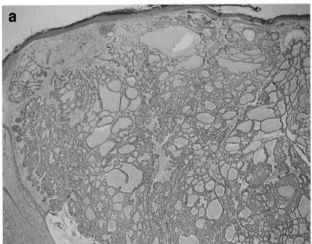

Fig. 3.1.14 (**a**) Adenoid BCC (H&E) 40×. (**b**) Nodular BCC with sebaceous differentiation (H&E) 200×

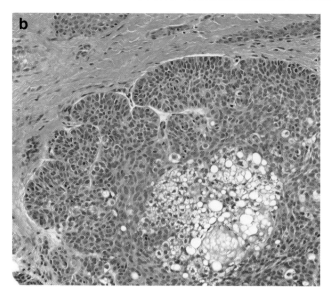

Fig. 3.1.14 (continued)

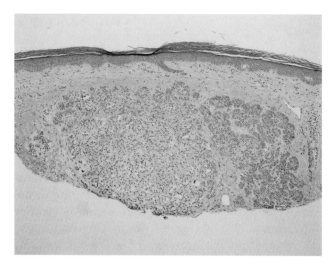

Fig. 3.1.15 Clear-cell BCC (H&E) 100×

it from sweat gland carcinomas which have an increased risk for metastases. A rare subtype, clear-cell BCC, was originally felt to be adnexal-related, but electron microscopy has shown it to result from lysosomal degeneration of a BCC [80] (Fig. 3.1.15).

Prognosis

Distinguishing this variant histologically from other forms of BCC is generally not considered clinically relevant, as treatment and prognosis appear to be similar to that of superficial and nodular BCC. However, BCC with sebaceous differentiation may be more common in Muir-Torre syndrome, and this may be clinically important as Muir-Torre syndrome is a genetic syndrome associated with internal malignancies.

There are no current studies describing a clinical profile and prognosis of these lesions.

3.1.1.7.10 Keratotic Basal Cell Carcinoma

ICD-O

8090/3

Clinical

This unusual subtype of BCC often appears as a pink pearly papule with small areas of keratin cysts or milia present on the surface [81].

Dermatopathology

Overall architecture is similar to that of nodular BCC with the exception of the extensive keratinization. The keratinization may be laminated and infundibular or more homogenous, cornified, and trichilemmal. Typically, the trichilemmal type is considered the most common form, though up to seven subclassifications have been identified with infundibular being the next most common keratin variant [82] (Fig. 3.1.16 a, b). Dystrophic calcium, apoptotic keratinocytes, and pale keratinocytes are also often present [80].

Prognosis

It is important to recognize this variant and distinguish it from basosquamous carcinoma, as the latter has a more aggressive clinical course and prognosis. Basosquamous carcinoma has the presence of differentiation of both BCC and

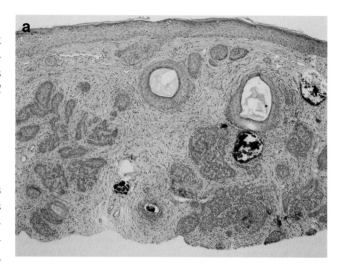

Fig. 3.1.16 (a) Trichoepithelioma-type BCC (H&E) 100× (b) Keratotic nodular BCC 200×

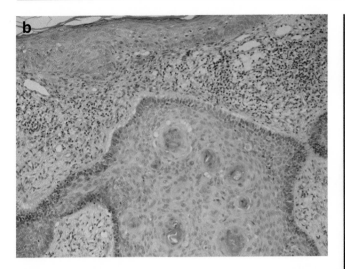

Fig. 3.1.16 (continued)

SCC, while keratotic BCC is entirely composed of BCC with numerous, small, keratin cysts.

3.1.1.8 Other Important Entities

3.1.1.8.1 Giant BCC

Giant BCCs are defined by the tumor having a diameter of greater than 5 cm regardless of histopathological architecture. They are quite rare and are thought to represent less than 1% of all BCCs [83]. These tumors are generally on the trunk and display aggressive behavior with an increased risk of local recurrence and metastases [84]. Some of these tumors are a result of long-term neglect, but they can also be due to recurrence of a previous cancer [85, 86] (Fig. 3.1.17). The treatment of choice for these tumors is surgical excision, though this can often be a complicated multistage operation as these tumors tend to invade surrounding nerve, bone, and soft tissue structures [83].

3.1.1.8.2 Pigmented BCC

Pigmentation can occur in several types of BCC including nodular, micronodular, superficial, and keratotic. Its presence does not affect prognosis, but gives pigmented BCCs an unusual clinical appearance with a more concerning initial diagnostic differential from their nonpigmented counterparts [87] (Fig. 3.1.18). Dermatoscopy reveals characteristic features of this distinctive subtype of BCC (Fig. 3.1.19). Typically, their histopathology is unchanged from nonpigmented BCC with the exception of scattered melanocytes in the tumor nests and pigmented macrophages in the dermis (Fig. 3.1.20). Treatment is governed by the subtype classification and is not dictated by the additional finding of increased pigment.

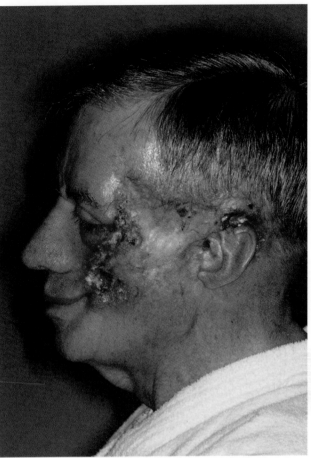

Fig. 3.1.17 Giant, recurrent BCC, left face

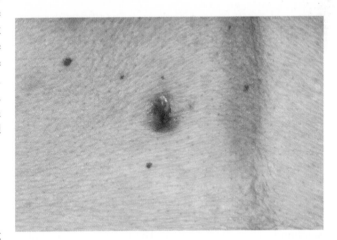

Fig. 3.1.18 Pigmented BCC, back

3.1.1.8.3 Metastatic

Metastasis of BCC has been reported, but the frequency is quite low, ranging from 0.03 to 0.5% of all BCC cases. Metastasis typically occurs in lymph node, lung, bone as well as skin [88, 89]. Factors that increase the risk of metastasis include location of the primary tumor on the scrotum, occurrence on the head and neck in patients with Celtic

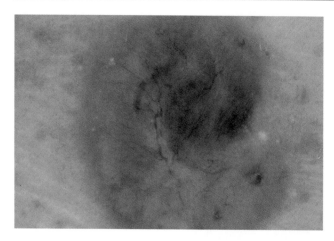

Fig. 3.1.19 Pigmented BCC, dermoscopy ×10

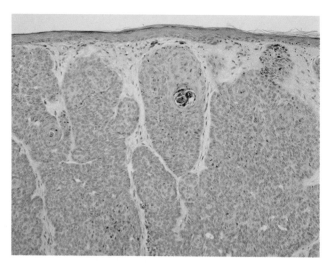

Fig. 3.1.20 Pigmented BCC (H&E) 200×

ancestry, and primary lesions that penetrate to a depth of greater than 1 cm and have a diameter of more than 3 cm. The vast majority of metastatic BCC occur in Caucasian males with a male/female ratio of 2:1–3:1. The median age of development of metastatic BCC is 59 years, and the time to onset of metastasis from the original tumor diagnosis is a median of 9 years. The rate of metastatic spread for BCC of scrotum is approximately 13%. The five-year survival after diagnosis of metastatic BCC is reportedly only 10%. Fortunately, the very low rate of metastasis is felt to be due to the dependence of the tumor mass on stromal interactions and support of tissues within the skin. Clearly, however, there are escape mechanisms that rarely are induced and overcome these limitations of growth. Treatments with retinoids, combination chemotherapy and, most recently, agents that target the hedgehog pathway show activity and can be used in combination with surgical approaches [90].

3.1.2 Squamous Cell Carcinoma

Mark A. Cappel, Michael B. Colgan, and Mark R. Pittelkow

3.1.2.1 Definition

Malignant neoplasm of epithelial keratinocytes displaying variable squamous differentiation.

3.1.2.2 ICD-O Code

8070/3

3.1.2.3 Synonyms

Recent terms – epidermoid carcinoma, squamous cell epithelioma.

Previously used/other terms – Soot warts, Marjolin's ulcer.

3.1.2.4 History

The term squamous cell carcinoma (SCC) is derived from the term squama or "the scale of a fish or serpent" referring to the flattened nature of the epithelial keratinocytes. Throughout most of its history, squamous cell carcinoma (SCC) has been recognized as a disease of occupational exposure. Sir Percival Pott is widely credited with the first description of SCC when he documented "soot warts" in adolescent British chimney sweeps [1]. SCC induced on the genitals of workers who exposed themselves to carcinogenic oil by straddling the turning axle of cotton-spinning machines (mules) was termed "Mule spinners disease" [2]. In 1828 French surgeon Jean-Nicholas Marjolin described SCC arising in traumatic scars and burns, the latter being termed a Marjolin's ulcer [3]. Later in 1887, Sir Jonathan Hutchinson noted a causal relationship of medicinal arsenic (Fowler's solution) in the treatment of asthma and psoriasis with the development of SCC [4]. In the early twentieth century SCC would be linked with X-ray exposure in technicians operating roentgen machines and later with Grenz rays in the treatment of acne and psoriasis [4–6]. Over the past century, as many of these occupations, chemicals, and medical treatments have become obsolete, ultraviolet (UV) radiation (light) has replaced them as the most prominent risk factor for the development of SCC [7].

3.1.2.5 SCC Epidemiology

Squamous cell carcinoma (SCC) is the second most common form of skin cancer [7]. In the United States nonmelanoma skin cancer(NMSC) was estimated to afflict over two million persons annually in 2006, and an incidence as high as 3.5 million cases per year in the US has been projected since direct incidence figures are not comprehensively recorded. Worldwide, these numbers are most likely greater than five million diagnosed cancers annually [8–10]. A worldwide increase is estimated at least 2.4% per year for the last several decades [11]. Though the occurrence of SCC is approximately 4 times less likely than basal cell carcinoma (BCC), SCC still accounts for roughly 15–25% of NMSCs, equating to 750,000–1,250,000 tumors diagnosed worldwide annually. Based on more limited date in 1994, there were between 135,000 and 250,000 SCCs diagnosed in the United states alone [12]. In some regions such as Australia, the incidence has been reported to be as high as 1% of the population [13]. Due to indolent course of cutaneous SCC and ability to be treated in an outpatient setting, it is likely that a large portion of SCC go unreported, making the documented incidence an underestimation [14].

SCCs tend to occur on photodistributed areas such as the face, ears, hands, and forearms. They are more common in the elderly and more frequent in men than women. SCCs metastasize at a much higher rate than BCCs contributing to a greater mortality and morbidity despite its reduced incidence. SCC metastasizes at rates estimated around 2.0–2.5% at less than 5 years and rates as high as 5% in greater than 5 years. Of the tumors that do metastasize, the prognosis is poor with around 40% survival with nodal metastasis and 25% survival with visceral organ involvement [15]. Extrapolating these rates to the number of tumors worldwide, between 6,750 and 14,000 will die of cutaneous SCC annually [16]. Though mortality is low, there is a significant medical and societal burden. In the U.S. medicare population it has been estimated that in 2001 alone 426 million dollars (US) was spent on BCCs and SCCs, making NMSCs one of the most costly skin cancers to treat [17, 18]. With an aging population and increasing health care costs, these numbers are likely to continue to increase.

Of all skin cancers, SCC is the one most closely linked with total and occupational UV radiation exposure [19]. In contrast to BCC where nonoccupational exposure and intermittent sunburns of typically nonexposed sites portend a higher risk, SCC is more closely linked to sites of maximum cumulative UV exposure. Similar to BCC, both intrinsic and extrinsic increases in a person's cumulative exposure to UV radiation increase a person's lifetime risk of SCC.

Those with an intrinsic predisposition to SCC are generally Fitzpatrick skin type I or II, Caucasian, and, in general, are people who get sunburnt but do not tan [8, 20, 21]. Darker pigmented individuals appear to be protected by greater amounts melanin in their skin [22, 23].

A person's genetic constitution can have a significant effect, especially with some syndromes associated with extreme numbers of SCCs. Examples are those with oculocutaneous albinism and xeroderma pigmentosum that lead to a lack of pigmented barrier protection and a defective DNA repair mechanism, respectively [7]. A patient's immune system also plays a critical role in their ability to suppress NMSC development with increased rates of SCC in transplant patients on immunosuppressive agents, those with chronic lymphocytic leukemia(CLL), and patients with HIV/AIDS [7, 24]. Similarly, epidermodysplasia verruciformis (EDV) is a rare, autosomal recessive disorder leading to decreased resistance and persistence of viral infection with human papillomavirus (HPV) and an associated increased risk of developing multiple SCC.

Extrinsic factors associated with SCC are similar to that of BCC with greater occurrence in people who have increased cumulative sun exposure through age, activities, occupations, hobbies, and lifestyle choices. There is increased incidence in quarrymen, masons, construction workers, farmers, and stationary equipment operators [25]. The incidence of SCC increases as genetically similar populations reside closer to the equator and as populations age [13, 21]. U.S. citizens living near the equator such as in Hawaii harbor a four times greater risk of developing NMSC compared to the mainland US [7, 26]. Japanese individuals living in Hawaii have a 45-fold increase vs. those living on mainland Japan, likely due secondary to both UV intensity and cultural lifestyle variances [27]. Few studies have been performed to link SCC association with altitude, but UV exposure is greatly increased in individuals who live, visit, or recreate at higher altitude [28, 29]. Therefore, populations living, working, or recreating at higher elevations likely have a greater risk of NMSC and SCC.

Non-UV exposure factors also have been documented and are strongly linked to SCC. Exposure to ionizing radiation such as nondiagnostic X-ray treatment for various skin conditions or chemicals such as arsenic, polycyclic aromatic hydrocarbons, insecticides, herbicides, and tobacco products appears to confer a greater risk of SCC [2, 30–32]. Infection with HPV is a well-documented and essentially required risk factor for the development of cervical cancer, and many investigations have postulated HPV to be involved in the development of SCC as well. These studies extend, in part, on the findings of increased risk of SCC among patients with the genodermatosis that harbors HPV, namely EDV. Recent studies have posited an increased risk of SCC among individuals infected with the beta subtypes of HPV, particularly HPV 5 [33, 34]. This association and the specific mechanisms leading to the increased risk of SCC development have yet to be fully defined, and many studies are currently pursuing

Table 3.1.2 Incidence rates of SCC in different geographic regions

SCC rates per 100,000
271 M and 112 F in Arizona 1985–1996 [35]
97 M and 32 F in New Hampshire 1993–1994 [36]
775 M and 501 F in western Australia 1987–1992 [37]
600 M and 298 F Australia Nambour 1985–1992 [38]
29 M and 18 F in Switzerland 1991–1992 [39]
7 M and 4 F in Finland 1991–1995 [40]
14.2 M and 6.2 F in Jordan 1997–2001 [41]
34 M and 16 F in New Brunswick 1992–2001 [42]
161.1 M and 99.7 F in Rochester, MN 1994 [20]

more sensitive and broad-based molecular techniques and the biologic approaches to determine detailed patho-mechanisms leading to virally induced skin carcinogenesis (Table 3.1.2).

3.1.2.6 Pathogenesis of SCC

Unlike BCC where the seminal research discoveries in pathogenesis stemmed from the identification of a specific genetic defect, namely, the autosomal dominant disorder basal cell nevus syndrome, SCC has always been implicated as a cutaneous malignancy due largely to environmental exposures. Therefore, research directed to SCC has followed a broader, multifactorial approach, with particular focus on the effects of UV radiation on induction of these tumors [43]. Nonetheless, genetic mechanisms underpinning development of SCC are beginning to be uncovered. The most widely examined genetic defects in SCC and its precursor lesions are the RAS family oncogenes as well as CDKN2A and p53 tumor suppressor genes. Not surprisingly, based on the range of risk factors identified, none of these genes is universally mutated in SCC. However, they are sufficiently frequent to be altered and provide insight into potential pathways that inevitably are critical in the pathogenesis of SCC. In this context, combinations of these more common mutations as well as specific additional mutations yet to be identified will eventually be delineated and assembled into specific genetic networks that underlie the more complex and multifactorial malignant development and progression of keratinocyte pathologies in SCC.

3.1.2.6.1 RAS

RAS defects are one of the most frequently identified genetic aberrations in human cancers. Products of activating RAS genetic mutations promote downstream activity in the MAPK-mediated signaling pathway, which play an important role in

upregulation of cell proliferation [44]. There are several members of RAS family, including K-RAS, H-RAS, and N-RAS, with H-RAS being the most frequently mutated in SCC. H-RAS mutations have been implicated in up to 46% of SCCs [45]. Other reports have lower frequencies of SCC-associated RAS mutations in the 12% range, but have identified RAS mutations in up to 16% of actinic keratosis (AK), generally considered to be the characteristic precursor lesion of SCC [46]. It is unlikely that a RAS mutation alone can induce unchecked proliferation, as several studies have shown that RAS mutations alone induce cell cycle arrest [47, 48]. However, given the frequency of the observed mutation in SCC, RAS is likely one of several important molecular mediators in the pathogenesis of SCC.

3.1.2.6.2 P53

P53 is the most commonly identified mutation in SCC. Similar to its potential role in the pathogenesis of BCC, the p53 tumor suppressor gene acts as a principle guardian of the genome and mediates induction of DNA repair mechanisms in those cells deemed to be only moderately damaged while also inducing apoptosis in severely damaged cells [43]. Depending on the study, p53 mutations have been identified in 41, 58, and 69 % of SCC, and 50–60% of AK, with many of these mutations displaying the characteristic UV-induced pyrimidine dimer signature [49–51]. Mouse models of cutaneous SCC have demonstrated that UV-damaged cells harboring p53 mutation fail to undergo apoptosis, thus making them much more susceptible to further mutation [52]. While a p53 mutation alone may not induce SCC, it likely represents one critical step in a series of mutations that leads to the development of SCC.

3.1.2.6.3 CDK2NA and Chromosome 9q21

Normally, the CDK2NA locus on the short arm of chromosome 9 functions in mediating tumor suppression through its specifically expressed protein regulators p14(ARF)/p16(INK4a) and their downstream activity on the p53 pathway. Mutations on chromosome 9, which correspond closely with CDK2NA, have been identified in SCC ranging from 30 to 50% of tumors [53, 54]. Specific analysis of the CDK2NA locus yields rates of mutation between 9 and 42% of sporadic SCC identified [54, 55]. In comparative analysis, loss of the CD2KNA locus has been identified in approximately 21% of AK and 46% of SCC [56]. This intriguing result suggests that a mutation within this locus may be critical in the malignant transformation of the precursor lesion, AK to SCC.

3.1.2.7 Clinico-Pathologic Features and Prognosis

3.1.2.7.1 Invasive Squamous Cell Carcinoma

ICD-O

8070/3

Clinical

The vast majority of the common types of invasive SCC have characteristic clinical and histologic features that distinguish them from the less common pathological features of the other types of SCC delineated below [7]. They typically develop scaling, erythematous papular to more irregular elevated hyperkeratotic plaques that progress to more nodular and eventually large tumor lesions (Fig. 3.1.21). Other presentations include more keratotic, horn-like lesions, ulcers, verrucous lesions, or smooth nodules. These features can overlap with the specific histologic types further described below. The features of invasive SCC also vary with the anatomic location (Fig. 3.1.22). They develop in sun-exposed regions most often, but can also occur where other carcinogenic insults, including burns, scars, chronic heat exposure, or inflammatory dermatoses as well as ionizing radiation have targeted the skin [2, 3, 5, 7].

Dermatopathology

Invasive SCC has as its hallmark feature penetration of dysplastic keratinocytes beyond the basement membrane and into the dermis. Cellular atypia, disrupted keratinocyte

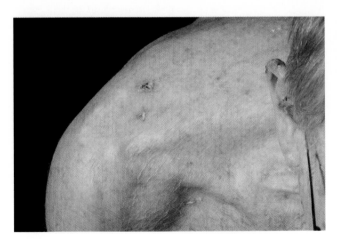

Fig. 3.1.21 SCCs of ear and shoulder

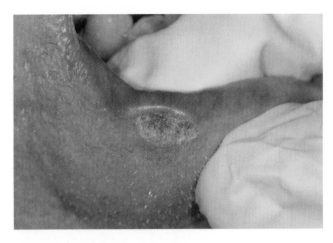

Fig. 3.1.22 Invasive SCC of lower lip

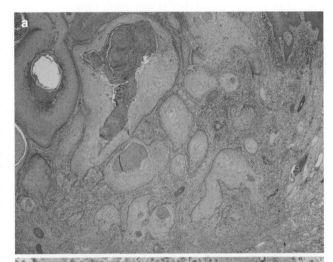

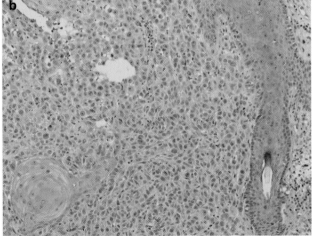

Fig. 3.1.23 (**a**) Invasive, well-differentiated SCC (H&E) 40×. (**b**) Invasive, moderately differentiated SCC (H&E) 200×

connections, and variable areas of keratinization are observed, depending on the grade of the tumor (Fig. 3.1.23a, b). A precursor lesion of invasive SCC is SCC in situ or Bowen's disease (Fig. 3.1.24).

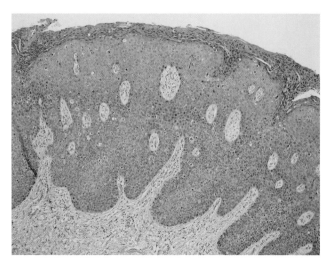

Fig. 3.1.24 Bowen's disease (SCC in situ) (H&E) 100×

Prognosis

As with the other types of SCC, traditional invasive SCC exhibits characteristic local growth and progression over time, but also harbors the potential for more aggressive invasion and metastasis as the malignancy advances. When it occurs, metastasis generally involves the regional lymph nodes. The likelihood of this event is fairly wide ranging for selected populations, being particularly high in immunosuppressed and solid organ transplant patients as well as patients with leukemias and lymphomas. Minimal or absent inflammatory response also appears to favor metastasis. Tumors arising in scars and higher grade lesions (Broders grade 3 or 4) as well as larger diameter (>2 cm) and deeper penetrating lesions (into reticular dermis and fat) also show greater propensity for metastasis [7].

3.1.2.7.2 Acantholytic (Adenoid) Squamous Cell Carcinoma

ICD-O

8075/3

Clinical

Acantholytic SCC typically accounts for approximately 2–4% of all cutaneous SCC [57, 58]. Similar to traditional SCC, it tends to occur on elderly men and presents clinically as a scaly to crusted, erythematous enlarging plaque typically developing on sun-exposed sites [58].

Dermatopathology

The defining characteristic of this subtype of SCC is the presence of acantholytic keratinocytes displaying the characteristic loosening of intercellular bridges and ballooning degeneration. Areas of acantholysis can range from small foci to quite large intraepidermal cavities, and these areas can even extend down follicles giving an almost pseudoglandular (adenoid) appearance [59] (Fig. 3.1.25). Under higher magnification, the typical features of SCC can be identified including dyskeratosis, keratinocyte atypia, increased cellular cytoplasm, increased mitotic figures, and altered maturation (Fig. 3.1.26a, b). Histopathologically, these lesions can look very similar to angiosarcoma (pseudovascular SCC), but it is important to make the distinction given the vastly different clinical and prognostic implications [59] (Fig. 3.1.27).

Prognosis

Distinguishing this variant of SCC has a twofold importance. Similar to traditional SCC, the overall prognosis is determined by depth and invasion. However, this variant has been postulated to be more aggressive than typical SCC, making this separate classification important [58, 60, 61]. The second reason to recognize this subtype is in distinguishing it from histologically similar, but very different lesions, such as angiosarcoma, adenocarcinoma, or several other benign acantholytic disorders [59].

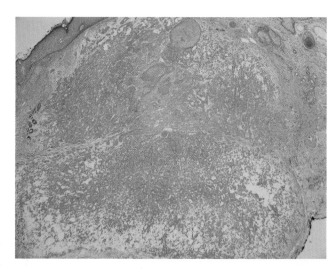

Fig. 3.1.25 Acantholytic/adenoid SCC (H&E) 20×

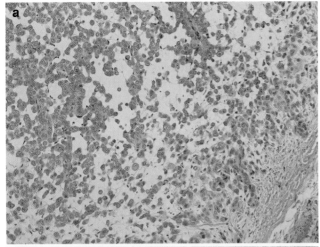

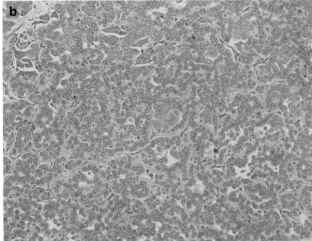

Fig. 3.1.26 (**a**) Acantholytic component (**b**) adenoid component of acantholytic/adenoid SCC (H&E) 200×

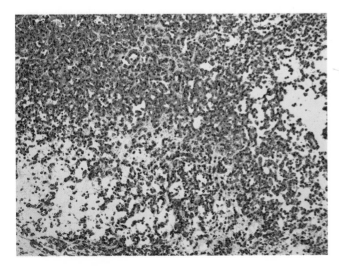

Fig. 3.1.27 Acantholytic/adenoid SCC (Cytokeratin) 200×

3.1.2.7.3 Spindle-Cell Squamous Cell Carcinoma

ICD-O

8074/3

Clinical

Spindle-cell SCC is a rare, high-risk subtype of SCC. It typically occurs in men on areas of sun damage, burn scars, and areas of previous radiation exposure [62]. Clinically, it typically appears as a fungating, exophytic mass and has a tendency to ulcerate and then become infected (Fig. 3.1.28). Rapid growth and aggressive invasion are hallmarks of this subtype [63].

Dermatopathology

Spindle-cell SCC derives its name from the histopathological appearance of poorly differentiated elongated oval cells with hyperchromatic nuclei infiltrating the underlying stroma

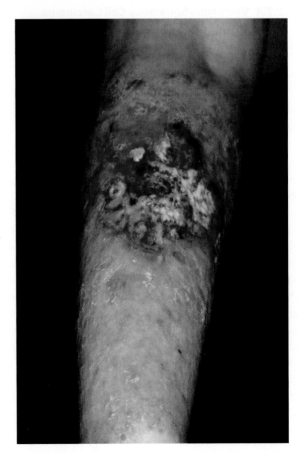

Fig. 3.1.28 Spindle-cell SCC. Fungating, infected tumor on posterior leg

and sometimes exhibiting a whorled pattern [62]. Histologic signs of keratinization are rarely seen. Occasionally, multinucleated pleomorphic giant cells can be found. It is important to differentiate these tumors from dermatofibroma sarcoma protuberans or spindle-cell malignant melanoma. Positive immunohistochemical stains for high molecular weight cytokeratin, variable staining with vimentin, and a negative stain for HMB-45 and S-100 can reliably exclude these other concerning entities and confirm a diagnosis of spindle-cell carcinoma [62].

Prognosis

These can have an aggressive appearance with a high rate of perineural invasion and an elevated risk for local recurrence. The risk for metastases, upwards of 10%, is thought to increase when these tumors arise in the sites of radiation, cutaneous scars, or burns. However, when not associated with a predisposing factor, these tumors are thought to have a very low risk of metastases [63, 64].

3.1.2.7.4 Verrucous Squamous Cell Carcinoma

ICD-O

8051/3

Clinical

Verrucous carcinoma accounts for about 2–12% of SCC and predominantly affects men in their fifth and sixth decade [65]. It typically has a much more malignant appearance clinically than histopathologically or by prognostic features. Part of the designated term, verrucous, derives from its clinical appearance as a cauliflower-like, exophytic, papillomatous growth similar to a large verruca vulgaris. It is most typically found on the oral mucosa, but is also located elsewhere and is subclassified by the location of the tumor: oral-Ackerman tumor or florid papillomatoses, genital-Buschke-Löwenstein, feet-epithelioma cuniculatum, or generalized-cutaneous verrucous carcinoma. Each of these subtypes has a distinctive clinical appearance, but each consistently demonstrates the unifying trait of a much worse clinical appearance than the actual prognosis or the histopathology demonstrates. Since these tumors are more frequently located in nonsun-exposed areas, multiple other subtype-dependent causative factors have been implicated in the development of these cancers including chronic irritation, local inflammation, poor hygiene, chemical carcinogens such as smokeless tobacco, long-standing ulceration, scars, and HPV(types 6 and 11) [65, 66].

Ackerman (Florid Papillomatosis)

First described by Ackerman in 1948, oral verrucous carcinoma is often referred to using the namesake of the pathologist who identified it or the newer term, florid papillomatosis [67]. These distinctive lesions account for approximately 2–12% of all oral carcinomas and tend to affect men in their fifth decade [65]. This variant is most frequently located on the buccal mucosa, but may also develop on the alveolar ridge, gingiva, and floor of the mouth (Fig. 3.1.29). Rare cases have been reported on the middle ear, maxillary antrum, nasal fossa, lacrimal duct, and bronchus [65]. It may initially appear as a soft, pale plaque, but often grows to form numerous keratinous papillary projections [67–69]. Tobacco is thought to be a major causative factor in the development of the oral variant of these tumors [65].

Epithelioma Cuniculatum

Epithelioma cuniculatum is an infrequent variant that often presents on the soles and initially may resemble a plantar wart, but slowly progresses to a boggy exophytic mass having a consistency described as an overripe orange [65, 70] (Fig. 3.1.30). There can be ulceration and sinus tracts with drainage of caseous material, and these tumors can be very painful or deforming [65, 70]. These tumors can also be found on the palms and digits with a similar presentation and prognosis.

Buschke-Löwenstein

Buschke-Löwenstein tumors account for approximately 5–24% of diagnosed penile cancers. Two-thirds of these tumors occur in men less than 50 and the majority of them are uncircumcised [71]. They are much more frequent on the penis than the vagina, cervix, vulva, rectum, or scrotum. Tumors in women are quite rare. There incidence has been difficult to estimate given their similar clinical appearance to that of a large condyloma acuminata [65]. They are often

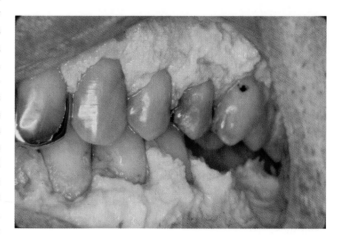

Fig. 3.1.29 Florid Papillomatosis (Ackerman tumor)

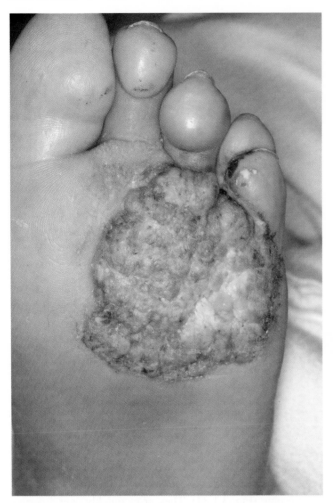

Fig. 3.1.30 Verrucous carcinoma or cuniculatum SCC of plantar foot

associated with HPV (types 6 and 11) infection and, therefore, have been considered to occupy a position along a developmental continuum of malignancy shared by viral warts [65]. Many define this variant as verrucal carcinoma on any anogenital mucosal including vagina, cervix, vulva, rectum, scrotum, or bladder, while others refer to it only when it occurs on the penis. In limited studies a poorer prognosis has been shown when these occur in the anorectal region [72].

Cutaneous Verrucous Carcinoma (Papillomatosis Cutis Carcinoids)

Cutaneous verrucous carcinoma or papillomatosis cutis carcinoids has generally been a historical term that refers to any verrucal carcinoma that does not fall into one of the other three main sight specific variants mentioned above. These are typically tumors that occur on areas such as the arms, legs, or trunk which by definition would exclude them from the other categories. Due to their rarity, there are few studies, and these have often been lumped in with the epithelioma cuniculatum variant [65].

Dermatopathology

Microscopically, these tumors display both an endophytic and exophytic growth pattern (Fig. 3.1.31). They tend to have blunt, deep, endophytic, pushing margins rather than infiltrative and destructive ones [73] (Fig. 3.1.32). They can form an extensive network of subepidermal extensions and sinuses that are cuniculate in their macroscopic appearance (rabbit-burrow-like) [65]. A hyperplastic epidermis is typical with vacuolated keratinocytes identical to the koilocytes of condylomata acuminata (Fig. 3.1.33). There is an edematous stroma with multiple inflammatory cells including neutrophils. Individual cells display very few mitotic figures, minimal atypia, and there is generally no foci of traditional SCC [73].

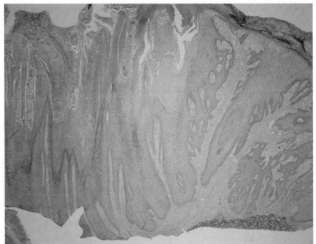

Fig. 3.1.31 Verrucous carcinoma

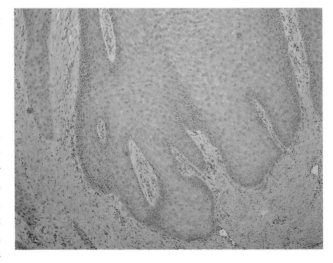

Fig. 3.1.32 Verrucous carcinoma with pushing borders (H&E) 100×

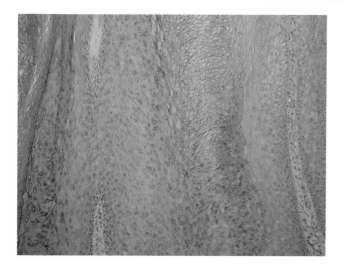

Fig. 3.1.33 Verrucous carcinoma with koilocytic change (H&E) 200×

Prognosis

Prognosis is typically that of a locally destructive tumor that has a low risk of metastasis, but a high risk of local recurrence if not completely excised. These tumors are known to infiltrate surrounding bone, muscle, and salivary glands -- in as many as 53% of tumors by some studies. If left untreated, the relentless local destruction can cause significant morbidity, and even mortality in the case of the difficult-to-detect esophageal variants. There have been several case reports of regional lymph node metastasis in epithelioma cuniculatum and other reports of tumors progressing into metastasizing SCC [65]. Generally with early detection and complete local excision, these tumors carry a very good prognosis.

3.1.2.7.5 Keratoacanthoma

ICD-O

8071/1

Clinical

Keratoacanthomas are commonly occurring lesions that have historically been categorized as a type of SCC, though this distinction still remains controversial [74]. Keratoacanthomas can share many features with typical invasive SCC, which has led to their association since their first description by Hutchinson in 1889 [63]. However, the biological and clinical evidence supports a separate classification of KA as a benign neoplasm, or at worst, a low-grade SCC [63].

Clinically, they present as eruptive pink to flesh-colored 1–2 cm dome-shaped nodule with a characteristic central

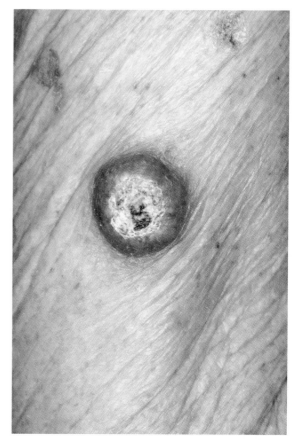

Fig. 3.1.34 Keratoacanthoma-SCC forearm

keratin plug (Fig. 3.1.34). They grow quickly over a period of 1–2 months and then spontaneously regress over a period of 4–6 months leaving a depressed scar. They typically occur on elderly men in their sixth or seventh decade on sun-exposed areas including the face and extremities, but can also occur on the trunk [63].

There are several recognized variants of KA including giant (>3 cm), KA centrifugum (characterized by peripheral growth and central healing), subungual KAs (rapid growth and local destruction), and multiple KA (Ferguson-Smith and Grzybowski types). KA of Ferguson-Smith is associated with internal malignancy and Muir-Torre syndrome. Grzybowski or eruptive type KA is distinguished by multiple (hundreds), rapidly appearing lesions, frequently involving the palms and soles. These eruptive KA lack any association with other syndromes or internal malignancy and follow a benign course in spite of their numbers [75].

Dermatopathology

Histopathologically, these tumors mimic well-differentiated SCC. On low power, these lesions have a characteristic well-circumscribed dome-shaped appearance with a centrally located keratin-filled crater surrounded by a mixed inflammatory infiltrate (Fig. 3.1.35). Like typical SCC, the cells are a proliferation of pale eosinophilic keratinocytes extending from an acanthotic epidermis in large buds and sheets displaying both an exophytic and endophytic growth pattern. The superficially located keratinocytes typically appear well differentiated, while those that are located deep or on the periphery can display prominent cytologic atypia and few mitoses [76, 77].

Prognosis

Much of the controversy surrounding this subtype of SCC centers on the argument that true KA is a benign, spontaneously resolving lesion and that any KA-like lesion that does not follow this benign course is actually an invasive SCC with very similar features histopathologically to a KA [74]. Others argue that, although rare, true KA has been observed to metastasize to the surrounding lymph nodes and tissue [76]. However, a recent review of these reports has disputed these findings on a case-by-case basis [63]. Definitive molecular testing has not yet been available to uniformly separate the two entities, SCC and KA; thus, morphology and histology remain the standard of identification [78]. With their similarity, the clinical standard of care remains to treat these lesions as SCC with local excision or destructive measures.

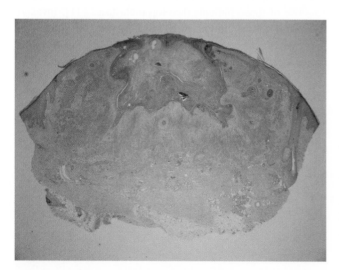

Fig. 3.1.35 Keratoacanthoma SCC (H&E) 20×

3.1.3 Bowen's Disease

Kazuyasu Fujii

Bowen's disease (BD) is a form of intraepidermal (in situ) squamous cell carcinoma of the skin and mucous membrane. It typically presents as a persistent, asymptomatic, scaly, or crusted erythematous plaque. Sun-exposed areas are the site of predilection, although any body part may be affected. Histopathologically, atypical cells are observed throughout the entire thickness of dermis. BD usually remains confined to epidermis; however, if it is left untreated, up to 5% of BD may become invasive.

3.1.3.1 Definition

Bowen's disease (BD) is a form of intraepidermal squamous cell carcinoma of the skin and mucous membrane with a low potential for invasive malignancy. BD can be distinguished from other precancerous conditions, such as actinic keratosis, as it presents with fullthickness involvement of large nonkeratinizing atypical keratinocytes.

3.1.3.2 ICD-O Code

8081/2

3.1.3.3 Synonyms

Morbus Bowen, squamous cell carcinoma in situ, carcinoma in situ of the skin

3.1.3.4 Clinical Features

BD represents a generally asymptomatic, extremely slowly growing and persistent plaque. Most affected individuals are in their sixth to eighth decade [13]. Typical BD lesions appear as a well-demarcated, irregularly bordered, slightly raised, scaly, erythematous plaque measuring a few millimeters to several centimeters in diameter (Fig. 3.1.36). Crusting, fissuring, and rarely pigmentation may be associated features.

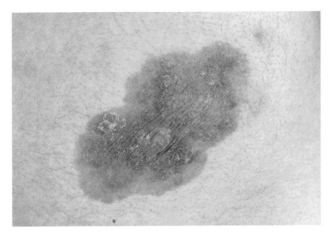

Fig. 3.1.36 Bowen's disease. A well-demarcated, irregular bordered, hyperkeratotic erythematous plaque on the buttock

Multiple lesions may be present. Ulceration is usually a sign of invasive carcinoma development. BD typically occurs in sun-exposed areas such as the head, neck, and lower legs [5, 8, 9, 12], though any part of the body may be affected. The actual cause of BD is unknown; however, chronic sun exposure has been established as a significant risk factor, especially for fair-complexioned people. Other etiologic factors include arsenic exposure, human papillomavirus (HPV), especially types 16, 18, and 31, immunosuppression, photodynamic therapy, and radiation therapy [6]. Because the morphology of the lesions is similar to that of other cutaneous disorders, BD is often not recognized initially. The clinical differential diagnosis includes psoriasis, nummular eczema, actinic keratosis, BCC, and amelanotic melanoma.

Erythroplasia of Queyrat is possibly the same entity of BD. It occurs exclusively under the foreskin of the penis and usually presents as a moist, glistening, slightly raised, well-defined, red plaque (Fig. 3.1.37). It has been overwhelmingly observed in uncircumcised males between 20 and 80 years old, most commonly in the fifth and sixth decade [7].

3.1.3.5 Histopathology

The typical histological features of the lesion are fullthickness replacement of the epidermis by atypical keratinocytes with loss of cellular polarity. Hyperkeratosis, parakeratosis, and irregular acanthosis are usually present. The atypical cells have large, hyperchromatic nuclei. Multinucleated keratinocytes and dyskeratotic cells are also frequently seen (Fig. 3.1.38). These cells are observed throughout the entire thickness of the epidermis, although the basement membrane remains intact. Adnexal structures are often involved, and this feature differentiates BD from actinic keratosis. A moderate to dense infiltrate of lymphocytes, histiocytes, and plasma cells is common in the superficial dermis. Increased vascularity and amyloid depositions also may be seen in the upper dermis. When the lesions are located in the sun-exposed areas, solar elastosis is prominent in the upper dermis.

In invasive Bowen's disease (Bowen's carcinoma), the findings consist of BD overlying an invasive tumor composed of large islands of squamoid and basaloid cells with central areas of necrosis and peripheral retraction artifact [2, 11].

3.1.3.6 Prognosis and Predictive Factors

While atypical cells are confined to the epidermis, the lesions do not demonstrate metastatic potential. However, if left untreated, up to 5% of BD may become invasive and up to 13–20% of those patients develop metastases [11]. Invasive squamous cell carcinoma in BD usually only develops after many years. The common presentation is a rapidly ulcerating tumor occurring in a preexisting scaly, erythematous, or

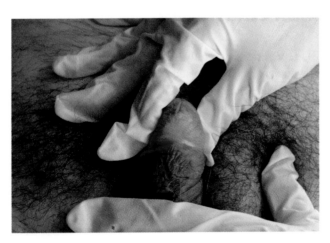

Fig. 3.1.37 Erythroplasia of Queyrat. A glistening, red plaque on the glans penis

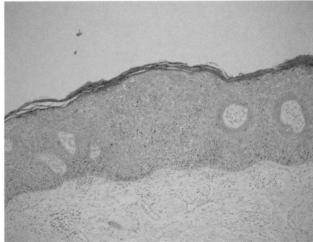

Fig. 3.1.38 Histological feature of Bowen's disease. Epidermal hyperplasia with atypical keratinocytes

pigmented patch [2]. Invasive BD occurs most commonly on the head and neck, followed by the extremities and trunk. Meanwhile, several cases of spontaneous complete or partial regression of BD also have been reported [3, 15, 17, 18].

In the past, this disease was thought to be a marker for internal cancers, although a significant number of recent investigations have shown no evidence for this association [1, 4, 10, 22]. Routine investigation for internal malignancy in patients with BD is not justified [6]. The exception is previous arsenic exposure. When there is good evidence of chronic arsenicalism, the possible evolution of a visceral malignancy, especially of the lung, should be kept in mind [16].

3.1.3.7 Bowenoid Papulosis

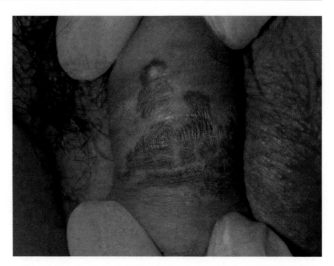

Fig. 3.1.39 Bowenoid papulosis. Flat-elevated, well-demarcated brownish plaques with a warty keratotic surface on the foreskin

Bowenoid papulosis (BP) typically appears as small, multiple, flat-top or verrucous, violaceous or red–brown papules (Fig. 3.1.39). It affects young, sexually active people in the 20–40-year age group. The genitalia are the site of predilection, although the perianal region may be the site of major involvement. The clinical differential diagnoses include condyloma acuminata, lichen planus, seborrheic keratoses, psoriasis, squamous cell carcinoma, basal cell carcinoma, and melanoma. Histologically, it bears resemblance to BD. It reveals hyperkeratosis, parakeratosis, irregular acanthosis, and papillomatosis. Dysplastic keratinocytes and mitotic figures are also present within the entire epidermis. The prognosis of BP is usually good. Spontaneous regression may occur within a few months, especially in young women, and development into invasive cancer is rare [20]. The transition from BP to invasive carcinoma usually occurs several

years after appearance of the primary lesion. High-risk HPVs, especially HPV 16 and 18, are regularly found in the lesions, and small number of cases with HPV 31, 32, 33, 34, 35, 39, 42, 48, 51, 52, 53, and 54 also have been reported [14, 24]. Moreover, the contributions of high-risk HPVs to the pathogenesis of BP have been indicated [14, 21]. Epidemiologic and virologic studies have established that BP can be sexually transmitted [23] and present a high risk for cervical carcinoma both for female patients and for sexual partners of male patients [19]. Therefore, sexual partners of patients are recommended to consult closely with their doctors. Because a strong association has been established between HPV type 16 and 18 and of the subsequent development of cervical cancer, HPV typing may be useful to identify patients at high risk.

3.1.4 Actinic Keratosis

Dorothea Terhorst and Eggert Stockfleth

3.1.4.1 Definition

Actinic keratoses (AKs) are proliferations of transformed, neoplastic keratinocytes confined to the epidermis and provoked by solar ultraviolet radiation. In 1896, Dubreuilh first described the special features of AK (keratosis senilis); Freudenthal illustrated its histological characteristics in 1926. Shortly after that, in 1931, Hookey elucidated that AKs may evolve into SCC or much less frequently into BCC. In 1958, Pinkus first introduced the term actinic keratosis [1].

For a long time, disagreement existed whether AK should be classified as precancerous lesions or carcinomas and a lively discussion still takes place. However, the literature leans toward a classification of AKs as in situ squamous cell carcinomas (SCCs) [2].

3.1.4.2 ICD-O Code

ICD code for AK is L57.0 (Version 2007).

3.1.4.3 Synonyms

Synonyms for actinic keratosis are numerous and include keratosis actinica, solar keratosis (keratosis solaris), and senile keratosis (keratosis senilis). As the appearance of AKs is not associated with old age per se, but rather with cumulative sun exposure, the term senile keratosis should be avoided. On lip mucosal surface, AK is known as actinic cheilitis. Keratinocytic intraepidermal neoplasia is a new term introduced, analogous to cervical intraepithelial neoplasia. Another name proposed is solar keratotic intraepidermal squamous cell carcinoma [1, 3].

3.1.4.4 Clinical Features

Typical AKs are skin-colored to reddish-brown scaly macules, papules, or plaques occurring in areas of chronic sun exposure, especially on face, forehead, scalp, ears, neck, décolleté, arms, dorsum of hands, and lower lips (Figs. 3.1.40–3.1.42). Lesions size ranges from a few millimeters up to 2 cm or more in diameter. It is characterized by a rough, scaly texture that resembles fine sandpaper. AKs can be classified into six clinical types: keratotic, atrophic, cornu

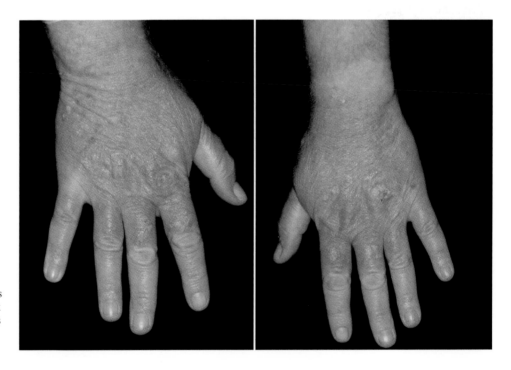

Fig. 3.1.40 Both hands of a 55-year-old patient show numerous hyperkeratotic plaques with partial confluence and thick adherent scaling. The patient has a history of long-standing occupational sun exposure

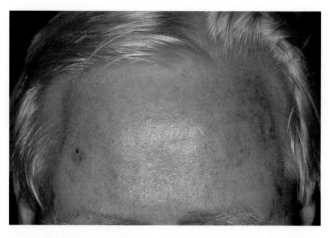

Fig. 3.1.41 The right forehead of the same patient shows a solitary scaly erythematous plaque which was rough on palpation

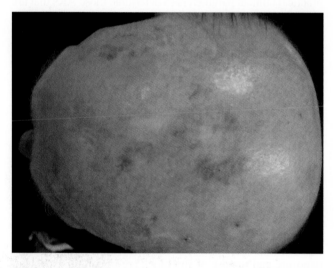

Fig. 3.1.42 The scalp of a kidney-transplanted patient receiving immunosuppressive therapy for 15 years. Multiple AKs and poikilodermia support the idea of field cancerisation

cutaneum, verrucous, pigmented, and lichenoid AK. Overlapping between subtypes is common. Similar to SCCs, a great majority of AKs are clinically asymptomatic, although sometimes local irritation and pruritus can be observed.

AKs rarely develop as solitary lesions; in fact, multiple lesions are commonly present (field cancerisation).

On the lips, AKs can present as actinic cheilitis with dryness, atrophy, and significant scaling or chapping; the lower lip is most commonly affected. Leukoplakia and focal hyperkeratosis may also be seen.

3.1.4.4.1 Risk Factors

AKs are mainly seen in older patients. However, in patients with genetically impaired UV-repair mechanisms such as albinism or xeroderma pigmentosum, AKs may already appear in childhood. The overall incidence is higher in men than in women, relating to a higher sun exposure in men [4].

3.1.4.4.2 Diagnostics

Diagnosis of AKs is generally based upon the typical clinical aspects. Histological confirmation is necessary to rule out invasive SCC, when clinical doubts exist, especially when the lesion is large, painful, pruritic, or bleeding. A cutaneous horn, for example, can result from AK, SCC, or verruca vulgaris. A biopsy that includes the dermis is required if deeper involvement needs to be excluded. Dermoscopy can be helpful in the differential diagnosis of pigmented AKs vs. lentigo maligna melanoma and superficial and/or pigmented basal cell carcinoma. Other techniques, including in vivo reflectance confocal microscopy (RCM), have been utilized in serial clinical investigations. RCM has recently been evaluated for diagnosis of AK with sensitivity rates of up to 97.7% in reference to histopathology as gold standard. In the context of "field cancerisation," repeated and multiple biopsies may not always be considered a practical approach. Therefore, evidence suggests that RCM may be a promising tool for the noninvasive evaluation, diagnosis, and monitoring of AKs [5]. Other new techniques such as the optical coherence tomography and high frequency ultrasound also show promising first results in detecting AKs [6].

3.1.4.5 Histopathology

AKs have been recognized as precursors of cancer or as precancerous lesions in the past. An ongoing discussion about its classification and definition shows that on histopathologic grounds alone, AK fulfills all criteria for SCC, thus being a very superficial SCC. AK and SCC are indistinguishable in the epidermal layer alone and may be contiguous with one another [7]. In a study of >1,000 SCC on sun-damaged skin, nearly 100% of these lesions contained histopathologic changes of AK at the periphery suggesting the concept of field cancerisation [8]. Early lesions are characterized by focally atypical keratinocytes (large pleomorphic nuclei, hyperchromatic nuclei) in the basal layer of the epidermis. The phenomenon of nuclear crowding describes nuclei packed closely together separated by little or no visible cytoplasm and often overlapping. In early and fully developed lesions the characteristic alternation of ortho- and parakeratosis can be found, sometimes referred to as flag sign. As further evidence for the actinic damage, actinic elastosis is depicted. Fully developed lesions may show hyperplasia (or sometimes atrophy) of the epidermis, rete ridges arranged in buds or columns, and a lymphocytic infiltrate of variable density. Atypical epidermal keratinocytes with dyskeratotic cells and mitotic figures involve mostly the lower half of the epidermis, sometimes with focal involvement of the full thickness of the epidermis.

The lichenoid subtype of AK is accompanied by dense band-like infiltrates of lymphocytes in the stratum papillare. Acantholytic dyskeratotic cells above suprabasal clefts are found in acantholytic AKs. Other histological types, modeled on the clinical types, are hypertrophic, bowenoid, acantholytic, lichenoid, and pigmented [9].

The degree of intraepidermal keratinocytic atypia is graded as either mild (AK I), moderate (AK II), or severe (AK III). In grade I the atypical keratinocytes are found in the basal and suprabasal layer, limited to the lower third of the epidermis, whereas in grade II atypical keratinocytes extend to the lower two-thirds of the epidermis and in grade III full thickness atypia of the epidermis is found, which is equivalent of changes previously called SCC in situ [10].

3.1.4.6 Prognosis and Predictive Factors

3.1.4.6.1 Prognosis

The risk of progression of AKs to invasive SCCs described in the literature ranges from 0.025 to 16%; extrapolation studies estimated the rate of progression at approximately 8–10% [11, 12].

One prospective study observed patients with the histopathologically confirmed diagnosis of AK. After an average of 2 years, an estimated 10% of the observed AKs developed into invasive SCCs [13].

An Australian survey estimated that approximately 60% of SCCs arise from AKs, the remainder coming from other predisposing conditions such as chronic wounds and radiation therapy [12].

AKs on mucosal surfaces carry a much greater risk for invasive SCC and SCC on mucosal surface also shows a higher metastatic potential [4, 7].

The risk of progression also depends on individual factors, such as drug therapy and acquired or iatrogenic immune suppression. High-risk AKs occur mainly in immunosuppressed patients [14]. Similarly, órgan-transplanted patients have a 250-fold higher risk to develop AKs and a 100-fold higher risk to develop invasive SCCs [15, 16]. About 40% of immunosuppressed patients with AKs develop an invasive SCC [15].

3.1.4.6.2 Predictive Factors

Clinically, it is not possible to determine with certainty whether or not and when an invasive SCC has developed. No distinct clinical boundaries exist between AKs and SCCs. It has been reported that before AKs progress to invasive SCCs, they may become inflamed and painful [17]. A systematic review of the literature was undertaken in order to obtain practical clinical parameters to determine those AKs that are at risk for becoming invasive SCCs. Major clinical parameters found were: induration (three studies), bleeding (three studies), enlargement in diameter (three studies), erythema (two studies), and ulceration (two studies). Minor criteria were pain, palpability, hyperkeratosis, pruritic lesions, and pigmentation [18].

3.1.4.6.3 Prevention

Prevention of AKs is an important part in AK management. Education of patients (UV-protection, self-examination, and detection of early lesions) is particularly important. AK is an ongoing disease that requires frequent follow-up (half-yearly to yearly) and long-term management. Avoiding sun exposure and the use of sun block are important aspects of preventing the development of AKs. Sun block has a combined emollient and photoprotective effect. Several studies showed that regularly applied sun block is effective not only in the prevention of AKs, but also in the reduction of AKs [19].

Preventive measures are invaluable and should be a major focus for those at risk, outdoor workers, patients with genetic UV-repair defects, fair skin phototypes, and immunocompromised patients. As cumulative solar exposure is a major risk factor for AKs, reducing sunlight exposure already in childhood may ultimately decrease the incidence of AKs later on.

In a recent single-center, matched-pairs, observational study, a group of 60 organ transplant recipients with daily application of a highly protective, liposomal sunscreen as part of their rigorous sun prevention behavior were compared with a control group with no explicit sun protective behavior. Within the duration of the study of 24 months, 42 of the 120 patients developed 82 new lesions of AK (all in the control group). Eight patients of the control group developed new invasive squamous cell carcinomas vs. none in the sunscreen group. In the sunscreen group, 102 preexisting AK-lesions went into spontaneous remission. Overall, the study concluded that sun protection measures have a positive impact on the high-risk group of organ transplant recipients [20].

3.1.4.7 Arsenic Keratosis

Arsenic has been known as both poison and medicine for a long time. In the 1700s, Thomas Fowler developed a solution of arsenic trioxide in potassium bicarbonate which has been used in the treatment of such different diseases as psoriasis, syphilis, eczema, and leprosy. Lacking benefits and manifesting health damage led to the abolition of Fowler's solution.

Nowadays, the absorption of arsenic takes place mainly through ingestion of water, food, beverage, and sometimes, swallowing of the inhaled particulate. Arsenic contamination of groundwater has led to a massive epidemic of arsenic poisoning and a global health problem, mostly in Bangladesh and Eastern India [21, 22].

Arsenic dermatosis appears after long years of intoxication and is composed of keratotic corns or warts on the palms and soles, generalized keratosis, and spotted melanosis interspersed with hypopigmentation on face, neck, back, palms, and soles. Solar elastosis is missing. When the diagnosis of chronic arsenicism is made, further cutaneous and internal neoplasms should be excluded.

The number and size of arsenic keratosis probably depend on the absorbed amount of arsenic. Arsenical keratoses are multiple and appear on areas not exposed to sunlight. Furthermore, skin cancers (M. Bowen, SCC, BCC) are associated with arsenic intoxication. Skin cancers can arise in the hyperkeratotic areas as well as appear on nonkeratotic areas of the trunk. In a study by Wong et al. the mean duration of Arsenic ingestion was 6.4 years and the latency period to the development of arsenical keratoses and squamous cell carcinoma of the skin was 28 and 41 years, respectively [23].

3.1.4.8 PUVA Keratosis

Psoralen plus ultraviolet-A radiation therapy (PUVA) has been utilized as a therapeutic modality for a variety of inflammatory proliferative skin conditions. Various types of hyperkeratotic lesions were described in psoriasis and vitiligo patients treated with photochemotherapy. PUVA keratoses appear as well-defined, discrete, gray–white, asymptomatic keratotic lesions,

approximately 4 mm in diameter, partly covered with adherend scales. PUVA keratoses are described to appear mostly on the extremities followed by the trunk. Histologically, lesions of PUVA keratosis showed marked hyperkeratosis with foci of incomplete parakeratosis in some lesions [24, 25].

These lesions are associated with an increased risk of SCC [26]. Well-defined and circular hand and foot keratoses have been described after high-dose PUVA treatment [27].

References

Basal Cell Carcinoma

1. Montgomery: Basal squamous cell epithelioma. Arch. Dermatol. Syphilol. **18**, 50–73 (1928)
2. Karpozilos, A., Pavlidis, N.: The treatment of cancer in Greek antiquity. Eur. J. Cancer **40**(14), 2033–2040 (2004)
3. Jacob, A.: An ulcer of peculiar character, which attacks the eye-lids and other parts of the face. Dublin Hosp. Rep. **4**, 232–239 (1827)
4. Weinstock, M.A., et al.: Nonmelanoma skin cancer mortality. A population-based study. Arch. Dermatol. **127**(8), 1194–1197 (1991)
5. Garner, K.L., Rodney, W.M.: Basal and squamous cell carcinoma. Prim. Care **27**(2), 447–458 (2000)
6. Rogers, H.W., et al.: Incidence Estimate of Nonmelanoma Skin Cancer in the United States, 2006. Arch Dermatol. **146**(3), 283–287 (2010)
7. Cancer.org. Cancer Org. [cited]; Available from: WWW.CANCER. ORG.
8. Crowson, A.N.: Basal cell carcinoma: biology, morphology and clinical implications. Mod. Pathol. **19**(Suppl 2), S127–S147 (2006)
9. Bastiaens, M.T., et al.: Differences in age, site distribution, and sex between nodular and superficial basal cell carcinoma indicate different types of tumors. J. Invest. Dermatol. **110**(6), 880–884 (1998)
10. Stang, A., et al.: Malignant melanoma and nonmelanoma skin cancers in Northrhine-Westphalia, Germany: a patient- vs. diagnosis-based incidence approach. Int. J. Dermatol. **46**(6), 564–570 (2007)
11. Scotto, J.F.T., Fraumeni, J.F.: Incidence of nonmelanocytic skin cancer in the United States. National Institutes of Health, Bethesda (1983)
12. Snow, S.N., et al.: Metastatic basal cell carcinoma. Report of five cases. Cancer **73**(2), 328–335 (1994)
13. Chen, J.G., et al.: Cost of nonmelanoma skin cancer treatment in the United States. Dermatol. Surg. **27**(12), 1035–1038 (2001)
14. Housman, T.S., et al.: Skin cancer is among the most costly of all cancers to treat for the Medicare population. J. Am. Acad. Dermatol. **48**(3), 425–429 (2003)
15. Armstrong, B.K., Kricker, A.: The epidemiology of UV induced skin cancer. J. Photochem. Photobiol. B Biol. **63**(1–3), 8–18 (2001)
16. Asuquo, M.E., et al.: Basal cell carcinoma in five albino Africans from the south-eastern equatorial rain forest of Nigeria. Int. J. Dermatol. **46**(7), 754–756 (2007)
17. Leiter, U., Garbe, C.: Epidemiology of melanoma and nonmelanoma skin cancer–the role of sunlight. Adv. Exp. Med. Biol. **624**, 89–103 (2008)
18. van Dam, R.M., et al.: Risk factors for basal cell carcinoma of the skin in men: results from the health professionals follow-up study. Am. J. Epidemiol. **150**(5), 459–468 (1999)

19. Gallagher, R.P., et al.: Sunlight exposure, pigmentary factors, and risk of nonmelanocytic skin cancer. I. Basal cell carcinoma. Arch. Dermatol. **131**(2), 157–163 (1995)

20. Lear, J.T., et al.: Risk factors for basal cell carcinoma in the UK: case-control study in 806 patients. J. R. Soc. Med. **90**(7), 371–374 (1997)

21. Marks, R.: Epidemiology of non-melanoma skin cancer and solar keratoses in Australia: a tale of self-immolation in Elysian fields. Australas. J. Dermatol. **38**(Suppl 1), S26–S29 (1997)

22. Kaidbey, K.H., et al.: Photoprotection by melanin–a comparison of black and Caucasian skin. J. Am. Acad. Dermatol. **1**(3), 249–260 (1979)

23. Yakubu, A., Mabogunje, O.A.: Skin cancer in Zaria, Nigeria. Trop. Doct. **25**(Suppl 1), 63–67 (1995)

24. Yakubu, A., Mabogunje, O.A.: Skin cancer in African albinos. Acta Oncol. **32**(6), 621–622 (1993)

25. Chuang, T.Y., et al.: Nonmelanoma skin cancer in Japanese ethnic Hawaiians in Kauai, Hawaii: an incidence report. J. Am. Acad. Dermatol. **33**(3), 422–426 (1995)

26. Suarez, B., et al.: Occupation and skin cancer: the results of the HELIOS-I multicenter case-control study. BMC Public Health **7**, 180 (2007)

27. Stone, J.L., et al.: Incidence of non-melanoma skin cancer in Kauai during 1983. Hawaii Med. J. **45**(8), 281–282 (1986) [erratum appears in Hawaii Med J 1986 Nov;45(11):378]

28. Allen, M., McKenzie, R.: Enhanced UV exposure on a ski-field compared with exposures at sea level. Photochem. Photobiol. Sci. **4**(5), 429–437 (2005)

29. Moehrle, M.: Outdoor sports and skin cancer. Clin. Dermatol. **26**(1), 12–15 (2008)

30. Ron, E., et al.: Skin tumor risk among atomic-bomb survivors in Japan. Cancer Causes Control **9**(4), 393–401 (1998)

31. Zak-Prelich, M., Narbutt, J., Sysa-Jedrzejowska, A.: Environmental risk factors predisposing to the development of basal cell carcinoma. Dermatol. Surg. **30**(2 Pt 2), 248–252 (2004)

32. Durrani, A.J., Miller, R.J., Davies, M.: Basal cell carcinoma arising in a laparoscopic port site scar at the umbilicus. Plast. Reconstr. Surg. **116**(1), 348–350 (2005)

33. Gurel, M.S., et al.: Basal cell carcinoma in a leishmanial scar. Clin. Exp. Dermatol. **30**(4), 444–445 (2005)

34. Kowal-Vern, A., Criswell, B.K.: Burn scar neoplasms: a literature review and statistical analysis. Burns **31**(4), 403–413 (2005)

35. Harris, R.B., Griffith, K., Moon, T.E.: Trends in the incidence of nonmelanoma skin cancers in southeastern Arizona, 1985–1996. J. Am. Acad. Dermatol. **45**(4), 528–536 (2001)

36. Karagas, M.R., et al.: Increase in incidence rates of basal cell and squamous cell skin cancer in New Hampshire, USA. New Hampshire Skin Cancer Study Group. Int. J. Cancer **81**(4), 555–559 (1999)

37. English, D.R., et al.: Incidence of non-melanocytic skin cancer in Geraldton, Western Australia. Int. J. Cancer **73**(5), 629–633 (1997)

38. Green, A., et al.: Skin cancer in a subtropical Australian population: incidence and lack of association with occupation. The Nambour Study Group. Am. J. Epidemiol. **144**(11), 1034–1040 (1996)

39. Levi, F., et al.: Trends in skin cancers in the Vaud canton, 1976–1992. Rev. Méd. Suisse Romande **115**(10), 739–746 (1995)

40. Hannuksela-Svahn, A., Pukkala, E., Karvonen, J.: Basal cell skin carcinoma and other nonmelanoma skin cancers in Finland from 1956 through 1995. [see comment]. Arch. Dermatol. **135**(7), 781–786 (1999)

41. Omari, A.K., Khammash, M.R., Matalka, I.: Skin cancer trends in northern Jordan. Int. J. Dermatol. **45**(4), 384–388 (2006)

42. Hayes, R.C., et al.: Incidence of nonmelanoma skin cancer in New Brunswick, Canada, 1992 to 2001. J. Cutan. Med. Surg. **11**(2), 45–52 (2007)

43. Lacour, J.P.: Carcinogenesis of basal cell carcinomas: genetics and molecular mechanisms. Br. J. Dermatol. **146**(Suppl 61), 17–19 (2002)

44. Halliday, G.M.: Inflammation, gene mutation and photoimmuno-suppression in response to UVR-induced oxidative damage contributes to photocarcinogenesis. Mutat. Res. **571**(1–2), 107–120 (2005)

45. Derry, W.B., Putzke, A.P., Rothman, J.H.: Caenorhabditis elegans p53: role in apoptosis, meiosis, and stress resistance. Science **294**(5542), 591–595 (2001)

46. Kogerman, P., et al.: Alternative first exons of PTCH1 are differentially regulated in vivo and may confer different functions to the PTCH1 protein. Oncogene **21**(39), 6007–6016 (2002)

47. Xie, J., et al.: Activating Smoothened mutations in sporadic basal-cell carcinoma. Nature **391**(6662), 90–92 (1998)

48. Scrivener, Y., Grosshans, E., Cribier, B.: Variations of basal cell carcinomas according to gender, age, location and histopathological subtype. Br. J. Dermatol. **147**(1), 41–47 (2002)

49. Hood, A.F., Kwan, T.H., Mihm, M.C., et al.: Primer of Dermatopathology, 3rd edn. Lippincott Williams and Wilkins, Philidelphia (2002)

50. Bolognia, J.L., Jorizzo, J.L., Rapini, R.P.: Dermatology, vol. 2, 2nd edn. Mosby/Elsevier, Philadelphia (2008)

51. Kirkham, N.: Lever's Histopathology of the Skin, 8th edn. Lippincott-Raven, Philidelphia (1997)

52. Nouri, K. (ed) Skin Cancer. McGraw-Hill. New York. (2008)

53. Sachs, D.L., Marghoob, A.A., Halpern, A.: Skin cancer in the elderly. Clin. Geriatr. Med. **17**(4), 715–38 (2001)

54. Wrone, D.A., et al.: Increased proportion of aggressive-growth basal cell carcinoma in the Veterans Affairs population of Palo Alto, California. J. Am. Acad. Dermatol. **35**(6), 907–910 (1996)

55. Goldberg, L.H., Leis, P., Pham, H.N.: Basal cell carcinoma on the neck. Dermatol. Surg. **22**(4), 349–353 (1996)

56. Ramdial, P.K., et al.: bcl-2 protein expression in aggressive and non-aggressive basal cell carcinomas. J. Cutan. Pathol. **27**(6), 283–291 (2000)

57. Zagrodnik, B., et al.: Superficial radiotherapy for patients with basal cell carcinoma: recurrence rates, histologic subtypes, and expression of p53 and Bcl-2. Cancer **98**(12), 2708–2714 (2003)

58. Farhi, D., et al.: Incomplete excision of basal cell carcinoma: rate and associated factors among 362 consecutive cases. Dermatol. Surg. **33**(10), 1207–1214 (2007)

59. Anthouli-Anagnostopoulou, F., Hatziolou, E.: Recurrent morphean basal cell carcinoma of the skin. A clinico-histopathological study of 97 cases. Adv. Clin. Pathol. **6**(1), 17–24 (2002)

60. Siegle, R.J., MacMillan, J., Pollack, S.V.: Infiltrative basal cell carcinoma: a nonsclerosing subtype. J. Dermatol. Surg. Oncol. **12**(8), 830–836 (1986)

61. Cohen, P.R., Schulze, K.E., Nelson, B.R.: Basal cell carcinoma with mixed histology: a possible pathogenesis for recurrent skin cancer. Dermatol. Surg. **32**(4), 542–551 (2006)

62. Hendrix Jr., J.D., Parlette, H.L.: Duplicitous growth of infiltrative basal cell carcinoma: analysis of clinically undetected tumor extent in a paired case-control study. Dermatol. Surg. **22**(6), 535–539 (1996)

63. Hendrix Jr., J.D., Parlette, H.L.: Micronodular basal cell carcinoma. A deceptive histologic subtype with frequent clinically undetected tumor extension. Arch. Dermatol. **132**(3), 295–298 (1996)

64. Sexton, M., Jones, D.B., Maloney, M.E.: Histologic pattern analysis of basal cell carcinoma. Study of a series of 1039 consecutive neoplasms. J. Am. Acad. Dermatol. **23**(6 Pt 1), 1118–1126 (1990)

65. Cherpelis, B.S., Marcusen, C., Lang, P.G.: Prognostic factors for metastasis in squamous cell carcinoma of the skin. Dermatol. Surg. **28**(3), 268–273 (2002)

66. Martin 2nd, R.C., et al.: Basosquamous carcinoma: analysis of prognostic factors influencing recurrence. Cancer **88**(6), 1365–1369 (2000)

67. Garcia, C., Poletti, E., Crowson, A.N.: Basosquamous carcinoma. J. Am. Acad. Dermatol. **1**(60), 137–143 (2009)

68. Maloney, M.L.: What is basosquamous carcinoma? Dermatol. Surg. **26**(5), 505–506 (2000)

69. Bowman, P.H.: Basosquamous carcinoma. Dermatol. Surg. **29**(8), 830–832 (2003). discussion 833
70. Sendur, N., et al.: Cutaneous basosquamous carcinoma infiltrating cerebral tissue. J. Eur. Acad. Dermatol. Venereol. **18**(3), 334–336 (2004)
71. de Faria, J.L., Navarrete, M.A.: The histopathology of the skin basal cell carcinoma with areas of intermediate differentiation. A metatypical carcinoma? Pathol. Res. Pract. **187**(8), 978–985 (1991)
72. Barnes, L., et al.: Basaloid squamous cell carcinoma of the head and neck: clinicopathological features and differential diagnosis. Ann. Otol. Rhinol. Laryngol. **105**(1), 75–82 (1996)
73. Saldanha, G., Fletcher, A., Slater, D.N.: Basal cell carcinoma: a dermatopathological and molecular biological update. Br. J. Dermatol. **148**(2), 195–202 (2003)
74. Walsh, N., Ackerman, A.B.: Infundibulocystic basal cell carcinoma: a newly described variant. Mod. Pathol. **3**(5), 599–608 (1990)
75. Kelly, S.C., Ermolovich, T., Purcell, S.M.: Nonsyndromic segmental multiple infundibulocystic basal cell carcinomas in an adolescent female. Dermatol. Surg. **32**(9), 1202–1208 (2006) [erratum appears in Dermatol. Surg. 2006 Oct;32(10):1308]
76. Pinkus, H.: Epithelial and fibroepithelial tumors. Arch. Dermatol. **91**, 24–37 (1965)
77. Bowen, A.R., LeBoit, P.E.: Fibroepithelioma of pinkus is a fenestrated trichoblastoma. Am. J. Dermatopathol. **27**(2), 149–154 (2005)
78. Heenan, P.J., Bogle, M.S.: Eccrine differentiation in basal cell carcinoma. J. Investig. Dermatol. **100**(3), 295S–299S (1993)
79. Sakamoto, F., et al.: Basal cell tumor with apocrine differentiation: apocrine epithelioma. J. Am. Acad. Dermatol. **13**(2 Pt 2), 355–363 (1985)
80. Oliver, G.F., Winkelmann, R.K.: Clear-cell, basal cell carcinoma: histopathological, histochemical, and electron microscopic findings. J. Cutan. Pathol. **15**(6), 404–408 (1988)
81. Aloi, F.G., Molinero, A., Pippione, M.: Basal cell carcinoma with matrical differentiation. Matrical carcinoma. Am. J. Dermatopathol. **10**(6), 509–513 (1988)
82. Misago, N., Satoh, T., Narisawa, Y.: Cornification (keratinization) in Basal cell carcinoma: a histopathological and immunohistochemical study of 16 cases. J. Dermatol. **31**(8), 637–650 (2004)
83. Takemoto, S., et al.: Giant basal cell carcinoma: improvement in the quality of life after extensive resection. Scand. J. Plast. Reconstr. Surg. Hand Surg. **37**(3), 181–185 (2003)
84. Sahl Jr., W.J., Snow, S.N., Levine, N.S.: Giant basal cell carcinoma. Report of two cases and review of the literature. J. Am. Acad. Dermatol. **30**(5 Pt 2), 856–859 (1994)
85. Randle, H.W.: Basal cell carcinoma. Identification and treatment of the high-risk patient. Dermatol. Surg. **22**(3), 255–261 (1996)
86. Kokavec, R., Fedeles, J.: Giant basal cell carcinomas: a result of neglect? Acta Chir. Plast. **46**(3), 67–69 (2004)
87. Maloney, M.E., Jones, D.B., Sexton, F.M.: Pigmented basal cell carcinoma: investigation of 70 cases. J. Am. Acad. Dermatol. **27**(1), 74–78 (1992)
88. Solyemani, A.D., et al.: Metastatic basal cell carcinoma presenting with unilateral upper extremity edema and lymphatic spread. J. Am. Acad. Dermatol. **59**(2), s1–s3 (2008)
89. Snow, S.N., et al.: Metastatic basal cell cancer. Report of five cases. Cancer **73**, 328–335 (1994)
90. Von Hoff, D.D., et al.: Inhibition of the hedgehog pathway in advanced basal-cell carcinoma. N. Engl. J. Med. **361**(12), 1164–1172 (2009)

Squamous Cell Carcinoma

1. Pott, P.: Chirurgical Observations Relative to the Cataract, the Polypus of the Nose, the Cancer of the Scrotum, and Different Kinds of Ruptures, and Mortification of the Toes and Feet. L. Hawes, W.Clarke and R. Collins. London (1775)
2. Waterhouse, J.A.: Cutting oils and cancer. Ann. Occup. Hyg. **14**(2), 161–170 (1971)
3. Horton, C.E., et al.: The malignant potential of burn scar. Plast. Reconstr. Surg. Transplant. Bull. **22**(4), 348–353 (1958)
4. Hutchinson, J.: Arsenic cancer. Br. Med. J. **2**, 1280–1281 (1887)
5. Traenkle, H.: X-ray induced skin cancer in man. Natl. Cancer Inst. Monogr. **10**, 423–432 (1963)
6. Dabski, K., Stoll Jr., H.L.: Skin cancer caused by grenz rays. J. Surg. Oncol. **31**(2), 87–93 (1986)
7. Garner, K.L., Rodney, W.M.: Basal and squamous cell carcinoma. Prim. Care **27**(2), 447–458 (2000)
8. Cancer.org. Cancer Org. [cited]; Available from: WWW.CANCER. ORG.
9. Rogers, H.W., et al.: Incidence Estimate of Nonmelanoma Skin Cancer in the United States, 2006. Arch Dermatol. **146**(3), 283–287 (2010)
10. Crowson, A.N.: Basal cell carcinoma: biology, morphology and clinical implications. Mod. Pathol. **19**(Suppl 2), S127–S147 (2006)
11. Demers, A.A., et al.: Trends of nonmelanoma skin cancer from 1960 through 2000 in a Canadian population. J. Am. Acad. Dermatol. **53**(2), 320–328 (2005)
12. Miller, D.L., Weinstock, M.A.: Nonmelanoma skin cancer in the United States: incidence. J. Am. Acad. Dermatol. **30**(5 Pt 1), 774–778 (1994)
13. Diepgen, T.L., Mahler, V.: The epidemiology of skin cancer. Br. J. Dermatol. **146**(Suppl 61), 1–6 (2002)
14. Stang, A., et al.: Malignant melanoma and nonmelanoma skin cancers in Northrhine-Westphalia, Germany: a patient- vs. diagnosis-based incidence approach. Int. J. Dermatol. **46**(6), 564–570 (2007)
15. Weinberg, A.S., Ogle, C.A., Shim, E.K.: Metastatic cutaneous squamous cell carcinoma: an update. Dermatol. Surg. **33**(8), 885–899 (2007)
16. Snow, S.N., et al.: Metastatic basal cell carcinoma. Report of five cases. Cancer **73**(2), 328–335 (1994)
17. Chen, J.G., et al.: Cost of nonmelanoma skin cancer treatment in the United States. Dermatol. Surg. **27**(12), 1035–1038 (2001)
18. Housman, T.S., et al.: Skin cancer is among the most costly of all cancers to treat for the Medicare population. J. Am. Acad. Dermatol. **48**(3), 425–429 (2003)
19. Armstrong, B.K., Kricker, A.: The epidemiology of UV induced skin cancer. J. Photochem. Photobiol. B Biol. **63**(1–3), 8–18 (2001)
20. Gray, D.T., et al.: Trends in the population-based incidence of squamous cell carcinoma of the skin first diagnosed between 1984 and 1992. Arch. Dermatol. **133**(6), 735–740 (1997)
21. Giles, G.G., Marks, R., Foley, P.: Incidence of non-melanocytic skin cancer treated in Australia. Br. Med. J. (Clin. Res. Ed.) **296**(6614), 13–17 (1988)
22. Kaidbey, K.H., et al.: Photoprotection by melanin–a comparison of black and Caucasian skin. J. Am. Acad. Dermatol. **1**(3), 249–260 (1979)
23. Gallagher, R.P., et al.: Sunlight exposure, pigmentary factors, and risk of nonmelanocytic skin cancer. I. Basal cell carcinoma. Arch. Dermatol. **131**(2), 157–163 (1995)

24. Jensen, P., et al.: Skin cancer in kidney and heart transplant recipients and different long-term immunosuppressive therapy regimens. [see comment]. J. Am. Acad. Dermatol. **40**(2 Pt 1), 177–186 (1999)
25. Suarez, B., et al.: Occupation and skin cancer: the results of the HELIOS-I multicenter case-control study. BMC Public Health **7**, 180 (2007)
26. Stone, J.L., et al.: Incidence of non-melanoma skin cancer in Kauai during 1983. Hawaii Med. J. **45**(8), 281–282 (1986) [erratum appears in Hawaii Med. J. 1986 Nov;45(11):378]
27. Chuang, T.Y., et al.: Nonmelanoma skin cancer in Japanese ethnic Hawaiians in Kauai, Hawaii: an incidence report. J. Am. Acad. Dermatol. **33**(3), 422–426 (1995)
28. Allen, M., McKenzie, R.: Enhanced UV exposure on a ski-field compared with exposures at sea level. Photochem. Photobiol. Sci. **4**(5), 429–437 (2005)
29. Moehrle, M.: Outdoor sports and skin cancer. Clin. Dermatol. **26**(1), 12–15 (2008)
30. De Hertog, S.A., et al.: Relation between smoking and skin cancer. J. Clin. Oncol. **19**(1), 231–238 (2001)
31. Gallagher, R.P., et al.: Chemical exposures, medical history, and risk of squamous and basal cell carcinoma of the skin. Cancer Epidemiol. Biomark. Prev. **5**(6), 419–424 (1996)
32. Everall, J.D., Dowd, P.M.: Influence of environmental factors excluding ultra violet radiation on the incidence of skin cancer. Bull. Cancer **65**(3), 241–247 (1978)
33. Masini, C., et al.: Evidence for the association of human papillomavirus infection and cutaneous squamous cell carcinoma in immunocompetent individuals. Arch. Dermatol. **139**(7), 890–894 (2003)
34. Karagas, M.R., et al.: Human papillomavirus infection and incidence of squamous cell and basal cell carcinomas of the skin. [see comment]. J. Natl. Cancer Inst. **98**(6), 389–395 (2006)
35. Harris, R.B., Griffith, K., Moon, T.E.: Trends in the incidence of nonmelanoma skin cancers in southeastern Arizona, 1985–1996. J. Am. Acad. Dermatol. **45**(4), 528–536 (2001)
36. Karagas, M.R., et al.: Increase in incidence rates of basal cell and squamous cell skin cancer in New Hampshire, USA. New Hampshire Skin Cancer Study Group. Int. J. Cancer **81**(4), 555–559 (1999)
37. English, D.R., et al.: Incidence of non-melanocytic skin cancer in Geraldton, Western Australia. Int. J. Cancer **73**(5), 629–633 (1997)
38. Green, A., et al.: Skin cancer in a subtropical Australian population: incidence and lack of association with occupation. The Nambour Study Group. Am. J. Epidemiol. **144**(11), 1034–1040 (1996)
39. Levi, F., et al.: Trends in skin cancers in the Vaud canton, 1976–1992. Rev. Méd. Suisse Romande **115**(10), 739–746 (1995)
40. Hannuksela-Svahn, A., Pukkala, E., Karvonen, J.: Basal cell skin carcinoma and other nonmelanoma skin cancers in Finland from 1956 through 1995.[see comment]. Arch. Dermatol. **135**(7), 781–786 (1999)
41. Omari, A.K., Khammash, M.R., Matalka, I.: Skin cancer trends in northern Jordan. Int. J. Dermatol. **45**(4), 384–388 (2006)
42. Hayes, R.C., et al.: Incidence of nonmelanoma skin cancer in New Brunswick, Canada, 1992 to 2001. J. Cutan. Med. Surg. **11**(2), 45–52 (2007)
43. Nataraj, A.J., Trent II, J.C., Ananthaswamy, H.N.: p53 gene mutations and photocarcinogenesis. Photochem. Photobiol. **62**(2), 218–230 (1995)
44. Shields, J.M., et al.: Understanding Ras: 'it ain't over 'til it's over'. Trends Cell Biol. **10**(4), 147–154 (2000)
45. Pierceall, W.E., et al.: Ras gene mutation and amplification in human nonmelanoma skin cancers. Mol. Carcinog. **4**(3), 196–202 (1991)
46. Spencer, J.M., et al.: Activated ras genes occur in human actinic keratoses, premalignant precursors to squamous cell carcinomas. Arch. Dermatol. **131**(7), 796–800 (1995)
47. Lazarov, M., et al.: CDK4 coexpression with Ras generates malignant human epidermal tumorigenesis. Nat. Med. **8**(10), 1105–1114 (2002)
48. Dajee, M., et al.: NF-kappaB blockade and oncogenic Ras trigger invasive human epidermal neoplasia.[see comment]. Nature **421**(6923), 639–643 (2003)
49. Brash, D.E., et al.: A role for sunlight in skin cancer: UV-induced p53 mutations in squamous cell carcinoma. Proc. Natl. Acad. Sci. USA **88**(22), 10124–10128 (1991)
50. Bolshakov, S., et al.: p53 mutations in human aggressive and nonaggressive basal and squamous cell carcinomas. Clin. Cancer Res. **9**(1), 228–234 (2003)
51. Campbell, C., et al.: p53 mutations are common and early events that precede tumor invasion in squamous cell neoplasia of the skin. J. Invest. Dermatol. **100**(6), 746–748 (1993)
52. Ziegler, A., et al.: Sunburn and p53 in the onset of skin cancer.[see comment]. Nature **372**(6508), 773–776 (1994)
53. Quinn, A.G., Sikkink, S., Rees, J.L.: Delineation of two distinct deleted regions on chromosome 9 in human non-melanoma skin cancers. Genes Chromosom. Cancer **11**(4), 222–225 (1994)
54. Saridaki, Z., et al.: Mutational analysis of CDKN2A genes in patients with squamous cell carcinoma of the skin. Br. J. Dermatol. **148**(4), 638–648 (2003)
55. Kreimer-Erlacher, H., et al.: High frequency of ultraviolet mutations at the INK4a-ARF locus in squamous cell carcinomas from psoralen-plus-ultraviolet-A-treated psoriasis patients. J. Invest. Dermatol. **120**(4), 676–682 (2003)
56. Mortier, L., et al.: Progression of actinic keratosis to squamous cell carcinoma of the skin correlates with deletion of the 9p21 region encoding the p16(INK4a) tumor suppressor. Cancer Lett. **176**(2), 205–214 (2002)
57. Johnson, W.C., Helwig, E.B.: Adenoid squamous cell carcinoma (adenoacanthoma). A clinicopathologic study of 155 patients. Cancer **19**(11), 1639–1650 (1966)
58. Nappi, O., Pettinato, G., Wick, M.R.: Adenoid (acantholytic) squamous cell carcinoma of the skin. J. Cutan. Pathol. **16**(3), 114–121 (1989)
59. Nappi, O., et al.: Pseudovascular adenoid squamous cell carcinoma of the skin. A neoplasm that may be mistaken for angiosarcoma. Am. J. Surg. Pathol. **16**(5), 429–438 (1992)
60. Cherpelis, B.S., Marcusen, C., Lang, P.G.: Prognostic factors for metastasis in squamous cell carcinoma of the skin. Dermatol. Surg. **28**(3), 268–273 (2002)
61. Ikegawa, S., et al.: Vimentin-positive squamous cell carcinoma arising in a burn scar. A highly malignant neoplasm composed of acantholytic round keratinocytes. Arch. Dermatol. **125**(12), 1672–1676 (1989)
62. Petter, G., Haustein, U.F.: Histologic subtyping and malignancy assessment of cutaneous squamous cell carcinoma. Dermatol. Surg. **26**(6), 521–530 (2000)
63. Cassarino, D.S., Derienzo, D.P., Barr, R.J.: Cutaneous squamous cell carcinoma: a comprehensive clinicopathologic classification–part two. J. Cutan. Pathol. **33**(4), 261–279 (2006)
64. Cassarino, D.S., Derienzo, D.P., Barr, R.J.: Cutaneous squamous cell carcinoma: a comprehensive clinicopathologic classification. Part one. J. Cutan. Pathol. **33**(3), 191–206 (2006)
65. Schwartz, R.A.: Verrucous carcinoma of the skin and mucosa. [see comment]. J. Am. Acad. Dermatol. **32**(1), 1–21 (1995). quiz 22–24. [erratum appears in J Am Acad Dermatol 1995 May;32(5 Pt 1):710]
66. Schon, M.P., et al.: Presternal verrucous carcinoma. Hautarzt **51**(10), 766–769 (2000)
67. Ackerman, L.: Verrucous carcinoma of the oral cavity. Surgery **23**(4), 670–678 (1948)
68. Kraus, F.T., Perezmesa, C.: Verrucous carcinoma. Clinical and pathologic study of 105 cases involving oral cavity, larynx and genitalia. Cancer **19**(1), 26–38 (1966)
69. Goethals, P.L., Harrison Jr., E.G., Devine, K.D.: Verrucous squamous carcinoma of the oral cavity. Am. J. Surg. **106**, 845–851 (1963)
70. Kao, G.F.: Carcinoma arising in Bowen's disease. Arch. Dermatol. **122**(10), 1124–1126 (1986)

71. Lawrence-Brown, M.M., et al.: Carcinoma cuniculatum of the abdominal wall. Med. J. Aust. **140**(11), 668–669 (1984)
72. Chu, Q.D., et al.: Giant condyloma acuminatum (Buschke-Lowenstein tumor) of the anorectal and perianal regions. Analysis of 42 cases. Dis. Colon Rectum **37**(9), 950–957 (1994)
73. Pindborg, J.J., Reichart, P.A., Smith, C.J.: Histological Typing of Cancer and Precancer of the Oral Mucosa, 2nd edn. Springer, Berlin (1997)
74. Kossard, S., Tan, K.-B., Choy, C.: Keratoacanthoma and infundibulocystic squamous cell carcinoma. Am. J. Dermatopathol. **30**(2), 127–134 (2008)
75. Schwartz, R.A., Blaszczyk, M., Jablonska, S.: Generalized eruptive keratoacanthoma of Grzybowski: follow-up of the original description and 50-year retrospect. Dermatology **205**(4), 348–352 (2002)
76. Hodak, E., Jones, R.E., Ackerman, A.B.: Solitary keratoacanthoma is a squamous-cell carcinoma: three examples with metastases.[see comment]. Am. J. Dermatopathol. **15**(4), 332–342 (1993). discussion 343–352
77. Rinker, M.H., et al.: Histologic variants of squamous cell carcinoma of the skin. Cancer Control **8**(4), 354–363 (2001)
78. Cain, C.T., Niemann, T.H., Argenyi, Z.B.: Keratoacanthoma versus squamous cell carcinoma. An immunohistochemical reappraisal of p53 protein and proliferating cell nuclear antigen expression in keratoacanthoma-like tumors.[see comment]. Am. J. Dermatopathol. **17**(4), 324–331 (1995)

Bowen's Disease

1. Arbesman, H., Ransohoff, D.F.: Is Bowen's disease a predictor for the development of internal malignancy? A methodological critique of the literature. JAMA **257**, 516–518 (1987)
2. Cassarino, D.S., Derienzo, D.P., Barr, R.J.: Cutaneous squamous cell carcinoma: a comprehensive clinicopathologic classification–part two. J. Cutan. Pathol. **33**, 261–279 (2006)
3. Chisiki, M., Kawada, A., Akiyama, M., Itoh, Y., Tajima, S., Ishibashi, A., Yudate, F.: Bowen's disease showing spontaneous complete regression associated with apoptosis. Br. J. Dermatol. **40**, 939–944 (1999)
4. Chute, C.G., Chuang, T.Y., Bergstralh, E.J., Su, W.P.: The subsequent risk of internal cancer with Bowen's disease. A population-based study. JAMA **266**, 816–819 (1991)
5. Cox, N.H.: Body site distribution of Bowen's disease. Br. J. Dermatol. **130**, 714–716 (1994)
6. Cox, N.H., Eedy, D.J., Morton, C.A.: Therapy Guidelines and Audit Subcommittee, British Association of Dermatologists. Guidelines for management of Bowen's disease: 2006 update. Br. J. Dermatol. **156**, 11–21 (2007)
7. Goette, D.K.: Review of erythroplasia of Queyrat and its treatment. Urology **8**, 311–315 (1976)
8. Foo, C.C., Lee, J.S., Guilanno, V., Yan, X., Tan, S.H., Giam, Y.C.: Squamous cell carcinoma and Bowen's disease of the skin in Singapore. Ann. Acad. Med. Singapore **36**, 189–193 (2007)
9. Hansen, J.P., Drake, A.L., Walling, H.W.: Bowen's Disease: a four-year retrospective review of epidemiology and treatment at a university center. Dermatol. Surg. **34**, 878–883 (2008)
10. Jaeger, A.B., Gramkow, A., Hjalgrim, H., Melbye, M., Frisch, M.: Bowen disease and risk of subsequent malignant neoplasms: a population-based cohort study of 1147 patients. Arch. Dermatol. **135**, 790–793 (1999)
11. Kao, G.E.: Carcinoma arising in Bowen's disease. Arch. Dermatol. **122**, 1124–1126 (1986)
12. Kossard, S., Rosen, R.: Cutaneous Bowen's disease. An analysis of 1001 cases according to age, sex, and site. J. Am. Acad. Dermatol. **27**, 406–410 (1992)
13. Lee, M.M., Wick, M.M.: Bowen's disease. Clin. Dermatol. **11**, 43–46 (1993)
14. Liu, H., Urabe, K., Moroi, Y., Yasumoto, S., Kokuba, H., Imafuku, S., Koga, T., Masuda, T., Aburatani, H., Furue, M., Tu, Y.: Expression of p16 and hTERT protein is associated with the presence of high-risk human papillomavirus in Bowenoid papulosis. J. Cutan. Pathol. **33**, 551–558 (2006)
15. Masuda, T., Hara, H., Shimojima, H., Suzuki, H., Tanaka, K.: Spontaneous complete regression of multiple Bowen's disease in the web-spaces of the feet. Int. J. Dermatol. **45**, 783–785 (2006)
16. Miki, Y., Kawatsu, T., Matsuda, K., Machino, H., Kubo, K.: Cutaneous and pulmonary cancers associated with Bowen's disease. J. Am. Acad. Dermatol. **6**, 26–31 (1982)
17. Murata, Y., Kumano, K., Sashikata, T.: Partial spontaneous regression of Bowen's disease. Arch. Dermatol. **132**, 429–432 (1996)
18. Nihei, N., Hiruma, M., Ikeda, S., Ogawa, H.: A case of Bowen's disease showing a clinical tendency toward spontaneous regression. J. Dermatol. **31**, 569–572 (2004)
19. Obalek, S., Jablonska, S., Beaudenon, S., Walczak, L., Orth, G.: Bowenoid papulosis of the male and female genitalia: risk of cervical neoplasia. J. Am. Acad. Dermatol. **14**, 433–444 (1986)
20. Park, K.C., Kim, K.H., Youn, S.W., Hwang, J.H., Park, K.H., Ahn, J.S., Kim, Y.G., Kim, S.D., Lee, D.Y., Choe, J.H., Chung, J.H., Cho, K.H.: Heterogeneity of human papillomavirus DNA in a patient with Bowenoid papulosis that progressed to squamous cell carcinoma. Br. J. Dermatol. **139**, 1087–1091 (1998)
21. Patterson, J.W., Kao, G.F., Graham, J.H., Helwig, E.B.: Bowenoid papulosis: a clinicopathologic study with ultrastructural observations. Cancer **57**, 823–836 (1986)
22. Reizner, G.T., Chuang, T.Y., Elpern, D.J., Stone, J.L., Farmer, E.R.: Bowen's disease (squamous cell carcinoma in situ) in Kauai, Hawaii. A population-based incidence report. J. Am. Acad. Dermatol. **31**, 596–600 (1994)
23. Rüdlinger, R., Buchmann, P.: HPV 16-positive bowenoid papulosis and squamous-cell carcinoma of the anus in an HIV-positive man. Dis. Colon Rectum **32**, 1042–1045 (1989)
24. Schwartz, R.A., Janniger, C.K.: Bowenoid papulosis. J. Am. Acad. Dermatol. **24**, 261–264 (1991)

Actinic Keratosis

1. Heaphy Jr., M.R., Ackerman, A.B.: The nature of solar keratosis: a critical review in historical perspective. J. Am. Acad. Dermatol. **43**(1 Pt 1), 138–150 (2000)
2. Ackerman, A.B.: Solar keratosis is squamous cell carcinoma. Arch. Dermatol. **139**(9), 1216–1217 (2003)
3. Fu, W., Cockerell, C.J.: The actinic (solar) keratosis: a 21st-century perspective. Arch. Dermatol. **139**(1), 66–70 (2003)
4. Schwartz, R.A., et al.: Actinic keratosis: an occupational and environmental disorder. J. Eur. Acad. Dermatol. Venereol. **22**(5), 606–615 (2008)
5. Ulrich, M., et al.: Actinic keratoses: non-invasive diagnosis for field cancerisation. Br. J. Dermatol. **156**(Suppl 3), 13–17 (2007)
6. Mogensen, M., Jemec, G.B.: Diagnosis of nonmelanoma skin cancer/keratinocyte carcinoma: a review of diagnostic accuracy of nonmelanoma skin cancer diagnostic tests and technologies. Dermatol. Surg. **33**(10), 1158–1174 (2007)
7. Ackerman, A.B., Mones, J.M.: Solar (actinic) keratosis is squamous cell carcinoma. Br. J. Dermatol. **155**(1), 9–22 (2006)
8. Guenthner, S.T., et al.: Cutaneous squamous cell carcinomas consistently show histologic evidence of in situ changes: a clinicopathologic correlation. J. Am. Acad. Dermatol. **41**(3 Pt 1), 443–448 (1999)

9. Roewert-Huber, J., Stockfleth, E., Kerl, H.: Pathology and pathobiology of actinic (solar) keratosis - an update. Br. J. Dermatol. **157**(Suppl 2), 18–20 (2007)

10. Rowert-Huber, J., et al.: Actinic keratosis is an early in situ squamous cell carcinoma: a proposal for reclassification. Br. J. Dermatol. **156**(Suppl 3), 8–12 (2007)

11. Glogau, R.G.: The risk of progression to invasive disease. J. Am. Acad. Dermatol. **42**(1 Pt 2), 23–24 (2000)

12. Marks, R., Rennie, G., Selwood, T.S.: Malignant transformation of solar keratoses to squamous cell carcinoma. Lancet **1**(8589), 795–797 (1988)

13. Fuchs, A., Marmur, E.: The kinetics of skin cancer: progression of actinic keratosis to squamous cell carcinoma. Dermatol. Surg. **33**(9), 1099–1101 (2007)

14. Schmook, T., Stockfleth, E.: Current treatment patterns in non-melanoma skin cancer across Europe. J. Dermatolog. Treat. **14**(Suppl 3), 3–10 (2003)

15. Stockfleth, E., et al.: Epithelial malignancies in organ transplant patients: clinical presentation and new methods of treatment. Recent Results Cancer Res. **160**, 251–258 (2002)

16. Ulrich, C., et al.: Skin diseases in organ transplant patients. Hautarzt **53**(8), 524–533 (2002)

17. Berhane, T., et al.: Inflammation is associated with progression of actinic keratoses to squamous cell carcinomas in humans. Br. J. Dermatol. **146**(5), 810–815 (2002)

18. Quaedvlieg, P.J., et al.: Actinic keratosis: how to differentiate the good from the bad ones? Eur. J. Dermatol. **16**(4), 335–339 (2006)

19. Thompson, S.C., Jolley, D., Marks, R.: Reduction of solar keratoses by regular sunscreen use. N. Engl. J. Med. **329**(16), 1147–1151 (1993)

20. Ulrich, C., et al.: Sunscreens in organ transplant patients. Nephrol. Dial. Transplant. **23**(6), 1805–1808 (2008)

21. Sengupta, S.R., Das, N.K., Datta, P.K.: Pathogenesis, clinical features and pathology of chronic arsenicosis. Indian J. Dermatol. Venereol. Leprol. **74**(6), 559–570 (2008)

22. Walvekar, R.R., et al.: Chronic arsenic poisoning: a global health issue – a report of multiple primary cancers. J. Cutan. Pathol. **34**(2), 203–206 (2007)

23. Wong, S.S., Tan, K.C., Goh, C.L.: Cutaneous manifestations of chronic arsenicism: review of seventeen cases. J. Am. Acad. Dermatol. **38**(2 Pt 1), 179–185 (1998)

24. Gupta, A.K., et al.: Keratoses in patients with psoriasis: a prospective study in fifty-two inpatients. J. Am. Acad. Dermatol. **23**(1), 52–55 (1990)

25. Hassab-El-Naby, H.M., et al.: PUVA keratosis in vitiligo. J. Eur. Acad. Dermatol. Venereol. **20**(8), 1013–1014 (2006)

26. van Praag, M.C., et al.: *PUVA keratosis.* A clinical and histopathologic entity associated with an increased risk of nonmelanoma skin cancer. J. Am. Acad. Dermatol. **28**(3), 412–417 (1993)

27. Turner, R.J., et al.: PUVA-related punctate keratoses of the hands and feet. J. Am. Acad. Dermatol. **42**(3), 476–479 (2000)

Non-Melanoma Skin Cancer: Appendageal Tumours

3.2

Jivko A. Kamarashev and Steven Kaddu

3.2.1 Tumours with Apocrine and Eccrine Differentiation

Jivko A. Kamarashev

Sudoriferous tumours represent approximately 1% of all primary cutaneous neoplasias. They have a variable, often unspecific clinical presentation and a wide histologic spectrum. According to their origin, cutaneous sweat gland tumours can be classified as eccrine, apocrine, eccrine and apocrine (mixed origin), or composite adnexal tumours. Further, they can be classified as benign or malignant, tumours of the sweat ducts or of the sweat glands secretory apparatus.

One or more distinct tumours arise from each of the several morphological regions of the sweat glands. The outer cells of the coiled intraepidermal eccrine excretory duct give rise to poroma. The intradermal straight duct is thought to give rise to syringoma and spiradenoma. There is evidence that the coiled part of the intradermal duct gives rise to cylindroma. Malignant transformation of these tumours is extremely rare.

The cells lining the inner aspect of the eccrine duct and those of the secretory coil are involved in active secretion and resorption processes, and their benign neoplasms are called hidradenomas. These are more susceptible to malignant transformation. Their malignant counterparts are termed hidradenocarcinomas. Most hidradenomas show a mixed differentiation towards both duct lining cells and secretory coil cells. In some hidradenomas, the outer cells differentiate to myoepithelial cells and induce a conspicuous stromal reaction with depositions of large quantities of stromal mucins. This compresses the epithelial component of the lesion and produces the characteristic mixed tumour of skin.

3.2.1.1 Malignant Tumours

Carcinomas of the eccrine and apocrine glands are neoplasms with infiltrative and metastatic potential. Primary malignant neoplasms of sweat glands are very rare, constituting less than 1% of all malignant primary skin lesions [3, 164]. Some malignancies, like cylindrocarcinoma, spiradenocarcinoma or malignant apocrine mixed tumour, have benign counterparts from which they must be differentiated. A malignant counterpart of most benign lesions has been described. Features that suggest malignancy include asymmetry of the lesion, invasion, irregular arrangement of neoplastic cells, cytonuclear atypia and pleomorphism, and significantly increased mitotic activity in the presence of abnormal mitotic figures. Other sweat gland carcinomas, such as adenoid cystic carcinoma (ACC), mucinous carcinoma, or apocrine carcinoma, present differently from any benign tumour. Most of these entities are exquisitely rare. Differentiating primary cutaneous sweat gland carcinomas from metastatic carcinoma can often pose a serious challenge. Clinical history, histomorphological features, and immunohistochemical stains are all very important.

3.2.1.1.1 Tubular Carcinoma

First reported by Stout and Cooley [189], tubular carcinoma is a rare malignancy of apocrine differentiation exhibiting prominent tubular structures.

Clinical features: Regarded as a malignant counterpart of tubular adenoma, tubular carcinoma most often affects middle-aged females and can occur everywhere where apocrine glands are found, with axilla being the most common location. It is typically a nodular lesion up to 5 cm in diameter that may be ulcerated or adherent to deeper tissues.

J.A. Kamarashev (✉)
Department of Dermatology, University Hospital Zurich,
Gloriastrasse 31, 8091 Zurich, Switzerland
e-mail: jivko.kamarachev@usz.ch

S. Kaddu
Department of Dermatology, Medical University of Graz,
Auenbruggerplatz 8, 8036, Graz, Austria
e-mail: steven.kaddu@meduni-graz.at

R. Dummer et al. (eds.), *Skin Cancer – A World-Wide Perspective*,
DOI: 10.1007/978-3-642-05072-5_3.2, © Springer-Verlag Berlin Heidelberg 2011

Histopathology: Tubular carcinoma is characterised by a proliferation of atypical tubular structures, varying largely in size and shape, with a tendency for size diminution towards the deep part of the tumour. The more superficial, larger tubules often exhibit papillary projections. The tumour is poorly circumscribed and infiltrates the surrounding tissue often extending to the subcutis or deeper.

The tumour cells have pleomorphic nuclei and abundant mostly eosinophilic cytoplasm often with signs of decapitational secretion. Mitoses are numerous. Sometimes, areas of solid sheets and cords of cells with cribriform formations are present [50, 100, 134, 145]. Necrosis en masse is a frequent finding; stroma is typically sparse.

Differential diagnosis: As implied by the histomorphology, the differential diagnosis of tubular carcinoma is, in fact, a metastatic deposit of ductal carcinoma of the breast, which can be distinguished with a clinical history in most cases.

Further, CK 5/6 is expressed by most skin adnexal carcinomas, but only in 33% of metastatic adenocarcinomas [156]. Epidermal growth factor receptor is expressed by 81% of sweat gland tumours, but only by 17% of metastatic breast cancers [23]. In one study, none of the metastatic adenocarcinomas to skin stained for p63, whereas virtually all the adnexal carcinomas were positive [88].

Prognosis and management: Primary tubular carcinoma is an aggressive tumour that has a high risk of metastatic dissemination. A wide local excision and thorough staging are recommended.

3.2.1.1.2 Microcystic Adnexal Carcinoma

Microcystic adnexal carcinoma (MAC; sclerosing sweat duct carcinoma) is a rare, malignant, locally aggressive cutaneous neoplasm often extending far beyond its clinical presentation, with a high recurrence rate but a low propensity to metastasize. First described as a distinct entity by Goldstein and colleagues in 1982 [65], MAC is believed to be of eccrine origin. However, the issue is complicated by the presence of keratinous cysts and the description of apocrine and sebaceous differentiation in some cases [158]. It has been suggested that the cell of origin is a pluripotent adnexal keratinocyte that remains capable of differentiating into both sweat ducts and hair follicles [99, 140, 201].

Clinical features (Fig. 3.2.1a):MAC occurs as a solitary lesion in middle-aged to elderly adults, commonly on the head and neck, with a predilection for the central area of the face [39]. Both sexes appear to be equally affected [171, 183]. Risk factors include excessive UV exposure and previous radiation therapy. MAC has been reported in association with other unrelated cancers [144], and there are anecdotal reports of MAC occurring in immunosuppressed patients [25, 183].

Clinically, MAC presents as a solitary, smooth, indurated, skin-coloured to yellow nodule or plaque; it grows slowly and may persist and remain asymptomatic for many years without metastasis [35]. Patients sometimes report numbness, paresthesia, burning, discomfort, or rarely pruritus of the affected area. Those symptoms are related to the frequent perineural invasion, typical of this tumour.

Histopathology (Fig. 3.2.1b): Histologic examination demonstrates a poorly circumscribed neoplasm not only reaching deep in the dermis but also often infiltrating in the subcutis, fascia, and facial muscle. MAC has a characteristic stratified architecture with an abundance of keratin-filled cysts in the superficial dermis, solid basaloid cell aggregations of variable size and shape resembling islands and infiltrating cords in the middle part of the tumour, and a predominance of ductal structures with one or

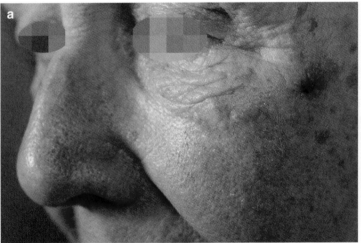
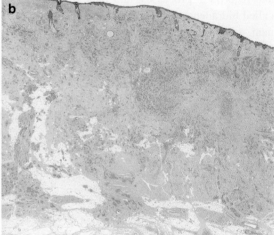

Fig. 3.2.1 (**a, b**) Microcystic adnexal carcinoma

two-cell-layer walls surrounding eosinophilic secretion in their lumen in the deep part of the tumour. There is no connection to the overlying epidermis. Perineural involvement is a common finding. Tumour cell morphology is deceptively inconspicuous without nuclear atypia. Mitotic figures, if present at all, are rare. Small granulomas indicating ruptured cornifying cysts are frequently seen in the upper dermis.

Cystic structures, solid cell aggregations, and ducts are packed closely and separated by dense, hyalinised stroma [112].

Differential diagnosis: MAC often bears similarity to desmoplastic trichoepithelioma and syringoma. Extensive tumour infiltration with perineural invasion, however, distinguishes MAC from these two other adnexal tumours. The histologic differential diagnosis includes further morpheaform basal cell carcinoma, squamous cell carcinoma, and metastatic breast carcinoma. The ductal elements are usually positive for epithelial membrane antigen (EMA) and carcinoembryonic antigen (CEA), which is helpful in differentiating MAC from desmoplastic trichoepithelioma [182]. The majority of MACs (92%) and desmoplastic trichoepitheliomas (100%) express CK15, while the infiltrative basal cell carcinoma and squamous cell carcinoma do not [81]. Negative Ber-EP4 staining was postulated to distinguish MAC from basal cell carcinoma, but it has been since shown that 38% of MACs stain positive for it [81]. Thus, though immunohistochemical stainings that can prove helpful are available, the evaluation of hematoxylin and eosin-stained sections of an adequate deep biopsy specimen remains the most reliable tool in the diagnosis of MAC.

Prognosis and management: Surgical excision is the only adequate therapy modality for this tumour. MAC is locally aggressive, and clear surgical margins are difficult to obtain. Reported margins for surgical excision vary from a few millimetres to 3–5 cm. Recurrence rates after surgical excision, even with wide margin, range from 40 to 60% [36]. Surgical control of MAC is more reliably achieved through Mohs micrographic surgery [104] with recurrence rates in the range of 0–12% [31, 113, 194]. Mohs micrographic surgery requires an average of 2–3 stages for complete removal. Average defect size/ lesion size ratios from 4 to 6.2 have been reported after Mohs surgery. [31, 194].

The role of radiotherapy, which has sometimes been applied in cases of multiple recurrences or in cases with microscopic residual tumour, is controversial since radioresistant cases of MAC and even recurrences in a clinically more extensive and histologically more aggressive form have been reported [188].

Despite possibility of extensive infiltration, only very few cases of metastases have been reported (2.1% incidence). Lifetime post-surgery monitoring is recommended in all cases.

3.2.1.1.3 Porocarcinoma

Eccrine porocarcinoma (EPC, malignant eccrine poroma) is a rare malignant tumour with metastatic potential arising from the intraepidermal portion of the eccrine sweat gland duct epithelium or acrosyringium. It was first described by Pinkus and Mehregan in 1963 [153]. The tumour usually develops from a pre-existing benign poroid tumour, and a benign component is reported in 18% of invasive eccrine carcinomas [135], but it may also arise de novo.

Clinical features: 60% of EPC are found on the lower extremities of middle-aged to elderly adults, but they also may occur on the head and neck, trunk, vulva, breast, nail bed, and upper extremity [129, 157, 166, 184]. Occurrence in males and females is equal. Porocarcinoma presents as a violaceous nodule usually less than 2 cm in size or a firm erythematous sometimes verrucous plaque. Signs of malignant transformation in an eccrine poroma include itching, pain, spontaneous bleeding, ulceration, and sudden growth over a period of time as short as a few weeks to a few months.

Histopathology (Fig. 3.2.2): Similar to its benign counterpart, primary porocarinoma may be contained entirely in the epidermis or may invade dermis. The in situ form of porocarcinoma, termed malignant hidroacanthoma simplex [10, 85], shows sharply demarcated nests of tumour cells within the epidermis (Borst–Jadassohn phenomenon). The distinction between malignant and benign hidroacanthoma simplex is based on the identification of cytologically malignant cells within tumour nests. When an in situ component coexists with an invasive dermal-based EPC, it clearly indicates a primary neoplasm. EPC is histologically characterised by an asymmetrical, solid, nodular growth pattern with infiltrative or pushing borders. The neoplastic cells are polygonal, may have basaloid features, resembling those of poroma, but show signs of atypia, pleomorphic, hyperchromatic nuclei, and prominent nucleoli [177, 207]. The malignant cells are

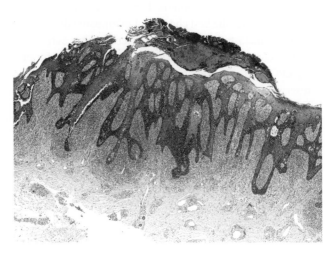

Fig. 3.2.2 Porocarcinoma

glycogen-rich and often contain several nuclei. Brisk mitotic activity, necrosis, and desmoplastic stromal reaction can be prominent. Foci of squamous and spindle cell differentiation are commonly seen. CEA-positive ductal structures are present in most cases, confirming the eccrine differentiation of the tumour. The stroma surrounding EPC may be highly myxoid, mucinous, hyalinized, or fibrotic.

Differential diagnosis: When the tumour is purely intra-epidermal or has a predominant intraepithelial component, distinction from clonal seborrhoeic keratosis with atypia, clonal Bowen's disease, melanoma in situ, and Paget disease is essential. The presence of an adjacent benign poroid component is a helpful feature in establishing the diagnosis. In clonal Bowen's disease, the tumour cells are more atypical, and there is more severe architectural abnormality. Clonal seborrhoeic keratosis and Bowen's disease are negative for CEA, cytokeratin 7, and S100, which are often positive in porocarcinoma. Melanoma in situ typically expresses S-100 protein but also expresses Melan-A and/or HMB-45; melanoma does not express CEA. In Paget's disease, the cells are large with clear PAS-positive cytoplasm.

Those tumours with dermal invasion must be distinguished from squamous cell carcinoma and other forms of malignant eccrine neoplasia. The presence of ductal structures and a PAS-positive cuticle in ECP often allows for differentiation from a cutaneous squamous cell carcinoma or an adenocarcinoma metastatic to the skin. Further, the cells and their nuclei in EPC are larger than those seen in the eccrine poroma but are, nonetheless, smaller than the tumour cells of squamous cell carcinoma.

Prognosis and management: Local recurrence of EPC is observed in 20% of cases, metastasis to regional lymph nodes in 20%, and solid organ metastases in 10% [166]. It has been suggested that tumour depth >7 mm, over14 mitoses per high power field, and the presence of lymphovascular invasion are associated with a more aggressive clinical course [197]. The survival for patients with metastatic EPC has been reported to be between 5 and 24 months. Early detection and definitive excision offer the best chances of minimising the mortality rate in metastatic EPC. Mohs micrographic surgery is currently considered the surgical treatment of choice for primary EPC [205]. Chemotherapy has a poor response rate and is reserved for the treatment of documented metastatic EPC. Response to radiation therapy is partial and inconsistent, and its use is reserved for palliative care.

It should be generally recommended that all benign poromas be removed in their entirety because of the possibility of malignant transformation.

3.2.1.1.4 Spiradenocarcinoma

Spiradenocarcinoma [41] is the malignant counterpart of spiradenoma and is extremely rare. Typically, spiradenocarcinomas originate from long pre-existing spiradenomas, but de novo spiradenocarcinomas have also been reported [66].

Clinical features: While eccrine spiradenoma is a fairly common benign sweat gland tumour usually presenting as a solitary tender nodule on the ventral aspect of the upper body of young adults, malignant transformation is extremely rare and may be related to traumas [6]. This transformation clinically manifests as a sudden change in tumour size or development of new symptoms such as pain or ulceration.

Both sexes are equally affected, and the peak incidence is in the sixth and seventh decade, though malignant eccrine spiradenoma may present in a wide age group. Tumours are usually large (average size-7.5 cm) at the time of excision. Patients report a pre-existing tumour from 7 months to 30 years before surgical removal, and any body site can be affected [176].

Spiradenocarcinomas are aggressive neoplasms with a high recurrence rate (up to 57%) and a propensity to metastasise to lymph nodes and distant organs including bones, lungs, liver, and brain (up to 39%) [191].

Histopathology: In most cases, there is continuity between benign eccrine spiradenoma and spiradenocarcinoma, but the malignant component comprises the bulk of the lesion. Histological evidence of malignant transformation includes loss of nodular growth pattern, infiltrative borders, loss of nested growth pattern, absence of a dual cell population, cytonuclear pleomorphism, hyperchromasia, increased mitotic activity, and tumour necrosis. At scanning magnification, spiradenocarcinoma typically localises in the dermis without contact with the epidermis; it is lobulated and has blunt "pushing-type" borders surrounded by a fibrous pseudocapsule. Ectatic blood vessels and haemorrhage are seen in most tumours. Necrosis can be prominent. Focal perineural invasion is an occasional finding. Almost all tumours contain a component of benign eccrine spiradenoma (see 3.2.1.2.6). Spiradenocarcinomas can show a variable degree of differentiation [66]. Well-differentiated spiradenocarcinomas resemble spiradenomas at low power but with closer inspection show areas of architectural disarrangement characterised by irregular and confluent strings and trabeculae. Moreover, the distinction between two cell populations, typical of the benign counterpart, is no longer evident, and the cells show an increased nuclear to cytoplasmic ratio, hyperchromasia, mild-to-moderate pleomorphism, small or inconspicuous nucleoli, and increased mitotic activity. Scattered lymphocytes permeate the neoplasm. The malignant elements often seem to merge imperceptibly with benign eccrine spiradenoma. In moderately differentiated tumours, oedema and vascular proliferation are more evident. Cellular and nuclear pleomorphism is more pronounced, and mitotic figures are more numerous. Areas of necrosis are more common, and there are usually no lymphocytes permeating the neoplasm. Sheets of large polygonal or spindled cells with high-grade nuclear atypia and conspicuous nucleoli constitute the undifferentiated spiradenocarcinomas. Numerous mitotic figures, some atypical, are found, and there may also be large zones of necrosis. In these cases, only a component associated with benign spiradenoma allows for an accurate diagnosis. The presence, at least focally within the lesion, of dual population (central basaloid cells and larger peripheral cells) is required for the diagnosis of spiradenocarcinoma.

Differential diagnosis: The main differential diagnosis of spiradenocarcinoma is its benign counterpart, especially in well-differentiated carcinomas. The p53 product gene has been reported to be strongly positive only in the malignant areas and negative in the benign areas [53].

Prognosis and management: Presently, a wide local excision is recommended as the only adequate therapy approach. The role, if any, of prophylactic lymph node dissection, postoperative adjuvant radiotherapy, or chemotherapy remains to be established.

3.2.1.1.5 Malignant Mixed Tumour

Malignant mixed tumour (MMT) [168], also known as malignant chondroid syringoma (CS)[124], is very rare and may arise de novo, or rarely, from a pre-existing benign mixed tumour of the skin that undergoes malignant transformation.

Clinical features: MMT has a female predilection, while their benign counterparts are more frequent in males. MMT often arises on the extremities and trunk as a rapidly growing nodule [70], whereas benign mixed tumours preferentially involve the head and neck. MMT is significantly larger than benign mixed tumours.

Histopathology: The diagnosis of MMT is based on morphologic criteria [70]. The tumour has both an epithelial and a mesenchymal component. Either eccrine or apocrine differentiation may be found in the epithelial component. Striking cellular atypia, nuclear pleomorphism, increased mitotic activity, infiltrative margins, satellite tumour nodules, and tumour necrosis are present only within the epithelial carcinomatous component of the tumour. The stroma has benign histologic features and may have a mucinous, cartilaginous, and osteoid differentiation. Thus, malignant CS may be classified as a sweat gland carcinoma with stromal induction.

Prognosis and management: MMT follows a seemingly unpredictable clinical course and has shown potential for lymphatic as well as hematogenous spread. According to one review, in 48% of reported cases, metastases to regional lymph nodes occurred, and in 45%, distant metastases were reported [11]. The two most common sites for distal metastases are the lung and bone.

The term "atypical mixed tumour of the skin" is used to describe tumours with histological features of malignancy as well as recurrence, local invasion, and satellite tumour nodules but without proven metastases [12].

3.2.1.1.6 Hidradenocarcinoma

The malignant counterpart of hidradenoma, hidradenocarcinoma (syn.: malignant nodular/clear cell hidradenoma, malignant clear cell acrospiroma, clear cell eccrine carcinoma, or primary mucoepidermoid cutaneous carcinoma), first described by Keasbey and Hadley in 1954 [102], is a very rare tumour with just over 50 cases reported, mostly as case reports with isolated small case series. In the past, these tumours were further subdivided into apocrine and eccrine, but it has recently been shown that features of both differentiations are simultaneously present in most lesions, and a combined "apoeccrine" differentiation has been proposed [107].

Clinical features: Hidradenocarcinoma most commonly arises de novo, but it may also arise in pre-existing hidradenoma and presents clinically as a rapidly growing dermal nodule, 1–5 cm in diameter, with or without superimposed ulceration, on the head and neck and the distal extremities of the elderly [15].

Histopathology: At scanning magnification, the neoplasm typically presents as a multinodular lesion, with areas of tumour necrosis. Architectural patterns include polypoid neoplasms, tumours with an infiltrative peripheral margin associated with stromal desmoplasia, and variants characterised by islands of neoplastic cells showing central necrosis. Often, more than one architectural pattern is present within the same lesion. The tumours consist of variable admixtures of basaloid, squamoid, and clear cells [147]. Ductal structures and intracytoplasmic tubular vacuoles are present and provide evidence of eccrine ductal differentiation at the light microscopic level. Signs of apocrine differentiation are frequently observed. Nodular hidradenoma remnants may be present [79]. Accepted histological criteria for diagnosing malignant transformation include the lack of circumscription, an infiltrative growth pattern, deep extension, nuclear pleomorphism, necrosis, vascular invasion, perineural invasion, and the presence of an increased number of mitoses.

The grade of differentiation in hidradenocarcinomas varies greatly. On one end of the spectrum, well-differentiated neoplasms show an invasive peripheral margin with stromal desmoplasia, increased mitotic rate, and metastatic potential in the absence of prominent cytologic atypia, and on the other end are overtly anaplastic cancers with evident nuclear features of malignancy.

The tumour cells stain positively for LMWK, and the ductal structures/luminal surfaces are highlighted by EMA and CEA.

Differential diagnosis: The differential diagnosis depends on the predominant cell morphology and differentiation grade. The main differential diagnosis of well-differentiated tumours is their benign counterpart. Clear cell hidradenocarcinoma must be differentiated from other malignant neoplasms with clear cell morphology – clear cell porocarcinoma, sebaceous carcinoma, trichilemmal carcinoma, clear cell basal cell carcinoma, and clear cell carcinomas metastatic to the skin including thyroid, lung, and renal cell carcinomas.

Prognosis and management: Despite the small number of cases and limited follow-up available, an aggressive clinical course of hidradenocarcinomas, characterised by repeated local recurrences and frequent systemic metastasis, has often been reported.

Early wide surgical excision of the lesions is the treatment of choice. Lymph node dissection, adjuvant chemotherapy, and radiotherapy remain controversial.

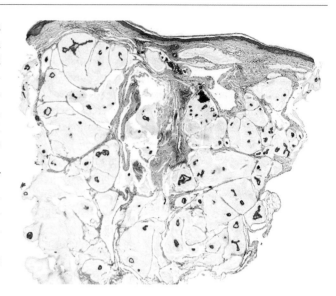

Fig. 3.2.3 Primary cutaneous mucinous carcinoma

3.2.1.1.7 Primary Cutaneous Mucinous Carcinoma

Primary cutaneous mucinous carcinoma (PCMC) (syn.: colloid carcinoma of the skin) is an extremely rare low-grade malignancy demonstrating frequent local recurrences but a low propensity to metastasise to regional lymph nodes and distant organs. Since its original description by Lennox et al. [115] in 1952, the number of reported cases has exceeded 150. It is believed to arise from the deepest portion of the eccrine secretory coil, the mucin-secreting dark cells.

Clinical features: PCMC presents clinically as a single pale, skin coloured, or violaceous nodule up to 3 cm in diameter involving the eyelids, face, head, neck, or axillary region of elderly patients (median age of onset 63 years). Telangiectases, lobulation, and ulceration may be present. Men are affected twice as often as women [130, 185].

Histopathology (Fig. 3.2.3)*:* Upon scanning magnification, a well-demarcated, lobular dermal tumour, with frequent extension into the subcutaneous tissue and no connection with the overlying epidermis, is observed. Small nests of variably cohesive neoplastic epithelia floating in large multilocular pools of PAS-positive, diastase-resistant mucin material that decorates with Alcian blue or Hale's colloidal iron are the histological hallmark of this entity [60, 130, 151, 210]. The tumour cells possess round, hyperchromatic nuclei, inconspicuous nucleoli, a moderate amount of pale eosinophilic to clear cytoplasm, and well-defined cell membranes. The cytoplasm is often vacuolated and may show signet ring. The degree of cytologic atypia varies from low grade to overtly anaplastic. Mitotic figures are rare. Tumour cells are typically positive for cytokeratins, α- lactalbumin, S-100, CEA, EMA, gross cystic disease fluid protein 15 (GCDFP-15), and oestrogen and progesterone receptors [2, 24]. As in the breast, PCMC may express synaptophysin and/or chromogranin, pointing to a neuroendocrine differentiation [160].

Differential diagnosis: It is of paramount importance to differentiate PCMC from metastasising mucinous carcinomas originating in the breast or gastrointestinal tract, which have an identical histomorphology [101]. However, metastases from breast or gastrointestinal tract carcinomas occur late in the disease process, and by this time, the clinical history and biological character of the neoplasm are almost always established. Further, location of the tumour on the chest wall, breast, or axillae can serve as clue to breast origin.

Prognosis and management: Treatment of PCMC requires complete tumour extirpation. Surgical excision with narrow margins is associated with a high (30–40%) local tumour recurrence rate [185]. Therefore, it should be removed with wide margins, reducing recurrence rates to 20%. Local tissue involvement can be assessed with magnetic resonance tomography. A fine-needle aspiration biopsy might also be useful in preoperative evaluation [163]. Many authors have advocated Mohs micrographic surgery as an effective treatment option [17, 122]. As the effectiveness of chemotherapy and radiotherapy has not been proved, surgery could also be indicated for the rare instances of metastatic lesions. Because local recurrence is of concern, regular follow-up examinations are warranted.

3.2.1.1.8 Digital Papillary Carcinoma

Digital papillary carcinomas (syn.: digital papillary adenocarcinoma, aggressive digital papillary tumour, aggressive digital papillary adenoma, aggressive digital papillary carcinoma) are rare sweat gland neoplasms of eccrine origin, first described by Helwig in 1979 and Kao et al. in 1984 [95].

They are generally regarded as low-grade malignant tumours of acral skin with no benign counterpart.

Clinical features: Digital papillary carcinomas occur most frequently on fingers but also on toes, palms, and soles. They present as a solitary solid or solid-cystic nodule in middle-aged adults, with a clear male predominance. They have aggressive local growth potential and a high recurrence rate, reported to be between 28 and 45% [96]. Some 14% of tumours metastasise, typically to lungs and lymph nodes.

Histopathology: The typical digital papillary carcinoma is a multinodular, solid, and cystic lesion with a characteristic pattern of fused back-to-back glands lined with cuboidal to low columnar epithelial cells in the solid portion of the tumour. There is no connection to the overlying epidermis. Areas of papillary projections protruding into cystically dilated lumina complement the picture. The cysts are formed either by central degeneration of solid areas or by eosinophilic secretory material [46]. Two types of papillary projections are found: pseudo-papillae formed by epithelial cells without associated fibrovascular cores in areas of central tumour degeneration and true papillae with fibrovascular cores in areas with eosinophilic secretory material. Cytological atypia, nuclear pleomorphism, increased mitotic activity, or tumour necrosis is frequently found. Rarely, decapitation secretion in parts of the lesion may be observed. The luminal tumour cells express CEA; other tumour cells express S100.

Initially, these tumours were subclassified on histologic grounds as aggressive digital papillary adenoma or aggressive digital papillary adenocarcinoma [96]. Poor glandular differentiation, necrosis, cytologic atypia, high mitotic rate, and invasion of soft tissue, bone, and blood vessels were defined as differentiating criteria typical of aggressive digital papillary adenocarcinoma. However, the distinction between adenoma and carcinoma on histological grounds alone does not seem to predict the clinical progression of these tumours, which often have a high rate of local recurrence and potential for metastasis.

Differential diagnosis: The histologic differential diagnosis includes spiradenocarcinoma (which shows at least foci of a two-cell population) and hidradenocarcinoma (usually not well circumscribed, with no papillary pattern, and back-to-back glandular differentiation). Papillary tubular adenoma is well circumscribed and lacks the back-to-back glandular differentiation and cystic component of digital papillary adenocarcinoma.

Prognosis and management: Since it has been shown that metastatic potential of these tumours cannot be predicted based on histology, all such tumours are best considered malignant and should be completely excised with or without amputation of the affected digit. Recurrences in incompletely excised tumours are observed in 50% of cases, compared with recurrence in 5% of patients who had an adequate re-excision or amputation. Sentinel lymph node biopsy has been suggested in the staging of these tumours [118]. Aggressive surgical therapy for limited metastatic disease seems warranted based on the limited number of cases studied. Still, no standard effective treatment exists for more extensive metastatic disease. All patients should be followed up, because local recurrences represent a major concern and metastases are possible.

3.2.1.1.9 Adenoid Cystic Carcinoma

First described by Boggio [20] in 1975, primary cutaneous ACC is an exceedingly rare low-grade malignant tumour of the skin, histologically indistinguishable from its more common salivary gland counterpart.

Clinical features: Primary cutaneous ACC is a tumour of the elderly, with female predominance. It develops most commonly in the scalp, but different anatomical sites can be affected [59, 175]. The tumour has a 50% local recurrence rate due to its characteristic perineural infiltration, but metastases to regional lymph nodes [32] and distant organs [28] seem to be much rarer than with the salivary gland counterpart.

Histopathology (Fig. 3.2.4)*:* Cutaneous ACC usually presents as a dermal tumour that consists of bland, monomorphous basaloid cells with hyperchromatic nuclei and indistinct nucleoli, arranged in tubuloalveolar structures with a solid, trabecular, or cribriform growth pattern [16]. Mitoses are typically inconspicuous. Mucinous material is present within the cystic lobules, and the stroma is fibrous. Globules of eosinophilic PAS-positive, diastase-resistant basement membrane-like material, similar to those seen in cylindroma, are a typical finding. The propensity of these tumours for perineural infiltration is striking and an important diagnostic criterion. The tumour cells express LMWK and pancytoker-

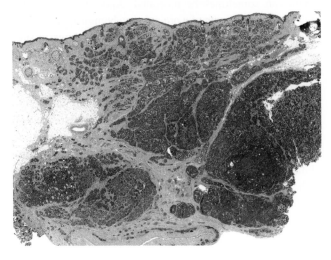

Fig. 3.2.4 Adenoid cystic carcinoma

atin (AE1/AE3), and the luminal cells are frequently immunoreactant with EMA and CEA.

Differential diagnosis: It is essential to clinically rule out the presence of salivary gland ACC and exclude other cutaneous basaloid tumours, especially adenoid basal cell carcinoma. The latter has a nodular architecture, without irregularly shaped tongues of tumour or stromal desmoplasia [202]. Apoptosis of individual cells and mitotic figures is typical of basal cell carcinoma but not of ACC. The lack of epidermal connection, absence of peripheral palisading of neoplastic cells and slit-like retraction from the adjacent stroma, as well as the presence of PAS-positive material, perineural space invasion, and EMA and CEA expression by tumour cells favour the diagnosis of ACC.

Prognosis and management: Complete excision with tumour-free margins, established with a permanent section biopsy, has been recommended as the standard treatment for ACC, since simple excision may result in frequent recurrence [109].

3.2.1.1.10 Apocrine Carcinoma

Apocrine carcinoma [200] is a rare primary cutaneous malignancy with a distinctive histologic appearance, originating from either normal or modified (ceruminous and Moll) apocrine glands.

Clinical features: Apocrine glands are distributed throughout the body but are present in greatest abundance in the axilla, followed by the anogenital region. The axilla is the most common site for these tumours accounting for some 65% of all cases [36], but apocrine carcinomas of the anogenital region, eyelid, ear, chest, wrist, lip, foot, toe, and finger have also been reported. There is a slight male preponderance (5:4) [36].These slow-growing tumours present as painless, reddish-to-purple solid, or cystic nodules, which can sometimes be ulcerated. Apocrine carcinomas may develop at the site of a pre-existing benign apocrine disease. Clinically, there are no characteristic findings to suggest that a particular nodule or cyst may represent an apocrine carcinoma. In fact, an axillary mass is much more likely to represent other neoplasms such as metastatic breast carcinoma, metastatic disease from other sites, lymphoma, benign apocrine disease, or even ectopic benign breast tissue than an apocrine carcinoma [27]. Because of their indolent nature, most apocrine carcinomas are between 1 and 3 cm at the time of diagnosis. Up to 50% have already lymph node metastases at the time of diagnosis.

Histopathology: Apocrine carcinoma is an asymmetric poorly demarcated dermal tumour, composed of irregular ductal and tubular structures that may extend to the subcutis [148, 172]. Papillary projections within the lumina and decapitation secretion, as a sign of apocrine differentiation,

are often present. The tumour cells are larger than normal apocrine cells, may contain iron-positive granules within their abundant eosinophilic cytoplasm, and demonstrate poor glandular formation with varying degrees of differentiation within the same tumour. Nuclear pleomorphism, increased mitotic activity, and areas of tumour necrosis are also noted. PAS-positive, diastase-resistant material is present in the cells or lumina. Histologic glandular patterns include papillary, complex glandular, and anastomosing tubular. In poorly differentiated areas, the tumour cells form solid strands or nests and sheets within a hyalinised fibrous stroma.

The tumour cells express LMWK, and the luminal cells are reactive for CEA, EMA, and GCDFP-15. S100 protein is also occasionally positive [136]. Apocrine carcinomas are usually positive for androgen receptors but negative for oestrogen and progesterone receptors and bcl-2. Calponin and SMA stain the peripheral myoepithelium and are helpful markers in delineating invasion.

Differential diagnosis: Highly differentiated malignant neoplasms are frequently difficult to differentiate from benign adnexal lesions. Less well-differentiated tumours must be differentiated from visceral adenocarcinoma metastases.

Prognosis and management: Grade of differentiation seems to have prognostic implications. It has been reported that patients with well-differentiated apocrine carcinomas did extremely well and achieved long-term remission with surgery alone [200]. In contrast, patients diagnosed with moderately or poorly differentiated tumours had higher local recurrence rates after resection and were far more likely to have metastatic disease.

Wide local excision is the standard therapy for these lesions. A margin of 1–2 cm is currently considered adequate. Small, well-differentiated apocrine carcinomas arising in functionally or cosmetically limiting locations, such as the eyelid, fingertip, or lip, may be effectively treated with Mohs micrographic surgery without compromising the oncologic outcome [180]. A therapeutic lymph node dissection is indicated for confirmed lymph node metastases. Apocrine carcinoma appears to spread via both lymphatic and vascular channels, with the lung being the most common site of metastatic disease [27]. The response of metastatic apocrine carcinoma to chemotherapy has generally been reported to be poor.

3.2.1.1.11 Paget Disease of Breast

Mammary Paget disease (PD), first described in 1874 by Sir James Paget in 15 women who presented with eczematous disease of the areola and nipple associated with carcinoma of the underlying mammary gland [146], accounts for 1–3% of all breast malignancies [8]. Neoplastic transformation of the breast ductal system with secondary extension to the skin manifests as PD of the breast. In contrast, extra-mammary PD is thought to represent a neoplasm arising in the germinative cells of the basal layer of the epidermis [110]. Both processes manifest apocrine differentiation but have different paths of lesional development. There are, however, cases of mammary PD lacking underlying ductal carcinoma of the breast [170], and there are lesions of extra-mammary PD with underlying sweat gland carcinoma. The clear cell of Toker, representing the termination of mammary and mammary-like ducts in the nipple and vulva, has been postulated as a potential alternative progenitor cell [30, 204].

Clinical features (Fig. 3.2.5a): Postmenopausal women are generally affected by PD of the breast, and the peak incidence lies in sixth decade [90, 170]. PD of the breast is extremely rare in male patients. Over 97% of patients with mammary PD have an underlying breast carcinoma.

Mammary PD typically presents as a slowly progressing, well-demarcated erythematous scaling or exudative patch or plaque, starting from the nipple, spreading to the areola, and eventually to the surrounding skin of the breast [170]. Early symptoms include itching and burning sensations. The lesion can initially improve or even temporarily resolve with topical corticosteroid treatment, which adds to a delay in diagnosis. Typically, 10–12 months transpire before PD is diagnosed correctly [170]. Later in its evolution, PD progresses to nipple crusting, skin erosion, and ulceration resulting in destruction of the nipple or areolar complex.

Risk factors for PD of the breast include age (exponential increase with age), factors related to abnormalities in oestrogen and androgen balance, benign breast conditions (nipple discharge, breast cysts, breast trauma), and radiation exposure. Risk factors related to a genetic predisposition include Klinefelter's syndrome (47, XXY karyotype), family history, and Jewish ancestry.

The disease can present in conjunction with an underlying invasive cancer, in conjunction with underlying ductal carcinoma in situ (DCIS), or without any underlying malignancy [29]. Patients may present with (54%) or without (46%) an underlying mass. Approximately 90% of patients presenting with a palpable or mammographic mass will have an underlying invasive carcinoma. On the other hand, 66–86% of patients without a clinical mass upon physical examination or mammography will have DCIS alone. Prognosis is determined primarily by the presence or absence of an invasive component, and recommendations for systemic therapy are given accordingly.

Histopathology (Fig. 3.2.5b): A proliferation of single and clustered neoplastic cells with evidence of glandular differentiation, in the form of intracytoplasmic lumina and ductal formations, is found in the epidermis of PD. The nuclei are round to oval with prominent nucleoli; the nuclear diameters are up to double those of adjacent keratinocyte nuclei [137]. The neoplastic cells have less well-defined intercellular bridges than keratinocytes and form loosely cohesive groups in a fashion that may mimic an acantholytic process. The tumour cells often spare the basal layer of the epidermis and appear to compress it from above. Anaplastic cases of PD have been described, in which there is full-thickness epidermal atypia, loss of nuclear polarity, marked cytologic anaplasia, and inconspicuous glandular differentiation [161].

The neoplastic cells contain cytoplasmic epithelial mucins that stain with alcian blue and mucicarmine. They express GCDFP-15 as well as CK 7 and CEA [75, 173]. Androgen receptors and Her2/neu are commonly expressed in both mammary and extra-mammary PD, while oestrogen and progesterone receptors are not.

Differential diagnosis: The clinical differential diagnosis includes eczema, contact dermatitis, and postradiation dermatitis.

Neoplasms that show pagetoid migration of malignant epithelia include Bowen's disease, sebaceous carcinoma, and melanomas. Melanomas express HMB-45 and Melan-A, as opposed to GCDFP-15, CK 7, and CEA in PD. Bowen's disease, in contrast, expresses high-molecular-weight

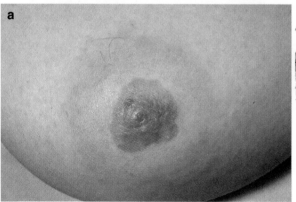
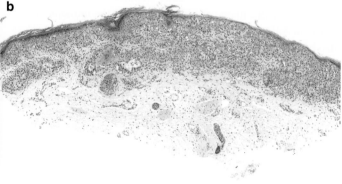

Fig. 3.2.5 (**a**, **b**) Paget disease of the breast

cytokeratins but not CK-7. In sebaceous carcinoma, the intraepidermal tumour cells are vacuolated, with a clear cytoplasm as opposed to PD, which reveals basophilic mucin-rich cytoplasm. It has been shown that CD5 will strongly decorate both mammary and extra-mammary PD but will not react with cells of Bowen's disease, melanoma in situ, or sebaceous carcinoma [21].

Prognosis and management: Prognosis and treatment are dependent on the presence or absence of palpable masses or axillary nodes and underlying invasive carcinoma. In every case, mammography and FNA or large needle biopsies of suspicious areas must be performed. Breast-conserving surgery seems to be a safe alternative to mastectomy, regarding both local control and breast cancer survival. As for postoperative radiotherapy of PD, it seems reasonable to use the same indications as for the underlying carcinoma. In patients with only nipple or areolar complex involvement, some experts recommend skin excision with consideration of adjunct radiation therapy [170]. In patients with a palpable mass and negative skin margins, lumpectomy with adjunctive radiation is recommended. The 5-year recurrence rate in this patient population was reported to be 28% if no post-surgery radiotherapy was performed. This recurrence rate can be diminished to 5% if surgery is followed by radiation therapy. Mastectomy should be reserved for relapses [121]. In patients with palpable mass and involved margins, complete mastectomy is recommended.

3.2.1.1.12 Extra-Mammary Paget Disease

Extra-mammary PD was first reported by Dubreilh in 1901 [45]. It is an uncommon cutaneous malignant neoplasm with an almost equal sex distribution arising in anatomical sites rich in apocrine glands, such as the vulva, scrotum, perineum, axillae, perineal region, eyelids, and the external auditory canals. Extension to anal, urethral, vaginal, and cervical mucosa has been observed [62, 91]. Apocrine differentiation of cells in extra-mammary PD has generally been accepted, although the histogenesis remains disputed. Some authors believe that extra-mammary PD arises from the intraepidermal stem cell [91]. An alternative origin from Toker cells has also been suggested [30, 204]. According to another intriguing hypothesis, extra-mammary PD may be a proliferation of adnexal stem cells residing in the infundibulo-sebaceous unit of hair follicles and adnexal structures [162]. Extra-mammary PD is a slowly progressing, usually intraepithelial tumour; it is only occasionally invasive and extremely rarely metastasizing. Only 20% of cases demonstrate a dermal invasive element [1]. When the invasive component is <1.0 mm in depth, the tumour is considered to be minimally invasive, and complete excision is usually curative [64]. Extra-mammary PD may also be associated with an underlying cutaneous adnexal carcinoma, usually an apocrine adenocarcinoma [155]. In up to 30% of cases, extra-mammary genital PD can be associated with a regional visceral malignancy such as cervical [127], rectal [13], prostate [4], or transitional cell carcinoma [203]. These cases are classified as secondary extra-mammary PD in contrast to primary extra-mammary PD without associated internal malignancy.

Clinical features (Fig. 3.2.6): Clinically, extra-mammary PD usually presents as an erythematous eczematoid patch or plaque, which may become erosive or ulcerated over time.

Histopathology: The histology is analogous to that of mammary Paget's disease. The tumour cells contain alcian blue, mucicarmine, and PAS-positive mucin in most cases. AE1/AE3, LMWK, and CK 7 are typically positive in primary extra-mammary PD; variable positivity is seen for EMA and CEA. GCDFP-15, androgen receptors, and Her2/neu are also commonly expressed in primary extra-mammary PD, whereas oestrogen receptors and progesterone receptors are not [44]. In secondary extra-mammary PD, the profile is similar to the original carcinoma. These cases are typically negative for GCDFP-15.

Differential diagnosis: Extra-mammary PD must be distinguished from Bowen's disease, metastatic visceral malignancy, and melanoma.

Prognosis and management: The prognosis for patients with extra-mammary PD is fairly good. A thorough examination for other tumours is recommended, with a minimum follow-up time of at least 5 years. After exclusion of an underlying tumour, a total lesion excision is the established

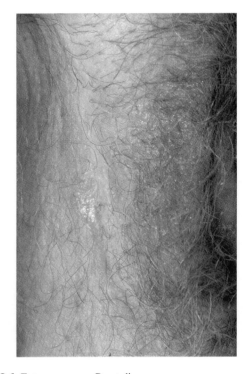

Fig. 3.2.6 Extra-mammary Paget disease

therapy. Extra-mammary PD has a highly irregular growth pattern, and subclinical microscopic extensions often result in marginal tumour persistence or recurrence. Mohs surgery with or without intra-operative CK 7 immunostaining has been shown to be useful [78]. Some encouraging results have been reported with topical imiquimod [73] and photodynamic therapy [179], but larger series are required.

3.2.1.2 Benign Tumours

3.2.1.2.1 Hidrocystoma

Hidrocystomas – benign, cystic sweat gland tumours of the skin – can be eccrine or apocrine and are often found on the head and neck. Hidrocystomas occur mostly in adults between 30 and 70 years of age.

Clinical features: Eccrine hidrocystomas (Fig. 3.2.7c) are small, tense, dome-shaped cysts, ranging from 1 to 6 mm in diameter. They may have an amber, brown, or bluish tint. During hot and humid weather, these lesions grow in size and may increase in number but usually do not involve the eyelid margin. Eccrine hidrocystomas usually result from cystic dilation due to retention of sweat and blockage of the sweat duct.

Robinson first described eccrine hidrocystoma in 1893 [165]. Most of his patients were women who worked in a hot, humid environment. Their lesions were reported as multiple small papules affecting the periorbital and malar areas. In 1973, Smith and Chernosky described another group of patients who most commonly had solitary lesions [181]. In their series, 40% of the patients were men. These two clinical presentations have become known as the Robinson (multiple) type and the Smith and Chernosky (solitary) type of eccrine hidrocystoma.

Apocrine hidrocystomas (Fig. 3.2.7a) arise from the proliferation of apocrine glands and are usually solitary, with a diameter of 3–15 mm. They appear as clear cystic nodules with a smooth surface, and the colour varies, ranging from flesh-coloured to blue–black. Multiple lesions on the face and neck have rarely been reported [43]. The cysts show no seasonal variations. Apocrine lesions can involve the eyelid margin near the inner canthus.

The inherited disorders most commonly associated with the presence of multiple hidrocystomas are Goltz-Gorlin syndrome (focal dermal hypoplasia) [7] and Schopf-Schulz-Passarge syndrome (multiple eyelid apocrine hidrocystoma, palmoplantar hyperkeratosis, hypodontia, and hypotrichosis) [63].

Graves' disease has also been associated with multiple eccrine hidrocystomas possibly due to hyperhidrosis [105].

Histopathology: Eccrine hidrocystoma (Fig. 3.2.7d) presents as a dermal unilocular cyst lined with one or two layers of small cuboidal cells. In most cases, eccrine secretory tubules and ducts are located below the cyst. There is no connection between the cyst and the overlying epidermis. There are no PAS-positive, diastase-resistant granules in the lining cells' cytoplasm.

Apocrine hidrocystomas (Fig. 3.2.7b) can be unilocular or multilocular. The epithelium is either a single or double layer of cuboidal-columnar epithelium, which lies above an outer myoepithelial cell layer. PAS-positive granules are observed in the cytoplasm of the inner lining cells, and sometimes, melanin and lipofuscin are also found. Apocrine secretion is observed but may be focal. Some apocrine hidrocystoma-like lesions exhibit florid papillary projections into the cystic cavity, consisting of vascular connective tissue, covered by the secretory epithelium. The designation "apocrine cystadenoma" has been suggested for these lesions. Different keratin and human milk fat globulin 1 expression patterns have been found in apocrine cystadenoma, apocrine hidrocystoma, and eccrine hidrocystoma, suggesting that they are distinct entities [42].

Differential diagnosis: Clinically, eccrine hidrocystomas and apocrine hidrocystomas must be distinguished from other head and neck cyst-like lesions such as epidermal cysts, mucoid cysts, hemangioma, lymphangioma, and basal cell carcinoma. Apocrine hidrocystomas, because of their typically blue–black colour, must be distinguished from melanocytic lesions, including nodular melanoma.

Prognosis and management: Treatment options include simple needle puncture, excision and drainage with cauterization and electrodesiccation of the cyst wall, and CO_2-laser vaporisation. Multiple-type lesions have been successfully treated with topical 1% atropine or scopolamine creams, although anticholinergic side effects could cause patients to discontinue the treatment [34].

3.2.1.2.2 Syringoma

Syringomas, first described in 1872 by Kaposi and Biesiadeki as lymphangioma tuberosum multiplex, are common benign tumours that arise from the straight segment of the intradermal eccrine sweat gland duct. They occur twice as often in women than in men, with adolescence being the most common time of onset [149].

Clinical features (Fig. 3.2.8a)*:* Syringomas appear as multiple skin-coloured to transparent papules 1–4 mm in diameter on the lower eyelids and malar areas but can also occur in the axillae, neck, chest, and occasionally on the abdomen or in the genital region. Distribution is usually symmetrical. Syringomas may rarely be familial, and in these cases, the mode of inheritance is autosomal dominant, suggesting a monogenetic entity [26, 131]. There is no

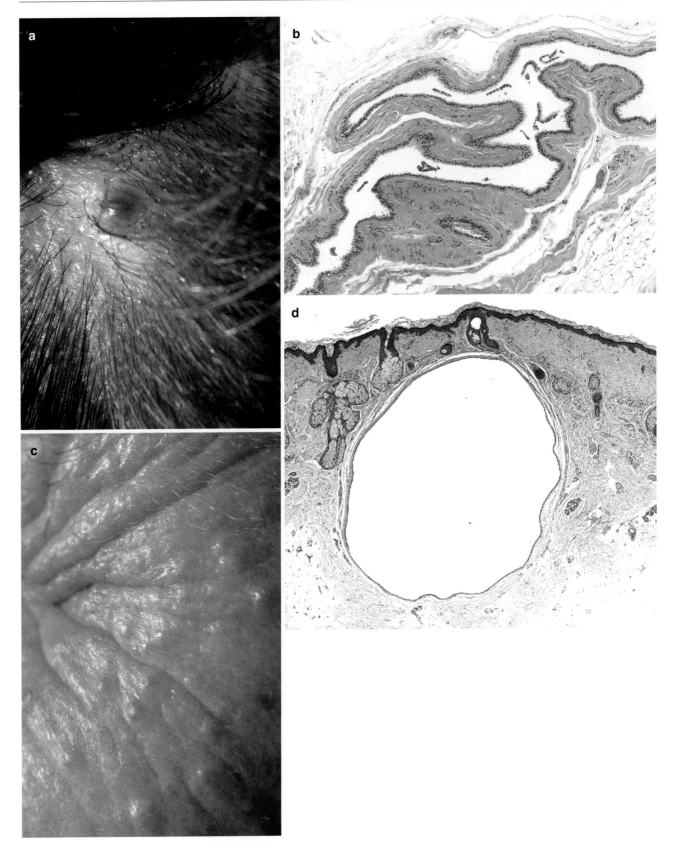

Fig. 3.2.7 (**a**, **b**) Apocrine hidrocystoma. (**c**, **d**) Eccrine hidrocystoma

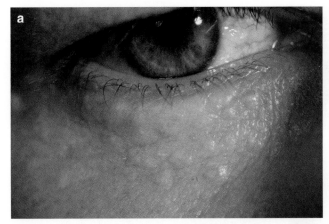

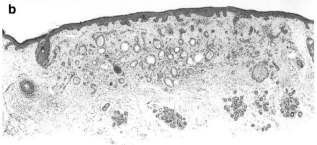

Fig. 3.2.8 (**a**, **b**) Syringoma

association with systemic diseases, but sometimes, syringoma can be associated with additional clinical findings in the context of genetic syndromes as, e.g., the syndrome of Nicolau and Balus (syringoma, milia, and atrophodermia vermiculata) [48] or Down syndrome [196]. In patients with Down syndrome, syringoma mostly manifests on or around the eyelids (18–64%), as is the case for syringoma observed in patients with Marfan and Ehlers-Danlos syndromes [47].

Rarely, numerous syringomas can develop in an eruptive fashion with no specific site predilection in young adults [186]. The pathogenesis of eruptive syringomas is controversial, and it has been suggested that they represent a reactive eccrine gland ductal proliferation provoked by cutaneous inflammatory conditions [67].

Histopathology (Fig. 3.2.8b): Syringomas are embedded in fibrous stroma complexes of small solid epithelial strands and colloid-material-containing cystic sweat ducts, confined to the upper dermis, and usually have no connection with the overlying normal epidermis. Some of the ducts are associated with epithelial cell cords, producing the typical "comma" or "tadpole" shape. The tubules are lined with a double layer of bland, monomorphous, cuboidal epithelial cells with small normochromic nuclei and little-to-moderate pale eosinophilic cytoplasm. In the clear cell variant of syringoma, the cytoplasm of the neoplastic cells is abundant and glycogen-rich, giving it a clear appearance [143]. PAS-positive eosinophilic material is often present within the tubular lumina.

Differential diagnosis: In the clinical differential diagnosis of syringoma of the eyelids and malar areas, milia and xanthelasma should be considered, while vulvar syringomas must be differentiated from Fox-Fordyce disease, epidermal cysts, senile angiomas, lichen simplex chronicus, and condyloma acuminata. Histologically, syringoma should be distinguished from its extremely rare malignant counterparts: syringoid eccrine carcinoma, MAC, and desmoplastic trichoepithelioma.

Prognosis and management: The treatment modalities include excision, electrodesiccation, laser, and cryotherapy [97, 199].

3.2.1.2.3 Poroma

Eccrine poroma, first described by Pinkus et al. in 1956 [154], is a fairly common cutaneous tumour, usually occurring as a solitary lesion. Eccrine poroma is thought to originate from the outer cells of the intraepidermal (acrosyringeal) excretory ducts of eccrine sweat glands [72].

Clinical features (Fig. 3.2.9a): In approximately two-thirds of cases, lesions occur on the soles or sides of the foot [82]. Its second most common localization is on the hands and fingers, but it can also be observed on the head, neck, and chest. Poroma can present as a dermal nodule or plaque, with a tendency to ulcerate and bleed.

Histopathology (Fig. 3.2.9b): According to their location in relation to the epidermis, there are four different entities within the poroma family of neoplasms: hidroacanthoma simplex, eccrine poroma, dermal duct tumour, and poroid hidradenoma [3, 93]. Hidroacanthoma simplex is an intraepidermal proliferation of poroid cells arranged in a nested fashion. Both dermal duct tumour and poroid hidradenoma are nodular, reticular dermal proliferations of poroid cells, showing no connection to the overlying epidermis. Dermal duct tumour consists of multiple nodules of poroid cells, while poroid hidradenoma represents a single large nodule with solid and cystic areas [159]. Classical eccrine poroma is characterised by a dermal proliferation of poroid cells with a lobular growth pattern and broad connections to the overlying epidermis. The tumour cells are uniform and cuboidal, somewhat smaller than epidermal keratinocytes, and have scant cytoplasm and small round-to-ovoid nuclei. Variable numbers of mitotic figures can be identified. The nested intraepidermal tumour cells are sharply demarcated from adjacent keratinocytes. Peripheral nuclear palisading is not found. Foci of squamous differentiation and clear cell change are frequent findings. A PAS-positive eosinophilic cuticle and small CEA-positive ducts lined with cuboidal cells are present in most cases and confirm the diagnosis. The tumour is supported by a stroma, which is characteristically highly vascularised.

Fig. 3.2.9 (a, b) Poroma

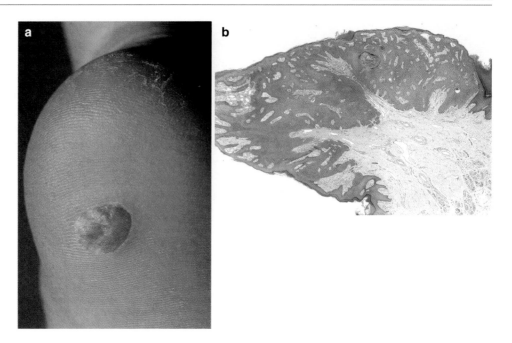

Differential diagnosis: Poroma must be differentiated from its rare malignant counterpart as well as from other sudoriferous tumours such as cylindroma and syringofibradenoma. Hidracanthoma simplex must be further differentiated from other tumours showing the "Borst–Jadassohn" phenomenon.

Prognosis and management: Poromas are treated with surgical excision. For hidracanthoma electrodesiccation and CO_2-laser ablation can be applied.

3.2.1.2.4 Syringofibroadenoma

Eccrine syringofibroadenoma (SFA)(syn. eccrine poromatosis, linear eccrine poroma, acrosyringeal nevus, nevus syringoadenomatosus papilliferus, and acrosyringeal adenomatosis) is a rare benign eccrine tumour of acrosyringeal origin, first described by Mascaro in 1963 [123].

The pathogenesis of the lesion is not clear, and it has been designated variously as a neoplasm, hamartoma, nevus, and reactive hyperplasia. It probably represents a group of heterogeneous disorders [57, 190]. Most authors consider eccrine SFA to be a benign tumour with eccrine ductal differentiation. Morphologically however, identical lesions have been reported in association with various dermatoses and cutaneous tumours such as burn, ulcer, stoma, chronic lymphedema, nevus sebaceus, lichen planus, bullous pemphigoid, and squamous cell carcinoma, suggesting a reactive nature of the process, termed "syringofibroadenomatous hyperplasia" [56, 61, 141, 167]. Squamous cell carcinoma in association with SFA has also been reported [19, 98, 114]. Whether SFA undergoes malignant degeneration or develops as a reaction to the squamous cell carcinoma remains unclear.

Clinical features: SFA usually occurs on the extremities of elderly patients as a slow-growing, solitary, flesh- or reddish-coloured nodule or plaque [84]. The lesion may also present as a verrucous nodule, ulcerative plaque, or nevoid lesion consisting of multiple papules or nodules arranged in a symmetrical or linear pattern, sometimes accompanied by hidrotic ectodermal dysplasia or palmoplantar keratoderma.

Five types of eccrine syingofibradenoma have been recognised: (1) solitary SFA; (2) multiple SFA associated with hidrotic ectodermal dysplasia (Schöpf syndrome); (3) multiple SFA without associated cutaneous findings (syringofibroadenomatosis); (4) non-familial unilateral linear SFA (nevoid SFA); and (5) reactive SFA, associated with inflammatory or neoplastic dermatoses [55].

Clinical findings are variable, but histological features are characteristic.

Histopathology (Fig. 3.2.10): Microscopic examination shows a proliferation of thin reticulated anastomosing strands and cords of monomorphous basophilic cuboidal epithelial cells, extending from the epidermis into the superficial dermis and embedded in a fibrovascular stroma. The cells are smaller than adjacent epidermal keratinocytes. They are PAS-positive and immunohistochemically reactive for EMA, HMWK, and cytokertain 14 [108]. The cords contain scattered ductal structures lined with CEA-positive cuboidal cells, resembling eccrine ducts. Areas of clear cell change may occur. Acrosyringial nevus is regarded by some authors as an identical lesion, but others consider it to be a different entity, showing prominent plasma cell infiltration.

Differential diagnosis: SFA must be differentiated from poroma and porocarcinoma, fibroepithelioma of Pinkus, and clear cell acanthoma.

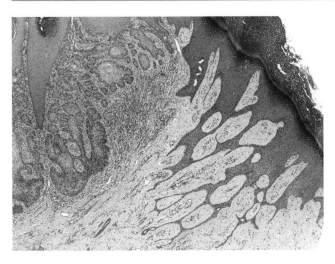

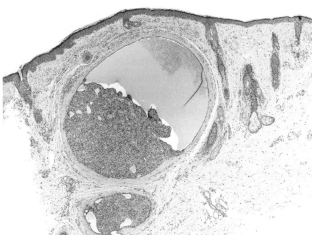

Fig. 3.2.10 Syringofibradenoma in association with squamous cell carcinoma

Fig. 3.2.11 Hidradenoma

3.2.1.2.5 Hidradenoma

Hidradenoma (syn.: nodular hidradenoma, eccrine acrospiroma, solid-cystic hidradenoma, clear cell hidradenoma, clear cell acrospiroma) was first described as a distinct clinical entity by Meyer in 1941 [125]. It is a benign sudoriferous tumour of uncertain histogenesis. In 1990, Abenoza and Ackerman [3] proposed subdividing hidradenomas into two groups: those with eccrine differentiation, composed mostly of poroid and cuticular cells, and those with apocrine differentiation, composed of clear, polygonal, and mucinous cells.

Clinical features: Hidradenoma is mostly seen between the fourth and eighth decades of life and is more common in females. It usually presents as a slowly growing, solitary, skin-coloured, reddish, bluish, or brown nodule, 1–2 cm in size. Multiple lesions are rare. The tumour may be located anywhere on the body, but there is a predilection for the scalp, face, thorax, and abdomen [174]. It is mostly asymptomatic. Only rarely do patients report tenderness, pruritus, burning, spontaneous oozing, or haemorrhage.

Histopathology (Fig. 3.2.11): Upon scanning magnification, hidradenoma is well circumscribed and has a characteristic pushy, but well-defined and regular, peripheral border. It consists of variably sized nests and lobulated nodules of epithelial cells, usually confined to the dermis. It may be connected to the epidermis and may extend into the subcutis. Cystic areas of varying proportions are often present. Small duct-like structures within the lobulated masses, usually lined with cuboidal epithelium, are found in most cases.

The tumour cells are usually small, monomorphous, and polyhedral, resembling the cells of poroma. Hidradenoma may have variable histomorphological patterns [126]. Clear cell change and squamous eddy formation may be prominent. Clear cell hidradenoma is characterised by the presence

of large pale to clear cells with small, monomorphous, round, often eccentrically located nuclei. The clear cells are rich in glycogen. In addition, they may show significant amount of PAS-positive, diastase-resistant material along their periphery [52]. Focal apocrine decapitation secretion may be observed in some hidradenomas.

Occasionally, benign-appearing tumours show focal, atypical features. The term atypical hidradenoma is used when there is prominent mitotic activity or nuclear atypia without evident signs of an infiltrating growth pattern [120].

Differential diagnosis: The clinical differential diagnosis includes basal cell and squamous cell carcinoma, melanoma, metastatic tumour, dermatofibroma, and pyogenic granuloma. Histologically, hidradenocarcinoma must be excluded. Malignancy is considered when there is increased mitotic activity, nuclear atypia, and angiolymphatic or perineural invasion.

Prognosis and management: Hidradenoma should be fully excised, as malignant transformation may occur. Furthermore, hidradenoma has a recurrence rate of approximately 12% if not fully excised [76]. Follow-up is advisable.

3.2.1.2.6 Spiradenoma

Spiradenomas are relatively common benign sudoriferous tumours of controversial origin, first described by Kersting and Helwig in 1956 [103]. Morphologic similarities between the spiradenomas cells and eccrine cells have been confirmed with ultrastructural studies, and it has been shown that spiradenomas have small quantities of the enzymes, phosphorylase and succinic dehydrogenase, present in eccrine glands [71]. Based on this evidence, spiradenomas are considered, by most authors, to originate from the straight intradermal eccrine duct. However, spiradenomas show similarities to cylindromas [132]. Further focal apocrine decapitation secretion may be present in the cells that surround the tubules of spiradenomas [119].

Clinical features: Spiradenomas are usually found on the ventral aspect of the head, trunk, and proximal limbs of adults in the third or fourth decade of life. However, they are slow-growing neoplasms ranging in size from 0.3 to 5 cm, and sometimes, patients report the presence of the tumour since childhood (9–15 years of age) [119]. Familial cases of autosomal dominant inheritance have been reported [193]. Clinically, it usually presents as a solitary, painful, firm, skin-coloured, or bluish nodule. Occasionally, multiple lesions may be present, sometimes arranged in a linear or segmental pattern [68], but in a study of 134 patients, only two had multiple tumours [103]. Spiradenomas can be associated with Brooke–Spiegler syndrome, a rare autosomal dominant inherited disorder, characterised by the development of multiple skin adnexal tumours [195].

Histopathology (Fig. 3.2.12): At scanning magnification, one or more large, sharply demarcated, encapsulated basophilic nodules in the dermis and subcutaneous tissue are observed, without connection to the epidermis. The neoplastic nodules are solid and vary in size, characteristically consisting of two epithelial cell types: small, dark, basaloid cells with hyperchromatic nuclei and cells with large, pale vesicular and ovoid nuclei. Pale cells tend to be at the centre of the lesions [119]. Cellular strings in a trabecular, reticular, or "petaloid" pattern may be observed, and formation of tubular structures is a characteristic finding of spiradenomas. Mitotic figures may be present. Globules of eosinophilic PAS-positive material are present within the tumour lobules. Typically, lymphocytes permeate the neoplasm. The prominent presence of lymphocytes in spiradenomas is helpful in their differentiation from cylindromas. Richly vascular edematous stroma with occasional thrombi, foci of squamous

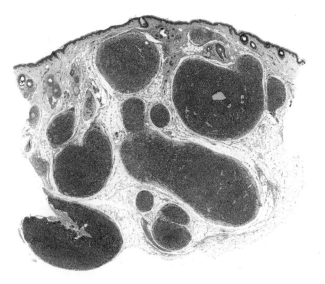

Fig. 3.2.12 Spiradenoma

differentiation, fibrosis, and cystic degenerative changes are commonly seen.

Dermal cylindromas are commonly associated with spiradenomas, and the growth stimulus for these two types of tumours appears to be identical [133].

Differential diagnosis: Clinically, other painful tumours such as leiomyoma, glomus tumour, neuroma, or angiolipoma must be considered [139]. Histologically, spiradenoma must be differentiated from cylindroma, hidradenoma, and spiradenocarcinoma.

Prognosis and management: The treatment of choice is surgical excision. Excision should be complete, because otherwise, recurrences are possible. CO_2-laser treatment has been reported to be of benefit in extensive nevoid cases [14, 193]. Malignant transformation is uncommon and occurs mostly in long-standing cases [54].

3.2.1.2.7 Cylindroma

Cylindromas are relatively uncommon benign neoplasms [37]. The histogenesis of cylindroma is controversial. There is some evidence favouring an eccrine origin from the coiled part of the intradermal duct [150], but arguments suggesting an apocrine differentiation have also been presented [164]. Cylindromas are most likely a very primitive sweat gland tumour of indeterminate differentiation. Cylindromas can occur in conjunction with spiradenomas. Cases of spiradeno-cylindromas demonstrating characteristics of both spiradenoma and cylindroma in the same tumour are no rarity, suggesting similar derivation of both tumours [133, 187].

Clinical features (Fig. 3.2.13a): Some 90% of cylindromas occur in the head and neck region, particularly on the scalp and face. Women are much more frequently affected than men, reported female-to-male ratios range between 6:1 and 9:1. Cylindromas can be sporadic and present as solitary, firm, rubbery nodules of pink, red, or bluish colour, varying in size from a few millimetres to several centimetres. When numerous nodules on the scalp enlarge and coalesce, they form the distinctive turban tumour feature. Rarely, multiple cylindromas can be associated with familial cylindromatosis (CYLD): an autosomal dominant disorder. The association of multiple trichoepitheliomas and cylindromas, the so-called Brooke–Spiegler syndrome, is also inherited in an autosomal dominant manner. In this case, there are multiple tumours that may also involve the trunk and extremities of children or young adults. The gene for familial CYLD has been localised to chromosome 16q12–13, and loss of gene function in tumours is consistent with the gene acting as a tumour suppressor [18]. The cause of sporadic, solitary cylindromas is unclear; however, genetic studies show loss of heterozygosity at and around the CYLD locus in a substantial proportion of sporadic cylindromas, suggesting that

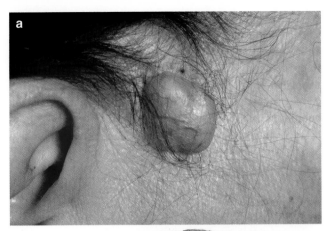

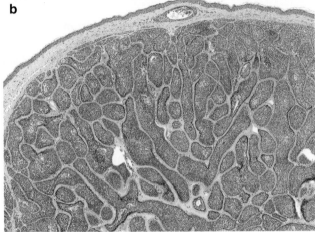

Fig. 3.2.13 (a, b) Cylindroma

this gene also plays a role in the development of the sporadic form [116].

Histopathology (Fig. 3.2.13b): Cylindroma is a dermal tumour, without attachment to the epidermis, composed of numerous well-defined, variably sized oval and polygonal nests and nodules of epithelial cells, lined with a thick PAS-positive basement membrane-like, hyalinised sheath and moulded into a characteristic "jigsaw puzzle" pattern. The hyaline sheaths, which surround tumour nests, are mostly composed of type IV collagen but also contain integrin $\alpha_4\beta_6$ and laminin 5. Fragments of anchoring fibrils, identical to type VII collagen, are also seen upon electron microscopy. Tumour islands are composed of two cell types: (1) large cells with pale-staining nuclei and moderate amount of amphophilic cytoplasm, located at the central zone, and (2) peripherally located, small, basaloid cells with dark-staining nuclei and scant cytoplasm that exhibit a palisading pattern. Small ductal lumina lined with cuboidal or columnar cells and containing intraluminal eosinophilic material are sometimes found. PAS-positive hyaline globules are present in the tumour islands. A lack of lymphoid tissue is a histological feature that differentiates cylindromas from spiradenomas. Cylindromas demonstrate a large number of prominent

dendritic cells that most likely represent Langerhans cells that permeate the tumour. Some tumours, termed spiradeno-cylindromas, have features of both cylindromas and eccrine spiradenomas [133, 187]. The existence of these combined tumours suggests that both entities may belong to a continuous morphological spectrum of a single entity. Both cylindroma and spiradenoma show immunopositivity for human milk fat globulin and lysosome in tubular cells, S100 protein within the tubular and large, pale-staining cells, SMA in small basaloid cells. Both tumours show identical cytokeratin patterns, with the expression of CK 7, 8, and 18 [132].

Differential diagnosis: The clinical differential diagnosis includes spiradenoma, follicular infundibular tumour, and pilar cyst. Histologically, cylindroma must be differentiated from spiradenoma and from its very rare malignant counterpart.

Prognosis and management: For solitary lesions, the treatment of choice is surgical excision. Multiple cylindromas usually require extensive plastic surgery that may be substituted by progressively excising groups of nodules in multiple procedures. Other treatments include electrodesiccation with curettage and cryotherapy. For small lesions, the CO_2-laser can be used.

Most cylindromas remain benign; however, malignant transformation has been reported. Malignant cylindroma is a rare tumour arising from pre-existing benign cylindroma, both in solitary sporadic and in autosomal dominant multiple forms. Malignant cylindroma is clinically characterised by rapid growth, long-standing ulceration or bleeding, and aggressive clinical behaviour, with local recurrence and the potential for distant metastases [49]. Malignant cylindromas demonstrate islands of cells displaying marked anaplasia and pleomorphism of nuclei. Mitotic figures are increased and abnormal. Besides invasion of surrounding tissue, loss of jigsaw appearance, loss of hyaline sheath, and loss of peripheral palisading occur.

Follow-up care of patients with multiple cylindromas is recommended. Genetic counselling for the multiple variant must be considered.

3.2.1.2.8 Tubular Adenoma and Tubular Papillary Adenoma

First described by Landry and Winkelmann in 1972 [111], tubular adenoma is a rare sweat gland tumour, and the discussion concerning its derivation is not yet completed. Rulon and Helwig [169] reported the first 14 cases of papillary eccrine adenoma in 1977. Many authors believe that tubular apocrine adenoma and papillary eccrine adenoma are likely the same neoplasm [33, 51, 94].

Clinical features: Tubular adenoma can arise de novo or in adjunction with an organoid nevus or syringocystadenoma papilliferum (SCAP). Women are affected twice as often as men. The scalp is by far the most common localization, although a variety of sites has been reported. The cases reported as papillary eccrine adenoma also showed a clear-cut female predilection and occurred mostly on the extremities.

Tubular adenoma presents usually as a deep-lying, skin-coloured nodule, 1–2 cm in diameter. Papillary eccrine adenoma has been reported as an erythematous, yellowish, or brownish nodule, 0.5–4.0 cm in diameter.

Histopathology: Tubular adenoma is composed of numerous tubular and cystic structures lined with two to several layers of monomorphous cells. The outer layer of tubules and cysts is composed of distinct, well-formed basal cuboidal or flattened myoepithelial cells. The lumens of the tubules may appear empty or contain granular eosinophilic material or cellular necrotic debris. Decapitation secretion is seen in a minority of the lumens. The tumour is centred in the deep dermis, sometimes communicating with the epidermis through dilated duct-like structures or involving the subcutis, and is embedded in a dense fibrous connective tissue stroma.

The luminal cells of the tubular lining express EMA and CEA. The myoepithelial cells are positive for S-100 and SMA [86].

The findings reported in papillary eccrine adenoma are very similar to those of tubular adenoma. In tubular papillary adenoma (Fig. 3.2.14), luminal cells form papillary projections of variable complexity.

There is a controversy about whether tubular adenoma and papillary eccrine adenoma represent two distinct entities or are the very same tumour, and if the latter, which lineage of differentiation it pursues [58, 86, 192]. Based on the histologic similarities, many authors believe that both tumours belong to the same entity, and as such, the designations "tubulopapillary hidradenoma" [192] and "papillary tubular

adenoma" [51] have been proposed. It has been suggested that the majority of these neoplasms exhibit apocrine differentiation. Arguments in favour of the apocrine origin include the presence of decapitation secretion, the association of the neoplasm with other apocrine lesions (SCAP, nevus sebaceous), a close proximity to hair follicular infundibulum, and appropriate ultrastructural features [5, 22, 86, 164]. Rare cases occurring in the sites normally devoid of apocrine glands may represent the eccrine counterpart.

Prognosis and management: The treatment of choice is surgical excision.

3.2.1.2.9 Syringocystadenoma Papilliferum

Syringocystadenoma papilliferum is a rare sweat gland tumour with a widely variable clinical appearance but with a distinct histology. Pinkus [152] and Helwig and Hackney [77] have provided detailed descriptions of this entity in early published case series.

Clinical features (Fig. 3.2.15a): Syringocystadenoma papilliferum is mostly a tumour of childhood; in about half of those affected, it is present at birth; and in an additional 15–30%, it develops before puberty. The lesions may evolve de novo or, in some 40% of cases, from a contiguous or pre-existing nevus sebaceous. In a series of 596 patients with nevus sebaceous lesions, 30 were found to have coexisting SCAP [38]. SCAP is most frequently found on the head and neck. In approximately 25% of cases, it is observed on other locations such as the trunk or the extremities.

SCAP usually presents as a hairless, single nodule or plaque on the scalp. A rare, small papular form has also been reported [138]. Larger nodules may ulcerate and acquire a crusted appearance. During puberty or pregnancy, SCAP grows in size and the smooth surface becomes warty.

Histopathology (Fig. 3.2.15b): Although SCAP has a varied clinical appearance, its histopathologic characteristics are distinctive. Duct-like invaginations and cyst-like cavities of various shapes and sizes extend from the epidermal surface into the dermis. Near the surface of the lesion, the invaginations are lined with keratinized stratified epithelium transitioning in the deeper portions of the tumour to ducts lined with a double-layered epithelium with an inner layer of tall columnar cells and an outer layer of small cuboidal ones. The connective tissue stroma surrounding these duct-like structures contains a chronic inflammatory infiltrate, rich in plasma cells.

Malignancies, which may be associated with SCAP, include, most commonly, basal cell carcinoma and, occasionally, squamous cell or sweat gland carcinoma. A rapid increase in size or number of SCAP lesions, ulceration, and pain are indicative of malignant transformation. Most reports

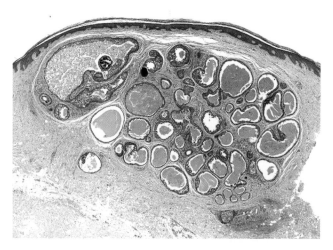

Fig. 3.2.14 Tubular papillary adenoma

Fig. 3.2.15 (a, b)
Syringocystadenoma
papilliferum

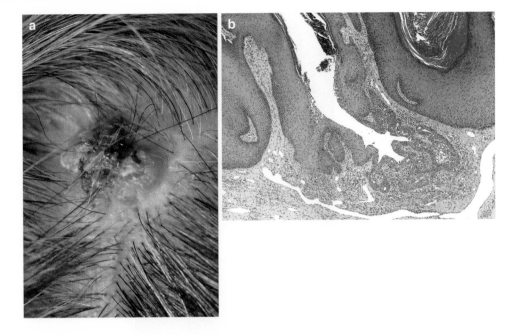

of SCAP-associated malignancy are in patients with nevus sebaceous. The length of time from onset of SCAP to malignant transformation has been reported to vary from 20 to 50 years [89].

Prognosis and management: The prophylactic excision of SCAP is of uncertain benefit, but in case of growing or ulcerating lesions, surgical removal should be performed. In anatomic areas where excision or grafting is problematic, CO_2-laser ablation is a treatment option [92].

3.2.1.2.10 Hidradenoma Papilliferum

Hidradenoma papilliferum (HP) [40] is a benign neoplasm involving anogenital mammary-like glands and may be considered an analogue of intraductal papilloma of the breast.

Clinical features: HP occurs almost exclusively in the anogenital region of adult women. Anecdotal cases of HP have been reported in males [117] and in extra-anogenital locations, particularly on the head and neck [198]. The tumour is solitary and is usually small and asymptomatic [206]. Only occasionally, a large, elevated, reddish-brown mass with an ulcerated and bleeding surface [69] is present.

Histopathology: Upon scanning magnification, the tumour appears as well-demarcated intradermal cystic-solid nodule with a complex pattern of branching and anastomizing tubular structures, interconnected in a complex labyrinth-like manner, with paths of fibrous tissue between them, focally forming papillae [128]. The tubules and papillae are lined with a luminal layer of monomorphic, clear or eosinophilic, tall columnar cells demonstrating focal decapitation secretion and a basal layer of small myoepithelial cells with hyperchromatic nuclei. Intracytoplasmic granules of PAS-positive,

diastase-resistant material are a common finding. The overlying epidermis may be normal, acanthotic, or ulcerated. Focal communication between tumour and epidermis is sometimes seen.

Luminal epithelial cells stain for cytokeratins (AE1/AE3), EMA, CEA, HMFG, and GCFP-15 [142]. The basal layer of myoepithelial cells shows positivity for SMA and S-100 protein.

Malignant variants of HP, characterised by tissue infiltration, nucleocellular atypia and pleomorphism, and brisk mitotic activity, are extremely rare [9, 178]. The term "hidradenocarcinoma papilliferum" has been used for those tumours [164].

Prognosis and management: Simple excision is curative for benign HP.

3.2.1.2.11 Mixed Tumour (Chondroid Syringoma)

After Billroth's first description of mixed tumour of the skin in 1859, as an entity analogous to the mixed tumours of the salivary glands, it was Hirsch and Helwig who, in 1961, first used the term "chondroid syringoma" because of the presence of sweat gland features in a cartilage-like stroma [80]. Headington classified chondroid syringomas as apocrine or eccrine based on their histologic appearances [74]. CS is a rare benign sudoriferous tumour. The incidence of CS is reported to be less than 0.01% among the primary skin tumours [106].

Clinical features (Fig. 3.2.16a): CS usually affects middle-aged or older male patients [209]. The male-to-female ratio is 2:1. The site of predilection for CS is the head and neck, but cases involving other sites including the hand, foot,

Fig. 3.2.16 (**a**, **b**) Mixed tumour
(chondroid syringoma)

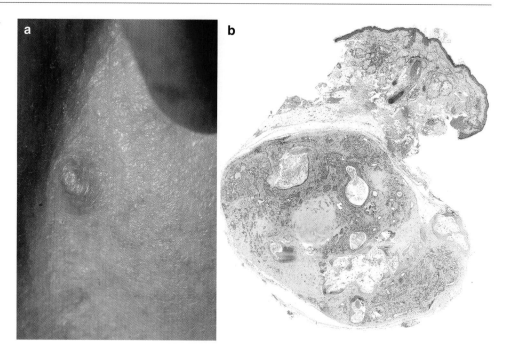

axillary region, abdomen, penis, vulva, and scrotum have
been documented. The typical clinical presentation is a solitary, small, slow-growing, firm, mobile nodule, usually
0.5–3 cm in diameter, localised in the dermis or subdermis.
The surface can be lobulated, and adnexal orifices have been
detected in some cases.

Histopathology (Fig. 3.2.16b): Histologically, CS is similar to the benign mixed tumour of the salivary glands, characteristically exhibiting an epithelial and a mesenchymal
stromal component. Epithelial chords, tubuloalveolar and
gland-like structures lined with two or more layers of cuboidal cells, islands of cuboidal or polygonal cells embedded in
a conspicuous stroma, in which myxoid, chondroid,
hyalinised, fibrous, fibroadipoid, or osteoid areas are variably combined, produce the typical pattern of this tumour
[83]. The inner layer of this tumour's epithelial cells stains
for cytokeratin, EMA, and CEA; the outer epithelial layer

stains for S-100 and vimentin [208]. In the mesenchymal
stromal component, large mucin-rich areas are highlighted
with alcian blue. CS is classified into apocrine and eccrine
types, based on the histopathological appearance of the glandular structures of the tumour. In apocrine-type lesions, areas
with pilar and sebaceous differentiation have been reported
[208], suggesting that some tumours represent hamartomatous lesions of the pilosebaceous-apocrine unit.

Prognosis and management: Surgical excision is curative,
and recurrences occur only if residual tumour is left. Rare
cases of more aggressive or malignant forms have been
reported. The malignant forms are more common in younger
patients, localised on the trunk or extremities [87], are often
larger than 3 cm in diameter, and upon histological evaluation, show infiltrative margins, satellite tumour nodules,
areas of necrosis, cytological atypia, and brisk mitotic
activity.

3.2.2 Tumours with Follicular Differentiation

Steven Kaddu

3.2.2.1 Pilomatrical Carcinoma

Definition: Pilomatrical carcinoma, the malignant counterpart of pilomatricoma, is an extremely rare malignant follicular tumour that may be locally aggressive or show metastatic spread to distant sites [2, 21, 35, 60, 119, 127, 135, 210, 215]. The diagnosis of pilomatrical carcinoma and its distinction from pilomatricoma depend mainly on the presence of a number of histopathologic features, including an infiltrative growth pattern, high mitotic activity, and features suggestive of vascular and perineural invasion. Rarely however, examples of clinically aggressive pilomatrical carcinomas may lack clear-cut histopathologic features of malignancy [153].

Synonyms: calcifying epitheliocarcinoma of Malherbe, invasive pilomatrixoma, malignant melanocytic matricoma, malignant pilomatrixoma, matrical carcinoma, matrix carcinoma, pilomatrix carcinoma.

Aetiology: The majority of pilomatrical carcinomas develop de novo, although malignant transformation from pre-existing pilomatricoma has been reported [170]. It is possible that proliferating pilomatricoma, a variant of pilomatricoma that presents mainly in middle-aged and elderly individuals, may represent an intermediate precursor lesion [84]. Recent studies have demonstrated mutations in CTNNB1, the gene encoding beta-catenin, in both benign pilomatricomas and pilomatrical carcinomas, suggesting a common initial pathogenesis and that pilomatrix carcinomas may at least on occasion arise from their benign counterparts [103]. A case of pilomatrical carcinoma arising in association with HIV and hepatitis C infections was recently reported [174].

Clinical features: Pilomatrical carcinoma presents mostly in adults with a broad age range. The mean age at the time of diagnosis is about 48 years. The male-to-female ratio is 2:1. Lesions occur commonly as asymptomatic, slowly growing, firm, non-tender nodules measuring 1–10 cm in diameter. Most cases localise on the head or neck [94]. Pilomatrical carcinomas also rarely develop on other anatomical sites including the upper and lower extremities [35, 118], the axilla [57] (Fig. 3.2.17), the chest [60], and the inguinal region [208].

Histopathology: Histopathologic examination shows irregularly sized and differently shaped cutaneous/subcutaneous epithelial islands of basaloid (matrical and supramatrical) cells with conspicuous foci of shadow cells (Fig. 3.2.18a–c) [13, 21]. The basaloid cells often reveal marked nuclear atypia and frequent mitoses. Large areas of geographical necrosis as well as foci of calcification and ossification may be observed. Sections may show tumour involvement of vascular lumina, subjacent deep soft tissues and bone. Rare cases reveal an

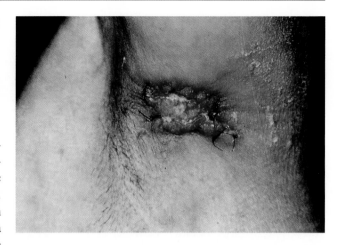

Fig. 3.2.17 Pilomatrical carcinoma located in the axilla

increased proliferation of melanocytes within the epithelial component (malignant melanocytic matricoma) [75].

Immunohistochemistry: Pilomatrical carcinoma may express cytokeratin in the basaloid component as well as in shadow cells [33].

Treatment and prognosis: The treatment of choice is surgical excision with adequate margins [105, 170]. A minimum of 5 mm has been recommended as an adequate margin for surgical treatment of pilomatrical carcinoma. Mohs micrographic surgery is useful in some cases [165]. Pilomatrical carcinomas are mainly locally aggressive neoplasms, though there are a number of well-documented cases with distant metastases [21, 35, 119, 127, 135]. Local recurrences following surgical excision have been recorded in up to 46% of patients and multiple recurrences in up to 22% [60]. Metastases mainly involve regional lymph nodes, lungs, and bone [21, 35, 60, 119, 127, 135].

3.2.2.2 Proliferating Tricholemmal Tumour

Definition: Proliferating tricholemmal tumour is a relatively uncommon follicular neoplasm predominantly characterised by features of differentiation toward the outer root sheath of a normal hair follicle at the level of the isthmus, variable cytologic atypia, and mitotic activity. Until recently, proliferating tricholemmal tumours were generally regarded as benign lesions; however, following reports of carcinomatous transformation with distant metastases in some examples of these neoplasms [7, 14, 63, 69, 106, 111, 117, 132, 133, 142, 199, 211], a number of authors have recently suggested that at least a subset of these tumours represents a type of squamous cell carcinoma [2, 47, 124, 220]. Accordingly, categorization of proliferating tricholemmal tumours into three groups, benign, low-grade malignancy, and high-grade malignancy, has been proposed [220].

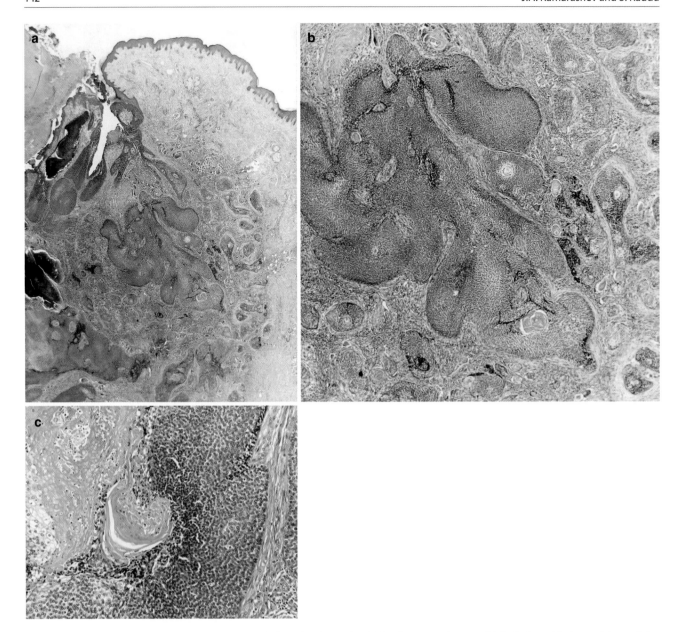

Fig. 3.2.18 (**a**) Pilomatrical carcinoma. Ulcerated lesion showing irregularly sized and variously shaped epithelial islands of basaloid cells with foci of cornification. (**b**) Irregular epithelial aggregations of basaloid cells are contiguous with foci of cornified material containing shadow cells. (**c**) Epithelial aggregations of atypical basaloid cells are contiguous with areas of shadow cells

Aetiology: It is uncertain whether proliferating tricholemmal tumours arise de novo or from pre-existing tricholemmal cysts [124, 149]. Observations of multiple proliferating tricholemmal tumours arising in association with trichilemmal cysts may suggest a common histogenesis of both lesions [68]. Human papillomavirus has been proposed as an etiological agent in some cases [3].

Synonyms: giant hair matrix tumour, invasive pilomatrixoma, pilar tumour of the scalp, proliferating epidermoid cyst, proliferating follicular cystic neoplasm, proliferating pilar tumour, proliferating trichilemmal cyst, proliferating trichilemmal tumour, trichilemmal pilar tumour, trichochlamydocarcinoma.

Clinical features: Proliferating tricholemmal tumours present mostly as solitary, slowly growing, cystic, lobulated, exophytic, and occasionally ulcerated nodules or tumours located mainly on the scalp (Fig. 3.2.19), trunk, or extremities of elderly individuals [2, 210, 215]. Lesions commonly measure

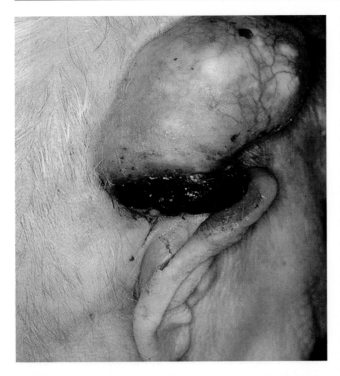

Fig. 3.2.19 Proliferating pilar tumour. An ulcerated giant nodule on the scalp

2–12 cm in diameter [106], but tumours up to 25 cm have been reported [28]. Women are about two times more commonly affected than men [172]. Rare examples occur as multiple, sometimes familial lesions [68], or as neoplasms arising in association with a pre-existing nevus sebaceus [154, 196].

Histopathology: Most proliferating tricholemmal tumours show a sharply circumscribed, round or oval, solid or solid-cystic, dermal or dermal/subcutaneous lesion with an epithelium lining nearly the whole lesion. The epithelial wall focally extends within the lesion in a radial fashion forming several partially interconnecting, solid, and cystic lobules (Fig. 3.2.20a, b). The epithelium reveals squamous cells with some areas of clear cells containing glycogen. A characteristic feature is the presence, in the centre of lobules, of tricholemmal cornification (abrupt formation of compact eosinophilic keratin without granular layer interposition) (Fig. 3.2.20c). Some lobules display a palisade arrangement of nuclei at the periphery. A zone of fibrous stroma with clefts between the stroma and surrounding normal tissue encompasses the lesion. Additional features of individual neoplasms include foci with keratohyaline granules, small horn pearls and squamous eddies, calcification, stromal calcium deposition, and ossification.

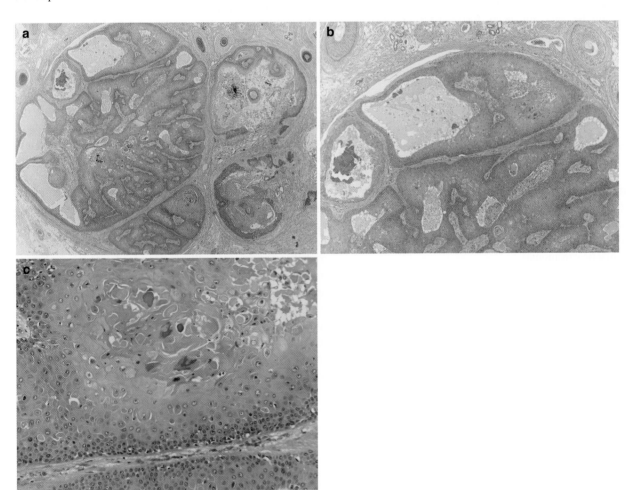

Fig. 3.2.20 (**a**) Proliferating pilar tumour. A deep dermal lesion consisting of several partially interconnected cystic epithelial lobules, surrounded by fibrous stroma with artifactual clefts. (**b**) The epithelium consists mainly of squamous cells. (**c**) An area of tricholemmal cornification

Some examples reveal a lymphohistiocytic inflammatory infiltration with foreign-body granulomas. Rare cases display features of hair matrix differentiation and shadow cells [134] or apocrine-acrosyringeal and sebaceous differentiation [167].

A minority of proliferating tricholemmal tumours reveal "atypical" features including local infiltration of tumour cells into the stroma, galea, and underlying cranium, a high mitotic activity, dyskeratotic cells, edema and cystic degeneration, as well as tumoural necrosis [220]. These changes are generally suggestive of aggressive behaviour.

Immunohistochemistry: Proliferating tricholemmal tumours express foetal hair root cytokeratin and cytokeratin 7 [56]. "Atypical" proliferating tricholemmal tumours may show an increase in staining in nucleolar organiser regions [184].

Treatment and prognosis: Total excision with clear margins is the treatment of choice, though there are presently no well-agreed-upon recommendations regarding the size of margins. Lesions without atypical features generally behave in a benign fashion. Tumours with an invasive growth pattern or cytologic atypia have an unpredictable course. They may be locally aggressive, recur, or metastasize [7, 14, 63, 69, 91, 111, 117, 130–133, 142, 199, 211]. Malignant proliferating tricholemmal tumours, particularly tumours larger than 5 cm or with spindle cell components, tend to have a poorer prognosis than the histopathologically similar "ordinary" cutaneous squamous cell carcinomas [171, 220]. Thorough follow-up is recommended in all cases, even in patients with neoplasms showing benign-appearing histopathologic features.

3.2.2.3 Trichoblastoma

Definition: Trichoblastoma represents a broad and heterogeneous group of benign follicular neoplasms with follicular germinative differentiation [2, 3, 64]. Trichoblastoma is regarded as the benign analogue of basal cell carcinoma (trichoblastic carcinoma).

Synonyms: trichoepithelioma, trichogenic trichoblastoma, trichoblastic fibroma, trichoblastic trichoblastoma, immature trichoepithelioma, trichogenic myxoma, trichogenic fibroma, lymphadenoma, adamantinoid trichoblastoma, trichogerminoma, sclerosing epithelial hamartoma, Brooke–Fordyce disease (multiple trichoblastomas), Brooke–Spiegler disease (familial multiple trichoblastomas and cylindromas) or epithelioma adenoides cysticum.

Clinical features: Trichoblastoma presents in all ages and tends to show no gender predilection. Lesions occur mostly as solitary, non-ulcerated, skin-coloured to brown, or bluish-black papules and nodules measuring 1–2 cm in diameter, located commonly on the head and neck, particularly on the scalp and face of adults and, occasionally, on

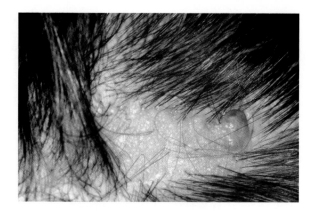

Fig. 3.2.21 Trichoblastoma arising in a nevus sebaceus

the extremities or trunk [2, 3, 37, 79, 81, 177, 205, 210]. They are thought to be dermal nevi at the time of excision but may be initially suspected to be basal cell carcinomas in older individuals. Less commonly, trichoblastomas present as giant lesions measuring up to 17 cm in diameter [136, 140]. Multiple trichoblastomas are a feature of Brooke–Fordyce and Brooke–Spiegler diseases. Multiple trichoblastomas arising in Brooke–Fordyce and Brooke–Spiegler diseases commonly present as centrofacial papules or nodules. Trichoblastomas sometimes develop in a pre-existing nevus sebaceus (Fig. 3.2.21) [34, 79, 81].

Histopathology: Trichoblastomas generally reveal dermal or dermal-subcutaneous lesions composed of relatively monomorphous basaloid cells (basophilic germinative cells) and variable eosinophilic cells, surrounded by a fibrous or fibromyxoid stroma. In some cases, areas of sclerosis may be observed. Epithelial aggregations typically reveal periphery palisading and foci with rudimentary follicular papillae and germs. Clefts may be observed within the stroma, especially around clusters of fibroepithelial units. Epithelial aggregations are arranged in different architectural patterns, including nodular, retiform, cribriform, racemiform, and columnar. A single pattern may predominate in individual lesions, but generally, more than one pattern is observed. Accordingly, trichoblastomas are further categorised into a number of morphological variants based mainly on the predominant architectural pattern, including nodular (small and large nodular), adamantinoid (lymphadenoma, lymphoepithelial tumour of the skin), retiform (giant solitary trichoepithelioma), cribriform (classic trichoepithelioma), racemiform (non-classic trichoepithelioma), and columnar (desmoplastic trichoepithelioma) [2, 3].

3.2.2.3.1 Nodular Trichoblastoma

Nodular trichoblastomas (small and large nodular) are characterised by well-circumscribed dermal or dermal-subcutaneous lesions consisting of solid epithelial aggregations of

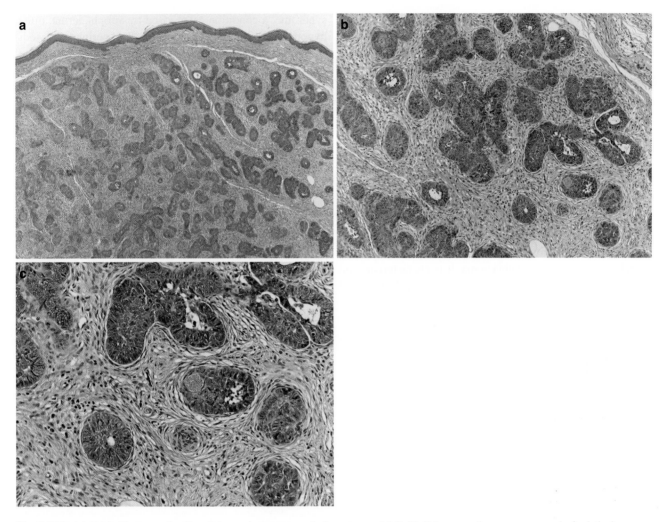

Fig. 3.2.22 (**a**) Trichoblastoma. Small nodular variant composed of numerous, solid, and solid-cystic aggregations of basaloid cells surrounded by a fibrous stroma. (**b**) Basaloid aggregations showing a palisade arrangement of cells at the periphery, surrounded by dense fibrous stroma. (**c**) Epithelial aggregations are composed of relatively monomorphous basaloid cells (basophilic germinative cells). Note the focal area with a rudimentary follicular papilla

relatively uniform cells, surrounded by a fibrous or fibromyxoid stroma (Fig. 3.2.22a-c). Both small and large nodular patterns are frequently observed in the same lesion, though neoplasms with a predominantly large nodular pattern are more common. Some tumours may be exclusively located in the subcutis (subcutaneous trichoblastoma) [80]. Nodular trichoblastomas may additionally show areas of melanin pigmentation, infundibulocystic structures (adenoid cystic trichoblastoma) [18], amyloid deposits, and features of differentiation toward other parts of the hair follicle, including bulbs, outer and inner sheath. Rare neoplasms may display a rippled-pattern (resembling Verocay bodies of a schwannoma) [5, 53], prominent pigmentation (pigmented trichoblastoma) [6], an increase of melanocytes, features of apocrine and/ sebaceous differentiation [207, 223], or a conspicuous clear cell change [203]. A distinctive superficial type of trichoblastoma (resembling superficial basal cell carcinoma) is sometimes observed in lesions of nevus sebaceus [34, 76, 79, 81, 203].

3.2.2.3.2   Adamantinoid Trichoblastoma

Adamantinoid trichoblastoma (cutaneous lymphadenoma) is a variant of small nodular trichoblastoma, histopathologically resembling the dental tumour "adamantinoma". Adamantinoid trichoblastomas are rare neoplasms that present mainly as solitary, skin-coloured nodules situated on the head and neck of adults in their fourth to fifth decades [2, 169]. They are usually clinically suspected to be basal cell carcinomas. Histopathologically, adamantinoid trichoblastomas typically show multiple, variably sized, dermal lobules of basaloid cells, surrounded by a fibrous stroma. The basaloid lobules display focal palisading of nuclei at the periphery. An infiltrate of T- and B-lymphocytes is typically observed within the basaloid lobules with a focal sprinkling of lymphocytes in the stroma. Epithelial aggregations sometimes display signs of follicular and sebaceous, rarely, ductal differentiation [159] or extracellular mucin deposition [209].

3.2.2.3.3 Retiform Trichoblastoma

Retiform trichoblastomas are usually large, dermal/subcutaneous neoplasms consisting of long cords and columns of follicular germinative cells, focally joined together to form a netlike pattern [2, 3]. Lesions may be located entirely in the subcutis (giant solitary trichoepithelioma). Other patterns such as cribriform and racemiform may also be observed in these neoplasms.

3.2.2.3.4 Cribriform Type Trichoblastoma (Conventional Trichoepithelioma)

Although a cribriform (lace-like reticular) pattern may be found in any type of trichoblastoma, it is characteristic for conventional trichoepithelioma (Fig. 3.2.23a) [2]. Two distinctive forms of conventional trichoepithelioma are recognised: solitary and multiple. Solitary trichoepithelioma occurs mainly as a small (5–8 mm in diameter), skin-coloured papule situated on the face, especially around the nose, upper lip, and cheeks of adults. Occasionally, lesions develop on the trunk, neck, scalp, and lower extremities. Multiple trichoepitheliomas usually present in adolescents as numerous, small papules distributed on the face, with a predilection for the area around the nasolabial folds, forehead, chin, and preauricular regions. A few patients reveal plaques, nodules, or tumours due to coalescing of several lesions. Multiple trichoepitheliomas are mostly transmitted as an autosomal dominant trait in patients with Brooke–Spiegler (epithelioma adenoides cysticum) disease [95, 213]. In these cases, patients have a predisposition for developing multifocal cylindromas, spiradenomas, basal cell carcinomas, and milia. Multiple trichoepitheliomas may rarely be associated with a number of other systemic conditions including systemic lupus erythematosus, myasthenia gravis, and Rombo

syndrome, a condition categorised by atrophoderma, milia, hypotrichosis, basal cell carcinomas, and peripheral vasodilatation [11, 122, 193]. Histopathologically, trichoepitheliomas reveal dome-shaped, sharply circumscribed lesions composed of aggregations of relatively monomorphic basaloid (germinative) cells in the upper dermis, surrounded by abundant fibrous stroma with intrastromal clefts. The basaloid aggregations are mainly arranged in a cribriform pattern but sometimes display other architectural patterns including nodular, racemiform, and retiform. They also characteristically reveal peripheral palisading and several foci with rudimentary follicular papillae and germs (Fig. 3.2.23b). Additional findings occasionally include infundibulocystic structures, shadow cells, sebaceous cells, amyloid, calcification, melanin pigmentation, giant and multinucleated cells [88], and mucin deposits. A lymphohistiocytic infiltrate with small foreign-body granulomas is observed in some lesions.

3.2.2.3.5 Racemiform Type Trichoblastoma

In contrast to cribriform trichoblastoma, racemiform type is mostly vertically oriented and shows foci with aggregations of epithelial (follicular germinative) cells resembling "clusters of grapes". This variant has therefore been regarded as an unconventional trichoepithelioma [2].

3.2.2.3.6 Columnar Type Trichoblastoma (Desmoplastic Trichoepithelioma)

Columnar type trichoblastoma (desmoplastic trichoepithelioma, sclerosing epithelial hamartoma) is a relatively uncommon tumour that commonly presents as a small (up to 1 cm in diameter), asymptomatic, firm, oval, oblong, or annular papule or plaque on the face, particularly around the angle of the lip

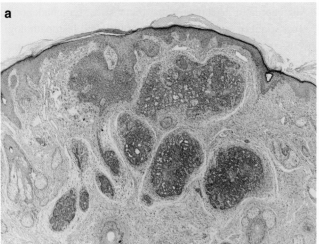
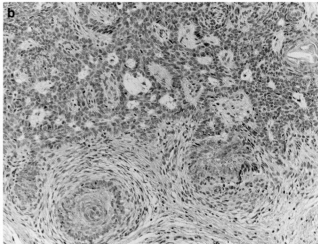

Fig. 3.2.23 (**a**) Cribriform type trichoblastoma (trichoepithelioma). (**b**) Cribriform trichoblastoma with rudimentary follicular papillae and germs

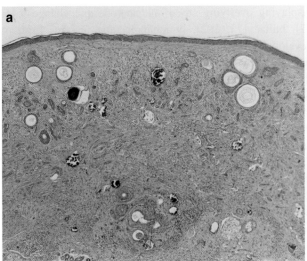
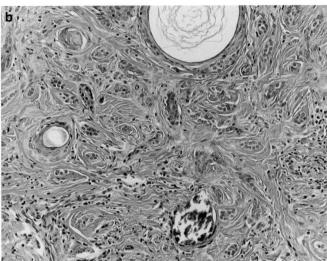

Fig. 3.2.24 (**a**) Columnar type trichoblastoma (desmoplastic trichoepithelioma) showing an upper dermal lesion with basaloid aggregations arranged predominantly in columns and cords, admixed with infundibulocystic structures and surrounded by a dense, desmoplastic stroma.

(**b**) Columns and cords of basaloid cells admixed with infundibulocystic structures and foci of calcification and surrounded by a dense, hypocellular desmoplastic stroma

[2]. Plaques often reveal a raised border and depressed centre. Lesions tend to occur in young and middle-aged adults. Women are about three times more commonly affected than men. Familial cases of solitary or multiple lesions have been reported. Histopathologically, the neoplasms reveal a relatively well-circumscribed lesion in the upper two-thirds of the dermis, rarely with extension to the lower dermis and subcutis. Lesions are composed of basaloid aggregations arranged predominantly in columns and cords, admixed with infundibulocystic structures and surrounded by a dense, hypocellular desmoplastic stroma (Fig. 3.2.24a, b). A focal connection to the epidermis is usually present. Additional features may include foci of sebaceous cells, shadow ("ghost") cells, foreign-body granulomas, calcification, and ossification. A subset of these neoplasms reveals an associated dermal melanocytic nevus.

Immunohistochemistry: Trichoblastomas show a pattern of cytokeratin expression similar to that of basal cell carcinomas [176, 219], supporting a common line of follicular differentiation. The presence of numerous Merkel cells tends to favour trichoblastoma over basal cell carcinoma [31, 98, 115].

Somatic genetics: Multiple trichoblastomas seen in Brooke–Fordyce disease are transmitted as an autosomal dominant trait linked to chromosome 9p21 [59]. Solitary (sporadic) trichoblastomas have occasionally been linked to 9q22.3, which is also the locus for nevoid basal cell carcinoma syndrome [112]. Familial multiple trichoblastomas and cylindromas (Brooke–Spiegler disease) have been linked to chromosome 16q12–q13 [46]. Mutations in the CYLD gene have been reported in individuals with Brooke–Spiegler disease, familial CYLD, and multiple familial trichoepithelioma, suggesting that all these disorders may represent phenotypic variations of a single defect [222].

Treatment: Surgery is usually effective in removing solitary lesions. However, surgical treatment of multiple trichoepitheliomas is generally disappointing. Alternative therapies for patients with multiple lesions include cryotherapy, electrodesiccation, and carbon dioxide laser [160]. Rare cases of basal cell carcinomas arising in trichoblastomas have been documented [157, 173]. Some of these neoplasms revealed features of high-grade trichoblastic carcinoma and eventually led to distant metastases and death.

3.2.2.4 Pilomatricoma

Definition: Pilomatricoma is a relatively common, benign adnexal tumour that predominantly shows differentiation toward the hair matrix cells of a normal hair follicle [2, 3, 83].

Aetiology: Pilomatricoma was first described by Malherbe and Chenantais as "l epitheliome calcifie des glandes sebacées" in 1880 [109]. In 1949, Lever and Griesemer noted that the proliferating cells of the neoplasm were similar to hair matrix cells [104]. Later, ultrastructural and histochemical studies provided further evidence of derivation of the neoplasm from hair matrix cells [62, 114]. Following these studies and others, subsequent authors suggested the name "pilomatrixoma" for this neoplasm [48]. The current term, "pilomatricoma", was eventually proposed as being more etymologically accurate [10, 218]. Recent studies of pilomatricomas have demonstrated mutations in CTNNB1, the gene encoding beta-catenin [50, 103]. Beta-catenin is a cytoplasmic protein believed to play a role in hair morphogenesis and regulation of the hair growth cycle [16].

Synonyms: calcifying epithelioma of Malherbe, piloma-trixoma, trichomatricoma.

Clinical features: Lesions occur commonly as solitary, asymptomatic, firm, 1–3 cm, skin-coloured, or bluish-to-red nodules, located mostly on the head, neck, and upper extremities [2, 210]. Pilomatricomas present mainly in children and young adults, though a second peak of onset has been observed in older adults (Fig. 3.2.25) [82]. Unusual cases occur as painful or tender nodules [78], rapidly growing or giant neoplasms sometimes associated with hypercalcaemia and elevated levels of parathyroid hormone-related protein [86, 107], exophytic lesions [200], or perforating/ulcerated neoplasms (Fig. 3.2.26) [224]. Rare cases of pilomatricoma

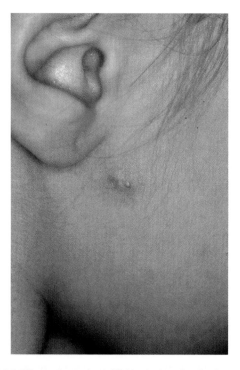

Fig. 3.2.25 Pilomatricoma in a child located on the cheek

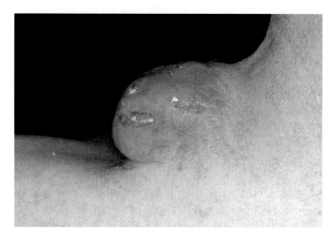

Fig. 3.2.26 A large, exophytic pilomatricoma located on the lower neck

displaying overlying striae and anetodermic changes [45, 77], bullae [73, 102], lymphangiectatic features [36], or developing in a pre-existing nevus sebaceus [123] or BCG scar [9] have been documented. Multiple (usually less than five) and sometimes familial pilomatricomas have been observed in patients with Gardner's syndrome [152, 210], myotonic dystrophy, Turner's syndrome, xeroderma pigmentosum, basal cell nevus syndrome, Soto's syndrome [51], and in cases of growth hormone deficiency [139].

Histopathology: Pilomatricomas display a spectrum of morphologic features, which probably reflects the different evolutionary stages of the neoplasm [2, 83]. Relatively less well-developed and well-developed pilomatricomas reveal variably sized, round-to-oval cystic lesions lined with basaloid epithelium (matrical cells and supramatrical cells) at the periphery and filled in the centre with masses of eosinophilic, faulty hair matrix material containing "shadow" ("ghost") cells (Fig. 3.2.27a, b). Basaloid cells may display variable numbers of mitotic figures. Foci of squamoid epithelium are sometimes observed within the epithelial lining. Regressing pilomatricomas reveal haphazardly arranged foci of basaloid and shadow cells, as well as an inflammatory infiltrate with scattered multinucleated histiocytic giant cells. Granulation tissue is sometimes noted. Old pilomatricomas show no basaloid component but exhibit irregularly shaped, partially confluent masses of shadow cells with foci of calcification or ossification. Melanin deposition, transepidermal elimination (perforating pilomatricoma), and extramedullary hematopoiesis have been described in some pilomatricomas. Rare lesions may reveal foci with hair follicular germinative cells [129].

Proliferating pilomatricoma is a peculiar variant, which usually presents in middle-aged and elderly individuals and is histopathologically characterised by relatively large areas of basaloid cells and small foci of shadow cells [58, 84, 166]. "Matricoma" represents another rare variant of pilomatricoma with numerous, discrete, small, solid aggregations of basaloid cells and foci of shadow cells. The basaloid aggregations in matricoma sometimes display connections to pre-existing infundibula at several points [2, 3].

Treatment: Complete surgical excision is the treatment of choice for pilomatricomas. Some lesions, especially those arising in children, may regress spontaneously. Local recurrences have occasionally been observed following incomplete excision. One case of malignant transformation has been documented [170].

3.2.2.5 Tricholemmoma

Definition: Tricholemmoma is a relatively common, benign follicular neoplasm that usually presents as a solitary papule

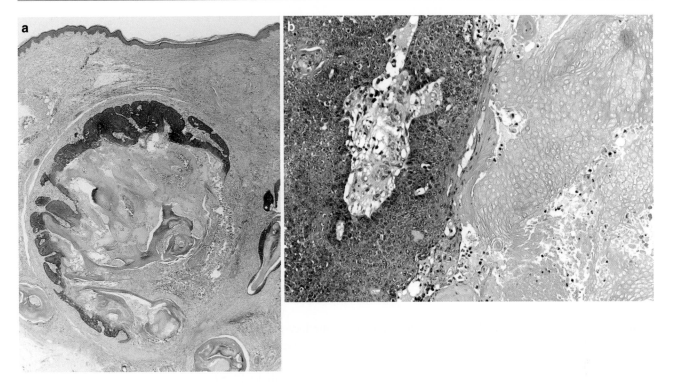

Fig. 3.2.27 (**a**) Pilomatricoma. A cystic lesion lined focally at the periphery with basaloid epithelium and filled with masses of eosinophilic, cornified material with shadow cells. (**b**) Basaloid (matrical and supramatrical cells) showing continuity with shadow cells

on the face of adults and shows histopathological differentiation toward the outer root (tricholemmal) sheath of a normal
hair follicle at the level of the bulb [66, 67, 70, 116]. Multiple
tricholemmomas represent an important cutaneous marker
for Cowden's disease [42, 168, 183, 192].

Aetiology: There is still considerable debate about whether
tricholemmomas are of hamartomatous/neoplastic [22, 65,
156, 161] or viral origin [2, 4]. In 1962, Headington and
French first described tricholemmoma as a benign neoplasm
with differentiation toward pilosebaceous follicular epithelium [67]. Based on the wart-like morphology, however,
some authors have proposed tricholemmoma to be an old
viral wart [2]. One study revealed HPV DNA in a subset tricholemmomas using PCR [162].

Synonyms: trichilemmoma

Clinical features: Tricholemmomas present mostly as
solitary, small (3–8 mm in diameter), asymptomatic, keratotic, or smooth-surfaced papules arising on the face, particularly around the nose and upper lip of adults [2, 210]. Lesions
are often excised either as basal cell carcinomas or as viral
warts. Tricholemmomas sometimes develop in association
with nevus sebaceus [79]. Multiple facial tricholemmomas
are important cutaneous markers for Cowden's disease (multiple hamartoma and neoplasia syndrome). Cowden's disease
is an autosomal dominant disorder characterised by a wide
array of abnormalities mainly including hamartomas of the
skin, breast, thyroid, and oral mucosa [24, 25, 191]. The
pathognomonic features of Cowden's disease include

multiple smooth facial tricholemmomas, acral keratosis, and
multiple oral papillomas [23, 194, 195]. An important feature of Cowden's disease is the tendency of these patients to
develop particular internal malignancies, especially involving the breast, colon, endometrium, and thyroid (particularly
follicular thyroid carcinoma) [25, 42, 168, 189]. Patients
with Cowden's disease also occasionally reveal a range of
central nervous system manifestations including macroceph-
aly, megalencephaly, epilepsy, and cerebellar tumours, e.g.
dysplastic gangliocytomas of the cerebellum (Lhermitte-
Duclos disease) [141, 206]. Approximately 80% of patients
with Cowden's disease have an identifiable germline mutation in the PTEN gene [146, 188].

Histopathology: Tricholemmomas in most cases show a
lobular, folliculocentric, exo-endophytic proliferation of
polygonal, pale-staining, glycogen-containing squamoid
cells (Fig. 3.2.28a, b). The epidermal surface often reveals
parakeratosis with scale crusts and, sometimes, a cutaneous
horn (tricholemmal horn). The periphery of the lobules is
bordered by columnar cells arranged in a palisade. Foci with
small squamous eddies are occasionally observed in the centre of the tumour lobules. A distinct PAS- and type IV colla-
gen-positive basement membrane generally surrounds the
lesions. Mitoses are usually not observed.

Desmoplastic tricholemmoma represents a histopathologic variant of tricholemmoma characterised by a central
prominent desmoplastic component [70, 201]. Lesions display typical histopathological features of conventional

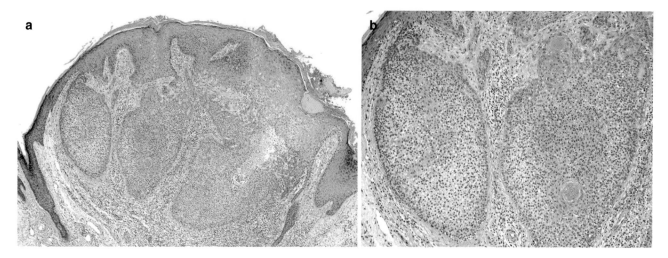

Fig. 3.2.28 (**a**) Tricholemmoma. A lobular, exo-endophytic proliferation of pale-staining squamoid cells in the upper dermis. (**b**) The cells at the periphery of the lobules show a palisade arrangement

tricholemmoma at the periphery. However, at the centre, the epithelial cells tend to cluster in narrow strands with distinctive artifactual clefts and are enclosed in dense, hypocellular, and fibrotic stroma. Epithelial cells in desmoplastic tricholemmoma may express CD34, a feature helpful in distinguishing this lesion from basal cell carcinoma [72].

Treatment: Complete surgical excision is curative. Patients with multiple tricholemmomas should be investigated for other systemic manifestations of Cowden's disease, especially internal malignancy.

3.2.2.6 Trichofolliculoma

Definition: Trichofolliculoma is a rare hamartoma, which generally presents in adults as a solitary papule or nodule on the face and is histopathologically characterised by a well-circumscribed, vertically oriented lesion with a prominent, central, dilated follicle connected to multiple secondary and tertiary follicles [2, 54].

Synonyms: hamartoma of hair follicle tissue, hair follicle tumour.

Clinical features: Trichofolliculoma usually presents in adults with a wide age range (11–77 years) and without any sex predilection. Lesions occur as small, solitary, dome-shaped papules or nodules measuring 0.5–1 cm in diameter, situated mainly on the face, particularly around the nose [2]. A central, dilated, keratin-plugged ostium with vellus hair(s) is often observed.

Histopathology: The dermal lesion is ordinarily centred on one or, less frequently, several contiguous, variably dilated, primary follicles lined with infundibular and isthmus-type epithelium, opening to the skin surface (Fig. 3.2.29a, b) [2].

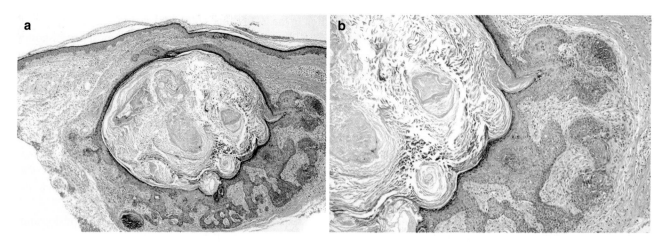

Fig. 3.2.29 (**a**) Trichofolliculoma showing a dilated infundibulocystic structure at the centre, contiguous with numerous vellus follicles. (**b**) The vellus hair follicles emanating from the dilated infundibulocystic structure are surrounded by a fibrous stroma

Numerous smaller, secondary (vellus) hair follicles bud from the wall of the central follicle in a radial fashion. The central follicle is commonly filled with cornified cells and sometimes contains vellus hairs. Secondary follicles often reveal differentiation toward germinative epithelium or hair formation [180]. They are surrounded by a prominent fibrous stroma, which is separated from adjacent normal dermis by clefts. Individual tumours display variable features of outer root sheath differentiation, especially at the level of the isthmus with tricholemmal cornification, basaloid or matrical cells or with features of sebaceous differentiation. Increased numbers of Merkel cells have been observed in trichofolliculomas [61].

Several histopathologic variants, some of which probably reflect the evolutionary stages of trichofolliculoma, have been described [179, 180]. Folliculo-sebaceous cystic hamartoma is regarded as a late-stage variant of trichofolliculoma; it displays nearly complete regression of transient follicular epithelium but concurrent proliferation of mature sebaceous elements [92, 179, 185]. Sebaceous trichofolliculoma is considered to be a variant characterised by large, sebaceous follicles connected to the central cavity but without vellus hair follicles radiating from the dilated follicular infundibulum [148]. Hair follicle nevus has been proposed to be a type of trichofolliculoma, with a predominance of mature vellus follicles and an absence of central infundibular lumen [2]. Collision tumours of trichofolliculoma and basal cell carcinoma [20] and superficial angiomyxoma [143] have been reported.

Treatment: Surgical excision is the treatment of choice. To date, there are no reports of recurrences.

3.2.2.7 Fibrofolliculoma/Trichodiscoma

Definition: Fibrofolliculloma and trichodiscoma were previously considered separate follicular neoplasms. Presently, however, these lesions are regarded as different developmental stages of a single follicular hamartoma, with variations in epithelial and mesenchymal tissue elements [2]. Accordingly, fibrofolliculoma is considered the early, and trichodiscoma the late, stage of development in this follicular hamartoma [2]. Consistent with this hypothesis, both fibrofolliculomas and trichodiscomas are frequently observed in patients with Birt-Hogg-Dubé syndrome. The stromal components in both fibrofolliculoma and trichodiscoma are similar and composed of variable fibrillary collagen, mucin, and fibrocytes, reminiscent of the peri-isthmic connective tissue in a normal hair follicle. Tumours with intermediate features between fibrofolliculoma and trichodiscoma have also been recorded [2, 99]. The clinicopathological spectrum of fibrofolliculoma and trichodiscoma has recently been expanded to include neurofollicular hamartoma [99].

Synonyms: Trichodiscoma was previously thought to arise from the hair disc (Haarscheibe) [147]. The term "mantleoma", reflecting the likely derivation from the sebaceous mantle, has been used for both fibrofolliculoma and trichodiscoma [2, 197].

Clinical features: Fibrofolliculomas and trichodiscomas show similar clinical presentations. They occur mainly as multiple, asymptomatic, small, skin-coloured papules measuring 2–4 mm in diameter, situated on the face, arms, trunk, and sometimes the legs. Lesions usually arise in the third and fourth decade of life and show no sex predilection. Rarely, fibrofolliculomas and trichodiscomas may occur as solitary lesions [182, 190]. Multiple fibrofolliculomas and trichodiscomas may be inherited in an autosomal dominant fashion in the setting of Birt-Hogg-Dubé syndrome [2, 27, 55, 90, 178, 210, 212]. This familial syndrome is characterised mainly by the presence of multiple fibrofolliculomas, trichodiscomas, and acrochordons. Patients with Birt-Hogg-Dubé syndrome may additionally show a range of other pathologies including multiple or bilateral renal carcinomas, particularly chromophobe renal carcinomas, renal oncocytomas, pulmonary cysts, spontaneous pneumothoraces, large connective-tissue nevi, parathyroid adenomas, flecked chorioretinopathy, bullous emphysema, lipomas, angiolipomas, parotid oncocytomas, multiple oral mucosal papules, neural tissue tumours, and multiple facial angiofibromas [97, 202]. Cutaneous lesions in patients with Birt-Hogg-Dubé syndrome often precede the development of renal neoplasia. The genetic alteration for Birt-Hogg-Dubé syndrome has been mapped to chromosome 17p12q11 [89].

Histopathology: Fibrofolliculomas are characterised by a dome-shaped lesion with a central, relatively well-formed hair follicle displaying a single or several, contiguous, dilated, keratin-filled infundibula. The infundibula are connected to several thin, focally anatomizing epithelial strands, which extend in a radial fashion into the connective tissue (Fig. 3.2.30a, b). Features of sebaceous differentiation are commonly observed within the epithelial strands. The lesion is often surrounded by a well-circumscribed, fibrillary collagenous or mucinous stroma with scant or no elastic tissue.

Trichodiscoma reveals a well-circumscribed, non-encapsulated, dome-shaped, or horizontally oriented dermal lesion consisting mainly of loose, fine, fibrillary connective tissue bundles of collagen, mucin, fibrocytes, and venules [2]. The fibrous tissue is encircled by collarettes of infundibular epithelium that are focally continuous with epithelial cords radiating into the stroma. The epithelial cords sometimes contain sebaceous cells. A hair follicle or nerve fibres may be noted at the edge of the lesion. Rare plaque-like variants with confluent single lesions have been described [178].

Neurofollicular hamartoma represents a variant of fibrofolliculoma and/or trichodiscoma with a highly cellular stromal component, displaying varying proportions of S100-positive dendritic and spindle cells [99].

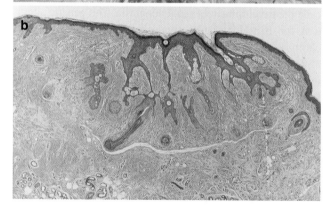

Immunohistochemistry: The stromal fibrocytes in fibrofolliculoma and trichodiscomas strongly express CD34 [30, 32].

Treatment: The treatment of choice is surgical excision. Carbon dioxide laser is useful in the removal of multiple lesions [49, 74, 85]. Patients should be screened and monitored for internal manifestations of Birt-Hogg-Dubé syndrome, specifically renal carcinomas, pulmonary cysts, and pneumothoraces.

Fig. 3.2.30 (**a**) Fibrofolliculoma. A dome-shaped lesion with infundibula connected to several thin, focally anatomizing epithelial strands extending in a radial fashion into the connective tissue. The lesion is separated from the adjacent normal dermis by artifactual clefts. (**b**) Epithelial cords anatomize to form a fenestrated pattern

3.2.3 Tumours with Sebaceous Differentiation

Steven Kaddu

3.2.3.1 Sebaceous Carcinoma

Definition: Sebaceous carcinomas represent a spectrum of malignant appendage tumours showing, predominantly, features of sebaceous differentiation and a propensity for locally invasive behaviour and/or metastasis [2, 198, 210]. Histopathologically, they are generally characterised by poorly circumscribed, non-encapsulated lesions composed of epithelial lobules of cells with variable features of sebaceous differentiation, including atypical basaloid cells and atypical sebocytes. Sebaceous carcinomas have traditionally been divided into ocular and extraocular types [110, 145, 151, 214, 225]. Of these, the ocular type is the most common.

Rarely, examples of sebaceous carcinomas may present in individuals with Muir-Torre syndrome [41, 187]. Muir-Torre syndrome represents an autosomal dominant disorder characterised by the presence of at least one sebaceous gland tumour (sebaceous adenoma, sebaceomas/sebaceous epithelioma, cystic sebaceous tumour, and/or sebaceous carcinoma) and a minimum of one visceral malignant neoplasm [1, 144, 150, 164, 181]. Internal malignancies generally include colorectal and genitourinary cancers [181], though a variety of other malignancies including head and neck, small bowel, and hematologic neoplasms may be observed. Microsatellite instability has been detected in tumours of Muir-Torre syndrome patients, and germline mutations in the hMSH2 and hMLH1 mismatch repair genes have also been reported in some of these cases [12, 43, 96]. The spectrum of cancers and germline mutations characteristic of Muir-Torre syndrome suggest that this disorder represents a phenotypic variant of hereditary non-polyposis colorectal cancer (HNPCC) or Lynch syndrome [108]. Rarely, cases of sebaceous carcinoma have also been observed in individuals infected with human immunodeficiency virus [100, 221].

Clinical features: Ocular-type sebaceous carcinoma usually presents in older adults aged 60–80 years, though tumours may be observed at any age, including childhood. Women are more commonly affected than men. Patients may report a history of radiation. In most cases, the neoplasm occurs as a relatively small, solitary, slowly enlarging papule or nodule on the eyelid, particularly around the Meibomian glands and glands of Zeiss on the upper eyelid. Upper lids are 2–3 times more commonly affected than lower lids. Lesions are often initially diagnosed as a chalazion, and patients may be treated for a long time for "recurrent chalazia" before a

biopsy is performed. Ocular type of sebaceous carcinomas may, also initially, clinically mimic blepharoconjunctivitis, keratoconjunctivitis, basal cell carcinoma, squamous cell carcinoma, cutaneous horn, sarcoidosis, and/or cicatricial pemphigoid [40, 52, 6].

Extraocular sebaceous carcinomas account for approximately 25% of all sebaceous carcinomas. Extraocular sebaceous carcinomas present mostly as yellowish, firm, often ulcerated nodules located on the head and neck (Fig. 3.2.31) and less frequently on the trunk, genitalia, and extremities. Lesions occur most commonly in adults (mean age, 63 years) and show an equal sex distribution. Some cases may present in the mouth and around the parotid and submandibular glands [38, 137].

Histopathology: Sebaceous carcinoma is normally characterised by an asymmetrical lesion centred in the dermis, consisting of variously sized and irregularly shaped aggregations of neoplastic cells (Fig. 3.2.32a) [198]. Involvement of the subcutaneous tissue and/or underlying muscle is observed in some cases. Neoplasms may be relatively well-differentiated with prominent sebaceous lobules and/or sebaceous ductal structures or show undifferentiated features with neither readily discernible cytoplasmic vacuoles

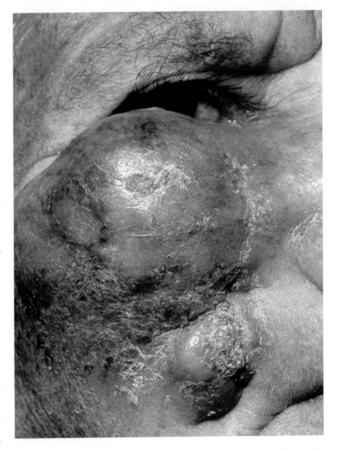

Fig. 3.2.31 Sebaceous carcinoma. A large tumour located on the cheek

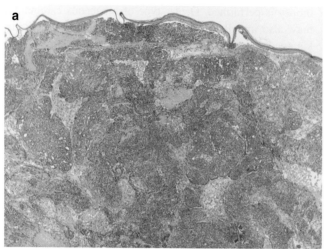
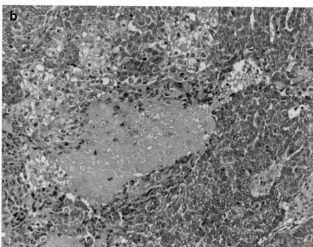

Fig. 3.2.32 (**a**) Sebaceous carcinoma. An asymmetrical lesion consisting of variously sized and irregularly shaped aggregations of atypical basaloid cells and atypical sebocytes. (**b**) Sebaceous carcinoma.

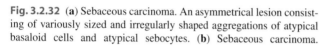
Epithelial aggregations displaying prominent atypia, increased mitotic figures, and areas of geographical necrosis

nor ductal differentiation. The nuclei of the neoplastic cells, especially along the periphery of the tumour nests, tend to be crowded and pleomorphic and may exhibit marked atypia as well as increased mitotic figures. Sections often reveal areas of geographical necrosis (Fig. 3.2.32b). Infiltrative lesions of sebaceous carcinomas may show features of carcinoma in situ or extra-mammary Paget disease in the overlying surface epithelium or surrounding skin appendages [29, 126].

Sebaceous carcinomas have previously been categorised into three grades based mainly on the predominant architectural pattern [155]. Grade I comprises neoplasms with well-demarcated, roughly equally sized lobules; grade II neoplasms display an admixture of well-defined nests with infiltrative profiles or confluent cell groups, and grade III tumours exhibit highly infiltrative growth or a medullary sheet-like pattern.

Several histopathologic variants of sebaceous carcinoma have previously been described. Intraepithelial sebaceous carcinoma represents a variant showing no invasive component in the dermis. Basaloid sebaceous carcinoma is a peculiar type characterised by areas of basaloid cells with periphery palisading and with few sebocytes. Squamoid sebaceous carcinoma reveals prominent squamous metaplasia often with horn pearls. Rare cases of sebaceous carcinoma may also display a pseudo-endocrine organoid pattern, mimicking "carcinoid tumours" [87].

Histochemistry and Immunohistochemistry: Intracellular vacuoles stain positive for oil-red-O and Sudan black [217]. Sebaceous carcinomas reveal positivity for various cytokeratins, including AE1/AE3 and low molecular weight cytokeratin, EMA, anti-breast carcinoma-associated antigen-225 antibody (CU18), anti-CA 15.3 antibody, and androgen receptor protein, and are negative for CEA, S100 protein, and GCDFP-15 [8, 15]. Immature as well as mature neoplastic sebocytes may express cytokeratin 14 [175].

Treatment: The treatment of choice is surgical excision with adequate margins or Mohs micrographic surgery [17]. Radiation therapy may be effective in some patients with eyelid neoplasms. In contrast to ocular tumours, extraocular sebaceous carcinomas very rarely reveal nodal or visceral metastases [125]. Sebaceous carcinomas arising in Muir-Torre syndrome seem to be less aggressive than their counterpart unassociated with the syndrome [181].

Up to one-third of patients with ocular type sebaceous carcinoma show lymph node metastases, particularly to the preauricular and cervical nodes, and the 5-year mortality rate is about 20%. Distant metastases have been observed in a number of sites, including the lungs, liver, and bone [71], and have been reported as late as 5 years after treatment of the eyelid carcinoma [71]. Histopathologic features suggestive of a poor prognosis include the presence of vascular and lymphatic invasion, orbital extension, poor differentiation, infiltrative growth pattern, and large tumour size. Treatment of metastatic disease may include a combination of chemotherapy, radiation, and surgical neck dissection [71].

3.2.3.2 Sebaceous Adenoma

Definition: Sebaceous adenoma is a relatively small neoplasm composed of basaloid cells and mature sebocytes. Sebaceous adenoma does not possess a potential for aggressive growth or metastasis. Multiple sebaceous adenomas are markers of Muir-Torre syndrome [198].

Clinical features: Sebaceous adenoma commonly presents as relatively small, yellowish tumour, sometimes showing an overlying scale crust [163]. Lesions develop in individuals over 40 years of age. They are usually located on chronically sun-damaged areas of the face and neck.

Sebaceous adenomas in patients with Muir-Torre syndrome occur as solitary or multiple, skin-coloured, yellowish, or reddish-brown, sometimes ulcerated papules and nodules, commonly situated on the face (Fig. 3.2.33a, b). Similar to other sebaceous neoplasms arising in Muir-Torre syndrome, sebaceous adenomas may precede or coincide with visceral malignancies, and their presence should prompt a thorough evaluation. In individuals with Muir-Torre syndrome, sebaceus adenomas may also coexist with keratoacanthomas and/or epidermal cysts. Colorectal and genitourinary cancers are the most common internal malignancies reported in these patients, though a variety of other malignant tumours including head and neck, small bowel, and hematologic malignancies may be observed.

Histopathology: Sebaceous adenomas are well-circumscribed, multilobulated, sometimes excoriated lesions with a frequent connection to the overlying epidermis. Individual lobules are composed of sebocytes of various sizes, with central portions showing larger, mature sebocytes and the periphery displaying relatively small, undifferentiated, germinative basaloid cells (Figs. 3.2.34a, b) [113]. The mature sebocytes contain pale-staining, foamy-to-bubbly cytoplasm and central, crenated, hyperchromatic nuclei. The smaller, basaloid cells reveal round-to-oval, vesicular nuclei and basophilic cytoplasm. Ductal structures with holocrine secretion are occasionally observed within the lobules. Nuclear hyperchromatism, prominent nucleoli, and mitotic activity are rarely seen in sebaceous adenomas. Immunohistologically, loss of MSH-2 and MLH-1 repair proteins may be exhibited in sebaceous adenomas arising in cases of Muir-Torre syndrome [186].

Prognosis and treatment: Sebaceous adenomas are benign neoplasms without potential for aggressive growth or metastasis. The treatment of choice is complete surgical excision. Local recurrences are occasionally reported following incomplete removal. The prognosis in individuals with Muir-Torre syndrome depends on that of the associated internal malignant neoplasm(s).

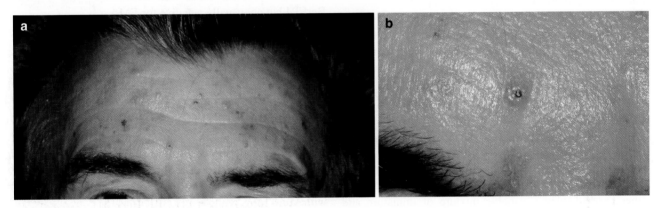

Fig. 3.2.33 (**a**) Sebaceous adenomas. Multiple small tumours on the face of a patient with Muir-Torre syndrome. (**b**) Sebaceous adenoma. A small, excoriated facial papule

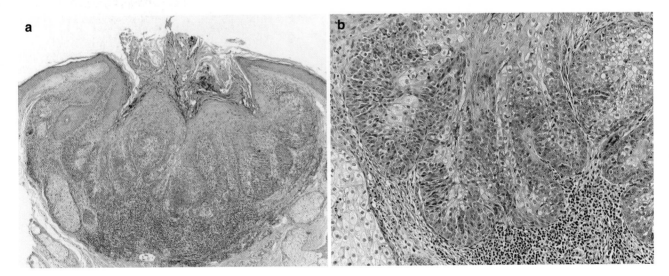

Fig. 3.2.34 (**a**) Sebaceous adenoma showing a well-circumscribed, multilobulated lesion in the upper dermis. (**b**) Lobules are composed of relatively large sebocytes in the centre and smaller, undifferentiated, germinative basaloid cells at the periphery

3.2.3.3 Sebaceoma

Definition: The term "sebaceoma" was first proposed by Troy and Ackerman in 1984 for a distinct benign neoplasm with sebaceous differentiation characterised by sharply circumscribed aggregations of monomorphous, small, basaloid cells (undifferentiated sebocytes) admixed with single or small clusters of large, mature vacuolated sebocytes and ductal structures [204]. Sebaceomas may be associated with Muir-Torre syndrome [181].

Synonyms: sebaceous epithelioma, basal cell carcinoma with sebaceous differentiation, sebomatricoma.

Clinical features: Sebaceoma commonly presents as a solitary, slowly growing, asymptomatic, yellowish papule or small nodule, on the face, scalp, or, rarely, trunk of older individuals (mean age, approximately 70 years) [19, 39, 128, 138, 158, 198, 204]. Women appear to be more commonly affected than men. Occasionally, tumours arise within a seborrheic keratosis [19] or pre-existing nevus sebaceus, sometimes in association with a trichoblastoma [81].

Histopathology: Lesions are centred in the dermis, with occasional involvement of the subcutis, and consist mainly of symmetrical, well-circumscribed, smoothly bordered, lobular aggregations of epithelial cells with focal connections to pre-existing infundibula [120, 198]. Epithelial aggregations are composed of basaloid cells with relatively monomorphous nuclei, admixed with variable foci of discernible sebocytes and sebaceous ductal structures (Fig. 3.2.35a, b). Rare cases have revealed almost entirely immature sebocytes (basaloid cells with small monomorphous nuclei and scant cytoplasm but without vacuoles). Other cases display a variable mixture of immature and mature sebocytes with highly vacuolated, abundant cytoplasm and nuclei exhibiting scalloped borders. There is no palisaded arrangement of nuclei at the periphery of epithelial aggregations, similar to that observed in basal cell carcinomas. Scattered mitoses are observed in some lesions. Some neoplasms display cystic and duct-like structures and relatively large foci of holocrine secretion. However, necrosis en masse of neoplastic cells is rarely seen.

A range of morphological patterns has been reported in sebaceomas, including neoplasms with reticulated, cribriform, glandular, and ripple-like features [87, 93, 121]. Unusual variants of sebaceoma include a pigmented type [158], sebaceoma arising in nevus sebaceus [81] or seborrheic keratosis [19], and a variant exhibiting eccrine differentiation [138]. Sebaceomas arising in Muir-Torre syndrome may display a keratoacanthoma-like architectural pattern [26].

Immunohistochemistry: The use of a combination of antibodies including Ber-EP4 and EMA is helpful in distinguishing sebaceomas from basal cell carcinoma [44]. Sebaceomas commonly stain positive for EMA but are negative for BER-EP4, whereas basal cell carcinomas may express BerEP4 but are usually negative for EMA.

Treatment: Simple surgical excision is curative in most cases. Electrodesiccation, curettage, and cryotherapy may be effective treatments for some lesions.

3.2.3.4 Cystic Sebaceous Tumour

Definition: Cystic sebaceous tumour is a large, well-circumscribed, deeply located dermal sebaceous neoplasm with a cystic architectural pattern, arising exclusively in patients with Muir-Torre syndrome [1, 101, 164, 181].

Synonyms: cystic sebaceous neoplasm.

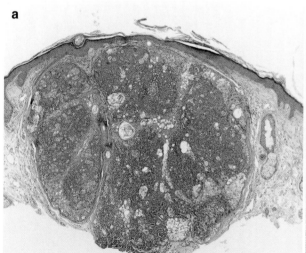
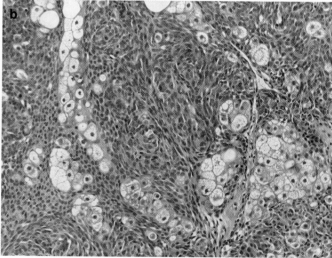

Fig. 3.2.35 (**a**) Sebaceoma. Well-circumscribed tumour composed of basaloid aggregations admixed with sebocytes and cystic structures. (**b**) Sebaceoma. Epithelial aggregations are composed of basaloid cells with relatively monomorphous nuclei and mature sebocytes

Epidemiology: Cystic sebaceous tumour is a diagnostic marker lesion of Muir-Torre syndrome. Muir-Torre syndrome, a phenotypic variant of the hereditary non-polyposis colon cancer syndrome (HNPCC), is a rare autosomal-dominant inherited genodermatosis, characterised by the occurrence of a wide range of sebaceous neoplasms and internal malignancies in the absence of other predisposing factors. Although most patients present with sebaceous adenomas, cystic sebaceous tumours have also been reported as specific markers of this syndrome. A model of tumour progression from clearly benign, cystic sebaceous adenoma to large, proliferating, atypical cystic sebaceous tumour and early cystic sebaceous carcinoma has been proposed [164]. Internal malignancies generally consist of gastrointestinal and genitourinary neoplasms, but patients may also develop neoplasms in a variety of other anatomical sites and organs. Sebaceous tumours in Muir-Torre syndrome typically reveal microsatellite instability and germline mutations in the DNA mismatch repair genes MutS homolog (MSH)-2 and MLH1. Notably, some cases of Muir-Torre syndrome have been reported to arise spontaneously [101].

Clinical features: Cystic sebaceous tumours usually present as solitary, rarely as multiple, large dermal nodules, commonly localising on the trunk of middle-aged and elderly individuals [1, 101, 164]. Similar to other sebaceous tumours arising in individuals with Muir-Torre syndrome, the diagnosis of cystic sebaceous tumours may come before or coincide with that of an internal malignancy.

Histopathology: Cystic sebaceous tumours show a spectrum of morphologic features, ranging from lesions with benign cystic features (sebaceous cystic adenomas) to "proliferative" lesions simulating sebaceous carcinomas (proliferative cystic sebaceous tumours) [164]. Lesions with benign features reveal a thin cyst wall lined with a rim of basaloid cells, exhibiting regular maturation into sebaceous cells toward the centre. They display few or no mitotic figures. Proliferative lesions are characterised by a lobulated growth pattern with an infolded epithelial lining, revealing a prominent proliferation of focally atypical basaloid cells (sebocytes). These cells exhibit relatively high mitotic activity, are located mainly at the periphery of the epithelial lobules of neoplastic cells, and are contiguous with the larger mature sebaceous cells towards the inner portion of the lobules [1, 164]. The mature sebaceous cells are typically immunoreactive for EMA.

Treatment and prognosis: Cystic sebaceous tumours generally show a benign course without recurrences or metastases after complete excision. However, since cystic sebaceous tumours are markers of Muir-Torre syndrome, overall prognosis of these patients depends on that of the associated internal malignant neoplasm. Regular monitoring and long-term screening for cutaneous and internal malignancy are, therefore, necessary in all of these patients.

References

Tumours with Apocrine and Eccrine Differentiation

1. Abbott, J.J., Ahmed, I.: Adenocarcinoma of mammary-like glands of the vulva: report of a case and review of the literature. Am. J. Dermatopathol. **28**, 127–133 (2006)
2. Abe, S., Matsumoto, Y., Fujita, T.: Primary mucinous carcinoma of the skin. Plast. Reconstr. Surg. **99**, 1160–1164 (1997)
3. Abenoza, P., Ackerman, A.B.: Neoplasms with Eccrine Differentiation – Ackerman's Histologic Diagnosis of Neoplastic Skin Diseases: A Method by Pattern Analysis. Lea & Febiger, Philadelphia (1989)
4. Allan, S.J., McLaren, K., Aldridge, R.D.: Paget's disease of the scrotum: a case exhibiting positive prostate-specific antigen staining and associated prostatic adenocarcinoma. Br. J. Dermatol. **138**, 689–691 (1998)
5. Ansai, S., Watanabe, S., Aso, K.: A case of tubular apocrine adenoma with syringocystadenoma papilliferum. J. Cutan. Pathol. **16**, 230–236 (1989)
6. Arslan, E., Unal, S., Cinel, L., et al.: Malignant eccrine spiradenoma occurring on a traumatized area. Plast. Reconstr. Surg. **110**, 365–367 (2002)
7. Knowles, A.J.A., SL, T.K.C.: Extensive facial clefting in a patient with Goltz syndrome: multidisciplinary treatment of a previously unreported association. Cleft Palate Craniofac. J. **39**, 469–473 (2002)
8. Ashikari, R., Park, K., Huvos, H.G., et al.: Paget's disease of the breast. Cancer **26**, 680–685 (1970)
9. Bannatyne, P., Elliott, P., Russell, P.: Vulvar adenosquamous carcinoma arising in a hidradenoma papilliferum, with rapidly fatal outcome: case report. Gynecol. Oncol. **35**, 395–398 (1989)
10. Bardach, H.: Hidroacanthoma simplex with in situ porocarcinoma. J. Cutan. Pathol. **5**, 236–248 (1978)
11. Barnett, M.D., Wallack, M.K., Zuretti, A., et al.: Recurrent malignant chondroid syringoma of the foot: a case report and review of the literature. Am. J. Clin. Oncol. **23**, 227–232 (2000)
12. Bates, A.W., Baithun, S.I.: Atypical mixed tumor of the skin: histologic, immunohistochemical, and ultrastructural features in three cases and a review of the criteria for malignancy. Am. J. Dermatopathol. **20**, 35–40 (1998)
13. Battles, O.E., Page, D.L., Johnson, J.E.: Cytokeratins, CEA, and mucin histochemistry in the diagnosis and characterization of extra-mammary Paget's disease. Am. J. Clin. Pathol. **108**, 6–12 (1997)
14. Bedlow, A.J., Cook, M.G., Kurwa, A.: Extensive naevoid eccrine spiradenoma. Br. J. Dermatol. **149**, 419–425 (1999)
15. Berg, J., McDivitt, R.W.: Pathology of sweat gland carcinoma. Pathol. Annu. **3**, 123–144 (1968)
16. Bergman, R., Lichtig, C., Moscona, R.A., et al.: A comparative immunohistochemical study of adenoid cystic carcinoma of the skin and salivary glands. Am. J. Dermatopathol. **13**, 162–168 (1991)
17. Bertagnoli, R., Cook, D.L., Goldman, G.D.: Bilateral primary mucinous carcinoma of the eyelid treated with Mohs surgery. Dermatol. Surg. **25**, 566–568 (1999)
18. Bignell, G.R., Warren, W., Seal, S., et al.: Identification of the familial cylindromatosis tumour-suppressor gene. Nat. Genet. **25**, 160–165 (2000)
19. Bjarke, T., Ternesten-Bratel, A., Hedblad, M., et al.: Carcinoma and eccrine syringofibroadenoma: a report of five cases. J. Cutan. Pathol. **30**, 382–392 (2003)
20. Boggio, R.: Letter: Adenoid cystic carcinoma of scalp. Arch. Dermatol. **111**, 793–794 (1975)

21. Bogner, P.N., Su, L.D., Fullen, D.R.: Cluster designation 5 staining of normal and non-lymphoid neoplastic skin. J. Cutan. Pathol. **32**, 50–54 (2005)

22. Burket, J.M., Zelickson, A.S.: Tubular apocrine adenoma with perineural invasion. J. Am. Acad. Dermatol. **11**, 639–642 (1984)

23. Busam, K.J., Tan, L.K., Granter, S.R., et al.: Epidermal growth factor, estrogen, and progesterone receptor expression in primary sweat gland carcinomas and primary and metastatic mammary carcinomas. Mod. Pathol. **12**, 786–793 (1999)

24. Cabell, C.E., Helm, K.F., Sakol, P.J., et al.: Primary mucinous carcinoma in a 54-year-old man. J. Am. Acad. Dermatol. **49**, 941–943 (2003)

25. Carroll, P., Goldstein, G.D., Brown Jr., C.W.: Metastatic microcystic adnexal carcinoma in an immunocompromised patient. Dermatol. Surg. **26**, 531–534 (2000)

26. Ceulen, R.P., Van Marion, A.M., Steijlen, P.M., et al.: Multiple unilateral skin tumors suggest type 1 segmental manifestation of familial syringoma. Eur. J. Dermatol. **18**, 285–288 (2008)

27. Chamberlain, R.S., Huber, K., White, J.C., et al.: Apocrine gland carcinoma of the axilla. Review of the literature and recommendations for treatment. Am. J. Clin. Oncol. **22**, 131–135 (1999)

28. Chang, S.E., Ahn, S.J., Choi, J.H., et al.: Primary adenoid cystic carcinoma of skin with lung metastasis. J. Am. Acad. Dermatol. **40**, 640–642 (1999)

29. Chen, C.Y., Sun, L.M., Anderson, B.O.: Paget disease of the breast: changing patterns of incidence, clinical presentation, and treatment in the U.S. Cancer **107**, 1448–1458 (2006)

30. Chen, Y.H., Wong, T.W., Lee, J.Y.Y.: Depigmented genital extramammary Paget's disease: a possible histogenetic link to Toker's clear cells and clear cell papulosis. J. Cutan. Pathol. **28**, 105–108 (2001)

31. Chiller, K., Passaro, D., Scheuller, M., et al.: Microcystic adnexal carcinoma: forty-eight cases, their treatment, and their outcome. Arch. Dermatol. **136**, 1355–1359 (2000)

32. Chu, S.S., Chang, Y.L., Lou, P.J.: Primary cutaneous adenoid cystic carcinoma with regional lymph node metastasis. J. Laryngol. Otol. **115**, 673–675 (2001)

33. Civatte, J., Belaich, S., Lauret, P.: Tubular apocrine adenoma (4 cases) (author's translation). Ann. Dermatol. Vénéréol. **106**, 665–669 (1979)

34. Clever, H.W., Sahl, W.J.: Multiple eccrine hidrocystomas: a non-surgical treatment. Arch. Dermatol. **127**, 422–424 (1991)

35. Cooper, P.H.: Sclerosing carcinomas of sweat ducts (microcystic adnexal carcinoma). Arch. Dermatol. **122**, 261–264 (1986)

36. Cooper, P.H.: Carcinoma of sweat glands. Pathol. Annu. **22**, 83–124 (1987)

37. Crain, R.C., Helwig, E.B.: Dermal cylindroma (dermal eccrine cylindroma). Am. J. Clin. Pathol. **35**, 504–515 (1961)

38. Cribier, B., Scrivener, Y., Grosshans, E.: Tumors arising in nevus sebaceus: a study of 596 cases. J. Am. Acad. Dermatol. **132**, 263–268 (2000)

39. Culhaci, N., Copcu, H.E., Dikicioglu, E.: Microcystic adnexal carcinoma: report of a case. J. Oral Maxillofac. Surg. **61**, 723–725 (2003)

40. Cunningham, J., Hardy, J.: Hidradenomas of the vulva. South Surg. **13**, 831–838 (1947)

41. Dabska, M.: Malignant transformation of eccrine spiradenoma. Pol. Med. J. **11**, 388–396 (1972)

42. De Viragh, P.A., Szeimies, R.M., Eckert, F.: Apocrine cystadenoma, apocrine hidrocystoma, and eccrine hidrocystoma: three distinct tumors defined by expression of keratins and human milk fat globulin 1. J. Cutan. Pathol. **24**, 249–255 (1997)

43. del Pozo, J., García-Silva, J., Peña-Penabad, C., et al.: Multiple apocrine hidrocystomas: treatment with carbon dioxide laser vaporization. J. Dermatolog. Treat. **12**, 97–100 (2001)

44. Diaz de Leon, E., Carcangiu, M.L., Prieto, V.G., et al.: Extramammary Paget disease is characterized by the consistent lack of estrogen and progesterone receptors but frequently expresses androgen receptor. Am. J. Clin. Pathol. **113**, 572–575 (2000)

45. Dubreuilh, W.: Paget's disease of the vulva. Br. J. Dermatol. **13**, 407–413 (1901)

46. Duke, W.H., Sherrod, T.T., Lupton, G.P.: Aggressive digital papillary adenocarcinoma (aggressive digital papillary adenoma and adenocarcinoma revisited). Am. J. Surg. Pathol. **24**, 775–784 (2000)

47. Dupré, A., Bonafe, J.L.: Syringomas mongolism, Marfan's disease and Ehlers Danlos' disease. Ann. Dermatol. Vénéréol. **104**, 224–230 (1977)

48. Dupré, A., Carrere, S., Bonafé, J.L.: Syringomes éruptifs généralisés, grains de milium et atrophodermie vermiculée: Syndrome de Nicolau et Balus. Dermatologica **162**, 281–286 (1981)

49. Durani, B.K., Kurzen, H., Jaeckel, A., et al.: Malignant transformation of multiple dermal cylindromas. Br. J. Dermatol. **145**, 653–656 (2001)

50. El-Domeiri, A.A., Brasfield, R.D., Huvos, A.G., et al.: Sweat gland carcinoma: a clinicopathologic study of 83 patients. Ann. Surg. **173**, 270–274 (1971)

51. Falck, V.G., Jordaan, H.F.: Papillary eccrine adenoma. A tubulo-papillary hidradenoma with eccrine differentiation. Am. J. Dermatopathol. **8**, 64–72 (1986)

52. Faulhaber, D., Worle, B., Trautner, B., et al.: Clear cell hidradenoma in a young girl. Am. Acad. Dermatol. **42**, 693–695 (2000)

53. Fernández-Aceñero, M.J., Manzarbeitia, F., Mestre, M.J., et al.: P53 expression in two cases of spiradenocarcinomas. Am. J. Dermatopathol. **22**, 104–107 (2000)

54. Fernandez-Acepero, M.J., Manzarbeitia, F., Mestre de Juan, M.J., et al.: Malignant spiradenoma: report of two cases and literature review. J. Am. Acad. Dermatol. **44**, 395–398 (2001)

55. French, L.E.: Reactive eccrine syringofibroadenoma: an emerging subtype. Dermatology **195**, 309–310 (1997)

56. French, L.E., Masgrau, E., Chavaz, P., et al.: Eccrine syringofibroadenoma in a patient with erosive palmoplantar lichen planus. Dermatology **195**, 399–401 (1997)

57. Fouilloux, B., Perrin, C., Dutoit, M., et al.: Clear cell syringofibroadenoma (of Mascaro) of the nail. Br. J. Dermatol. **144**, 625–627 (2001)

58. Fox, S.B., Cotton, D.W.: Tubular apocrine adenoma and papillary eccrine adenoma. Entities or unity? Am. J. Dermatopathol. **14**, 149–154 (1992)

59. Fueston, J.C., Gloster, H.M., Mutasim, D.F.: Primary cutaneous adenoid cystic carcinoma: a case report and literature review. Cutis **77**, 157–160 (2006)

60. Fukamizu, H., Tomita, K., Inoue, K., et al.: Primary mucinous carcinoma of the skin. J. Dermatol. Surg. Oncol. **19**, 625–628 (1993)

61. Gambini, C., Rongioletti, F., Semino, M.T., et al.: Solitary eccrine syringofibroadenoma (or eccrine syringofibroadenomatous hyperplasia?) and diabetic polyneuropathy. Dermatology **193**, 68–69 (1996)

62. Geisler, J.P., Gates, R.W., Shirrel, W.: Extramammary Paget's disease with diffuse involvement of the lower female genito-urinary system. Int. J. Gynecol. Cancer **7**, 84–87 (1997)

63. Gira, A.K., Robertson, D., Swerlick, R.A.: Multiple eyelid cysts with palmoplantar hyperkeratosis–quiz case. Arch. Dermatol. **140**, 231–236 (2004)

64. Goldblum, J.R., Hart, W.R.: Vulvar Paget's disease: a clinicopathologic and immunohistochemical study of 19 cases. Am. J. Surg. Pathol. **21**, 1178–1187 (1997)

65. Goldstein, D.J., Barr, R.J., Santa Cruz, D.J.: Microcystic adnexal carcinoma: a distinct clinicopathologic entity. Cancer **50**, 566–572 (1982)

66. Granter, S.R., Seeger, K., Calonje, E., et al.: Malignant eccrine spiradenoma (spiradenocarcinoma): a clinicopathologic study of 12 cases. Am. J. Dermatopathol. **22**, 97–103 (2000)

67. Guitart, J., Rosenbaum, M.M., Requena, L.: "Eruptive syringoma": a misnomer for a reactive eccrine gland ductal proliferation? J. Cutan. Pathol. **30**, 202–205 (2003)

68. Gupta, S., Jain, V.K., Singh, U., et al.: Multiple eccrine spiradenomas in zosteriform distribution in a child. Pediatr. Dermatol. **17**, 384–386 (2000)

69. Handa, Y., Yamanaka, N., Inagaki, H., et al.: Large ulcerated perianal hidradenoma papilliferum in a young female. Dermatol. Surg. **29**, 790–792 (2003)

70. Harrist, T.J., Aretz, T.H., Mihm Jr., M.C., et al.: Cutaneous malignant mixed tumor. Arch. Dermatol. **117**, 719–724 (1981)

71. Hashimoto, K., Gross, B.G., Nelson, R.G., et al.: Eccrine spiradenoma: histochemical and electron microscopic studies. J. Invest. Dermatol. **46**, 347–365 (1966)

72. Hashimoto, K., Lever, W.F.: Eccrine poroma: histochemical and electron microscopic studies. J. Invest. Dermatol. **43**, 237–247 (1964)

73. Hatch, K.D., Davis, J.R.: Complete resolution of Paget disease of the vulva with imiquimod cream. J. Low. Genit. Tract Dis. **12**, 90–94 (2008)

74. Hedington, J.T.: Mixed tumors of the skin: eccrine and apocrine types. Arch. Dermatol. **84**, 989–996 (1961)

75. Helm, K.F., Goellner, J.R., Peters, M.S.: Immunohistochemical stains in extramammary Paget's disease. Am. J. Dermatopathol. **14**, 402–407 (1992)

76. Helwig, E.B.: Eccrine acrospiroma. J. Cutan. Pathol. **11**, 415–420 (1984)

77. Helwig, E.B., Hackney, V.C.: Syringadenoma papilliferum: lesions with and without naevus sebaceus and basal cell carcinoma. Arch. Dermatol. **71**, 361–372 (1955)

78. Hendi, A., Brodland, D.G., Zitelli, J.A.: Extramammary Paget's disease: surgical treatment with Mohs micrographic surgery. J. Am. Acad. Dermatol. **51**, 767–773 (2004)

79. Hernandez-Parez, E., Cestoni-Parducci, R.: Nodular hidradenoma and hidradenocarcinoma. A 10-year review. J. Am. Acad. Dermatol. **12**, 15–20 (1985)

80. Hirsch, P., Helwig, E.B.: Chondroid syringoma-mixed tumor of skin, salivary gland type. Arch. Dermatol. **84**, 835–847 (1961)

81. Hoang, M.P., Dresser, K.A., Kapur, P., et al.: Microcystic adnexal carcinoma: an immunohistochemical reappraisal. Mod. Pathol. **21**, 178–185 (2008)

82. Hyman, A.B., Brownstein, M.H.: Eccrine poroma: an analysis of forty-five new cases. Dermatologica **138**, 29–38 (1969)

83. Iglesias, F.D., Forcelledo, F.F., Sanchez, T.S., et al.: Chondroid syringoma: a histological and immunohistochemical study of 15 cases. Histopathology **17**, 311–317 (1990)

84. Ishida-Yamamoto, A., Iizuka, H.: Eccrine syringofibroadenoma (Mascaro): an ultrastructural and immunohistochemical study. Am. J. Dermatopathol. **18**, 207–211 (1996)

85. Ishikawa, K.: Malignant hidroacanthoma simplex. Arch. Dermatol. **104**, 529–532 (1971)

86. Ishiko, A., Shimizu, H., Inamoto, N., et al.: Is tubular apocrine adenoma a distinct clinical entity? Am. J. Dermatopathol. **15**, 482–487 (1993)

87. Ishimura, E., Iwamoto, H., Kobashi, Y., et al.: Malignant chondroid syringoma: report of a case with widespread metastasis and review of pertinent literature. Cancer **52**, 1966–1973 (1983)

88. Ivan, D., Hafeez Diwan, A., et al.: Expression of p63 in primary cutaneous adnexal neoplasms and adenocarcinoma metastatic to the skin. Mod. Pathol. **18**, 137–142 (2005)

89. Jones, E.W., Heyl, T.: Naevus sebaceus: a report of 140 cases with special regard to the development of secondary malignant tumours. Br. J. Dermatol. **82**, 99–117 (1970)

90. Jones, R.E.: Mammary Paget's disease without underlying carcinoma. Am. J. Dermatopathol. **7**, 361–365 (1985)

91. Jones, R.E., Austin, C., Ackerman, A.B.: Extramammary Paget's disease. A critical reexamination. Am. J. Dermatopathol. **1**, 101–131 (1979)

92. Jordan, J.A., Brown, O.E., Biavati, M.J., et al.: Congenital syringocystadenoma papilliferum of the ear and neck treated with the CO_2-laser. Int. J. Pediatr. Otorhinolaryngol. **38**, 81–87 (1996)

93. Kakinuma, H., Miyamoto, R., Iwasawa, U., et al.: Three subtypes of poroid neoplasia in a single lesion: eccrine poroma, hidroacanthoma simplex, and dermal duct tumor. Histologic, histochemical, and ultrastructural findings. Am. J. Dermatopathol. **16**, 66–72 (1994)

94. Kanitakis, J., Hermier, C., Thivolet, J.: Tubular apocrine adenoma: apropos of a case. Dermatologica **169**, 23–28 (1984)

95. Kao, G.F., Graham, J.H., Helwig, E.B.: Aggressive digital papillary adenoma and adenocarcinoma. [Abstract]. Arch. Dermatol. **120**, 1612 (1984)

96. Kao, G.F., Helwig, E.B., Graham, J.H.: Aggressive digital papillary adenoma and adenocarcinoma. A clinicopathological study of 57 patients, with histochemical, immunopathological, and ultra-structural observations. J. Cutan. Pathol. **14**, 129–146 (1987)

97. Karam, P., Benedetto, A., Karma, P.: Intralesional electrodesiccation of syringomas. Dermatol. Surg. **23**, 921–924 (1997)

98. Katane, M., Akiyama, M., Ohnishi, T., et al.: Carcinomatous transformation of eccrine syringofibroadenoma. J. Cutan. Pathol. **30**, 211–214 (2003)

99. Kato, H., Mizuno, N., Nakagawa, K., et al.: Microcystic adnexal carcinoma: a light microscopic immunohistochemical and ultrastructural study. J. Cutan. Pathol. **17**, 87–95 (1990)

100. Kay, S., Hall, W.E.B.: Sweat gland carcinoma with proved metastases. Cancer **7**, 373–376 (1954)

101. Kazakov, D.V., Suster, S., LeBoit, P.E., et al.: Mucinous carcinoma of the skin, primary, and secondary: a clinicopathologic study of 63 cases with emphasis on the morphologic spectrum of primary cutaneous forms: homologies with mucinous lesions in the breast. Am. J. Surg. Pathol. **29**, 764–782 (2005)

102. Keasbey, L.E., Hadley, G.G.: Clear-cell hidradenoma: report of three cases with widespread metastases. Cancer **7**, 934–952 (1954)

103. Kersting, E., Helwig, E.B.: Eccrine spiradenoma. Arch. Dermatol. **73**, 199–227 (1956)

104. Khachemoune, A., Olbricht, S.M., Johnson, D.S.: Microcystic adnexal carcinoma: report of four cases treated with Mohs' micrographic surgical technique. Int. J. Dermatol. **44**, 507–512 (2005)

105. Kim, Y.D., Lee, E.J., Song, M.H., et al.: Multiple eccrine hidrocystomas associated with Graves' disease. Int. J. Dermatol. **41**, 295–297 (2002)

106. Kitazawa, T., Hataya, Y., Matsuo, K.: Chondroid syringoma of the orbit. Ann. Plast. Surg. **42**, 100–102 (1999)

107. Ko, C.J., Cochran, A.J., Eng, W., et al.: Hidradenocarcinoma: a histological and immunohistochemical study. J. Cutan. Pathol. **33**, 726–730 (2006)

108. Komine, M., Hattori, N., Tamaki, K.: Eccrine syringofibroadenoma (Mascaro): an immunohistochemical study. Am. J. Dermatopathol. **22**, 171–175 (2000)

109. Krunic, A.L., Kim, S., Medenica, M., et al.: Recurrent adenoid cystic carcinoma of the scalp treated with Mohs micrographic surgery. Dermatol. Surg. **29**, 647–649 (2003)

110. Kuan, S.F., Montag, A.G., Hart, J., et al.: Differential expression of mucin genes in mammary and extramammary Paget's disease. Am. J. Surg. Pathol. **25**, 1469–1477 (2001)

111. Landry, M., Winkelmann, R.K.: An unusual tubular apocrine adenoma. Arch. Dermatol. **105**, 869–879 (1972)

112. LeBoit, P.E., Sexton, M.: Microcystic adnexal carcinoma of the skin: a reappraisal of the differentiation and differential diagnosis of an under recognized neoplasm. J. Am. Acad. Dermatol. **29**, 609–618 (1993)

113. Leibovitch, I., Huilgol, S.C., Selva, D., et al.: Microcystic adnexal carcinoma: treatment with Mohs micrographic surgery. J. Am. Acad. Dermatol. **52**, 295–300 (2005)

114. Lele, S.M., Gloster, E.S., Heilman, E.R., et al.: Eccrine syringofibroadenoma surrounding a squamous cell carcinoma: a case report. J. Cutan. Pathol. **24**, 193–196 (1997)

115. Lennox, B., Pearse, A.G., Richards, H.G.: Mucin-secreting tumours of the skin with special reference to the so-called mixed-salivary tumour of the skin and its relation to hidradenoma. J. Pathol. Bacteriol. **64**, 865–880 (1952)

116. Leonard, N., Chaggar, R., Jones, C., et al.: Loss of heterozygosity at cylindromatosis gene locus, CYLD, in sporadic skin adnexal tumours. J. Clin. Pathol. **54**, 689–692 (2001)

117. Loane, J., Kealy, W.F., Mulcahy, G.: Perianal hidradenoma papilliferum occurring in a male: a case report. Ir. J. Med. Sci. **167**, 26–27 (1998)

118. Malafa, M.P., McKesey, P., Stone, S., et al.: Sentinel node biopsy for staging of aggressive digital papillary adenocarcinoma. Dermatol. Surg. **26**, 580–583 (2000)

119. Mambo, N.C.: Eccrine spiradenoma: clinical and pathologic study of 49 tumors. J. Cutan. Pathol. **10**, 312–330 (1983)

120. Mambo, N.C.: The significance of atypical nuclear changes in benign eccrine acrospiromas: a clinical and pathological study of 18 cases. J. Cutan. Pathol. **11**, 35–44 (1984)

121. Marcus, E.: The management of Paget's disease of the breast. Curr. Treat. Options Oncol. **5**, 153–160 (2004)

122. Marra, D.E., Schanbacher, C.F., Torres, A.: Mohs micrographic surgery of primary cutaneous mucinous carcinoma using immuno-histochemistry for margin control. Dermatol. Surg. **30**, 799–802 (2004)

123. Mascaro, J.M.: Considérations sur les tumeurs fibro-épithéliales. Le syringofibroadénome eccrine. Ann. Dermatol. Syphiligr. **90**, 143–153 (1963)

124. Matz, L.R., McCully, D.J., Stokes, B.A.R.: Metastasizing chondroid syringoma: case report. Pathology **1**, 77–81 (1969)

125. Mayer, I.: Zur Histologie der Hidroadenome. Frankfurt Z Pathol. **55**, 548–580 (1941)

126. McKee, P., Calonje, E., Granter, S.: Pathology of the Skin: With Clinical Correlations, pp. 1632–1636. Elsevier, Mosby, Edinburgh (2005)

127. McKee, P.H., Hertogs, K.T.: Endocervical adenocarcinoma and vulval Paget's disease: a significant association. Br. J. Dermatol. **103**, 443–448 (1980)

128. Meeker, J., Neubecker, R., Helwig, E.: Hidradenoma papilliferum. Am. J. Clin. Pathol. **37**, 182–195 (1962)

129. Mehregan, A.H., Hasimoto, K., Homayoon, R.: Eccrine adenocarcinoma – a clinicopathologic study of 35 cases. Arch. Dermatol. **119**, 104–114 (1983)

130. Mendoza, S., Helwig, E.B.: Mucinous (adenocystic) carcinoma of the skin. Arch. Dermatol. **103**, 68–78 (1971)

131. Metze, D., Wigbels, B., Hildebrand, A.: Familial syringoma: a rare clinical variant. Hautarzt **52**, 1045–1048 (2001)

132. Meybehm, M., Fischer, H.P.: Spiradenoma and dermal cylindroma: comparative immunohistochemical analysis and histogenetic considerations. Am. J. Dermatopathol. **19**, 154–161 (1997)

133. Michal, M.: Spiradenocylindroma of the skin: tumors with morphological features of spiradenoma and cylindroma in the same lesion: report of 12 cases. Pathol. Int. **49**, 419–425 (1999)

134. Miller, W.L.: Sweat gland carcinoma: a clinicopathologic problem. Am. J. Clin. Pathol. **47**, 767–780 (1967)

135. Mishima, Y., Morioka, S.: Oncogenic differentiation of the intraepidermal eccrine sweat duct: eccrine poroma, poroepithelioma and porocarcinoma. Dermatologica **138**, 238–250 (1969)

136. Miyamoto, T., Hagari, Y., Inoue, S., et al.: Axillary apocrine carcinoma with benign apocrine tumours: a case report involving a pathological and immunohistochemical study and review of the literature. J. Clin. Pathol. **58**, 757–761 (2005)

137. Nadji, M., Morales, A.R., Girtanner, R.E., et al.: Paget's disease of the skin: a unifying concept of histogenesis. Cancer **50**, 2203–2206 (1982)

138. Narang, T., De, D., Dogra, S., Saikia, U.N., et al.: Linear papules and nodules on the neck. Syringocystadenoma papilliferum (SP). Arch. Dermatol. **144**, 1509–1514 (2008)

139. Naversen, D.N., Trask, D.M., Watson, F.H., et al.: Painful tumors of the skin, 'LEND AN EGG'. J. Am. Acad. Dermatol. **28**, 298–300 (1993)

140. Nickoloff, B.J., Fleischmann, H.E., Carmel, J., et al.: Microcystic adnexal carcinoma. Immunohistologic observations suggesting dual (pilar and eccrine) differentiation. Arch. Dermatol. **122**, 290–294 (1986)

141. Nomura, K., Kogawa, T., Hashimoto, I., et al.: Eccrine syringofibroadenomatous hyperplasia in a patient with bullous pemphigoid: a case report and review of the literature. Dermatologica **182**, 59–62 (1991)

142. Offidani, A., Campanati, A.: Papillary hidradenoma: immunohistochemical analysis of steroid receptor profile with a focus on apocrine differentiation. J. Clin. Pathol. **52**, 829–832 (1999)

143. Ohnishi, T., Watanabe, S.: Immunohistochemical analysis of keratin expression in clear cell syringoma. A comparative study with conventional syringoma. J. Cutan. Pathol. **24**, 370–376 (1997)

144. Ohtsuka, H., Nozawa, R., Kushida, Y.: Synchronous microcystic adnexal carcinoma and gastric cancer with review of the literature. J. Dermatol. **32**, 43–47 (2005)

145. Okada, N., Ota, J., Sato, K., et al.: Metastasizing sweat gland carcinoma. Arch. Dermatol. **120**, 768–769 (1984)

146. Paget, J.: On disease of the mammary areola preceding cancer of the mammary gland. St. Barth. Hosp. Rep. **10**, 87–89 (1874)

147. Park, H.J., Kim, Y.C., Cinn, Y.W.: Nodular hidradenocarcinoma with prominent squamous differentiation: case report and immunohistochemical study. J. Cutan. Pathol. **27**, 423–427 (2000)

148. Paties, C., Taccagni, G.L., Papotti, M., et al.: Apocrine carcinoma of the skin. A clinicopathologic, immunocytochemical, and ultrastructural study. Cancer **71**, 375–381 (1993)

149. Patrizi, A., Neri, I., Marzaduri, S., et al.: Syringoma: a review of twenty-nine cases. Acta Derm. Venereol. **78**, 460–462 (1998)

150. Penneys, N.S., Kaiser, M.: Cylindroma expresses immunohistochemical markers linking to eccrine coil. J. Cutan. Pathol. **20**, 40–43 (1993)

151. Pilgram, J.P., Kloss, S.G., Wolfish, P.S., et al.: Primary mucinous carcinoma of the skin with metastases to the lymph nodes. Am. J. Dermatopathol. **7**, 461–469 (1985)

152. Pinkus, H.: Life history of naevus syringadenomatosus papilliferus. AMA Arch. Derm. Syphilol. **63**, 305–322 (1954)

153. Pinkus, H., Mehregan, A.H.: Epidermotropic eccrine carcinoma: a case combining features of eccrine poroma and Paget's disease. Arch. Dermatol. **88**, 597–606 (1963)

154. Pinkus, H., Rogin, J.R., Goldman, P.: Eccrine poroma: tumors exhibiting features of the epidermal sweat duct unit. Arch. Dermatol. **74**, 511–521 (1956)

155. Piura, B., Zirkin, H.J.: Vulvar Paget's disease with an underlying sweat gland adenocarcinoma. J. Dermatol. Surg. Oncol. **14**, 533–537 (1988)

156. Plumb, S.J., Argenyi, Z.B., Stone, M.S., et al.: Cytokeratin 5/6 immunostaining in cutaneous adnexal neoplasms and metastatic adenocarcinoma. Am. J. Dermatopathol. **26**, 447–451 (2004)

157. Poiares, B.A., Tellechea, O., Reis, J.P., et al.: Eccrine porocarcinoma: a review of 24 cases. Ann. Dermatol. Vénéréol. **120**, 107–115 (1993)

158. Pujol, R.M., LeBoit, P.E., Su, W.P.: Microcystic adnexal carcinoma with extensive sebaceous differentiation. Am. J. Dermatopathol. **19**, 358–362 (1997)

159. Pylyser, K., Dewolf-Peeters, C., Marlen, K.: The histology of eccrine poromas: a study of 14 cases. Dermatologica **167**, 243–249 (1983)

160. Rahilly, M.A., Beattie, G.J., Lessells, A.M.: Mucinous eccrine carcinoma of the vulva with neuroendocrine differentiation. Histopathology **27**, 82–86 (1995)

161. Rayne, S.C., Santa Cruz, D.J.: Anaplastic Paget's disease. Am. J. Surg. Pathol. **16**, 1085–1091 (1992)

162. Regauer, S.: Extramammary Paget's disease-a proliferation of adnexal origin? Histopathology **48**, 723–729 (2006)

163. Reid-Nicholson, M., Iyengar, P., Friedlander, M.A., et al.: Fine needle aspiration biopsy of primary mucinous carcinoma of the skin: a case report. Acta Cytol. **50**, 317–322 (2006)

164. Requena, L., Kiryu, H., Ackerman, A.B.: Neoplasms with Apocrine Differentiation – Ackerman's Histologic Diagnosis of Neoplastic Skin Disease: A Method by Pattern Analysis. Lippincott-Raven, Philadelphia (1998)

165. Robinson, A.R.: Hidrocystoma. J. Cutan. Genitourin. Dis. **11**, 293–303 (1893)

166. Robinson, A., Greene, J., Ansari, N., et al.: Eccrine porocarcinoma (malignant eccrine poroma): a clinicopathologic study of 69 cases. Am. J. Surg. Pathol. **25**, 710–720 (2001)

167. Rongioletti, F., Gambini, C., Parodi, A., et al.: Mossy leg with eccrine syringofibroadenomatous hyperplasia resembling multiple eccrine syringofibroadenoma. Clin. Exp. Dermatol. **21**, 454–456 (1996)

168. Rosborough, D.: Malignant mixed tumours of skin. Br. J. Surg. **50**, 697–699 (1963)

169. Rulon, D.B., Helwig, E.B.: Papillary eccrine adenoma. Arch. Dermatol. **113**, 596–598 (1977)

170. Sakorafas, G.H., Blanchard, D.K., Sarr, M.G., et al.: Paget's disease of the breast: a clinical perspective. Langenbecks Arch. Surg. **386**, 444–450 (2001)

171. Salerno, S., Terrill, P.: Will MAC be back? Aust. NZ. J. Surg. **73**, 830–832 (2003)

172. Santa Cruz, D.J.: Sweat gland carcinomas: a comprehensive review. Semin. Diagn. Pathol. **4**, 38–74 (1987)

173. Satoh, F., Umemura, S., Osamura, R.Y.: Immunohistochemical analysis of GCDFP-15 and GCDFP-24 in mammary and non-mammary tissue. Breast Cancer **7**, 49–55 (2000)

174. Schweitzer, W.J., Goldin, H.M., Bronson, D.M., et al.: Ulcerated tumor on the scalp. Clear-cell hidradenoma. Arch. Dermatol. **125**, 985–986 (1989)

175. Seab, J.A., Graham, J.H.: Primary cutaneous adenoid cystic carcinoma. J. Am. Acad. Dermatol. **17**, 113–118 (1987)

176. Seyhan, T., Borman, H., Bal, N.: Malignant eccrine spiradenoma of the scalp. J. Craniofac. Surg. **19**, 1608–1612 (2008)

177. Shaw, M., McKee, P.H., Lowe, D., et al.: Malignant eccrine poroma: a study of twenty-seven cases. Br. J. Dermatol. **107**, 675–680 (1982)

178. Shenoy, Y.: Malignant perianal papillary hidradenoma. Arch. Dermatol. **83**, 119–121 (1961)

179. Shieh, S., Dee, A.S., Cheney, R.T., et al.: Photodynamic therapy for the treatment of extramammary Paget's disease. Br. J. Dermatol. **146**, 1000–1005 (2002)

180. Shintaku, M., Tsuta, K., Yoshida, H., et al.: Apocrine adenocarcinoma of the eyelid with aggressive biological behavior: report of a case. Pathol. Int. **52**, 169–173 (2002)

181. Smith, J.D., Chernosky, M.E.: Hidrocystomas. Arch. Dermatol. **108**, 676–679 (1973)

182. Smith, K.J., Williams, J., Corbett, D., et al.: Microcystic adnexal carcinoma: an immunohistochemical study including markers of proliferation and apoptosis. Am. J. Surg. Pathol. **25**, 464–471 (2001)

183. Snow, S., Madjar, D.D., Hardy, S., et al.: Microcystic adnexal carcinoma: report of 13 cases and review of the literature. Dermatol. Surg. **27**, 401–408 (2001)

184. Snow, S.N., Reizner, G.T.: Eccrine porocarcinoma of the face. J. Am. Acad. Dermatol. **27**, 306–312 (1992)

185. Snow, S., Reizner, G., Dudley, C., et al.: Eccrine mucinous carcinoma. In: Miller, S., Maloney, M. (eds.) Cutaneous Oncology, pp. 758–762. Blackwell Science, Malden) (1998)

186. Soler-Carrillo, J., Estrach, T., Mascaro, J.M.: Eruptive syringoma: 27 new cases and review of the literature. J. Eur. Acad. Dermatol. Venereol. **15**, 242–246 (2001)

187. Soyer, H.P., Kerl, H., Ott, A.: Spiradenocylindroma - more than a coincidence? Am. J. Dermatopathol. **20**, 315–317 (1998)

188. Stein, J.M., Ormsby, A., Esclamado, R., et al.: The effect of radiation therapy on microcystic adnexal carcinoma: a case report. Head Neck **25**, 251–254 (2003)

189. Stout, A.P., Cooley, S.G.: Carcinoma of sweat glands. Cancer **4**, 521–536 (1951)

190. Takeda, H., Mitsuhashi, Y., Hayashi, M., et al.: Eccrine syringofibroadenoma: case report and review of the literature. J. Eur. Acad. Dermatol. Venereol. **15**, 147–149 (2000)

191. Tay, J.S., Tapen, E.M., Solari, P.G.: Malignant eccrine spiradenoma. Case report and review of the literature. Am. J. Clin. Oncol. **20**, 552–557 (1997)

192. Tellechea, O., Reis, J.P., Marques, C., et al.: Tubular apocrine adenoma with eccrine and apocrine immunophenotypes or papillary tubular adenoma? Am. J. Dermatopathol. **17**, 499–505 (1995)

193. Ter Poorten, M.C., Barrett, K., Cook, J.: Familial eccrine spiradenoma: a case report and review of literature. Dermatol. Surg. **29**, 411–414 (2003)

194. Thomas, C.J., Wood, G.C., Marks, V.J.: Mohs micrographic surgery in the treatment of rare aggressive cutaneous tumors: the Geisinger experience. Dermatol. Surg. **33**, 333–339 (2007)

195. Uede, K., Yamamoto, Y., Furukawa, F.: Brooke-Spiegler syndrome associated with cylindroma, trichoepithelioma, spiradenoma and syringoma. J. Dermatol. **31**, 32–38 (2004)

196. Urban, C.D., Cannon, J.R., Cole, R.D.: Eruptive syringomas in Down's syndrome. Arch. Dermatol. **117**, 374–375 (1981)

197. Urso, C., Bondi, R., Paglierani, M., et al.: Carcinomas of sweat glands: report of 60 cases. Arch. Pathol. Lab. Med. **125**, 498–505 (2001)

198. Vang, R., Cohen, P.R.: Ectopic hidradenoma papilliferum: a case report and review of the literature. J. Am. Acad. Dermatol. **41**, 115–118 (1999)

199. Wang, J., Roenigk, H.J.: Treatment of multiple facial syringomas with the carbon dioxide laser. Dermatol. Surg. **25**, 136–139 (1999)

200. Warkel, R.L., Helwig, E.B.: Apocrine gland adenoma and adenocarcinoma of the axilla. Arch. Dermatol. **114**, 198–203 (1978)

201. Wick, M.R., Cooper, P.H., Swanson, P.E., et al.: Microcystic adnexal carcinoma: an immunohistochemical comparison with other cutaneous appendage tumors. Arch. Dermatol. **126**, 189–194 (1990)

202. Wick, M.R., Swanson, P.E.: Primary adenoid cystic carcinoma of the skin. A clinical, histological, and immunocytochemical comparison with adenoid cystic carcinoma of salivary glands and adenoid basal cell carcinoma. Am. J. Dermatopathol. **8**, 2–13 (1986)

203. Wilkinson, E.J., Brown, H.M.: Vulvar Paget disease of urothelial origin: a report of three cases and a proposed classification of vulvar Paget disease. Hum. Pathol. **33**, 549–554 (2002)

204. Willman, J.H., Golitz, L.E., Fitzpatrick, J.E.: Vulvar clear cells of Toker. Precursors of extramammary Paget's disease. Am. J. Dermatopathol. **27**, 185–188 (2005)

205. Wittenberg, G., Rovertson, D., Solomon, A.: Eccrine porocarcinoma treated with Mohs micrographic surgery: a report of five cases. Dermatol. Surg. **21**, 911–913 (1999)

206. Woodworth, H., Dockerty, M., Wilson, R.B.: Papillary hidradenoma of the vulva: a clinicopathologic study of 69 cases. Am. J. Obstet. Gynecol. **10**, 501–508 (1971)

207. Yamamoto, O., Haratake, J., Yokoyama, S., et al.: A histopathological and ultrastructural studay of eccrine porocarcinoma with special reference to its subtypes. Virchos Arch. A Pathol. Anat. Histopathol. **420**, 395–401 (1992)

208. Yamamoto, O., Yasuda, H.: An immunohistochemical study of the apocrine type of cutaneous mixed tumors with special reference to their follicular and sebaceous differentiation. J. Cutan. Pathol. **26**, 232–241 (1999)

209. Yavuzer, R., Basterzi, Y., Sari, A., et al.: Chondroid syringoma: a diagnosis more frequent than expected. Dermatol. Surg. **29**, 179–181 (2003)
210. Yeung, K.Y., Stinson, J.C.: Mucinous (adenocystic) carcinoma of sweat glands with widespread metastasis. Cancer **39**, 2556–2562 (1977)

Tumours with Follicular Differentiation

1. Abbott, J.J., Hernandez-Rios, P., Amirkhan, R.H., Hoang, M.P.: Cystic sebaceous neoplasms in Muir-Torre syndrome. Arch. Pathol. Lab. Med. **127**, 614–617 (2003)
2. Ackerman, A.B., Reddy, V.B., Soyer, H.P.: Neoplasms with Follicular Differentiation. Ardor Scribendi, New York (2001)
3. Ackerman, A., De Viragh, P., Chongchitnant, N.: Neoplasms with Follicular Differentiation. Lea & Febiger, Philadelphia (1993)
4. Ackerman, A.B., Wade, T.R.: Tricholemmoma. Am. J. Dermatopathol. **2**, 207–224 (1980)
5. Akasaka, T., Imamura, Y., Mori, Y., Iwasaki, M., Kon, S.: Trichoblastoma with rippled-pattern. J. Dermatol. **24**, 174–178 (1997)
6. Aloi, F., Tomasini, C., Pippione, M.: Pigmented trichoblastoma. Am. J. Dermatopathol. **14**, 345–349 (1992)
7. Amaral, A.L., Nascimento, A.G., Goellner, J.R.: Proliferating pilar (trichilemmal) cyst. Report of two cases, one with carcinomatous transformation and one with distant metastases. Arch. Pathol. Lab. Med. **108**, 808–810 (1984)
8. Ansai, S., Mitsuhashi, Y., Kondo, S., Manabe, M.: Immuno-histochemical differentiation of extra-ocular sebaceous carcinoma from other skin cancers. J. Dermatol. **31**, 998–1008 (2004)
9. Aquilina, S., Gatt, P., Boffa, M.J.: Pilomatricoma arising at a BCG vaccination site. Clin. Exp. Dermatol. **31**, 296–297 (2006)
10. Arnold, H.: Pilomatricoma (Letter to the Editor). Arch. Dermatol. **113**, 998–1008 (1977)
11. Ashinoff, R., Jacobson, M., Belsito, D.V.: Rombo syndrome: a second case report and review. J. Am. Acad. Dermatol. **28**, 1011–1014 (1993)
12. Bapat, B.V., Madlensky, L., Temple, L.K., Hiruki, T., Redston, M., Baron, D.L., Xia, L., Marcus, V.A., Soravia, C., Mitri, A., Shen, W., Gryfe, R., Berk, T., Chodirker, B.N., Cohen, Z., Gallinger, S.: Family history characteristics, tumor microsatellite instability and germline MSH2 and MLH1 mutations in hereditary colorectal cancer. Hum. Genet. **104**, 167–176 (1999)
13. Bassarova, A., Nesland, J.M., Sedloev, T., Danielsen, H., Christova, S.: Pilomatrix carcinoma with lymph node metastases. J. Cutan. Pathol. **31**, 330–335 (2004)
14. Batman, P.A., Evans, H.J.: Metastasising pilar tumour of scalp. J. Clin. Pathol. **39**, 757–760 (1986)
15. Bayer-Garner, I.B., Givens, V., Smoller, B.: Immunohistochemical staining for androgen receptors: a sensitive marker of sebaceous differentiation. Am. J. Dermatopathol. **21**, 426–431 (1999)
16. Behrens, J., von Kries, J.P., Kuhl, M., Bruhn, L., Wedlich, D., Grosschedl, R., Birchmeier, W.: Functional interaction of beta-catenin with the transcription factor LEF-1. Nature **382**, 638–642 (1996)
17. Berlin, A.L., Amin, S.P., Goldberg, D.J.: Extraocular sebaceous carcinoma treated with Mohs micrographic surgery: report of a case and review of literature. Dermatol. Surg. **34**, 254–257 (2008)
18. Betti, R., Cerri, A., Moneghini, L., Inselvini, E., Crosti, C.: Adenoid-zystisches cribriformes Trichoblastom. Hautarzt **48**, 417–419 (1997)
19. Betti, R., Inselvini, E., Vergani, R., Moneghini, L., Crosti, C.: Sebaceoma arising in association with seborrheic keratosis. Am. J. Dermatopathol. **23**, 58–61 (2001)
20. Boran, C., Parlak, A.H., Erkol, H.: Collision tumour of tricho-folliculoma and basal cell carcinoma. Australas. J. Dermatol. **48**, 127–129 (2007)
21. Bremnes, R.M., Kvamme, J.M., Stalsberg, H., Jacobsen, E.A.: Pilomatrix carcinoma with multiple metastases: report of a case and review of the literature. Eur. J. Cancer **35**, 433–437 (1999)
22. Brownstein, M.H.: Trichilemmoma. Benign follicular tumor or viral wart? Am. J. Dermatopathol. **2**, 229–231 (1980)
23. Brownstein, M.H., Mehregan, A.H., Bikowski, J.B., Lupulescu, A., Patterson, J.C.: The dermatopathology of Cowden's syndrome. Br. J. Dermatol. **100**, 667–673 (1979)
24. Brownstein, M.H., Shapiro, L.: Trichilemmoma. Analysis of 40 new cases. Arch. Dermatol. **107**, 866–869 (1973)
25. Brownstein, M.H., Wolf, M., Bikowski, J.B.: Cowden's disease: a cutaneous marker of breast cancer. Cancer **41**, 2393–2398 (1978)
26. Burgdorf, W.H., Pitha, J., Fahmy, A.: Muir-Torre syndrome. Histologic spectrum of sebaceous proliferations. Am. J. Dermatopathol. **8**, 202–208 (1986)
27. Camarasa, J.G., Calderon, P., Moreno, A.: Familial multiple tricho-discomas. Acta Derm. Venereol. **68**, 163–165 (1988)
28. Casas, J.G., Woscoff, A.: Giant pilar tumor of the scalp. Arch. Dermatol. **116**, 1395 (1980)
29. Chao, A.N., Shields, C.L., Krema, H., Shields, J.A.: Outcome of patients with periocular sebaceous gland carcinoma with and without conjunctival intraepithelial invasion. Ophthalmology **108**, 1877–1883 (2001)
30. Chartier, M., Reed, M.L., Mandavilli, S., Fung, M., Grant-Kels, J., Murphy, M.: CD34-reactive trichodiscoma. J. Cutan. Pathol. **34**, 808 (2007)
31. Collina, G., Eusebi, V., Capella, C., Rosai, J.: Merkel cell differentiation in trichoblastoma. Virchows Arch. **433**, 291–296 (1998)
32. Collins, G.L., Somach, S., Morgan, M.B.: CD-34-reactive tricho-discoma. J. Cutan. Pathol. **33**, 709 (2006)
33. Cribier, B., Asch, P.H., Regnier, C., Rio, M.C., Grosshans, E.: Expression of human hair keratin basic 1 in pilomatrixoma. A study of 128 cases. Br. J. Dermatol. **140**, 600–604 (1999)
34. Cribier, B., Scrivener, Y., Grosshans, E.: Tumors arising in nevus sebaceus: A study of 596 cases. J. Am. Acad. Dermatol. **42**, 263–268 (2000)
35. De Galvez-Aranda, M.V., Herrera-Ceballos, E., Sanchez-Sanchez, P., Bosch-Garcia, R.J., Matilla-Vicente, A.: Pilomatrix carcinoma with lymph node and pulmonary metastasis: report of a case arising on the knee. Am. J. Dermatopathol. **24**, 139–143 (2002)
36. del Pozo, J., Martinez, W., Yebra-Pimentel, M.T., Fonseca, E.: Lymphangiectatic variant of pilomatricoma. J. Eur. Acad. Dermatol. Venereol. **18**, 575–576 (2004)
37. Delfino, M., D'Anna, F., Ianniello, S., Donofrio, V.: Multiple hereditary trichoepithelioma and cylindroma (Brooke-Spiegler syndrome). Dermatologica **183**, 150–153 (1991)
38. Diedhiou, A., Cazals-Hatem, D., Rondini, E., Sterkers, O., Degott, C., Wassef, M.: Sebaceous carcinoma of the submandibular gland: a case report. Ann. Pathol. **21**, 348–351 (2001)
39. Dinneen, A.M., Mehregan, D.R.: Sebaceous epithelioma: a review of twenty-one cases. J. Am. Acad. Dermatol. **34**, 47–50 (1996)
40. Dogru, M., Matsuo, H., Inoue, M., Okubo, K., Yamamoto, M.: Management of eyelid sebaceous carcinomas. Ophthalmologica **211**, 40–43 (1997)
41. Dores, G.M., Curtis, R.E., Toro, J.R., Devesa, S.S., Fraumeni Jr., J.F.: Incidence of cutaneous sebaceous carcinoma and risk of associated neoplasms: insight into Muir-Torre syndrome. Cancer **113**, 3372–3381 (2008)
42. Elston, D.M., James, W.D., Rodman, O.G., Graham, G.F.: Multiple hamartoma syndrome (Cowden's disease) associated with non-Hodgkin's lymphoma. Arch. Dermatol. **122**, 572–575 (1986)
43. Entius, M.M., Keller, J.J., Drillenburg, P., Kuypers, K.C., Giardiello, F.M., Offerhaus, G.J.: Microsatellite instability and expression of hMLH-1 and hMSH-2 in sebaceous gland carcinomas as markers for Muir-Torre syndrome. Clin. Cancer Res. **6**, 1784–1789 (2000)
44. Fan, Y.S., Carr, R.A., Sanders, D.S., Smith, A.P., Lazar, A.J., Calonje, E.: Characteristic Ber-EP4 and EMA expression in

sebaceoma is immunohistochemically distinct from basal cell carcinoma. Histopathology **51**, 80–86 (2007)

45. Fender, A.B., Reale, V.F., Scott, G.A.: Anetodermic pilomatricoma with perforation. J. Am. Acad. Dermatol. **58**, 535–536 (2008)

46. Fenske, C., Banerjee, P., Holden, C., Carter, N.: Brooke-Spiegler syndrome locus assigned to 16q12–q13. J. Invest. Dermatol. **114**, 1057–1058 (2000)

47. Folpe, A.L., Reisenauer, A.K., Mentzel, T., Rutten, A., Solomon, A.R.: Proliferating trichilemmal tumors: clinicopathologic evaluation is a guide to biologic behavior. J. Cutan. Pathol. **30**, 492–498 (2003)

48. Forbis Jr., R., Helwig, E.B.: Pilomatrixoma (calcifying epithelioma). Arch. Dermatol. **83**, 606–618 (1961)

49. Gambichler, T., Wolter, M., Altmeyer, P., Hoffman, K.: Treatment of Birt-Hogg-Dube syndrome with erbium:YAG laser. J. Am. Acad. Dermatol. **43**, 856–858 (2000)

50. Gat, U., DasGupta, R., Degenstein, L., Fuchs, E.: De Novo hair follicle morphogenesis and hair tumors in mice expressing a truncated beta-catenin in skin. Cell **95**, 605–614 (1998)

51. Gilaberte, Y., Ferrer-Lozano, M., Olivan, M.J., Coscojuela, C., Abascal, M., Lapunzina, P.: Multiple giant pilomatricoma in familial Sotos syndrome. Pediatr. Dermatol. **25**, 122–125 (2008)

52. Gloor, P., Ansari, I., Sinard, J.: Sebaceous carcinoma presenting as a unilateral papillary conjunctivitis. Am. J. Ophthalmol. **127**, 458–459 (1999)

53. Graham, B.S., Barr, R.J.: Rippled-pattern sebaceous trichoblastoma. J. Cutan. Pathol. **27**, 455–459 (2000)

54. Gray, H., Helwig, E.B.: Trichofolliculoma. Arch Dermatol **86**, 99–105 (1962)

55. Grosshans, E., Dungler, T., Hanau, D.: Pinkus' trichodiscoma (author's transl). Ann. Dermatol. Vénéréol. **108**, 837–846 (1981)

56. Haas, N., Audring, H., Sterry, W.: Carcinoma arising in a proliferating trichilemmal cyst expresses fetal and trichilemmal hair phenotype. Am. J. Dermatopathol. **24**, 340–344 (2002)

57. Haferkamp, B., Bastian, B.C., Brocker, E.B., Hamm, H.: Pilomatrixkarzinom in ungewöhnlicher Lokalisation. Fallnericht und Literaturübersicht. Hautarzt **50**, 355–359 (1999)

58. Hague, J.S., Maheshwari, M., Ryatt, K.S., Abdullah, A.: Proliferating pilomatricoma mimicking pyogenic granuloma. J. Eur. Acad. Dermatol. Venereol. **21**, 688–689 (2007)

59. Harada, H., Hashimoto, K., Ko, M.S.: The gene for multiple familial trichoepithelioma maps to chromosome 9p21. J. Invest. Dermatol. **107**, 41–43 (1996)

60. Hardisson, D., Linares, M.D., Cuevas-Santos, J., Contreras, F.: Pilomatrix carcinoma: a clinicopathologic study of six cases and review of the literature. Am. J. Dermatopathol. **23**, 394–401 (2001)

61. Hartschuh, W., Schulz, T.: Immunohistochemical investigation of the different developmental stages of trichofolliculoma with special reference to the Merkel cell. Am. J. Dermatopathol. **21**, 8–15 (1999)

62. Hashimoto, K., Nelson, R.G., Lever, W.F.: Calcifying epithelioma of Malherbe. Histochemical and electron microscopic studies. J. Invest. Dermatol. **46**, 391–408 (1966)

63. Hashimoto, Y., Matsuo, S., Iizuka, H.: A DNA-flow cytometric analysis of trichilemmal carcinoma, proliferating trichilemmal cyst and trichilemmal cyst. Acta Derm. Venereol. **74**, 358–360 (1994)

64. Headington, J.T.: Differentiating neoplasms of hair germ. J. Clin. Pathol. **23**, 464–471 (1970)

65. Headington, J.T.: Tricholemmoma. To be or not to be? Am. J. Dermatopathol. **2**, 225–226 (1980)

66. Headington, J.T.: Tumors of the hair follicle. A review. Am. J. Pathol. **85**, 479–514 (1976)

67. Headington, J.T., French, A.J.: Primary neoplasms of the hair follicle. Histogenesis and classification. Arch. Dermatol. **86**, 430–441 (1962)

68. Hendricks, D.L., Liang, M.D., Borochovitz, D., Miller, T.: A case of multiple pilar tumors and pilar cysts involving the scalp and back. Plast. Reconstr. Surg. **87**, 763–767 (1991)

69. Herrero, J., Monteagudo, C., Ruiz, A., Llombart-Bosch, A.: Malignant proliferating trichilemmal tumours: an histopathological and immunohistochemical study of three cases with DNA ploidy and morphometric evaluation. Histopathology **33**, 542–546 (1998)

70. Hunt, S.J., Kilzer, B., Santa Cruz, D.J.: Desmoplastic trichilemmoma: histologic variant resembling invasive carcinoma. J. Cutan. Pathol. **17**, 45–52 (1990)

71. Husain, A., Blumenschein, G., Esmaeli, B.: Treatment and outcomes for metastatic sebaceous cell carcinoma of the eyelid. Int. J. Dermatol. **47**, 276–279 (2008)

72. Illueca, C., Monteagudo, C., Revert, A., Llombart-Bosch, A.: Diagnostic value of CD34 immunostaining in desmoplastic trichilemmoma. J. Cutan. Pathol. **25**, 435–439 (1998)

73. Inui, S., Kanda, R., Hata, S.: Pilomatricoma with a bullous appearance. J. Dermatol. **24**, 57–59 (1997)

74. Jacob, C.I., Dover, J.S.: Birt-Hogg-Dube syndrome: treatment of cutaneous manifestations with laser skin resurfacing. Arch. Dermatol. **137**, 98–99 (2001)

75. Jani, P., Chetty, R., Ghazarian, D.M.: An unusual composite pilomatrix carcinoma with intralesional melanocytes: differential diagnosis, immunohistochemical evaluation, and review of the literature. Am. J. Dermatopathol. **30**, 174–177 (2008)

76. Jaqueti, G., Requena, L., Sanchez Yus, E.: Trichoblastoma is the most common neoplasm developed in nevus sebaceus of Jadassohn: a clinicopathologic study of a series of 155 cases. Am. J. Dermatopathol. **22**, 108–118 (2000)

77. Jones, C.C., Tschen, J.A.: Anetodermic cutaneous changes overlying pilomatricomas. J. Am. Acad. Dermatol. **25**, 1072–1076 (1991)

78. Julian, C.G., Bowers, P.W.: A clinical review of 209 pilomatricomas. J. Am. Acad. Dermatol. **39**, 191–195 (1998)

79. Kaddu, S., Schaeppi, H., Kerl, H., Soyer, H.P.: Basaloid neoplasms in nevus sebaceus. J. Cutan. Pathol. **27**, 327–337 (2000)

80. Kaddu, S., Schaeppi, H., Kerl, H., Soyer, H.P.: Subcutaneous trichoblastoma. J. Cutan. Pathol. **26**, 490–496 (1999)

81. Kaddu, S., Schappi, H., Kerl, H., Soyer, H.P.: Trichoblastoma and sebaceoma in nevus sebaceus. Am. J. Dermatopathol. **21**, 552–556 (1999)

82. Kaddu, S., Soyer, H.P., Cerroni, L., Salmhofer, W., Hodl, S.: Clinical and histopathologic spectrum of pilomatricomas in adults. Int. J. Dermatol. **33**, 705–708 (1994)

83. Kaddu, S., Soyer, H.P., Hodl, S., Kerl, H.: Morphological stages of pilomatricoma. Am. J. Dermatopathol. **18**, 333–338 (1996)

84. Kaddu, S., Soyer, H.P., Wolf, I.H., Kerl, H.: Proliferating pilomatricoma. A histopathologic simulator of matrical carcinoma. J. Cutan. Pathol. **24**, 228–234 (1997)

85. Kahle, B., Hellwig, S., Schulz, T.: Multiple Mantleome bei Birt-Hogg-Dube-Syndrom Erfolgreiche Therapie mit dem CO$_2$-Laser. Hautarzt **52**, 43–46 (2001)

86. Kambe, Y., Nakano, H., Kaneko, T., Aizu, T., Ikenaga, S., Harada, K., Nakajima, N., Moritsugu, R., Hanada, K.: Giant pilomatricoma associated with hypercalcaemia and elevated levels of parathyroid hormone-related protein. Br. J. Dermatol. **155**, 208–210 (2006)

87. Kazakov, D.V., Kutzner, H., Rutten, A., Mukensnabl, P., Michal, M.: Carcinoid-like pattern in sebaceous neoplasms: another distinctive, previously unrecognized pattern in extraocular sebaceous carcinoma and sebaceoma. Am. J. Dermatopathol. **27**, 195–203 (2005)

88. Kazakov, D.V., Michal, M.: Trichoepithelioma with giant and multinucleated neoplastic epithelial cells. Am. J. Dermatopathol. **28**, 63–64 (2006)

89. Khoo, S.K., Bradley, M., Wong, F.K., Hedblad, M.A., Nordenskjold, M., Teh, B.T.: Birt-Hogg-Dube syndrome: mapping of a novel hereditary neoplasia gene to chromosome 17p12–q11.2. Oncogene **20**, 5239–5242 (2001)

90. Kim, E.H., Jeong, S.Y., Kim, H.J., Kim, Y.C.: A case of Birt-Hogg-Dube syndrome. J. Korean Med. Sci. **23**, 332–335 (2008)

91. Kim, Y.C., Vandersteen, D.P., Park, H.J., Cinn, Y.W.: A case of giant proliferating trichilemmal tumor with malignant transformation. J. Dermatol. **27**, 687–688 (2000)

92. Kimura, T., Miyazawa, H., Aoyagi, T., Ackerman, A.B.: Folliculosebaceous cystic hamartoma. A distinctive malformation of the skin. Am. J. Dermatopathol. **13**, 213–220 (1991)

93. Kiyohara, T., Kumakiri, M., Kuwahara, H., Saitoh, A., Ansai, S.: Rippled-pattern sebaceoma: a report of a lesion on the back with a review of the literature. Am. J. Dermatopathol. **28**, 446–448 (2006)

94. Kondo, T., Tanaka, Y.: Malignant pilomatricoma in the parietal area. Pathol. Oncol. Res. **12**, 251–253 (2006)

95. Korting, H.C., Konz, B.: Koinzidenz multipler Zylindrome mit Trichoepitheliomen (Brooke-Spiegler-Syndrom. Hautarzt **33**, 34–46 (1982)

96. Kruse, R., Rutten, A., Lamberti, C., Hosseiny-Malayeri, H.R., Wang, Y., Ruelfs, C., Jungck, M., Mathiak, M., Ruzicka, T., Hartschuh, W., Bisceglia, M., Friedl, W., Propping, P.: Muir-Torre phenotype has a frequency of DNA mismatch-repair-gene mutations similar to that in hereditary nonpolyposis colorectal cancer families defined by the Amsterdam criteria. Am. J. Hum. Genet. **63**, 63–70 (1998)

97. Kupres, K.A., Krivda, S.J., Turiansky, G.W.: Numerous asymptomatic facial papules and multiple pulmonary cysts: a case of Birt-Hogg-Dube syndrome. Cutis **72**, 127–131 (2003)

98. Kurzen, H., Esposito, L., Langbein, L., Hartschuh, W.: Cytokeratins as markers of follicular differentiation: an immunohistochemical study of trichoblastoma and basal cell carcinoma. Am. J. Dermatopathol. **23**, 501–509 (2001)

99. Kutzner, H., Requena, L., Rutten, A., Mentzel, T.: Spindle cell predominant trichodiscoma: a fibrofolliculoma/trichodiscoma variant considered formerly to be a neurofollicular hamartoma: a clinicopathological and immunohistochemical analysis of 17 cases. Am. J. Dermatopathol. **28**, 1–8 (2006)

100. Kuwahara, R.T., Rudolph, T.M., Skinner Jr., R.B., Rasberry, R.D.: A large ulcerated tumor on the back. Diagnosis: solitary giant sebaceous carcinoma in a human immunodeficiency virus-positive patient. Arch. Dermatol. **137**, 1367–1372 (2001)

101. Lachiewicz, A.M., Wilkinson, T.M., Groben, P., Ollila, D.W., Thomas, N.E.: Muir-Torre syndrome. Am. J. Clin. Dermatol. **8**, 315–319 (2007)

102. Lao, L.M., Kumakiri, M., Kiyohara, T., Sakata, K., Takeuchi, A.: Papillary endothelial hyperplasia and dilated lymphatic vessels in bullous pilomatricoma. Acta Derm. Venereol. **85**, 160–163 (2005)

103. Lazar, A.J., Calonje, E., Grayson, W., Dei Tos, A.P., Mihm Jr., M.C., Redston, M., McKee, P.H.: Pilomatrix carcinomas contain mutations in CTNNB1, the gene encoding beta-catenin. J. Cutan. Pathol. **32**, 148–157 (2005)

104. GR, L.W.F.: Calcifying epithelioma of Malherbe: report of 15 cases, with comments on its differentiation from calcified epidermal cyst and on its histogenesis. Arch. Dermatol. **59**, 506–518 (1949)

105. Lineaweaver, W.C., Wang, T.N., Leboit, P.L.: Pilomatrix carcinoma. J. Surg. Oncol. **37**, 171–174 (1988)

106. Lopez-Rios, F., Rodriguez-Peralto, J.L., Aguilar, A., Hernandez, L., Gallego, M.: Proliferating trichilemmal cyst with focal invasion: report of a case and a review of the literature. Am. J. Dermatopathol. **22**, 183–187 (2000)

107. Lozzi, G.P., Soyer, H.P., Fruehauf, J., Massone, C., Kerl, H., Peris, K.: Giant pilomatricoma. Am. J. Dermatopathol. **29**, 286–289 (2007)

108. Lynch, H.T., Fusaro, R.M., Roberts, L., Voorhees, G.J., Lynch, J.F.: Muir-Torre syndrome in several members of a family with a variant of the Cancer Family Syndrome. Br. J. Dermatol. **113**, 295–301 (1985)

109. CJ, M.A.: Note sur l'epitheliome calcifie des glandes sebacées. Prog. Med. **8**, 826–828 (1880)

110. Margo, C.E., Mulla, Z.D.: Malignant tumors of the eyelid: a population-based study of non-basal cell and non-squamous cell malignant neoplasms. Arch. Ophthalmol. **116**, 195–198 (1998)

111. Mathis, E.D., Honningford, J.B., Rodriguez, H.E., Wind, K.P., Connolly, M.M., Podbielski, F.J.: Malignant proliferating trichilemmal tumor. Am. J. Clin. Oncol. **24**, 351–353 (2001)

112. Matt, D., Xin, H., Vortmeyer, A.O., Zhuang, Z., Burg, G., Boni, R.: Sporadic trichoepithelioma demonstrates deletions at 9q22.3. Arch. Dermatol. **136**, 657–660 (2000)

113. McBride, S.R., Leonard, N., Reynolds, N.J.: Loss of p21(WAF1) compartmentalisation in sebaceous carcinoma compared with sebaceous hyperplasia and sebaceous adenoma. J. Clin. Pathol. **55**, 763–766 (2002)

114. McGavran, M.H.: Ultrastructure of pilomatrixoma (calcifying epithelioma). Cancer **18**, 1445–1456 (1965)

115. McNiff, J.M., Eisen, R.N., Glusac, E.J.: Immunohistochemical comparison of cutaneous lymphadenoma, trichoblastoma, and basal cell carcinoma: support for classification of lymphadenoma as a variant of trichoblastoma. J. Cutan. Pathol. **26**, 119–124 (1999)

116. Mehregan, A.H.: Infundibular tumors of the skin. J. Cutan. Pathol. **11**, 387–395 (1984)

117. Mehregan, A.H., Lee, K.C.: Malignant proliferating trichilemmal tumors–report of three cases. J. Dermatol. Surg. Oncol. **13**, 1339–1342 (1987)

118. Migirov, L., Fridman, E., Talmi, Y.P.: Pilomatrixoma of the retroauricular area and arm. J. Pediatr. Surg. **37**, E20 (2002)

119. Mir, R., Cortes, E., Papantoniou, P.A., Heller, K., Muehlhausen, V., Kahn, L.B.: Metastatic trichomatricial carcinoma. Arch. Pathol. Lab. Med. **110**, 660–663 (1986)

120. Misago, N., Mihara, I., Ansai, S., Narisawa, Y.: Sebaceoma and related neoplasms with sebaceous differentiation: a clinicopathologic study of 30 cases. Am. J. Dermatopathol. **24**, 294–304 (2002)

121. Misago, N., Narisawa, Y.: Rippled-pattern sebaceoma. Am. J. Dermatopathol. **23**, 437–443 (2001)

122. Miyakawa, S., Araki, Y., Sugawara, M.: Generalized trichoepitheliomas with alopecia and myasthenia gravis. J. Am. Acad. Dermatol. **19**, 361–362 (1988)

123. Miyake, H., Hara, H., Shimojima, H., Suzuki, H.: Follicular hybrid cyst (trichilemmal cyst and pilomatricoma) arising within a nevus sebaceus. Am. J. Dermatopathol. **26**, 390–393 (2004)

124. Mones, J.M., Ackeman, A.B.: Proliferating trichilemmal cyst is a squamous-cell carcinoma. Dermatopathol. Pract Concept. **4**, 295–310 (2003)

125. Moreno, C., Jacyk, W.K., Judd, M.J., Requena, L.: Highly aggressive extraocular sebaceous carcinoma. Am. J. Dermatopathol. **23**, 450–455 (2001)

126. Nguyen, G.K., Mielke, B.W.: Extraocular sebaceous carcinoma with intraepidermal (pagetoid) spread. Am. J. Dermatopathol. **9**, 364–365 (1987)

127. Niedermeyer, H.P., Peris, K., Hofler, H.: Pilomatrix carcinoma with multiple visceral metastases. Report of a case. Cancer **77**, 1311–1314 (1996)

128. Nielsen, T.A., Maia-Cohen, S., Hessel, A.B., Xie, D.L., Pellegrini, A.E.: Sebaceous neoplasm with reticulated and cribriform features: a rare variant of sebaceoma. J. Cutan. Pathol. **25**, 233–235 (1998)

129. Nishie, W., Kimura, T.: Follicular germinative cells in pilomatricoma. Am. J. Dermatopathol. **28**, 510–513 (2006)

130. Noto, G.: 'Benign' proliferating trichilemmal tumour: does it really exist? Histopathology **35**, 386–387 (1999)

131. Noto, G.: Re: Malignant transformation of a giant proliferating trichilemmal tumor of the scalp. Ann. Plast. Surg. **43**, 574–575 (1999)

132. Noto, G., Pravata, G., Arico, M.: Malignant proliferating trichilemmal tumor. Am. J. Dermatopathol. **19**, 202–204 (1997)

133. Noto, G., Pravata, G., Arico, M.: Proliferating tricholemmal cyst should always be considered as a low-grade carcinoma. Dermatology **194**, 374–375 (1997)

134. Noto, G., Pravata, G., Arico, M.: "Shadow" cells in proliferating trichilemmal tumors. Am. J. Dermatopathol. **12**, 319–320 (1990)

135. O'Donovan, D.G., Freemont, A.J., Adams, J.E., Markham, D.E.: Malignant pilomatrixoma with bone metastasis. Histopathology **23**, 385–386 (1993)

136. Ogata, T., Tanaka, S., Goto, T., Iijima, T., Kawano, H., Sasaki, M., Ishida, T., Nakamura, K.: Giant trichoblastoma mimicking malignancy. Arch. Orthop. Trauma. Surg. **119**, 225–227 (1999)

137. Ohara, N., Taguchi, K., Yamamoto, M., Nagano, T., Akagi, T.: Sebaceous carcinoma of the submandibular gland with high-grade malignancy: report of a case. Pathol. Int. **48**, 287–291 (1998)

138. Okuda, C., Ito, M., Fujiwara, H., Takenouchi, T.: Sebaceous epithelioma with sweat gland differentiation. Am. J. Dermatopathol. **17**, 523–528 (1995)

139. Oswiecimska, J.M., Ziora, K.T., Ziora, K.N., Pindycka-Piaszczynska, M., Zajecki, W., Pikiewicz-Koch, A., Stojewska, M.: Growth hormone therapy in boy with panhypopituitarism may induce pilomatricoma recurrence: case report. Neuro Endocrinol. Lett. **29**, 51–54 (2008)

140. Oursin, C., Kruger, H.J., Sigmund, G., Hellerich, U.: MR imaging of a giant solitary trichoepithelioma of the skin. Radiologe **31**, 574–576 (1991)

141. Padberg, G.W., Schot, J.D., Vielvoye, G.J., Bots, G.T., de Beer, F.C.: Lhermitte-Duclos disease and Cowden disease: a single phakomatosis. Ann. Neurol. **29**, 517–523 (1991)

142. Park, B.S., Yang, S.G., Cho, K.H.: Malignant proliferating trichilemmal tumor showing distant metastases. Am. J. Dermatopathol. **19**, 536–539 (1997)

143. Perez Tato, B., Saez, A.C., Fernandez, P.R.: Superficial angiomyxoma with trichofolliculoma. Ann. Diagn. Pathol. **12**, 375–377 (2008)

144. Peris, K., Onorati, M.T., Keller, G., Magrini, F., Donati, P., Muscardin, L., Hofler, H., Chimenti, S.: Widespread microsatellite instability in sebaceous tumours of patients with the Muir-Torre syndrome. Br. J. Dermatol. **137**, 356–360 (1997)

145. Pickford, M.A., Hogg, F.J., Fallowfield, M.E., Webster, M.H.: Sebaceous carcinoma of the periorbital and extraorbital regions. Br. J. Plast. Surg. **48**, 93–96 (1995)

146. Pilarski, R.: Cowden syndrome: a critical review of the clinical literature. J. Genet. Couns. **18**, 13–27 (2008)

147. Pinkus, H., Coskey, R., Burgess, G.H.: Trichodiscoma. A benign tumor related to haarscheibe (hair disk). J. Invest. Dermatol. **63**, 212–218 (1974)

148. Plewig, G.: Sebaceous trichofolliculoma. J. Cutan. Pathol. **7**, 394–403 (1980)

149. Poiares Baptista, A., Garcia, E.S.L., Born, M.C.: Proliferating trichilemmal cyst. J. Cutan. Pathol. **10**, 178–187 (1983)

150. Ponti, G., Ponz de Leon, M.: Muir-Torre syndrome. Lancet Oncol. **6**, 980–987 (2005)

151. Pricolo, V.E., Rodil, J.V., Vezeridis, M.P.: Extraorbital sebaceous carcinoma. Arch. Surg. **120**, 853–855 (1985)

152. Pujol, R.M., Casanova, J.M., Egido, R., Pujol, J., de Moragas, J.M.: Multiple familial pilomatricomas: a cutaneous marker for Gardner syndrome? Pediatr. Dermatol. **12**, 331–335 (1995)

153. Rabkin, M.S., Wittwer, C.T., Soong, V.Y.: Flow cytometric DNA content analysis of a case of pilomatrix carcinoma showing multiple recurrences and invasion of the cranial vault. J. Am. Acad. Dermatol. **23**, 104–108 (1990)

154. Rahbari, H., Mehregan, A.H.: Development of proliferating trichilemmal cyst in organoid nevus. Presentation of two cases. J. Am. Acad. Dermatol. **14**, 123–126 (1986)

155. Rao, N.A., Hidayat, A.A., McLean, I.W., Zimmerman, L.E.: Sebaceous carcinomas of the ocular adnexa: a clinicopathologic study of 104 cases, with five-year follow-up data. Hum. Pathol. **13**, 113–122 (1982)

156. Reed, R.J.: Tricholemmoma. A cutaneous hamartoma. Am. J. Dermatopathol. **2**, 227–228 (1980)

157. Regauer, S., Beham-Schmid, C., Okcu, M., Hartner, E., Mannweiler, S.: Trichoblastic carcinoma ("malignant trichoblastoma") with lymphatic and hematogenous metastases. Mod. Pathol. **13**, 673–678 (2000)

158. Requena, L., Kuztner, H., Farina, M.C.: Pigmented and nested sebomatricoma or seborrheic keratosis with sebaceous differentiation? Am. J. Dermatopathol. **20**, 383–388 (1998)

159. Requena, L., Sanchez Yus, E.: Cutaneous lymphadenoma with ductal differentiation. J. Cutan. Pathol. **19**, 429–433 (1992)

160. Retamar, R.A., Stengel, F., Saadi, M.E., Kien, M.C., Della Giovana, P., Cabrera, H., Chouela, E.N.: Brooke-Spiegler syndrome – report of four families: treatment with CO2 laser. Int. J. Dermatol. **46**, 583–586 (2007)

161. Richfield, D.F.: Tricholemmoma. True and false types. Am. J. Dermatopathol. **2**, 233–234 (1980)

162. Rohwedder, A., Keminer, O., Hendricks, C., Schaller, J.: Detection of HPV DNA in trichilemmomas by polymerase chain reaction. J. Med. Virol. **51**, 119–125 (1997)

163. Rulon, D.B., Helwig, E.B.: Cutaneous sebaceous neoplasms. Cancer **33**, 82–102 (1974)

164. Rutten, A., Burgdorf, W., Hugel, H., Kutzner, H., Hosseiny-Malayeri, H.R., Friedl, W., Propping, P., Kruse, R.: Cystic sebaceous tumors as marker lesions for the Muir-Torre syndrome: a histopathologic and molecular genetic study. Am. J. Dermatopathol. **21**, 405–413 (1999)

165. Sable, D., Snow, S.N.: Pilomatrix carcinoma of the back treated by mohs micrographic surgery. Dermatol. Surg. **30**, 1174–1176 (2004)

166. Sakai, A., Maruyama, Y., Hayashi, A.: Proliferating pilomatricoma: a subset of pilomatricoma. J. Plast. Reconstr. Aesthet. Surg. **61**, 811–814 (2008)

167. Sakamoto, F., Ito, M., Nakamura, A., Sato, Y.: Proliferating trichilemmal cyst with apocrine-acrosyringeal and sebaceous differentiation. J. Cutan. Pathol. **18**, 137–141 (1991)

168. Salem, O.S., Steck, W.D.: Cowden's disease (multiple hamartoma and neoplasia syndrome). A case report and review of the English literature. J. Am. Acad. Dermatol. **8**, 686–696 (1983)

169. Santa Cruz, D.J., Barr, R.J., Headington, J.T.: Cutaneous lymphadenoma. Am. J. Surg. Pathol. **15**, 101–110 (1991)

170. Sassmannshausen, J., Chaffins, M.: Pilomatrix carcinoma: a report of a case arising from a previously excised pilomatrixoma and a review of the literature. J. Am. Acad. Dermatol. **44**, 358–361 (2001)

171. Satyaprakash, A.K., Sheehan, D.J., Sangueza, O.P.: Proliferating trichilemmal tumors: a review of the literature. Dermatol. Surg. **33**, 1102–1108 (2007)

172. Sau, P., Graham, J.H., Helwig, E.B.: Proliferating epithelial cysts. Clinicopathological analysis of 96 cases. J. Cutan. Pathol. **22**, 394–406 (1995)

173. Sau, P., Lupton, G.P., Graham, J.H.: Trichogerminoma. Report of 14 cases. J. Cutan. Pathol. **19**, 357–365 (1992)

174. Scheinfeld, N.: Pilomatrical carcinoma: a case in a patient with HIV and hepatitis C. Dermatol. Online J. **14**, 4 (2008)

175. Schirren, C.G., Jansen, T., Lindner, A., Kind, P., Plewig, G.: Diffuse sebaceous gland hyperplasia. A case report and an immunohistochemical study with cytokeratins. Am. J. Dermatopathol. **18**, 296–301 (1996)

176. Schirren, C.G., Rutten, A., Kaudewitz, P., Diaz, C., McClain, S., Burgdorf, W.H.: Trichoblastoma and basal cell carcinoma are neoplasms with follicular differentiation sharing the same profile of

cytokeratin intermediate filaments. Am. J. Dermatopathol. **19**, 341–350 (1997)

177. Schirren, C.G., Worle, B., Kind, P., Plewig, G.: A nevoid plaque with histological changes of trichoepithelioma and cylindroma in Brooke-Spiegler syndrome. An immunohistochemical study with cytokeratins. J. Cutan. Pathol. **22**, 563–569 (1995)

178. Schulz, T., Ebschner, U., Hartschuh, W.: Localized Birt-Hogg-Dube syndrome with prominent perivascular fibromas. Am. J. Dermatopathol. **23**, 149–153 (2001)

179. Schulz, T., Hartschuh, W.: Folliculo-sebaceous cystic hamartoma is a trichofolliculoma at its very late stage. J. Cutan. Pathol. **25**, 354–364 (1998)

180. Schulz, T., Hartschuh, W.: The trichofolliculoma undergoes changes corresponding to the regressing normal hair follicle in its cycle. J. Cutan. Pathol. **25**, 341–353 (1998)

181. Schwartz, R.A., Torre, D.P.: The Muir-Torre syndrome: a 25-year retrospect. J. Am. Acad. Dermatol. **33**, 90–104 (1995)

182. Scully, K., Bargman, H., Assaad, D.: Solitary fibrofolliculoma. J. Am. Acad. Dermatol. **11**, 361–363 (1984)

183. Shapiro, S.D., Lambert, W.C., Schwartz, R.A.: Cowden's disease. A marker for malignancy. Int. J. Dermatol. **27**, 232–237 (1988)

184. Shet, T., Modi, C.: Nucleolar organizer regions (NORs) in simple and proliferating trichilemmal cysts (pilar cysts and pilar tumors). Indian J. Pathol. Microbiol. **47**, 469–473 (2004)

185. Simon, R.S., de Eusebio, E., Alvarez-Vieitez, A., Sanchez Yus, E.: Folliculo-sebaceous cystic hamartoma is but the sebaceous end of tricho-sebo-folliculoma spectrum. J. Cutan. Pathol. **26**, 109 (1999)

186. Singh, R.S., Grayson, W., Redston, M., Diwan, A.H., Warneke, C.L., McKee, P.H., Lev, D., Lyle, S., Calonje, E., Lazar, A.J.: Site and tumor type predicts DNA mismatch repair status in cutaneous sebaceous neoplasia. Am. J. Surg. Pathol. **32**, 936–942 (2008)

187. Southey, M.C., Young, M.A., Whitty, J., Mifsud, S., Keilar, M., Mead, L., Trute, L., Aittomaki, K., McLachlan, S.A., Debinski, H., Venter, D.J., Armes, J.E.: Molecular pathologic analysis enhances the diagnosis and management of Muir-Torre syndrome and gives insight into its underlying molecular pathogenesis. Am. J. Surg. Pathol. **25**, 936–941 (2001)

188. Stambolic, V., Suzuki, A., de la Pompa, J.L., Brothers, G.M., Mirtsos, C., Sasaki, T., Ruland, J., Penninger, J.M., Siderovski, D.P., Mak, T.W.: Negative regulation of PKB/Akt-dependent cell survival by the tumor suppressor PTEN. Cell **95**, 29–39 (1998)

189. Starink, T.M.: Cowden's disease: analysis of fourteen new cases. J. Am. Acad. Dermatol. **11**, 1127–1141 (1984)

190. Starink, T.M., Brownstein, M.H.: Fibrofolliculoma: solitary and multiple types. J. Am. Acad. Dermatol. **17**, 493–496 (1987)

191. Starink, T.M., Hausman, R.: The cutaneous pathology of extrafacial lesions in Cowden's disease. J. Cutan. Pathol. **11**, 338–344 (1984)

192. Starink, T.M., Hausman, R.: The cutaneous pathology of facial lesions in Cowden's disease. J. Cutan. Pathol. **11**, 331–337 (1984)

193. Starink, T.M., Lane, E.B., Meijer, C.J.: Generalized trichoepitheliomas with alopecia and myasthenia gravis: clinicopathologic and immunohistochemical study and comparison with classic and desmoplastic trichoepithelioma. J. Am. Acad. Dermatol. **15**, 1104–1112 (1986)

194. Starink, T.M., Meijer, C.J., Brownstein, M.H.: The cutaneous pathology of Cowden's disease: new findings. J. Cutan. Pathol. **12**, 83–93 (1985)

195. Starink, T.M., van der Veen, J.P., Arwert, F., de Waal, L.P., de Lange, G.G., Gille, J.J., Eriksson, A.W.: The Cowden syndrome: a clinical and genetic study in 21 patients. Clin. Genet. **29**, 222–233 (1986)

196. Stavrianeas, N.G., Katoulis, A.C., Stratigeas, N.P., Karagianni, I.N., Patertou-Stavrianea, M., Varelzidis, A.G.: Development of multiple tumors in a sebaceous nevus of Jadassohn. Dermatology **195**, 155–158 (1997)

197. Steffen, C.: Mantleoma. A benign neoplasm with mantle differentiation. Am. J. Dermatopathol. **15**, 306–310 (1993)

198. Steffen, C., Ackerman, A.B.: Neoplasms with Sebaceous Differentiation. Lea & Febiger, Philadelphia (1994)

199. Takata, M., Rehman, I., Rees, J.L.: A trichilemmal carcinoma arising from a proliferating trichilemmal cyst: the loss of the wild-type p53 is a critical event in malignant transformation. Hum. Pathol. **29**, 193–195 (1998)

200. Tay, Y.K.: Exophytic pilomatricoma. Pediatr. Dermatol. **20**, 373 (2003)

201. Tellechea, O., Reis, J.P., Baptista, A.P.: Desmoplastic trichilemmoma. Am. J. Dermatopathol. **14**, 107–4 (1992)

202. Toro, J.R., Glenn, G., Duray, P., Darling, T., Weirich, G., Zbar, B., Linehan, M., Turner, M.L.: Birt-Hogg-Dube syndrome: a novel marker of kidney neoplasia. Arch. Dermatol. **135**, 1195–1202 (1999)

203. Tronnier, M.: Clear cell trichoblastoma in association with a nevus sebaceus. Am. J. Dermatopathol. **23**, 143–145 (2001)

204. Troy, J.L., Ackerman, A.B.: Sebaceoma. A distinctive benign neoplasm of adnexal epithelium differentiating toward sebaceous cells. Am. J. Dermatopathol. **6**, 7–13 (1984)

205. Uede, K., Yamamoto, Y., Furukawa, F.: Brooke-Spiegler syndrome associated with cylindroma, trichoepithelioma, spiradenoma, and syringoma. J. Dermatol. **31**, 32–38 (2004)

206. Uppal, S., Mistry, D., Coatesworth, A.P.: Cowden disease: a review. Int. J. Clin. Pract. **61**, 645–652 (2007)

207. Usmani, A.S., Rofagha, R., Hessel, A.B.: Trichoblastic neoplasm with apocrine differentiation. Am. J. Dermatopathol. **24**, 358–360 (2002)

208. van der Walt, J.D., Rohlova, B.: Carcinomatous transformation in a pilomatrixoma. Am. J. Dermatopathol. **6**, 63–69 (1984)

209. Wechsler, J., Fromont, G., Andre, J.M., Zafrani, E.S.: Cutaneous lymphadenoma with focal mucinosis. J. Cutan. Pathol. **19**, 142–144 (1992)

210. Weedon, D.: Skin Pathology, 2nd edn. Churchill Livingstone, Edinburgh (2002)

211. Weiss, J., Heine, M., Grimmel, M., Jung, E.G.: Malignant proliferating trichilemmal cyst. J. Am. Acad. Dermatol. **32**, 870–873 (1995)

212. Welsch, M.J., Krunic, A., Medenica, M.M.: Birt-Hogg-Dube Syndrome. Int. J. Dermatol. **44**, 668–673 (2005)

213. Weyers, W., Nilles, M., Eckert, F., Schill, W.B.: Spiradenomas in Brooke-Spiegler syndrome. Am. J. Dermatopathol. **15**, 156–161 (1993)

214. Wick, M.R., Goellner, J.R., Wolfe 3rd, J.T., Su, W.P.: Adnexal carcinomas of the skin. II. Extraocular sebaceous carcinomas. Cancer **56**, 1163–1172 (1985)

215. Wick, M.R., Swanson, P.E.: Cutaneous Adnexal Tumors: A guide to Pathologic Diagnosis. ASCP Press, Chicago (1991)

216. Wolfe III, J.T., Yeatts, R.P., Wick, M.R., Campbell, R.J., Waller, R.R.: Sebaceous carcinoma of the eyelid. Errors in clinical and pathologic diagnosis. Am. J. Surg. Pathol. **8**, 597–606 (1984)

217. Wolfe, J.T., Wick, M.R., Campbell, R.J.: Sebaceous carcinoma of the oculo-cutaneous adnexa and extraocular skin. In: Wick, M.R. (ed.) Pathology of unusual malignant cutaneous tumours, pp. 77–106. Marcel Dekker, New York (1985)

218. Wong, W.K., Somburanasin, R., Wood, M.G.: Eruptive, multicentric pilomatricoma (calcifying epithelioma). Roentgenographic detection of fine tumor calcification. Arch. Dermatol. **106**, 76–78 (1972)

219. Yamamoto, O., Asahi, M.: Cytokeratin expression in trichoblastic fibroma (small nodular type trichoblastoma), trichoepithelioma and basal cell carcinoma. Br. J. Dermatol. **140**, 8–16 (1999)

220. Ye, J., Nappi, O., Swanson, P.E., Patterson, J.W., Wick, M.R.: Proliferating pilar tumors: a clinicopathologic study of 76 cases with a proposal for definition of benign and malignant variants. Am. J. Clin. Pathol. **122**, 566–574 (2004)

221. Yen, M.T., Tse, D.T.: Sebaceous cell carcinoma of the eyelid and the human immunodeficiency virus. Ophthal. Plast. Reconstr. Surg. **16**, 206–210 (2000)
222. Young, A.L., Kellermayer, R., Szigeti, R., Teszas, A., Azmi, S., Celebi, J.T.: CYLD mutations underlie Brooke-Spiegler, familial cylindromatosis, and multiple familial trichoepithelioma syndromes. Clin. Genet. **70**, 246–249 (2006)
223. Yu, D.K., Joo, Y.H., Cho, K.H.: Trichoblastoma with apocrine and sebaceous differentiation. Am. J. Dermatopathol. **27**, 6–8 (2005)
224. Zulaica, A., Peteiro, C., Quintas, C., Pereiro Jr., M., Toribio, J.: Perforating pilomatricoma. J. Cutan. Pathol. **15**, 409–411 (1988)
225. Zurcher, M., Hintschich, C.R., Garner, A., Bunce, C., Collin, J.R.: Sebaceous carcinoma of the eyelid: a clinicopathological study. Br. J. Ophthalmol. **82**, 1049–1055 (1998)

Melanocytic Tumors

Jivko A. Kamarashev, Leo Schärer, Marie C. Zipser,
Lauren L. Lockwood, Reinhard Dummer, and Sven Krengel

3.3.1 Disease Entities: Malignant Melanoma

**Jivko A. Kamarashev, Leo Schärer, Marie C. Zipser,
Lauren L. Lockwood, and Reinhard Dummer**

3.3.1.1 Malignant Melanoma: Introduction

3.3.1.1.1 Definition

Melanoma is a tumor derived from melanocytes. As such, it can originate from the retina, meninges or even the bronchi, but in the overwhelming majority of cases the primary tumor arises in the skin.

3.3.1.1.2 Clinical Features

The undoubtedly increasing incidence of melanoma coupled with its high malignant potential has rendered it a major issue in contemporary medical science. Every available approach has been mobilized to the end of solving the enigma of melanoma. Although front-line research has already produced some important insights and carries a lot of promise, the major success in fighting melanoma has come in increased awareness, early diagnosis, and prevention.

J.A. Kamarashev (✉), L.L. Lockwood, and R. Dummer
Department of Dermatology, University Hospital of Zurich,
Zurich, Switzerland
e-mail: jivko.kamarachev@usz.ch; reinhard.dummer@usz.ch

L. Schärer
Dermatopathologische Gemeinschaftspraxis,
Friedrichshafen, Germany

M.C. Zipser
University Hospital of Zürich, Department of Dermatology F2,
Gloriastrasse 31, 8091 Zürich, Switzerland
e-mail: marie.zipser@usz.ch

S. Krengel
Dermatologische Gemeinschaftspraxis, Moislinger Allee 95,
23558 Lübeck
e-mail: sven.krengel@uk-sh.de

Major Subtypes

Melanoma has an enormous molecular complexity. Clinical diagnosis might cover a variety of molecularly and mechanistically distinct entities. Adequate means of properly defining disease subtypes, allowing for the development of individually tailored therapeutic strategies, are still evolving [16]. Four main clinical variants have been recognized, which show certain epidemiological and histological differences: superficial spreading melanoma (SSM), nodular malignant melanoma (NMM), lentigo maligna melanoma (LMM), and acrolentiginous melanoma (ALM).

Melanoma may also be classified as to the nature of its vertical growth phase, e.g., as expansile nodules composed of epithelioid cells, spindle cells, or smaller nevus-like cells supervening on one of the previously mentioned radial growth components or developing de novo. Less common variants include desmoplastic and desmoplastic neurotropic melanomas (often arising within lentigo maligna).

Sites of Involvement

In both sexes, the most commonly affected sites are the face [25], shoulder, and upper arm [11]. Melanoma is also more common on the back for men and leg for women [11, 22]. In older patients, frequently affected body sites are those experiencing continuous sun exposures [23].

Age Distribution

Melanoma predominantly affects young and middle-aged people. The median age of diagnosis is around the sixth decade of life. However, the incidence of melanoma in children is increasing at an alarming pace [57]. Any changing pigmented lesion regardless of the age of the patient should, therefore, arouse suspicion.

R. Dummer et al. (eds.), *Skin Cancer – A World-Wide Perspective*,
DOI: 10.1007/978-3-642-05072-5_3.3, © Springer-Verlag Berlin Heidelberg 2011

3.3.1.1.3 Diagnosis

The recognition of a number of risk factors has helped to identify individuals at high risk and put them under regular surveillance. The diagnosis of full blown melanoma poses no problems. Early diagnosis, on the other hand, is often very difficult but is essential for a favorable outcome. The clinical and histological criteria for the diagnosis of early melanoma have significantly improved. The introduction of specific diagnostic procedures, e.g., dermoscopy, has further contributed significantly to the timely recognition of early lesions.

ABCD Rule

Early diagnosis cannot be overemphasized, and therefore, recognition of the clinical characteristics of early malignant melanoma is of extreme importance. The ABCD acronym for melanoma screening was established in 1985 [26] and revised in 2005 with a change of D from diameter to dynamics [19, 20], because today many melanomas get detected before they reach a diameter of 5 mm. ABCD is an easily remembered mnemonic for clinical recognition. A is encoding for asymmetry, B for border irregularity, C for multiple colors, and D for dynamics (change over time) (Table 3.3.1).

A minority of melanomas develop in precursor pigmentary lesions, of which atypical, junctional, and compound naevi are most important.

However, there are pitfalls concerning sensitivity of ABCD criteria. Very small pigmented lesions represent a diagnostic challenge, only D might alert the patient and the physician (Fig. 3.3.1).

Nodular melanoma frequently lack changes in the first three criteria, only showing noticeable changes in dynamics. The ABCDs, therefore, have the greatest accuracy when used in combination [1]. On the other hand, benign melanocytic naevi may have atypical features when assessed with ABCD rule, thus decreasing its specificity.

Dermoscopy

See Chap. 26.

Histopathology

A variety of architectural patterns, cytologic features, and stromal changes may be observed in melanoma [7]. The

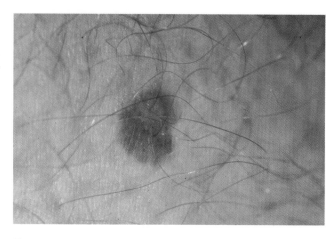

Fig. 3.3.1 Small melanoma. Small irregular melanocytic lesions on the upper leg of a 28-year-old male. Dimensions: 0.6×0.4 mm. Histology revealed a superficial spreading melanoma (SSM), tumor thickness 0.25 mm, level III

histologic features of melanoma may mimic those of several carcinomas, sarcomas, lymphomas, and germ cell tumors [7] (Fig. 3.3.2, Table 3.3.2).

Immunohistochemistry

Melanoma expresses a variety of antigens, which can be detected with immunohistochemistry. Sometimes melanoma presents histologically as an undifferentiated tumor, of which distinction from epithelial or mesenchymal tumors using morphological criteria is impossible. In these cases, stainings, which are nowadays quite routinely used, S100 and melanocytic differentiation antigens, e.g., Melan A and HMB45, are especially useful. The S100 antigen is mainly expressed in nerve sheath cells, myoepithelial cells, adipocytes, chondrocytes, Langerhans cells, and melanocytes. The expression of S100 is also preserved in tumors originating from these normal cells. Although S100 immunoreactivity is by no means specific for melanocytic lesions, it is highly sensitive. Very few anecdotal cases of S100 negative melanomas have been reported to date. Furthermore, S100 reactivity has been reported in the serum of patients with metastatic melanoma but not of patients with early melanoma. It has been shown that measurements of serum S100 can be used as a clinical marker for progression of the disease as well as a marker for response to treatment [35].

More specific immunohistochemical markers are used to distinguish between melanoma from other S100 positive malignancies. HMB45 is a monoclonal antibody against the cytoplasmic premelanosomal glycoprotein group 100 protein (gp100) [14]. It was first raised in mice by Gown et al. using hybridoma technology [29]. They reported it to produce a highly specific but less sensitive cytoplasmic staining in melanoma and junctional naevus cells, but not in dermal melanocytes. There are however certain exceptions, as occasional cells in the dermal component of dysplastic naevi and

Table 3.3.1 ABCD clinical criteria for melanoma

A – asymmetry in shape and color distribution
B – border irregularity with coastlike outlines
C – color variegation
D – dynamics (with respect to size, shape, shades of color, surface features, or symptoms)

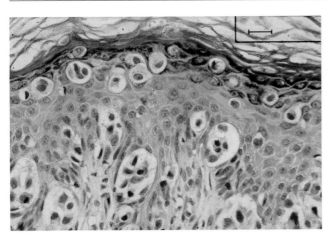

Fig. 3.3.2 Histological features of melanoma: pagetoid spread. Close-up of pagetoid cells transmigrating to the epidermis. Some large cells are solitary; others are still arranged in nests (magnification 400×)

Table 3.3.2 Histological criteria for establishing the diagnosis of melanoma (after Ackerman [2])

Architectural pattern
Asymmetric
Poorly circumscribed
No maturation of melanocytes with progressive descent into the dermis
Nests of melanocytes within the epidermis are not equidistant from one another
Nests of melanocytes vary markedly in size and shape
Some nests of melanocytes become confluent
Melanocytes in some "nests" are not cohesive
A dispersion of melanocytes above the dermo-epidermal junction
Melanocytes arranged as solitary units more commonly than as nests in some high-power fields
Melanocytes arranged as solitary units are not equidistant from one another
Melanocytes extend deep into the epithelial structures of the adnexa, in the same pattern as they are arrayed within the epidermis
Melanin is not distributed symmetrically within the epidermis, adnexa, and dermis
Cytologic features
Melanocytes may be atypical
Melanocytes in mitosis
Melanocytes may be necrotic

some Spitz naevi have been reported to stain positive. On the other hand, desmoplastic and metastatic melanoma may sometimes be nonreactive with the antibody. Because melanocytes in fetal skin stain positive with HMB45, it has been surmised that the antibody reacts with a fetal cytoplasmic protein that is also expressed later in life upon activation of the melanocytes [55].

A103 is a monoclonal IgG antibody against Melan-A, and M2-7C10 detects melanoma antigen recognized by T-cells-1 (MART-1). A correlation of almost 100% has been established between the two clones using melanoma staining, however A103 additionally stains tumors derived from

steroid hormone producing cells such as adrenocortical carcinomas [12, 24].

Tyrosinase hydroxylates tyrosine in the first step of melanin-synthesis. T311, a monoclonal antibody against tyrosinase showed a sensitivity of 94% for melanoma, with very high specificity for melanocytic cells in paraffin embedded sections [36].

Interestingly it has been observed, that the monoclonal antibody 57B, which reacts specifically with MAGE 4A, stains formalin-fixed, paraffin-embedded melanoma material, but stains neither normal melanocytes nor naevus cells. Particular naevus subtypes, e.g., balloon cell as well as Reed and Spitz naevus, were also negative. Although, the sensitivity of the staining was 44, 100% specificity seemed to be very promising for the differentiation of malignant cells [37]. However, activated melanocytes, e.g., in clonal populations, may demonstrate immunoreactivity.

Additionally, Ki-67, a nuclear antigen present during cell cycle proliferation, is a commonly used adjunct in distinguishing benign naevi from melanoma.

3.3.1.1.4 Staging

The American Joint Committee (AJCC) Staging system for cutaneous melanoma [5], is based on the tumor thickness, mitotic rate (histologically defined as mitoses/mm²) and ulceration (T), the number of lymph nodes involved and their clinically occult or apparent nature (N), the site of distant metastases, and serum lactate dehydrogenase level (M) (Table 3.3.3).

T Classification

The T-category is mainly based on Breslow tumor thickness [10], with thresholds of 1.0, 2.0, and 4.0 mm, mitotic rate (histologically defined as mitoses/mm²) and ulceration. The measurement of tumor thickness is made from the top of the granular layer to the deepest point of invasion [46]. Classification, ranging from T1 to T4, is based on the extent of melanoma thickness (Table 3.3.3). Tx includes nonassessable tumors, shave biopsies, and regressed melanomas.

Melanoma ulceration, "the absence of an intact epidermis overlying a major portion of the primary tumor," in histopathological evaluation is appended to the T numerical subset as "b." No microscopic signs of ulceration is classified as "a."

In the revised 2009 AJCC staging system, primary tumor mitotic rate replaces Clark level of invasion for defining T1b. T1a melanoma are restricted to those whose tumor thickness is ≤1.0 mm and that have no ulceration, and less than one mitosis per square millimeter. T1b melanomas are defined as those whose tumor thickness is ≤1.0 mm in combination with at least one mitosis per square millimeter or tumor ulceration [5].

Table 3.3.3 The 2009 staging system for cutaneous melanoma according to the AJCC [5]

Classification	Thickness (mm)	Ulceration status/mitoses
T		
Tis	NA	NA
T1	≤1.00	Without ulceration and mitosis <1/mm^2
		With ulceration or mitoses ≥1/mm^2
T2	1.01–2.00	Without ulceration
		With ulceration
T3	2.01–4.00	Without ulceration
		With ulceration
T4	>4.00	Without ulceration
		With ulceration
N	*Number of metastatic nodes*	*Nodal metastatic burden*
No	0	NA
N1	1	Micrometastasis[a]
		Macrometastasis[b]
N2	2–3	Micrometastasis[a]
		Macrometastasis[b]
		In-transit metastases/satellites without metastatic nodes
N3	4+ metastatic nodes, or matted nodes, or in-transit metastases/satellites with metastatic nodes	
M	*Site*	*Serum LDH*
Mo	No distant metastases	NA
M1a	Distant skin, subcutaneous, or nodal metastases	Normal
M1b	Lung metastases	Normal
M1c	All other visceral metastases	Normal
	Any distant metastasis	elevated

NA not applicable; *LDH* lactate dehydrogenase

[a]Micrometastases are diagnosed after sentinel lymph node biopsy

[b]Macrometastases are defined as clinically detectable nodal metastases which are confirmed pathologically

N Classification

The number of infiltrated regional lymph nodes as well as their tumor burden (micrometastasis vs. macrometastases) and the presence or absence of satellite and in-transit metastases, delineates the N category. Lymph node involvement is defined as isolated tumor cells or tumor deposits meeting the criteria of histologic or immunohistochemical detection. Immunohistochemistry must include at least one melanoma-associated maker (e.g., HMB-45, Melan-A, MART-1) and malignant morphologic features detected in the immunohistochemistry stained tissue. If one node is involved, the classification is N1. N2 designates involvement of two or three and N3 of four or more lymph nodes. Micrometastases are diagnosed histopathologically after sentinel node biopsy or elective lymphadenectomy. They are classified as "b" and appended to the N numerical subset. A clinically and/or radiologically assessed and pathologically confirmed regional lymph node macrometastases designates "a" and is appended to the N numerical subset. When a micrometastasis exhibits gross extracapsular extension, it is also considered a macrometastasis.

Satellites are located up to 5 cm from the primary tumor. When a regional metastasis is over 5 cm away from the primary tumor, but remains in the same lymph node drainage area, it is referred to as an in-transit metastasis. In the absence of regional lymph node metastases, satellites and in-transit metastases are both classified as N2c, and if present with any number of micro- or macrometastases they are classified as N3.

Every fifth patient with intermediate-thickness (1.2–3.5 mm), the primary melanoma develops infiltration of the regional nodes [48]. Clinical diagnosis and imaging techniques usually fail to detect small tumor foci [48]. Complete lymph-node dissection exposes patients to morbidity, even in patients who would not develop regional lymph node infiltration [48]. Sentinel-node biopsy after wide excision of the primary tumor allows for avoidance of unnecessary complete lymph-node dissections [48]. The first multicenter selective lymphadenectomy trial revealed fewer local, regional, and distant recurrences in the sentinel-node biopsy group when compared to patients that were simply observed after wide excision [49]. Nevertheless, sentinel-node biopsy was not able to improve overall survival [49]. Furthermore, sentinel-node biopsy allows for better prognostic assessment than primary tumor thickness [49]. Patients with tumor-negative sentinel-nodes require no further nodal surgery and show a prolonged survival [49]. This also plays an important role in recommended follow-up visits [49].

M Classification

Two important prognostic factors gave rise to the current M categories: anatomic site of distant metastases and serum lactate dehydrogenase level (LDH). Distant metastases in the skin, subcutaneous tissue, or distant lymph nodes with normal LDH levels are defined as M1a. Normal LDH with pulmonary metastases is classified as M1b, and any other distant metastases with elevated LDH are designated as M1c.

Stage Grouping

TNM classification determines staging. Clinical staging is comprised of pathological staging of the primary tumor and clinical/radiologic evaluation of metastases. Patients with localized melanoma, without any evidence of metastases, are categorized into stage I and II. They are subdivided by the different T criteria into IA/B and IIA/B/C. Patients with regional lymph node metastases and or satellite or in-transit metastases are categorized as stage III. If detailed histological lymph node staging has been performed, this stage is subdivided in III from A to C depending on the N classification. Distant metastasized melanoma is defined as stage IV without any further subdivisions. For more details please see Table 3.3.4 [5]

3.3.1.1.5 Prognosis

The majority of lesions, with the exception of NMM, first grow horizontally. In this so-called radial growth phase, melanoma does not form a tumor or metastasize. If diagnosed in this phase and if the entire tumor is removed with surgery, the prognosis is excellent [30]. Only in the phase of vertical growth, when an invading tumor is formed the prognosis does become dubious. Advanced melanoma is associated with a very poor prognosis, especially when metastatic disease has spread to visceral sites.

Cox proportional hazards regression was used to study factors that predict melanoma-specific survival rates (Fig. 3.3.3) [4]. The study revealed T category melanoma thickness according to Breslow [10] and ulceration of the primary lesion as the most powerful predictors of survival. "Thick" melanomas, with depth of infiltration more than 4.0 mm, have a 5-year survival rate of 45.1% when they are ulcerated, while the 5-year survival rate for melanomas less than 1 mm thick without ulceration is 95.3%. As for the nodal status, only the number of metastatic nodes, regardless of whether they were clinically apparent, and primary tumor ulceration demonstrated prognostic influence. A clinically occult micrometastasis in one lymph node reveals a 5-year survival rate of 69.5%, whereas the 5-year survival of a patient with 4 or more metastatic nodes is 26.7%. In the M category, patients without visceral metastases (involvement of distant skin, subcutaneous, or distant lymph nodes) showed significantly better survival. Within the visceral metastasized patients, those with lung metastases were associated with a better 1-year survival [6].

Other factors with alleged prognostic value are male gender and more advanced age. The localization of the tumor also has some predictive value [3]. Lesions on the scalp, neck, thorax, upper arms, hands, and feet are generally associated with a worse prognosis than lesions on the lower arms, thighs, and lower legs.

3.3.1.1.6 Prevention

Though the etiology of melanoma is unclear, certain factors are well recognized. This allows for development of strategies opposing the increase in incidence. The most important preventive measures concern efficient sun protection. Sun protection is a necessity in modern life for everybody, it is especially important for children and teenagers. Sunburn in the first years of life implies a particularly high risk for developing melanoma, although the latent period may be several decades. Skin phototypes I and II are especially prone to acute and chronic sun damage, including an increased risk for developing melanoma and nonmelanoma skin cancers and therefore require more stringent sun protection. Today

Table 3.3.4 Stage grouping for cutaneous melanoma [5]

	Clinical staging[a]				Pathologic staging[b]		
	T	N	M		T	N	M
0	Tis	No	Mo	0	Tis	No	Mo
IA	T1a	No	Mo	IA	T1a	No	Mo
IB	T1b	No	Mo	IB	T1b	No	Mo
	T2a	No	Mo		T2a	No	Mo
IIA	T2b	No	Mo	IIA	T2b	No	Mo
	T3a	No	Mo		T3a	No	Mo
IIB	T3b	No	Mo	IIB	T3b	No	Mo
	T4a	No	Mo		T4a	No	Mo
IIC	T4b	No	Mo	IIC	T4b	No	Mo
III	Any T	N > No	Mo	IIIA	T1-4a	N1a	Mo
					T1-4a	N2a	Mo
				IIIB	T1-4b	N1a	Mo
					T1-4b	N2a	Mo
					T1-4a	N1b	Mo
					T1-4a	N2b	Mo
					T1-4a	N2c	Mo
				IIIC	T1-4b	N1b	Mo
					T1-4b	N2b	Mo
					T1-4b	N2c	Mo
					Any T	N3	Mo
IV	Any T	Any N	M1	IV	Any T	Any N	M1

[a]Clinical staging includes microstaging of the primary melanoma and clinical/radiologic evaluation for metastases. By convention, it should be used after complete excision of the primary melanoma with clinical assessment for regional and distant metastases

[b]Pathological staging includes microstaging of the primary melanoma and pathologic information about the regional lymph nodes after partial (i.e., sentinel node biopsy) or complete lymphadenectomy. Pathologic stage O or stage IA patients are the exception; they do not require pathologic evaluation of their lymph nodes

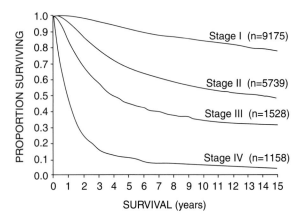

Fig. 3.3.3 Survival in patients with malignant melanoma [4]. Ten year survival of patients with malignant melanoma. The *first* and *second line* shows survival of patients with localized melanoma (stage I and II). The *third line* shows the survival of patients with regional metastases (stage III) and the *fourth line,* the survival of patients with distant metastases (stage IV)

there is an abundance of sun-screens in the market. It should be stressed that only those with sun-protection factor (SPF) of 20 and more are recommended. It is not yet certain which wavelengths of the electromagnetic spectrum are most caus-ative for melanoma, and thus, broad spectrum sunscreens are preferred. It has been suggested that UVA-rays are important for the induction of melanoma. Therefore, it is essential that the sunscreen applied covers as much of this part of the spec-trum as possible. Another requirement good sunscreens should fulfill is to be water resistant, especially in hot weather when excessive perspiration and swimming are likely. Every product should provide information as to the rules of appli-cation and, most importantly, the conditions which necessi-tate its reapplication (period of time, scrubbing, friction, sweating, bathing). These instructions should be followed stringently by the user. Nowadays, there are products avail-able claiming to offer all-day-long protection. These are cer-tainly more convenient, but even they must be reapplied under certain conditions. A problem which often arises with sunscreens is that the user fails to apply it on the whole skin surface, and some areas remain unprotected and, therefore, get burnt. Another problem is sparse use; the average applier uses only 25% of the amount used for determination of the SPF. To minimize these risks, it is necessary that the product be easy to spread and that the user applies it scrupulously everywhere.

A sunscreen, even when optimally chosen and applied, does not provide sufficient protection and should be used in combination with other sun protective measures. In this respect, clothing plays an important role. Nowadays, special textile materials have been introduced, which provide high-grade sun protection. Otherwise, it should be known that dark, thick clothes offer better protection than light transparent ones. Long sleeved shirts, long legged trousers, and long skirts belong undoubtedly to sensible summer fashion. A broad brimmed hat and effective sun-glasses complete the beach-look for the beginning of the twenty-first century.

People with large congenital naevi, with multiple naevi larger than 5 mm irregular in shape and color, with or without a personal or family history of melanoma are considered to be at high risk, and should be put under regular clinical and, if necessary, histological surveillance. All suspicious lesions should be promptly excised. Good photodocumentation plays an important part in this respect. Lately, more stress has been placed on self-examination, which requires adequate public education programs and a high level of public awareness.

3.3.1.2 Superficial Spreading Melanoma

3.3.1.2.1 ICD-O Code

8743/3

3.3.1.2.2 Synonyms

Pagetoid melanoma.

3.3.1.2.3 Clinical Features

Superficial spreading melanoma (SSM) is the variant most commonly encountered in phototypes I, II, and III. In females, the most common localization is on the legs, in men – the back. The patients are usually in their 50s, but may be much younger. The lesion may arise de novo or in a preexisting benign melanocytic lesion. Although there is an undoubtable correlation with UV-exposure, it is not linear but rather biphasic. Intermittent sun exposure (associated with weekend or holiday tourism) carries a much higher risk for the development of melanoma than professional-associated, daily exposure. In Australia, where the intensity of the UV-rays is very high, a second peak associated with high-intensity, everyday exposure has been reported. The clinical picture of SSM is that of an irregular patch, with highly variable color distribution within the lesion, encompassing different shades of brown, red, and gray. Areas of regression are often visible. The borders are sharply demarcated, palpable, and irregular.

3.3.1.2.4 Histopathology and Immunohistochemistry

Histologically, atypical tumor cells are found predominantly in not only the lower portion of the epidermis, but also higher up. While at the dermoepidermal junction, tumor cells tend to be grouped in nests, in the upper epidermis they are mostly singular, contributing to a pagetoid pattern of infiltration. Atypical cells have a large nucleus to cytoplasm ratio, coarse nuclear chromatin, prominent eosinophilic nucleoli, and fine dusty pigment in the cytoplasm. Mitoses are often detected, some of which are atypical. In the dermis, an inflammatory reaction is present, which is more pronounced below the epidermal portion of the tumor than beneath the dermal portion. Fibrosis is often found in the upper dermis.

The histological equivalent of the regression phenomenon consists of focal absence of tumor cells and a pronounced inflammatory reaction accompanied by fibrosis and pigment incontinence (Fig. 3.3.4, Tables 3.3.5 and 3.3.6).

3.3.1.3 Nodular Melanoma

3.3.1.3.1 ICD-O Code

8721/3

3.3.1.3.2 Clinical Features

Nodular melanoma (NM) is characterized by the lack of discernible horizontal growth phase. It may arise de novo in a naevus but, from the start, grows vertically and is capable of tumor formation and metastasizing. Localization is indiscriminate. Clinically, it presents as a tumor, which is often symmetrical, well demarcated, and may be poorly pigmented or even amelanotic, thus delaying adequate recognition. The lesion grows quickly and is usually advanced at the point of initial diagnosis. For this reason, the prognosis is often poorer than that of the variants with a horizontal growth phase. The rapid tumor growth and the inadequate vasculature account for the frequent development of ulceration and bleeding.

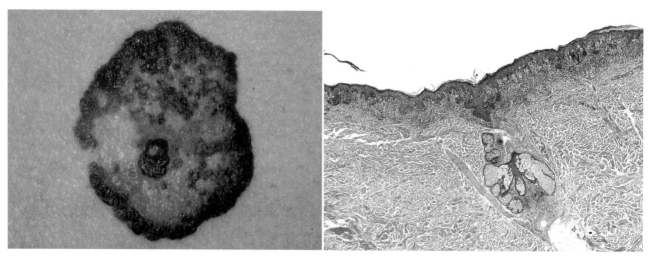

Fig. 3.3.4 Clinical and histological findings of SSM

Table 3.3.5 Clinical features of SSM

Occurrence – up to 70% of all cases (most common variant in Caucasians)
Localization – predominantly on intermittently exposed skin
Size – 1 to several centimeters
Shape – round or irregular with angular indentations
Borders – slightly elevated, may be palpable
Color – variable, often with areas of regression
Surface – smooth, rarely hyperkeratotic

Table 3.3.6 Differential diagnosis of SSM

Junctional or compound naevus
Recurrent naevus (pseudomelanoma)
Lentigo maligna melanoma
Pigmented actinic keratosis
Flat seborrheic keratosis
Superficial basal cell carcinoma
Kaposi sarcoma
Paget`s disease

3.3.1.3.3 Histopathology and Immunohistochemistry

Histologically NM presents as a bottom heavy tumor lying predominantly in the dermis. The overlying but not the adjacent epidermis is involved, often with a pagetoid pattern of infiltration. There is no "shoulder" formation. Cell atypia is usually uniform within one nest or even area, but different areas show distinct cell morphology, with presence of both major cell types (epithelioid and spindle-shaped). Deep mitoses, some of which are atypical, are a characteristic finding. Inflammation is scarce and patchy (Fig. 3.3.5, Tables 3.3.7 and 3.3.8).

3.3.1.4 *Lentigo Maligna and Lentigo Maligna Melanoma*

3.3.1.4.1 ICD-O Code

8742/2

3.3.1.4.2 Synonyms

Hutchinson melanotic freckle.

3.3.1.4.3 Clinical Features

Lentigo maligna (LM) and lentigo maligna melanoma (LMM) are usually encountered on the sun damaged skin of the face (rarely the back of the hand) of people in their 60s and 70s. Unlike the other variants of melanoma, LMM shows a linear correlation to cumulative UV-exposure, similar to those characteristic of basal and squamous-cell carcinomas. LMM arises from LM after many years, and actually only about half of all LM lesions evolve into an invasive tumor. That is the main reason for preserving the term LM, which is actually equivalent to level I LMM. LM starts as a small pigmentary macule, which grows slowly into an irregular noninfiltrated patch up to 10 cm in diameter, with uneven pigmentation and unclear borders. Finally as invasive growth develops, part of the lesion becomes infiltrated and nodules may arise.

3.3.1.4.4 Histopathology and Immunohistochemistry

Histologically, atrophy of the epidermis and solar elastosis are typical features. Most atypical cells are confined to the basal layer of the epidermis, and epidermal transmigration is

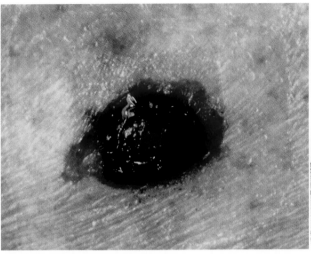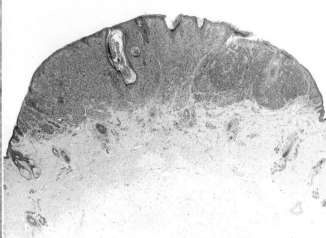

Fig. 3.3.5 Clinical and histological findings of NMM

Table 3.3.7 Clinical features of NMM

Occurrence – up to 20% of all cases
Localization – predominantly on the trunk
Size – indiscriminate
Shape – flat or hemispheric papule or nodule
Border – often sharply demarcated
Color – from blue–black through dark red to that of the normal skin (amelanotic)
Surface – smooth, shiny, with loss of the normal skin relief, or ulcerated

Table 3.3.8 Differential diagnosis of NMM

Dermal or compound melanocytic naevus
SPITZ naevus
Cellular blue naevus
Halo naevus
Metastatic melanoma
Granuloma pyogenicum
Angiokeratoma
Hemangioma
KAPOSI sarcoma
Angiosarcoma
Seborrheic keratosis
Basal cell carcinoma
Squamous cell carcinoma
Adnexal tumor
Merkel cell carcinoma
Pigmented histiocytoma
Atypical fibroxanthoma
Malignant fibrous histiocytoma
Cutaneous lymphoma
Tumor metastasis

less pronounced than in acral-lentiginous melanoma. Cell atypia is more discrete, with a predominance of small pleiomorphic spindle-shaped cells, often preserving their dendrites; pigment granules are coarse, and mitoses are not prominent. The dermal portion of the tumor develops after many years. Desmoplasia can sometimes be an associated feature (Fig. 3.3.6, Tables 3.3.9 and 3.3.10).

3.3.1.5 Acral-Lentiginous Melanoma

3.3.1.5.1 ICD-O Code

8744/3

3.3.1.5.2 Synonyms

Acral melanoma, palmar-plantar-subungual-mucosal melanoma (P-S-M melanoma), unclassified plantar melanoma.

3.3.1.5.3 Clinical Features

Acral-lentiginous melanoma (ALM) is a rare variant with approximately equal incidence in all skin phototypes and ethnicities. It accounts for most of the melanoma cases in patients of Asian or African descent. There is no correlation with UV-exposure. The localization is on the nonhairbearing

Fig. 3.3.6 Clinical finding of LM and histological findings of LMM

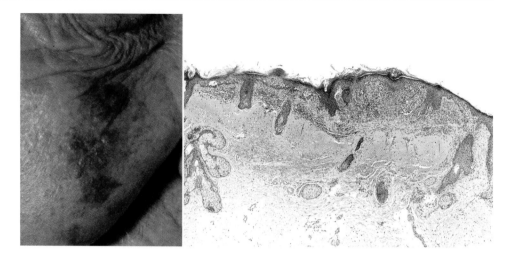

Table 3.3.9 Clinical features of LMM

Occurrence – up to 10% of all cases (most common variant in elderly people)
Localization – predominantly on chronically sun exposed skin
Size – 1 to several centimeters
Shape – irregular, geographic map-like
Borders – indistinct, flat, nonpalpable
Color – variable within the lesion (light brown to black), often with areas of regression (blue–white or white)
Surface – flat, often scaly

Table 3.3.10 Differential diagnosis of LMM

SSM
Lentigo solaris
Actinic keratosis
Seborrheic keratosis
Basal cell carcinoma
Junctional naevus
Postinflammatory pigmentation

skin of the palms and soles as well as the volar surface of the fingers and toes, sub- or periungually. Clinically, the lesion presents as an unevenly pigmented patch. Even in the vertical growth phase, the surface often remains flat, because of the thickness of the overlying epidermis.

Mucosal melanoma is also a rare variant, similar in many respects to ALM; many authors regard these two as a single melanoma type. Mucosal melanoma lesions are localized in the oral cavity, or on the nasal mucosa, sinuses, conjunctiva, pharynx, vagina, distal part of the urethra etc. These sites are associated with a quick transition to invasive growth phase and metastatic dissemination and consequently a poor prognosis.

3.3.1.5.4 Histopathology and Immunohistochemistry

Histologically, ALM and mucosal melanomas are somewhat intermediate between SMM and LMM, with significant epidermal transmigration of atypical cells and pigment in the center of the lesion and more lentiginous pattern in the periphery. Cell atypia is prominent in both large epithelioid and smaller spindle-shaped cells. Mitoses, some of which are atypical, are often prominent (Fig. 3.3.7, Tables 3.3.11–3.3.13).

3.3.1.6 Desmoplastic Melanoma

3.3.1.6.1 ICD-O Code

8745/3

3.3.1.6.2 Clinical Features

Signs of desmoplasia are usually observed in LMM, more rarely in ALM. Clinically, desmoplastic melanoma carries the features of the main variant from which it developed, but pigment content is usually low, and the surface of the tumor may be almost amelanotic. Another specific sign is the induration, which may be sufficiently pronounced as to suggest a fibroma or a fibrosarcoma.

3.3.1.6.3 Histopathology and Immunohistochemistry

The term desmoplastic refers to the vertical growth phase of the tumor, which is present by definition; a horizontal growth phase may or may not be present. Desmoplastic melanoma is characterized by a sarcomatous pattern of the tumor/stroma distribution. The tumor cells, which are predominantly spindle-shaped, are dispersed throughout the collagen-rich connective tissue. Thus, collagen production is a prominent

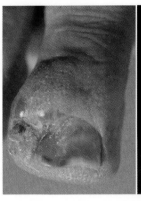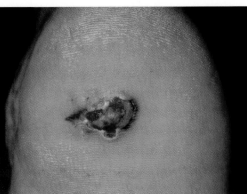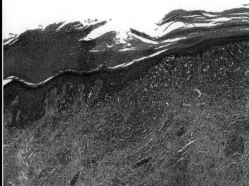

Fig. 3.3.7 Clinical and histological findings of ALM

Table 3.3.11 Clinical features of ALM

Occurrence – rare (most common variant in darker ethnic and racial groups – skin type > III)
Localization – hairless skin – palms, soles, flexural surfaces of fingers and toes, subungual and periungual areas; no relation to sun exposure
Size – 6 mm to several centimeters
Shape – irregular
Borders – irregular, ill-defined, nonpalpable
Color – variable – brown to blue–black
Surface – often remains flat even in lesions with a significant vertical growth component due to the thickness of the epidermis

Table 3.3.12 Clinical features of mucosal melanoma

Occurrence – rare; up to 5% of all cases
Localization – oral cavity, nasopharynx, sinuses, vulva, anus, urethra
Size – often significantly larger than clinically apparent
Shape – irregular
Border – not clearly demarcated
Color – often amelanotic, stimulating an inflammatory process
Surface – flat, impalpable or protruding and ulcerated, depending on the growth phase

Table 3.3.13 Differential diagnosis of ALM

Melanocytic naevus
Subcorneal or subungual hemorrhage
Granuloma pyogenicum
Kaposi sarcoma
Angiosarcoma
Squamous cell carcinoma
Trophic ulcer
Chronic paronychia
Panaritium

feature of this variant. Because of their shape, it may be impossible to distinguish the tumor cells from fibroblasts on a HE-slide, which can seriously hinder diagnosis. Sometimes the histological picture is very similar to that of a scar or to that of a histiocytic tumor. In such cases, immunohistochemistry is often required. It is advisable to use more than one antibody, because both S100 and HMB45 give a lower yield of positive results than in other melanoma types. The characteristic epidermal involvement and the presence of a patchy round cell inflammatory infiltrate in the dermal part of the tumor are associate features which can significantly help in recognizing the lesion for what it is. Although single mitoses are a common finding, the mitotic rate is usually very low.

3.3.1.6.4 Desmoplastic Neurotropic Melanoma

Desmoplastic neurotropic melanoma is distinguished from desmoplastic melanoma on the basis of evidence of peri- and intraneural infiltration (neurotropism). Similar to the desmoplastic melanoma, most tumor cells in desmoplastic neurotropic melanoma are spindle-shaped. Therefore, neurotropism should be carefully sought after in all lentiginous melanomas and especially in those with a predominance of spindle cells or features of desmoplasia. Interestingly, although neurotropism is often histologically pronounced, pain and sensitivity changes have only been clinically observed in very few cases.

Prognosis is considered to be poor, not only because of the thickness of these lesions, which is in most cases considerable, but also because of the treacherous peri- or endoneural spread, the extent of which is difficult to estimate, and therefore the chance of local recurrence is quite high. It should also be noted that neural involvement within the tumor mass (contiguous neurotropism) is far more common than involvement beyond the tumor borders, but the latter has a much larger impact as far as the risk of local recurrence is concerned (Fig. 3.3.8, Tables 3.3.14 and 3.3.15).

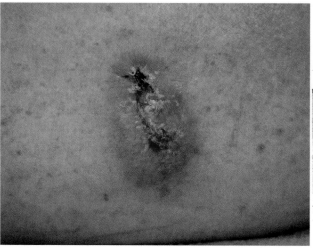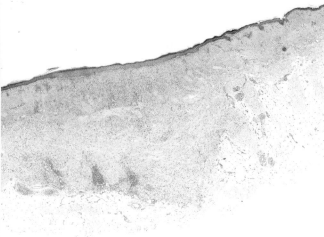

Fig. 3.3.8 Clinical and histological findings of desmoplastic melanoma

Table 3.3.14 Desmoplastic melanoma particular features

Vertical growth phase – present by definition
Horizontal growth phase – may be present or not; when present it is of LMM type, rarely of ALM or MLM type
Pigment production – low, with large amelanotic areas
Cell atypia – spindle-shaped cells with wavy nuclei forming thin fascicles separated by collagen fibers (sarcomatous pattern); some epithelioid or cuboidal cells are often present but mainly in the epidermis and the papillary dermis; mitoses – rare; often neurotropic growth
Patchy lymphocytic inflammatory reaction within the tumor

Table 3.3.15 Differential diagnosis of desmoplastic melanoma

Desmoplastic Spitz naevus
Neurotized naevus
Neurofibroma
Cellular dermatofibroma
Keloid
Dermatofibrosarcoma protuberans
Malignant schwannoma

3.3.1.7 Melanoma Arising from Blue Naevus

3.3.1.7.1 ICD-O Code

8780/3

3.3.1.7.2 Synonyms

Malignant blue naevus, blue naevus-like melanoma.

3.3.1.7.3 Clinical Features

Melanoma arising from blue naevus, malignant blue naevus (MBN), or blue naevus-like melanoma is a very rare entity. Its place in the taxonomy of pigmented tumors is not precisely clarified. While some authors regard it as subtype of melanoma, in which malignant transformation initiates in the dermis, others regard it as a separate entity, their major argument being the lack of junctional activity. MBN most often arises in cellular blue naevus, but it can also develop in any other recognized form of blue naevus – common, combined, or plaque type [61]. Anecdotal cases of MBN developing in a giant congenital naevus, naevus of Ota, or even de novo in normal skin have been reported. Typically however, there is a history of blue naevus, present since birth or childhood, which recently enlarged quickly. The patients are usually in their 40s or 50s, and there is a female predilection [28].

The most common localization is the scalp, but lesions on the trunk and extremities have also been reported. At the time of initial diagnosis, the lesion is already significant in size and presents with a blue to black nodule, which may be multilobulated. A lesion with similar characteristics should always be suspected to be MBN, and clinical suspicion is very important, as the histological features, though distinct, are not sufficiently specific. Thus, a strong correlation between the clinical and histological data is essential for a correct diagnosis.

3.3.1.7.4 Histopathology and Immunohistochemistry

Histologically, melanoma arising from blue naevus is composed of thick fascicles of closely aggregated, spindle-shaped, bipolar cells in the dermis and usually also in the hypodermis. The epidermis is never involved. The pigment content of the cells varies significantly between different parts of the lesion. An admixture of plumper, even epithelioid looking cells is often observed, whose cytoplasm is often clear. Large, multinucleated cells may also be detected. An important feature is the presence of mitoses, some of which are atypical. These are a constant finding, although the mitotic index may vary within broad limits. Necrosis, when present, is highly suggestive of the diagnosis. However, its absence does not exclude the diagnosis, as it is detected in only about half of all cases. In most lesions, parts are detected whose histological characteristics correspond to those of a benign cellular blue naevus. When properly interpreted, this feature may actually assist the diagnosis, but it may also lead to confusion through a sample error.

Upon immunohistochemistry, MBN stains positive for S100 and HMB45. Interestingly, increased proportions of Ki-67 (MIB-1) positive cells have been reported. Ki-67 is a nuclear antigen, expressed by proliferating cells. Benign cellular blue naevi have been shown to be Ki-67–negative, and it has been suggested that the change from negative to positive Ki-67 reactivity may be a valuable marker of malignant and metastatic potential in cellular blue naevi [9].

3.3.1.7.5 Prognosis

The prognosis of MBN is generally considered to be poor, which probably correlates with the late stage of development at which most of these lesions are diagnosed. However, measurement of Breslow thickness, as in melanoma, is impossible, as the epidermis is not involved, and the whole lesion lies in the dermis and deeper. MBN most often produces regional lymph node metastases, which do not necessarily mean a pessimistic prognosis. On the other hand, the presence of distant hematogenic metastases, when present, is a strong negative prognostic factor.

As in melanoma, the only curative measure is surgical removal of the tumor in toto as early as possible. Criteria which could assist the timely recognition of malignant transformation of a cellular blue naevus have been proposed [28]. These are: (1) diameter of greater than 2 cm in a solitary lesion; (2) presence of multiple lesions in a multinodular or plaque form; or (3) history of rapid or progressive growth or sudden change. The presence of any one of these features should indicate excisional biopsy with serial section evaluation, to avoid sampling error (Tables 3.3.16 and 3.3.17).

Table 3.3.16 Clinical features of melanoma arising from blue naevus

Occurrence – very rare
Localization – predominantly on the scalp
Size – 1–3 cm or more
Shape – hemispheric or multilobulated nodule
Border – sharply demarcated
Color – blue-black
Surface – smooth, rarely ulcerated

Table 3.3.17 Differential diagnosis of melanoma arising from blue naevus

Primary melanoma
Metastatic melanoma
Malignant combined naevus
Cellular blue naevus
Histiocytoma

3.3.1.8 Melanoma Arising in a Giant Congenital Naevus

3.3.1.8.1 ICD-O Code

8761/3

3.3.1.8.2 Synonyms

Malignant melanoma arising in a garment naevus, malignant melanoma arising in a bathing trunk naevus, malignant melanoma arising in a giant hairy naevus.

3.3.1.8.3 Clinical Features

Congenital melanocytic naevi are visible at birth or shortly after in approximately 1% of all infants. The simplest definition of giant congenital naevus (GCN) is a melanocytic naevus larger than 20 cm in diameter [58]. GCN are rare, but they are a risk factor for malignant melanoma. However, the magnitude of risk for malignant transformation is still unknown and a matter of ongoing debate [41]. Five prospective studies addressed the issue of melanoma arising in congenital naevi [17, 21, 31, 39, 53]. Follow-up ranged between 2 and 7.3 years. Inclusion criteria also varied greatly between studies. Some explored congenital melanocytic nevi of all sizes [17], while others used defined criteria (e.g., ≥5% of the body surface or ≥20 cm diameter [21]). The melanoma proportion was identified as 4.3% (3 melanomas in 2/46 patients) [21], 3.75% (3/80) [53], 2.4% (4/170) [31], 1.5% (2/133) [17] and 0 [39]. It is postulated that the risk of melanoma development within a congenital nevus increases with increasing size.

Melanoma arising in small congenital naevi presents at the dermal-epidermal junction, similar to usual melanoma. Up to two-thirds of melanomas associated with larger and GCN arise in the dermis, subcutaneous fat, or deeper as a nodule [8, 58]. They present as a rapidly-growing, asymmetrical nodule, plaque, or as a cystic lesion [40].

Other tumor entities arising from GCN include poorly differentiated, small round cell cancer, malignant cellular blue nevus, spindle-cell malignant tumor with lamellar cell (pseudomeissnerian) differentiation, so-called "minimal deviation melanoma," heterologous malignant mesenchymal differentiation, including rhabdomyosarcoma and liposarcoma, and undifferentiated spindle-cell cancer [34].

3.3.1.8.4 Histopathology and Immunohistochemistry

As described in the clinical section, it is crucial to interpret histological sections in a clinical-pathological context, carefully considering the age of the patient and the size of the lesion. There are significant differences between melanomas developing in giant congenital nevi and those developing in small congenital nevi or tardive congenital nevi. Whereas, melanomas developing in small congenital or tardive congenital nevi initially show a pagetoid, mostly intraepidermal pattern, similar to the radial growth phase of melanomas, those developing in giant congenital nevi show a more nodular dermal pattern of melanomatous dedifferentiation [62].

This pattern is also seen in the most important differential diagnosis: the proliferative nodule.

Proliferative nodules are considered benign. Cytomorphologically, they can display features of all known nevi (usually only one at a time): blue nevus, cellular blue nevus, deep penetrating nevus, Spitz nevus, and small cell nevus.

Proliferative nodules usually show a monomorphous cytological pattern with rare mitosis. In contrast, atypical mitotic figures are a feature of a melanoma.

Interspersed collagen bundles and a focal blending of melanocytes with the surrounding nevus, usually at the base of the nodule, speak in favor of a benign proliferation.

In contrast, melanomatous nodules in giant congenital nevi show a considerable degree of nuclear pleomorphism as well as mitotic activity, and atypical mitotic figures are usually found.

In 2007, Massi summarized the differences between proliferative nodules and dermal melanoma in the congenital nevus (Table 3.3.18) [47].

Table 3.3.18 Histological findings of congenital nevi and melanoma in a congenital melanoma (according to [47])

Proliferative nodule in congenital nevi	Intradermal melanoma in a congenital melanoma
Frequent	Rare
Cellular monomorphism	Cellular pleomorphism
Low mitotic rate	High mitotic rate
Roundish silhouette	Irregularly shaped silhouette
Collagen fibers interposed	Growth in solid pattern, collagen fibers obliterated

There is no clear immunohistochemical marker that differentiates proliferative nodules from dermal melanoma in giant congenital nevi.

However, the heightened proliferative rate (ki67/Mib1) and heightened number of mitoses (Ser 10/MPM2) observed in melanoma can be useful in differentiating the two entities.

In larger congenital nevi, there is a considerable risk, especially in partial excisions, to miss the "hot spot" due to a sampling error. A very accurate macropathological workup, close clinical-pathological correlation, and sometimes multiple sections are required to address this important issue [15, 27, 42, 51].

3.3.1.9 Melanoma of Childhood

3.3.1.9.1 Clinical Features

Melanoma of childhood is rare but potentially fatal [38], and its incidence is rising. The definition of melanoma of childhood varies. Some authors define it as melanoma developing prior to the onset of puberty, and some authors include patients aged from 15 to 20 years. It is important to recognize that melanoma occurs in children and to appreciate the particular clinical morphological criteria since melanoma of childhood may show an aggressive course with metastases. Conversely, Spitz naevi and atypical nodular proliferations developing in congenital naevi must be excluded in order to avoid overdiagnosis. Melanomas in children tend to be large and clinically striking, but they can also present as only a subcutaneous mass beneath a pigmented lesion or as regional lymphadenopathy [13]. At time of diagnosis they are usually thicker compared to those of adults [50]. This might be due to a delayed diagnosis and the higher incidence of nodular melanomas in children. Melanoma in children can be associated with pain and pruritus.

3.3.1.9.2 Histopathology and Immunohistochemistry

The pathological diagnosis of childhood melanoma is difficult. Useful criteria to distinguish melanomas from benign naevi are: large size, ulceration, high mitotic activity (>4 mitoses/mm^2), mitoses in the lower third of the lesion, asymmetry, poorly demarcated lateral borders, lack of maturation, dusty melanin, and marked nuclear polymorphism [56]. According to their predominant cellular population, melanoma of children can be subdivided [56]. The conventional epithelioid-cell type presents similar histological findings to melanoma in adults. Most of these melanoma present as superficial spreading type [59]. However, there is a higher fraction of nodular melanoma in children compared to adults. Small cell melanoma is composed of monomorphous small cells similar to benign naevi or lymphoma. Melanoma simulating Spitz naevus exhibits architectural and cytological features reminiscent of Spitz naevus. The differential diagnosis of childhood melanoma with benign Spitz naevus is extremely difficult and misdiagnosis seems to be common [60]. On the other hand, there are cases of metastasized melanoma initially diagnosed as Spitz naevus.

3.3.1.10 Naevoid Melanoma

3.3.1.10.1 ICD-O Code

8720/3

3.3.1.10.2 Synonyms

Minimal deviation melanoma.

3.3.1.10.3 Clinical Features

It has been known for many years that there is a small subset of malignant melanoma closely resembling banal nevi.

In Levene's classification of melanoma, where he included "verrucous and pseudonevoid" variants of melanoma, he first recognized these tumors as true melanomas due to their biological behavior [44]. The term "nevoid melanoma" was first coined by Schmoeckel et al. [54].

Nevoid melanomas resemble benign nevi in both clinical aspect and histology because of its architectural similarity to a compound-type nevus or papillomatous nevus.

The correct clinical and histological assessment of this rather rare melanoma is of particular importance.

Less than 100 cases of nevoid melanoma are described in the literature. This rare variant of malignant melanoma comprises less than 1% of malignant melanomas.

Zembowicz et al. published a series of twenty nevoid melanoma [63]. This study found nevoid melanoma only in Caucasian patients, with an equal gender distribution (10 males/10 females). At the time of diagnosis, patients had an average age of 40 (age range 19–81 years).

Of these 20 tumors, 6 recurred locally, and 3 metastasized with a fatal outcome. The mortality rate varies in published studies from 15 to 37.5% (with an average of 24%) for lesions with an average Breslow thickness of 2.1 mm.

While the site of predilection for male patients was the back, tumors were most often located on the extremities (mostly arms) in females.

Clinically, nevoid melanomas closely resemble a papillomatous or compound-type nevus. None of the nevoid melanomas were diagnosed clinically.

3.3.1.10.4 Histopathology and Immunohistochemistry

Nevoid melanomas resemble a benign nevus upon scanning magnification. Superficially, they show a nevoid cell type, a high degree of symmetry, and sometimes (pseudo-) maturation.

The epidermis presents with either a verrucous or a dome-shaped pattern. Similar to the histological features of nevi in young children, nevoid melanomas exhibit "filled papillae" with sheets and cords of melanocytes subjacent to the epidermis between the rete-ridges, extending into deeper parts of the dermis.

Usually, there is no significant involvement of the junctional zone and no prominent pagetoid spread. Adnexal epithelia may occasionally be infiltrated.

In the dermis, a mostly sheet-like growth pattern is observed. Some cases also show a more cord-like growth pattern with interspersed irregular nests of atypical melanocytes between collagen bundles.

Upon high-power magnification, one may observe partially epithelioid melanocytes with moderate to severe pleomorphism, thickened nuclear membranes, uneven distribution of chromatin or hyperchromasia, and enlarged nucleoli. Usually, these atypical melanocytes are seen both in superficial and deep areas of the tumor. Occasionally, the melanocytes may show a gradual decrease in size of the cytoplasmic rim from superficial to deep parts, while maintaining an atypically large nucleus, imitating maturation (so-called pseudomaturation).

Mitotic figures can be identified in all parts of the tumor, showing no gradient to the depth. The presence of mitotic figures at the base of the tumor is an especially strong indicator for nevoid melanoma [45, 47].

Strong and even Melan-A (MART-1) and S100 staining patterns are observed. In contrast to banal nevi, in which

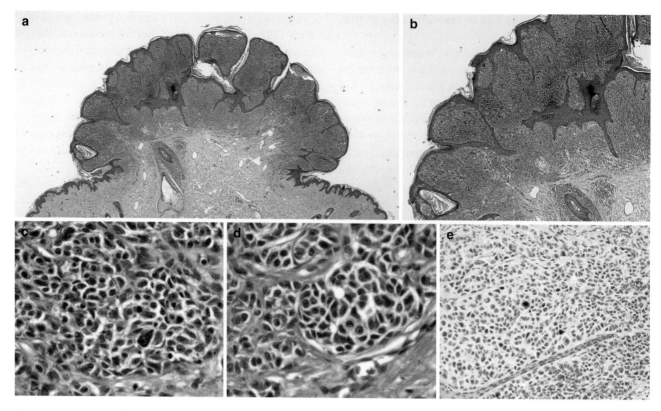

Fig. 3.3.9 Histological findings of nevoid melanoma. (**a**) In scanning power, nevoid melanomas closely resemble a papillomatous nevus. (**b**) Nevoid nelanomas grow, unlike banal nevi, in large sheets rather than in a nested pattern. There is usually no intraepidermal component or pagetoid spread. (**c**) Atypical melanocytes with an uneven pigment distri- bution showing considerable nuclear pleomorphism, uneven chromatin distribution, and atypically enlarged nucleoli. (**d**) In almost every high-power field there is at least one mitotic figure, many of them atypical. (**e**) Immunohistochemical detection of mitotic figures (MPM2)

Table 3.3.19 Differential diagnosis of banal nevus and nevoid melanoma

Banal nevus	Nevoid melanoma
Melanocytes mostly organized in nest	Melanocytes in sheets and chords ("filled papillae")
Monomorphous small melanocytes	Pleomorphic melanocytes with nuclear atypia
If visible, small nucleoli	Enlarged, eosinophilic nucleoli
Usually no mitotic figures	Numerous mitotic figures (1–2/high-power field)

hmb45-reactivity is usually present in the functional component and superficial dermal areas, hmb45 reactive cells may also be seen in deeper parts of nevoid melanoma. Proliferative activity (ki67/MiB1) and mitotic figures (i.e., Serin 10, MPM 2) are augmented and show no gradient to the depth. As in the diagnosis of more common types of melanoma (e.g., nodular melanoma), no single criterion in immunohistochemistry can prove or exclude the diagnosis of nevoid melanoma. Immunohistochemistry is considered to be a useful aid in the diagnosis of nevoid melanoma, but it must be interpreted in close relation to the histomorphological findings (Fig. 3.3.9, Table 3.3.19).

3.3.1.11 Persistent Melanoma and Local Metastasis of Melanoma

3.3.1.11.1 Synonyms

Local recurrence of melanoma.

3.3.1.11.2 Clinical Features

Persistent melanoma is identified as growth of the residual primary tumor within the site continuous with the scar after incomplete excision [33]. It clinically presents as a variably pigmented macule or patch in the area of the primary excision. In desmoplastic melanoma, nodule formation can also be a clinical sign of recurrence [33].

The skin is not only the most common localization for primary melanoma but is often the site of metastases. Skin metastases can arise as a consequence of lymphatic dissemination. These are called satellites when they are located up to 5 cm from the primary tumor. When the distance between such a regional metastasis and the primary tumor exceeds 5 cm, but the lesions remain in the same lymph node drainage area, it is referred to as an in transit metastasis. Distant skin metastases are the result of hematogenous dissemination. Clinically, cutaneous metastases often resemble nodular melanoma. They can be situated in the papillary or reticular dermis as well as in the hypodermis.

Invasive melanoma shows an aggressive course with a great capacity for metastasizing initially to the regional lymph nodes and, consequently, hematogenically in distant organs. Sometimes, multiple melanoma metastases are diagnosed while no primary tumor is detected. Although an extracutaneous localization of the primary tumor in these cases is possible, often it is the case that the primary cutaneous tumor has undergone complete regression. Sometimes in such cases, a discrete hypopigmented or hyperpigmented macule is detected, as the only residue of the primary tumor.

3.3.1.11.3 Histopathology and Immunohistochemistry

Persistent melanoma may present histologically as the original tumor. More commonly, it presents as in situ melanoma with or without focal dermal involvement [33]. Histologically, the main criteria for differentiating metastases from primary and persistent melanoma are the lack of epidermal involvement and inflammatory infiltrate in metastases [32]. However, these criteria are relative, as they can rarely also be met in cases of primary tumors.

Special attention should be paid to the epidermotropic melanoma metastasis – a particular variant, in which the papillary dermis is primarily infiltrated, and the overlying epidermis is secondarily engaged. The fact that only the part of the epidermis directly overlying the dermal portion of the tumor is affected and that there is no "shoulder" formation may help to differentiate this kind of lesion from the types of primary melanomas with a horizontal growth phase. Additionally, the epidermis is flattened and pushed by dermal aggregates of atypical melanocytic cells. Differentiation from nodular melanoma, which does not show any horizontal growth phase, is still possible, because in epidermotropic metastatic melanoma, the tumor infiltration is confined to the upper dermis, while in nodular melanoma it involves the deeper parts of the reticular dermis.

3.3.1.11.4 Rare Manifestations of Metastatic Melanoma

There are some rare but interesting manifestations of metastatic melanoma which deserve attention and are associated with disturbances of the pigmentation. These include generalized melanosis and vitiligo. First described by Legg over a 100 years ago [43], diffuse melanosis in metastatic melanoma is characterized by a diffuse, slate-blue discoloration, accentuated by exposure to UV-light. In addition to the skin,

the mucous membranes are affected. A pronounced darkening of the urine is an associated feature. Very few cases have been reported since the initial description, and the pathogenesis remains unclear. The possible explanations for this striking phenomenon include dissemination of melanosomes produced at the site of the tumor and its metastases, deposition of oxydated melanin precursors, and virtual hematogenous spread of single melanoma cells, which are then deposited in different tissues, including the skin.

Vitiligo-like manifestations, on the other hand, are not so rare in melanoma patients. Many authors prefer the term melanoma-associated hypopigmentation (MAH). The extent of these manifestations varies broadly within the range between a halo naevus and disseminated hypopigmentation, with involvement of the iris and the retina. Analogous changes occur not only spontaneously, but also in the course of chemoimmunotherapy [52]. It is believed that hypopigmentation occurs as a result of the immune response to melanoma antigens. Cytotoxic cellular response with involvement of the NK, by means of circulating antibodies, allegedly plays a major role. Correlation of MAH with a better prognosis has been reported [18] (Fig. 3.3.10).

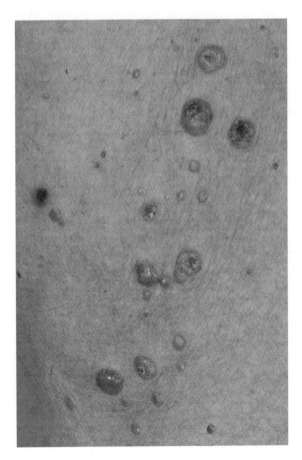

Fig. 3.3.10 Epidermotropic metastases. Multiple skin-colored papules. Histology revealed epidermotropic metastases of an acrolentiginous melanoma arising in the big toe

3.3.2 Benign Melanocytic Tumors

Sven Krengel

The current WHO concept classifies benign melanocytic skin tumors through a mixture of anamnestic ("congenital," "persistent"), clinico-morphologic ("acral," "blue"), and histomorphologic criteria ("lentiginous," "dysplastic"). A drawback of this system is that the entities partly lack a clear-cut definite distinction. Secondly, the currently established clinical and histological criteria to distinguish benign and (pre-) malignant changes ("dysplasia") are morphological and therefore, often imprecise. Thirdly, histological pictures are only snapshots of a dynamic pathogenesis. Therefore, every statement about the sequence of events in one single lesion is hypothetical (e.g., development from a junctional to a compound naevus or from a common to a dysplastic naevus).

Clinicians will miss the *common acquired melanocytic naevus* in this classification. Common melanocytic naevi are commonly subdivided into junctional, compound, and dermal types. Of these, only junctional naevi easily find a new place in the WHO system ("lentiginous naevi"). Compound and dermal naevi seem to remain orphan entities. Surprisingly, however, new insights into naevogenesis probably allow to categorize the majority of them as variants of lentiginous, dysplastic, or (tardive) superficial congenital naevi, respectively.

Better understanding of naevogenesis will in the future allow an improved reclassification of benign melanocytic tumors. However, until more specific molecular markers and (hopefully noninvasive) diagnostic methods are available, the current classification provides a reasonable working classification for clinical dermatologists and dermatopathologists.

3.3.2.1 Congenital Melanocytic Naevi

Congenital melanocytic naevi (CMN) are usually defined as melanocytic proliferations which are visible at birth or shortly thereafter, i.e., in the neonatal period ("tardive CMN"). Pathogenetically, larger CMN most likely represent hamartomas which originate from defective migratory, differentiational and/or proliferative properties of a subset of neural crest cells due to postzygotic (somatic) mutations (paradominant inheritance) [31]. The earlier in embryogenesis the mutational events occur, the larger and deeper the resulting CMN will be, in many cases extending into epidermal appendages, subcutaneous fat, peripheral nerves, or the central nervous system (neurocutaneous melanocytosis, NCM). A very important clinical hallmark of large CMN is the presence of so-called satellite naevi, i.e., sometimes hundreds of smaller naevi spreading from the neural crest over the whole body. CMN with a diameter of less than 20 cm at birth only rarely have satellite naevi [44]. Conceivably, all larger CMN presenting with satellites (whether with CNS involvement or without) represent neurocristopathies, which we suggest to designate as *deep type CMN*, analogous to the WHO category of *superficial type CMN*. In line with this concept are cytogenetic findings of frequent NRAS mutations in larger CMN, whereas small CMN like most acquired naevi exhibit BRAF mutations [12, 26].

In contrast to deep type CMN, superficial type CMN evolve after the neural crest stage and therefore lack satellite naevi. These CMN are smaller and probably represent benign neoplasms arising from melanocytes (or late-stage melanocytic precursor cells, respectively) which have already completed their ontogenetic pathway and reside in the epidermis or in the upper dermis, mostly in the vicinity of epidermal appendages. The transition between superficial "neoplastic" CMN and larger "hamartomatous" CMN seems to be gradual; however, the presence of satellite naevi is a good indicator of a neural crest origin. Recent studies have shown that only deep type CMN, i.e., large CMN with multiple satellites, have a measurably elevated risk of transforming into melanoma and NCM [19, 32]. Even in these "hamartomatous" CMN, the melanoma risk is probably smaller than previously expected (estimated 3–5% lifetime risk for giant CMN, [32]). Melanomas arising in large CMN tend to develop already in childhood and may start from dermal or even deeper tissue compartments rather than from epidermal melanocytes. In small and medium-sized CMN without satellites ("superficial type CMN"), the melanoma risk is much lower and, if elevated at all, might reflect the increased numbers of melanocytes rather than genuine biological features of congenitalness.

Although the above pathogenetic considerations favor the distinction between deep and superficial type CMN, a common and useful clinical classification is based on the largest diameter of the largest naevus (projected adult size). A recently modified version of the original Kopf' classification defines small (<1.5 cm), medium (1.5–10 cm), large (>10–20 cm), and giant CMN (>20 cm; G1 >20–30 cm; G2 >30–40 cm; G3 >40 cm; the presence of >50 satellites leads to the next higher category) [43].

Clinically, small CMN are found in about 1% of all newborns [48]. In contrast, large and giant CMN are found in only 1:20,000–1:500,000 newborns, the incidence inversely reflecting naevus size [13]. CMN (at least large and giant CMN) seem to have no racial predilection. Some studies show a slight female preponderance and a low-grade familial predisposition [29]. CMN can be found on any anatomic site. They mostly present as a homogeneous, light to dark brown papule or plaque. Inhomogeneous pigmentation, nodules, hairiness and a coarse, rugated surface are common features of large and giant CMN. The color of CMN often lightens to a certain degree in the first years of life.

On histologic examination, small and medium-sized CMN show dense, diffuse infiltrates of small monomorphous melanocytes only in the upper third of the dermis. By contrast, large and giant CMN extend deep into the dermis and subcutaneous fat, the melanocytes often infiltrating epidermal appendages, vessels, and nerves (for a review, see [31]). The epidermal component overlying CMN occasionally shows focal lentiginous or pagetoid spread of melanocytes. Similar features, mimicking severe atypia or even early melanoma, are also observed in acquired naevi of childhood, making childhood naevi facultative melanoma simulators.

Prophylactic excision of larger CMN is widely recommended, though not always achievable in giant CMN [54]. When counseling parents of children with CMN, melanoma prevention and cosmetic improvement should be discussed as separate issues. In the view of skin elasticity and wound healing properties and for psychological reasons, surgical intervention should be started in the first 2 years of life, either by serial excision, flaps with or without previous tissue expansion, or autologous transplants. In view of the relatively low incidence of melanoma, the decision of many parents, who refuse to let their child be operated, must be respected. Alternatively, superficial treatments (dermabrasion, laser treatment) are available and should be considered especially in facial nevi. They may lead to cosmetic improvement; however, partial repigmentation in the first 5–10 years is common. As melanoma in CMN may arise from deep tissue structures, these treatments are much less efficient to prevent malignancy.

Infants with large and giant CMN and/or multiple satellites should undergo MR imaging of the head and spine to rule out NCM. The prognosis of NCM varies widely, reaching from asymptomatic MR findings to severe neurological defects (seizures, hydrocephalus) with a possibly fatal outcome [19, 34].

3.3.2.1.1 Superficial Type

The clinical and histological features of superficial type CMN have been mentioned above. The fact that these lesions are histologically indistinguishable from a subset of acquired, "congenital-type" melanocytic naevi lends support to the view that they, even if in part not arising before adolescence or adulthood, probably share a similar pathogenesis. The classical concept of common acquired melanocytic naevi, proclamating a sequence from UV-induced epidermal ("junctional") to epidermo-dermal ("compound") to dermal naevus cell nests ("Abtropfung"), has expired [31]. All strings of evidence point to the existence of dermally located melanocytic precursor cells, from which dermal naevi arise. However, these precursor cells have not yet been sufficiently characterized in postnatal skin. Possibly, these cells are identical with the pluripotent stem cells of the hair follicle bulge region [52]. In favor of this view is the common adnexotropism of dermal naevus cells. Interestingly, Dadzie et al. [17] recently reported clinically inapparent, incidental foci of naevus cells in the dermis, mostly of the head and neck region.

Clinically, dermal melanocytic naevi represent brown to skin-colored papules or small plaques. On the face, they mostly appear in childhood or adolescence as small brown papules, and, gradually lightening, may grow to elevated, sometimes firm, dome-shaped papules ("Miescher naevus," [2]). In adulthood, growth of one or several thick hairs is common. Another variant of dermal naevi is more often located on the neck and trunk, presenting as a papillomatous, brown plaque ("Unna naevus," [2]). Histological examination of dermal melanocytic naevi shows symmetrically arranged, dense sheets or fascicles of small naevus cells in the upper to midreticular dermis, often surrounding (but not infiltrating) adnexa. "Unna type" naevi typically have a more papillomatous, irregular epidermal relief and varying numbers of melanophages in the papillary dermis. A low extent of lentiginous melanocytic hyperplasia in the overlying epidermis is a common finding.

As already mentioned, cytogenetic analysis revealed frequent BRAF mutations in small CMN as well as in acquired "congenital-pattern" naevi [12, 26]. Future research will reveal if the concept to classify these naevi together as "superficial type congenital naevi" holds through.

3.3.2.1.2 Proliferative Nodules in Congenital Melanocytic Nevi

Nodular proliferations in a preexisting CMN that are histologically atypical but behave in a benign fashion are denominated proliferative nodules (PN).

In giant CMN, single or multiple dark nodules may develop during the first months of life or even later. After an initial phase of rapid growth, the nodules stop growing and partially regress with neurotized histological changes over the following years.

On histological examination, a PN represents a sharply demarcated area with epithelioid or spindle-shaped melanocytes in the upper and middermis, embedded in the background masses of smaller melanocytes. Frequent numerical aberrations of whole chromosomes have been demonstrated in PN. By contrast, melanomas more likely carry cytogenetic alterations involving only partial chromosomes [10].

PN may be misinterpreted as melanoma arising in CMN. Therefore, and in view of the melanoma-mimicking histological changes of childhood naevi in general, the diagnosis of melanoma arising in CMN should be very carefully evaluated. Earlier reports on a high incidence of melanoma in CMN may be partly due to the interpretation of these histological changes as "minimal deviation melanoma" (for a review, see [32]). However, melanoma *may* arise from CMN, as well as from superficial and from deeper tissue components. A rapidly growing nodule arising in a CMN should be excised to rule out melanoma.

3.3.2.2 Dermal Melanocytic Lesions

Dermal melanocytoses are flat areas with blue discoloration which are often present at birth [49]. They show a predilection for Asian and Black races.

3.3.2.2.1 Mongolian Spot

Mongolian spots represent a trace of the ontogenetic pathway of melanocytic cells. Given to the temporo-spatial sequence of this process, they are mostly located on the lower back and in the gluteal region [28]. Mongolian spots are very frequent in newborns of Black and Oriental races, but are only rarely found in Caucasian children [15].

Usually present at birth or becoming visible in the newborn period, the blue-green to blue-gray areas of up to 10 cm tend to fade away until adolescence. Tumorous growth or malignant degeneration has not been noticed.

Histologically, mongolian spots show only a few pigmented dendritic cells orientated between the collagen fibers of the lower dermis. Possibly, such cells also exist in Caucasian newborns, but are not visible due to their much lower melanin production.

3.3.2.2.2 Naevus of Ota and Ito

Naevus of Ota is a rare condition, usually in Oriental or Black, mostly Japanese patients, with a slight female preponderance [49]. However, it also has repeatedly been reported in Caucasian individuals. The lesions are visible at birth in 50% of the cases, becoming apparent at the latest during adolescence. Naevus of Ito is even rarer and differs from naevus of Ota mainly by its anatomical localization.

Following the ophthalmic and maxillary branch of the trigeminal nerve, naevus of Ota presents with one large, unilateral blue or blue-gray macule in the periorbital, zygomatic, and temporal area, mostly including parts of the conjunctiva and sclera (naevus of Ito: supraclavicular, deltoid or scapular area, following the lateral branchial and posterior supraclavicular nerves). Sometimes, the lesions are speckled.

Importantly, meningeal involvement, mostly asymptomatic, may be found in naevus of Ota, supporting the concept of a neurocristopathy.

On histological examination, scattered dendritic or spindle-shaped, heavily pigmented cells are present in the superficial and middermis, often including some degree of basal epidermal hyperpigmentation.

In contrast to mongolian spots, naevus of Ota and Ito do not tend to regress spontaneously. Malignant degeneration of naevus of Ota, involving the skin, eye (uveal melanoma), or meninges is rare, but has repeatedly been reported in the literature. It seems to be slightly more common in Caucasians [46].

Laser has become a therapeutic standard in naevus of Ota [24].

3.3.2.3 Blue Naevus

Blue naevi are defined as acquired, papular or nodular dermal melanocytic proliferations [57]. Congenital occurrence has been described, exceptionally presenting as a large plaque with leptomeningeal involvement (Fig. 3.3.11).

Clinically, blue naevi are characterized by a single circumscribed, flat to dome-shaped blue or black papule that develops in the second to fourth decade of life, somewhat more frequently in females. Blue naevi are preferentially

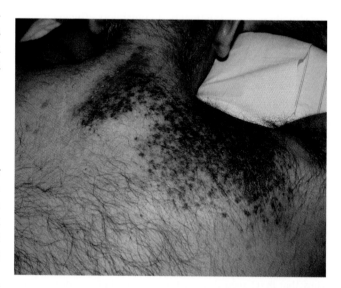

Fig. 3.3.11 Congenital, extensive plaque-type blue naevus on the shoulder of a 41-year-old male of Persian origin. Sudden, severe neurological problems led to the diagnosis of a diffuse leptomeningeal involvement. A spinal tumor was excised by laminectomy and revealed a melanocytic tumor of uncertain malignant potential. Following irradiation and 20 courses of temozolomide chemotherapy, the patient remained stable for 3 years. Then, a rapid deterioration with diffuse meningeal metastasis resulted in death

located on the extremities, especially the distal upper limbs, face, and scalp [53].

On histological examination, the number of pigmented, spindle-shaped or dendritic cells in the upper reticular and mid-dermis is variable, ranging from only a few cells interspersed between thickened collagen bundles to dense aggregates, concentrating around the adnexa. Blue naevus melanocytes nearly always react with HMB45, an antibody against early-stage melanosomes, which is also used as a nonspecific marker of melanoma.

It is tempting to speculate that blue naevi and cellular blue naevi (*vide infra*), analogous to superficial and deep congenital melanocytic naevi, represent neoplastic or hamartomatous proliferations of a special melanocyte subset, respectively. This subset is characterized by the ability to produce melanin independent from the presence of epidermal keratinocytes. Most recently, an oncogenic mutation of GNAQ, a protein involved in the protein kinase C pathway, has been identified as a common feature of blue naevus, naevus of Ota, and uveal melanoma [8].

3.3.2.3.1 Cellular Blue Naevus

Cellular blue naevi are usually larger than common blue naevi and are histologically characterized by dense dermal proliferations of oval or spindle-shaped cells growing in a tumor-like fashion [41, 51]. Congenital, very large plaques with leptomeningeal involvement are exceptional and probably represent neural crest hamartomas [27].

Cellular blue naevi have a predilection for the buttocks and the sacral region, but may occur on any site of the body. They develop in adolescence or young adulthood as blue–brown nodules or plaques, slowly growing to a size of one to several centimeters. In addition to the increased cellularity, cellular blue naevi differ from common blue naevi by the depth of invasion, often reaching the subcutaneous fat and even deeper tissue levels, including draining to regional lymph nodes. Epithelioid cellular blue naevi are recognized as a rare variant.

Although usually behaving in a benign fashion, cases with atypical histological features have been reported to result in systemic metastasis and death [4, 22]. Therefore, a complete excision should be performed.

The histopathological entity of "deep penetrating naevus" shares with blue naevi the presence of predominantly dermal, often deeply pigmented melanocytes. The cells are arranged in bundles or nests without maturation and exhibit a short spindle-shaped or rounded morphology. Sometimes, the cytological appearance focally reminds of Spitz naevi. Junctional naevus nests are a frequent finding, raising the differential diagnosis of a combined naevus. Malignant transformation has not been described.

3.3.2.4 Combined Naevus

A combined naevus in the narrow sense combines findings of a common acquired naevus with dermal changes of a blue naevus in one single lesion. The term has been extended to describe each intralesional combination of one or more distinct melanocytic naevus components [6]. These potentially include histological features of common naevi, dysplastic naevi, congenital-type naevi, blue naevi, Spitz naevi, and other rare variants. Histopathologically, combinations of different naevus types are infrequently, but regularly seen and do not necessarily raise suspicion of malignancy, unless clearly atypical changes are present. The main differential diagnosis is a focus of atypically differentiated cells in an otherwise normal naevus.

The clinical variability reflects the underlying histological patterns. Usually, combined naevi are excised under the diagnosis of atypical naevi in order to exclude melanoma.

3.3.2.5 Melanotic Macule, Simple Lentigo and Lentiginous Naevus

Melanotic macules, simple lentigines, and lentiginous naevi represent acquired, persistent, circumscribed melanocytic macules [45]. They all result from increased activity or proliferation of epidermal melanocytes and are histologically mostly confined to the epidermis. Multiple melanotic macules/lentigines occasionally point to distinct genetic syndromes (Peutz–Jeghers syndrome, LEOPARD syndrome, Carney complex) [11].

Melanotic macules may be found on the skin, the mucous membranes, and in the nail unit. Depending on anatomic location and UV factors, different clinical and histological entities have been defined.

One or multiple brown macules with irregular borders can be found on the vulvar and other female genital sites, most often the labia minora, on the glans penis or the penile shaft, and on the vermilion border of the lip. Similar macules may develop on the palms and soles of Black patients. Pigmented longitudinal streaks of the nail plate in mostly younger, dark-skinned persons represent a variant of melanotic macules.

UV-induced melanotic macules are persistent, brown to black spots with ragged borders that are found on the trunk after repeated and intense sun-exposure (reticulated black solar lentigines, PUVA lentigines [following Psoralen UVA-therapy, e.g., in psoriasis]).

Simple lentigines and lentiginous melanocytic naevi develop during childhood, adolescence or young adulthood as circumscribed brown macules with a diameter of 1–5 mm, mostly on the trunk and extremities.

Histologically, melanotic macules exhibit intense hyperpigmentation of the epidermis but only a slight, if at all perceptible increase in the number of melanocytes. Melanophages are often seen in the papillary dermis. In UV-induced melanotic macules, the basal hyperpigmentation is concentrated at the tips of the slightly elongated rete ridges and may show slight to moderate melanocytic hyperplasia with atypical nuclei, especially after prolonged PUVA therapy [40].

Differential diagnosis of melanotic macules in genital areas sometimes includes melanoma in situ. Clues to the diagnosis are derived from the degree of basal horizontal (lentiginous) spread and confluency of melanocytes, from an additional vertical ascension of melanocytes, and from the degree of cytological atypia.

Simple lentigines and lentiginous melanocytic naevi also exhibit intense hyperpigmentation of the epidermis, often including the stratum corneum, and melanophages in the papillary dermis. The number of basal melanocytes is increased, but as per definition, there is no horizontal confluency of basal melanocytes. The appearance of small nests of melanocytes ("naevus cells") at the tips of the rete ridges hallmarks the transition from a lentigo to a melanocytic naevus.

Melanotic macules, simple lentigines, and lentiginous naevi should be excised only if gross clinical examination or dermoscopy raise suspicion of melanoma.

3.3.2.6 Dysplastic Naevus

"Dysplasia" and "dysplastic naevi" represent ill-defined histopathological terms which are attributed to a group of benign melanocytic naevi with low malignant potential (for a review, see [39]). Besides the definitory problems with "congenital" naevi, this entity appears to be the WHO category with the highest potential for controversy. Due to the imprecise histomorphological definition, nearly every melanocytic naevus with fully developed junctional or dermoepidermal nests might be considered slightly "dysplastic" by some dermatopathologists. A significant level of discordance regarding the diagnosis of dysplasia and cytologic atypia has been repeatedly shown even among experienced dermatopathologists [20, 37]. Moreover, there is a lack of any other suitable WHO category for those (nonlentiginous) acquired melanocytic naevi formerly known as common melanocytic naevi. Consequently, though paradoxically, these naevi must be looked at as normal variants of dysplastic naevi. As a provisional term, the "dysplastic naevus" may be useful until new molecular markers allow a better distinction of naevus subtypes. The term "atypical naevus" is often used synonymously and highlights abnormal *clinical* findings. Atypical nevi and

melanomas share similar morphological features, which are commonly described by the ABCD rule (asymmetry, borders ill-defined or "fuzzy," color inhomogenous, diameter ≥5 mm). The presence of several of these parameters in a pigmentary lesion raises an increasing degree of suspicion for melanoma.

Dermoscopy offers a valuable additional source of morphological information. Several algorithms have been developed that allow a significantly better discrimination between naevi and melanoma than macroscopic clinical examination alone. Important features of dermoscopically atypical naevi (and possibly melanoma) include: (i) irregularities of the pigment network, (ii) simultaneous presence of different pigmented structures (network, globules, dots, homogeneous areas), (iii) presence of a blue–white veil, and iv) atypical vascular patterns [50].

Most individuals have essentially one or only a few different morphological "prototypes" of melanocytic naevi. The presence of a single pigmentary lesion that differs significantly from these prototypes has been called "ugly duckling sign" and is an independent, both clinically and dermoscopically valuable feature that should raise the attention of the clinician [25].

Naevi with histologically dysplastic features do not necessarily exhibit any of the mentioned atypical features and may look clinically normal [39]. However, compared to clinically normal naevi, the probability to find histological dysplasia is significantly higher in macroscopically and especially in dermoscopically atypical naevi. Moreover, the presence of >100 naevi and/or more than two clearly atypical, larger naevi (mostly on the back) correlates with a higher incidence of histological dysplasia in the naevi of an individual [36]. These features lack a clear mode of inheritance and are designated the "sporadic type" of the dysplastic naevus syndrome. The much rarer "familial type" affects families with germline mutations of the CDKN2a or CDK4 genes and carries an extremely high risk of melanoma [55].

Under the above premises, the clinical features of (histologically) dysplastic naevi may only be vaguely outlined. One single patient may have few to hundreds of mostly brown, red, or bicolored flat papules or plaques. They typically develop between childhood and the age of 30 and afterwards tend to persist or to gradually regress [31]. Dysplastic naevi may be present at any anatomic site, however, dysplasia is more frequently found in naevi from the trunk, scalp, buttocks, and the female breast.

By histology, dysplastic naevi show junctional melanocytic nests and single melanocytes at the tips and sides of elongated rete ridges, often adjacent to nests of naevus cells in the papillary dermis. Concentric fibrosis of the papillary dermis may be present ("stromal reaction"). The hallmarks of dysplasia are: i) atypical architecture (slight asymmetry, extension of a junctional "shoulder" beyond a dermal component, bridging of junctional nests and/or confluence of single basal melanocytes), and ii) facultative cytological abnormalities [42].

Genetic predisposition (in part reflected by skin color and sunburn sensitivity) and exposure to UV light are the most important etiologic determinants of dysplastic naevi as well as of lentiginous naevi [31]. Increased proliferation of junctional melanocytes due to BRAF mutations is the best characterized cytogenetic pathway associated with naevus development and appears to be a pathogenetic event shared by lentiginous and dysplastic naevi [38]. However, it has been assumed that both types of naevi significantly differ in their risk of transformation to melanoma. Whereas, this risk has been considered minimal for lentiginous naevi, the incidence of melanoma arising from any given dysplastic naevus has been estimated at 1:3,000 per year. It is well known that patients with melanoma have a significantly higher naevus count than matched controls [21]. Moreover, there is evidence that a higher degree of histopathological atypia in any excised naevus represents a marker of a higher individual melanoma risk [5]. However, until a more precise definition of the term "dysplasia" is available, any quantification of the risk meets definitory problems. Individuals with more than 50 melanocytic naevi, clinically or histologically atypical naevi or positive family history of melanoma should undergo a yearly macroscopic and dermoscopic whole-body examination. Any naevus with gross clinical or dermoscopic evidence of severe atypia should be excised.

3.3.2.7 Site-Specific and Meyerson Naevi

3.3.2.7.1 Acral Naevus

Acral naevi arise on the palms and soles. They are regarded as a separate entity because naevi on these body sites differ significantly from other types of naevi with respect to epidemiology, clinico-dermoscopic appearance and by their relationship to acral lentiginous melanoma.

By contrast to common melanocytic naevi in other locations, there is no clear racial predilection [16]. Acral naevi are present in 3–5% of the Caucasian population and are more commonly found in the second and third decades [33]. Incidences from some studies were higher in dark-skinned races [14], however, without histological confirmation acral naevi may be confounded with volar melanotic macules.

Following the dermatoglyphic pattern of volar skin, acral naevi clinically present as irregular brown macules. Dermoscopy greatly facilitates the differentiation of acral

naevi from acral melanoma, whereas, pigment is distributed in the dermal glyphic furrows in benign lesions, it is often accentuated along the dermatoglyphic ridges in melanoma [50].

Besides the typical histopathological features of volar skin, acral naevi often show asymmetry and intraepidermal upward spread of melanocytes, making these lesions facultative melanoma simulators. Severe cytological dysplasia and a dense lymphocytic infiltrate are important clues to the diagnosis of melanoma.

Even if acral naevi share epidemiological findings with acral-lentiginous melanoma, there is yet no indication that any single acral naevus has a higher risk to turn malignant than naevi at other locations. However, regarding their role as risk indicators [23] and in view of the serious prognosis of acral melanoma, regular monitoring of acral naevi is necessary. Excision is recommended if atypical clinical features raise the suspicion of melanoma.

3.3.2.7.2 Genital Naevus

Genital and perineal naevi, as well as flexural naevi and naevi of the phylogenetic "milk-line" from the axilla to the inner aspects of the thighs, often exhibit worrisome histological features [1]. These include an inhomogeneous distribution of nested or single melanocytes at the dermoepidermal junction, moderate asymmetry, and an intraepidermal ascent of melanocytic cell. However, these changes are usually situated above a well-maturating dermal naevus component. The lateral borders of genital naevi tend to be well-circumscribed.

Clinically, genital naevi present as dark-brown papules during the first three decades. Their incidence is higher in females. Routine prophylactic removal is not recommended.

3.3.2.7.3 Meyerson Naevus

Circumscribed spongiotic dermatitis affecting melanocytic naevi is a rare, but specific finding (Fig. 3.3.12). The changes may coincide with more widespread inflammatory skin diseases ("naevocentric dermatoses"), e.g., eczema, pityriasis rosea, and erythema multiforme. It is unknown why naevi are targeted by the inflammatory reaction.

One or several common melanocytic naevi get surrounded by a vesicular, later scaly erythema. Unlike in halo naevi, no reactive regression of the naevus cells is observed. Histopathology typically reveals changes of spongiotic dermatitis in the area of the naevus, including a considerable lymphocytic infiltrate.

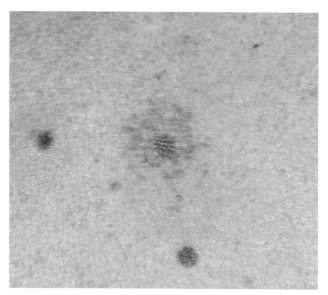

Fig. 3.3.12 Meyerson naevus on the back of a 39-year-old male with constitutive dry skin, clinically diagnosed as eczema

3.3.2.8 Persistent (Recurrent) Melanocytic Naevus

The well-known phenomenon of naevi recurring after incomplete excision or tissue destruction (e.g., by laser) is based on the persistence of mostly dermally located melanocytic cells. The recurrence of clinically visible changes is a dynamic process requiring active pigment production and proliferation of melanocytic cells, possibly originating from naevus remnants in the hair follicle.

Normally, the changes are observed about 6 months after the first excision. An irregularly outlined, speckled or striated brown macule or papule develops at the site of the scar. On histological examination, junctional hyperplasia of single melanocytes and small, often horizontally confluent melanocytic nests of different shapes are seen above an area of fibroplasia. Sometimes, dermal remnants of the former naevus are seen. The appearance may be very similar to regressive melanoma and has therefore been named "pseudomelanoma" [30]. The histopathological sections of the excised naevus should be revised in any case of doubt. A sharp lateral circumscription confined to the area of the scar is an important clue to the diagnosis of a benign, persistent naevus.

3.3.2.9 Spitz Naevus

Spitz naevi are predominant in children and adolescents and are characterized by a benign biological behavior despite of their atypical cytomorphological appearance.

Spitz naevi have been documented in all racial groups, mostly in the first two decades of life [47]. The prevalence of these naevi in adulthood might be underestimated because most pathologists assume Spitz naevi pediatric tumors and prefer the diagnosis of spitzoid melanoma in adults.

They clinically present as rapidly growing, dome-shaped, often reddish nodules on the face of children or on the proximal extremities of adolescents, although any anatomic site may be affected. Different degrees of pigmentation may be found. Growth stops typically at a diameter of 4–10 mm. Cases of a simultaneous eruption of several Spitz naevi in one region of the body have been repeatedly reported (agminated or eruptive Spitz naevi), raising suspicion of melanoma with satellite metastases.

On histologic examination, nests of large epithelioid, spindle-shaped or oval melanocytes with considerable cytological atypia are present at the dermoepidermal junction. The cells often exhibit abundant eosinophilic cytoplasm and large nuclei. The whole lesion is typically symmetrical and shows epidermal hyperplasia with intraepidermal eosinophilic globules ("Kamino bodies"). The histological spectrum of Spitz naevi includes compound and purely dermal forms as well as varying degrees of hyperpigmentation and desmoplasia. The differential diagnosis to melanoma in the absence of a classical clinical and pathological setting is often difficult. Criteria for melanoma are: i) asymmetry of the lesion, ii) pagetoid spread of atypical melanocytic cells, iii) absence of maturation at the dermal pole, iv) ulceration, and v) a high mitotic index [35].

Mutations of the HRAS gene have been demonstrated in a subset of Spitz naevi, whereas mutations of the BRAF gene are rarely found [9]. The unique histological characteristics point to the presence of one or several specific cytogenetic switches. The identification of such molecular markers would greatly facilitate the work of dermatopathologists.

Even if the lesion appears absolutely typical, the clinical suspicion of a Spitz naevus warrants complete excision.

3.3.2.10 Pigmented Spindle Cell Naevus (Reed)

Pigmented spindle cell naevi are commonly regarded as a heavily pigmented variant of Spitz naevi [7]. However, typical clinical and histological characteristics make these naevi a separate entity.

Reed naevi are most common in young adults and predominantly located on the limbs. A female predominance has been shown. Usually, the patients report rapid growth. On clinical examination, a dark brown, almost black papule up to 10 mm is seen. The dermoscopic picture shows radially arranged, pigmented streaks ("starburst pattern").

Histologically, spindle-shaped cells with abundant melanin deposits form vertically arranged nests at the dermo-epidermal junction, sometimes contiguous to nests in the papillary dermis. The epidermis may be thickened. Marked epidermal hyperpigmentation and melanophages are typical findings.

Reed naevi do not have malignant potential, however, due to the dark color and sometimes rapid growth an excision is usually the treatment of choice.

3.3.2.11 Halo Naevus

Halo naevi are induced by inflammatory changes in otherwise normal compound melanocytic naevi. They are frequently found in children, adolescents, and young adults. One or several melanocytic naevi begin to exhibit a rim of symmetrical peripheral whitening. After several weeks or months, the process leads to the disparition of the naevus, leaving an area of depigmentation behind.

At the site of depigmentation, the melanocytic cell nests of the upper dermis are intensely intermingled with a dense infiltrate of small, monomorphous lymphocytic cells. The inflammatory infiltrate is composed of T lymphocytes, including CD8+ T cells, and antigen presenting cells, suggesting a cytotoxic reaction against the naevus cells [56]. It is unknown why this response is limited to only one or few naevi of an individual. Especially in older patients, the histological differential diagnosis of melanoma with reactive inflammatory changes must be considered when severe cytological atypia and pagetoid intraepidermal ascension of atypical melanocytic cells is observed.

References

Disease Entities: Malignant Melanoma

1. Abbasi, N.R., Shaw, H.M., et al.: Early diagnosis of cutaneous melanoma: revisiting the ABCD criteria. JAMA **292**(22), 2771–2776 (2004)
2. Ackerman, A.B.: Criteria for histopathologic diagnosis of melanoma, including melanoma in situ, in historical perspective. J. Dermatol. **21**(11), 872–874 (1994)
3. Balch, C.M.: Cutaneous melanoma: prognosis and treatment results worldwide. Semin. Surg. Oncol. **8**(6), 400–414 (1992)
4. Balch, C.M., Buzaid, A.C., et al.: Final version of the American Joint Committee on Cancer staging system for cutaneous melanoma. J. Clin. Oncol. **19**(16), 3635–3648 (2001)
5. Balch, C.M., Gershenwald, J.E., et al.: Final version of 2009 AJCC melanoma staging and classification. J. Clin. Oncol. **20**, 6199–6206 (2009)
6. Balch, C.M., Soong, S.J., et al.: Prognostic factors analysis of 17,600 melanoma patients: validation of the American Joint Committee on Cancer melanoma staging system. J. Clin. Oncol. **19**(16), 3622–3634 (2001)
7. Banerjee, S.S., Harris, M.: Morphological and immunophenotypic variations in malignant melanoma. Histopathology **36**(5), 387–402 (2000)
8. Barnhill, R.L., Rabinovitz, H.: Benign melanocytic neoplasms. In: Bolognia, J.L., Jorizzo, J.L., Rapini, R.P. (eds.) Dermatology, 2nd edn. Mosby Elsevier, Philadelphia (2008)
9. Boni, R., Panizzon, R., et al.: Malignant blue naevus with distant subcutaneous metastasis. Clin. Exp. Dermatol. **21**(6), 427–430 (1996)
10. Breslow, A.: Thickness, cross-sectional areas and depth of invasion in the prognosis of cutaneous melanoma. Ann. Surg. **172**(5), 902–908 (1970)
11. Bulliard, J.L., De Weck, D., et al.: Detailed site distribution of melanoma and sunlight exposure: aetiological patterns from a Swiss series. Ann. Oncol. **18**(4), 789–794 (2007)
12. Busam, K.J., Jungbluth, A.A.: Melan-A, a new melanocytic differentiation marker. Adv. Anat. Pathol. **6**(1), 12–18 (1999)
13. Ceballos, P.I., Ruiz-Maldonado, R., et al.: Melanoma in children. N. Engl. J. Med. **332**(10), 656–662 (1995)
14. Clarkson, K.S., Sturdgess, I.C., et al.: The usefulness of tyrosinase in the immunohistochemical assessment of melanocytic lesions: a comparison of the novel T311 antibody (anti-tyrosinase) with S-100, HMB45, and A103 (anti-melan-A). J. Clin. Pathol. **54**(3), 196–200 (2001)
15. Crowson, A., Magro, C., et al.: The Melanocytic Proliferations: A Comprehensive Textbook of Pigmented Lesions. Wiley, New York (2001)
16. Curtin, J.A., Fridlyand, J., et al.: Distinct sets of genetic alterations in melanoma. N. Engl. J. Med. **353**(20), 2135–2147 (2005)
17. Dawson, H.A., Atherton, D.J., et al.: A prospective study of congenital melanocytic naevi: progress report and evaluation after 6 years. Br. J. Dermatol. **134**(4), 617–623 (1996)
18. Duhra, P., Ilchyshyn, A.: Prolonged survival in metastatic malignant melanoma associated with vitiligo. Clin. Exp. Dermatol. **16**(4), 303–305 (1991)
19. Dummer, R., Hauschild, A., et al.: Cutaneous malignant melanoma: ESMO clinical recommendations for diagnosis, treatment and follow-up. Ann. Oncol. **19**(suppl 2), ii86–ii88 (2008)
20. Dummer, R., Panizzon, R., et al.: Updated Swiss guidelines for the treatment and follow-up of cutaneous melanoma. Dermatology **210**(1), 39–44 (2005)
21. Egan, C.L., Oliveria, S.A., et al.: Cutaneous melanoma risk and phenotypic changes in large congenital nevi: a follow-up study of 46 patients. J. Am. Acad. Dermatol. **39**(6), 923–932 (1998)
22. Elwood, J.M., Gallagher, R.P.: Site distribution of malignant melanoma. Can. Med. Assoc. J. **128**(12), 1400–1404 (1983)
23. Elwood, J.M., Gallagher, R.P.: Body site distribution of cutaneous malignant melanoma in relationship to patterns of sun exposure. Int. J. Cancer **78**(3), 276–280 (1998)
24. Fetsch, P.A., Marincola, F.M., et al.: The new melanoma markers: MART-1 and Melan-A (the NIH experience). Am. J. Surg. Pathol. **23**(5), 607–610 (1999)
25. Franceschi, S., Levi, F., et al.: Site distribution of different types of skin cancer: new aetiological clues. Int. J. Cancer **67**(1), 24–28 (1996)
26. Friedman, R.J., Rigel, D.S., et al.: Early detection of malignant melanoma: the role of physician examination and self-examination of the skin. CA Cancer J. Clin. **35**(3), 130–151 (1985)
27. Gach, J.E., Carr, R.A., et al.: Multiple congenital melanocytic naevi presenting with neurofibroma-like lesions complicated by malignant melanoma. Clin. Exp. Dermatol. **29**(5), 473–476 (2004)

28. Goldenhersh, M.A., Savin, R.C., et al.: Malignant blue nevus. Case report and literature review. J. Am. Acad. Dermatol. **19**(4), 712–722 (1988)

29. Gown, A.M., Vogel, A.M., et al.: Monoclonal antibodies specific for melanocytic tumors distinguish subpopulations of melanocytes. Am. J. Pathol. **123**(2), 195–203 (1986)

30. Haffner, A.C., Garbe, C., et al.: The prognosis of primary and metastasising melanoma. An evaluation of the TNM classification in 2,495 patients. Br. J. Cancer **66**(5), 856–861 (1992)

31. Hale, E.K., Stein, J., et al.: Association of melanoma and neurocutaneous melanocytosis with large congenital melanocytic naevi–results from the NYU-LCMN registry. Br. J. Dermatol. **152**(3), 512–517 (2005)

32. Heenan, P.J., Ghaznawie, M.: The pathogenesis of local recurrence of melanoma at the primary excision site. Br. J. Plast. Surg. **52**(3), 209–213 (1999)

33. Heenan, P.J., Maize, J.C., et al.: Persistent melanoma and local metastasis of melanoma. In: LeBoit, E., Burg, G., Weedon, D., Sarasin, A. (eds.) World Health Organisation Classification of Tumors. Pathology and Genetics Skin Tumors. IARC, Lyon (2006)

34. Hendrickson, M.R., Ross, J.C.: Neoplasms arising in congenital giant nevi: morphologic study of seven cases and a review of the literature. Am. J. Surg. Pathol. **5**(2), 109–135 (1981)

35. Henze, G., Dummer, R., et al.: Serum S100–a marker for disease monitoring in metastatic melanoma. Dermatology **194**(3), 208–212 (1997)

36. Hofbauer, G.F., Kamarashev, J., et al.: Tyrosinase immunoreactivity in formalin-fixed, paraffin-embedded primary and metastatic melanoma: frequency and distribution. J. Cutan. Pathol. **25**(4), 204–209 (1998)

37. Hofbauer, G.F., Schaefer, C., et al.: MAGE-3 immunoreactivity in formalin-fixed, paraffin-embedded primary and metastatic melanoma: frequency and distribution. Am. J. Pathol. **151**(6), 1549–1553 (1997)

38. Huynh, P.M., Grant-Kels, J.M., et al.: Childhood melanoma: update and treatment. Int. J. Dermatol. **44**(9), 715–723 (2005)

39. Ka, V.S., Dusza, S.W., et al.: The association between large congenital melanocytic naevi and cutaneous melanoma: preliminary findings from an Internet-based registry of 379 patients. Melanoma Res. **15**(1), 61–67 (2005)

40. Kerl, H., Clemente, C., et al.: Melanoma arising in giant congenital naevi. In: LeBoit, E., Burg, G., Weedon, D., Sarasin, A. (eds.) World Health Organisation Classification of Tumors. Pathology and Genetics Skin Tumors. IARC, Lyon (2006)

41. Krengel, S., Hauschild, A., et al.: Melanoma risk in congenital melanocytic naevi: a systematic review. Br. J. Dermatol. **155**(1), 1–8 (2006)

42. Leech, S.N., Bell, H., et al.: Neonatal giant congenital nevi with proliferative nodules: a clinicopathologic study and literature review of neonatal melanoma. Arch. Dermatol. **140**(1), 83–88 (2004)

43. Legg, G.M.: Multiple melanoic sarcomata beginning in the choroid followed by pigmentation of the skin of the face and hands. Trans. Pathol. Soc. **35**, 367–372 (1984)

44. Levene, A.: On the histological diagnosis and prognosis of malignant melanoma. J. Clin. Pathol. **33**(2), 101–124 (1980)

45. Magro, C.M., Crowson, A.N., et al.: Unusual variants of malignant melanoma. Mod. Pathol. **19**(suppl 2), S41–S70 (2006)

46. Markovic, S.N., Erickson, L.A., et al.: Malignant melanoma in the 21st century, part 2: staging, prognosis, and treatment. Mayo Clin. Proc. **82**(4), 490–513 (2007)

47. Massi, G.: Melanocytic nevi simulant of melanoma with medicolegal relevance. Virchows Arch. **451**(3), 623–647 (2007)

48. Morton, D.L., Cochran, A.J., et al.: The rationale for sentinel-node biopsy in primary melanoma. Nat. Clin. Pract. Oncol. **5**(9), 510–511 (2008)

49. Morton, D.L., Thompson, J.F., et al.: Sentinel-node biopsy or nodal observation in melanoma. N. Engl. J. Med. **355**(13), 1307–1317 (2006)

50. Rao, B.N., Hayes, F.A., et al.: Malignant melanoma in children: its management and prognosis. J. Pediatr. Surg. **25**(2), 198–203 (1990)

51. Rose, C., Kaddu, S., et al.: A distinctive type of widespread congenital melanocytic nevus with large nodules. J. Am. Acad. Dermatol. **49**(4), 732–735 (2003)

52. Rosenberg, S.A., White, D.E.: Vitiligo in patients with melanoma: normal tissue antigens can be targets for cancer immunotherapy. J. Immunother. Emphasis Tumor Immunol. **19**(1), 81–84 (1996)

53. Ruiz-Maldonado, R., Tamayo, L., et al.: Giant pigmented nevi: clinical, histopathologic, and therapeutic considerations. J. Pediatr. **120**(6), 906–911 (1992)

54. Schmoeckel, C., Castro, C.E., et al.: Nevoid malignant melanoma. Arch. Dermatol. Res. **277**(5), 362–369 (1985)

55. Smoller, B.R., McNutt, N.S., et al.: HMB-45 recognizes stimulated melanocytes. J. Cutan. Pathol. **16**(2), 49–53 (1989)

56. Spatz, A., Avril, M.F.: Melanoma in childhood: review and perspectives. Pediatr. Dev. Pathol. **1**(6), 463–474 (1998)

57. Strouse, J.J., Fears, T.R., et al.: Pediatric melanoma: risk factor and survival analysis of the surveillance, epidemiology and end results database. J. Clin. Oncol. **23**(21), 4735–4741 (2005)

58. Tannous, Z.S., Mihm Jr., M.C., et al.: Congenital melanocytic nevi: clinical and histopathologic features, risk of melanoma, and clinical management. J. Am. Acad. Dermatol. **52**(2), 197–203 (2005)

59. Tate, P.S., Ronan, S.G., et al.: Melanoma in childhood and adolescence: clinical and pathological features of 48 cases. J. Pediatr. Surg. **28**(2), 217–222 (1993)

60. Wechsler, J., Bastuji-Garin, S., et al.: Reliability of the histopathologic diagnosis of malignant melanoma in childhood. Arch. Dermatol. **138**(5), 625–628 (2002)

61. Wlotzke, U., Hohenleutner, U., et al.: Malignant infiltrating blue nevus of the plaque type. Case report and literature review. Hautarzt **46**(12), 860–864 (1995)

62. Xu, X., Bellucci, K.S., et al.: Cellular nodules in congenital pattern nevi. J. Cutan. Pathol. **31**(2), 153–159 (2004)

63. Zembowicz, A., McCusker, M., et al.: Morphological analysis of nevoid melanoma: a study of 20 cases with a review of the literature. Am. J. Dermatopathol. **23**(3), 167–175 (2001)

Benign Melanocytic Tumors

1. Ackerman, A.B., Cerroni, L., Kerl, H.: Pitfalls in Histopathologic Diagnosis of Malignant Melanoma. Lea & Febiger, Philadelphia (1994)

2. Ackerman, A.B., Magana-Garcia, M.: Naming acquired melanocytic nevi. Unna's, Miescher's, Spitz's Clark's. Am. J. Dermatopathol. **12**, 193–209 (1990)

3. Akasu, R., Sugiyama, H., Araki, M., Ohtake, N., Furue, M., Tamaki, K.: Dermatoscopic and videomicroscopic features of melanocytic plantar nevi. Am. J. Dermatopathol. **18**(1), 10–18 (1996)

4. Aloi, F., Pich, A., Pippione, M.: Malignant cellular blue nevus: a clinicopathological study of 6 cases. Dermatology **192**, 36–40 (1996)

5. Arumi-Uria, M., McNutt, N.S., Finnerty, B.: Grading of atypia in nevi: correlation with melanoma risk. Mod. Pathol. **16**, 764–771 (2003)

6. Barnhill, R.L.: Melanocytic nevi with phenotypic heterogeneity. In: Barnhill, R.L., Piepkorn, M., Busam, K. (eds.) Pathology of Melanocytic Nevi and Malignant Melanoma, pp. 223–237. Springer, New York (2004)

7. Barnhill, R.L., Barnhill, M.A., Berwick, M., Mihm Jr., M.C.: The histologic spectrum of pigmented spindle cell nevus: a review of 120 cases with emphasis on atypical variants. Hum. Pathol. **22**, 52–58 (1991)

8. Bastian, B.C.: Frequent somatic mutations of GNAQ in uveal melanoma and intradermal melanocytic proliferations (abstract). In: Proceedings of the Annual Meeting of the American Association for Cancer Research, San Diego, CA (2008)

9. Bastian, B.C., LeBoit, P.E., Pinkel, D.: Mutations and copy number increase of HRAS in Spitz nevi with distinctive histopathological features. Am. J. Pathol. **157**, 967–972 (2000)

10. Bastian, B.C., Xiong, J., Frieden, I.J., Williams, M.L., Chou, P., Busam, K., Pinkel, D., LeBoit, P.E.: Genetic changes in neoplasms arising in congenital melanocytic nevi: differences between nodular proliferations and melanomas. Am. J. Pathol. **161**, 1163–1169 (2002)

11. Bauer, A.J., Stratakis, C.A.: The lentiginoses: cutaneous markers of systemic disease and a window to new aspects of tumorigenesis. J. Med. Genet. **42**, 801–810 (2005)

12. Bauer, J., Curtin, J.A., Pinkel, D., Bastian, B.C.: Congenital melanocytic nevi frequently harbor NRAS mutations but no BRAF mutations. J. Invest. Dermatol. **127**, 179–182 (2007)

13. Castilla, E.E., da Graça, D.M., Orioli-Parreiras, I.M.: Epidemiology of congenital pigmented naevi: I. Incidence rates and relative frequencies. Br. J. Dermatol. **104**, 307–315 (1981)

14. Coleman III, W.P., Gately III, L.E., Krementz, A.B., Reed, R.J., Krementz, E.T.: Nevi, lentigines, and melanomas in blacks. Arch. Dermatol. **116**, 548–551 (1980)

15. Cordova, A.: The Mongolian spot: a study of ethnic differences and a literature review. Clin. Pediatr. (Phila). **20**, 714–719 (1981)

16. Cullen, S.I.: Incidence of nevi. Report of survey of the palms, soles, and genitalia of 10,000 young men. Arch. Dermatol. **86**, 40–43 (1962)

17. Dadzie, O.E., Goerig, R., Bhawan, J.: Incidental microscopic foci of nevic aggregates in skin. Am. J. Dermatopathol. **30**, 45–50 (2008)

18. DeDavid, M., Orlow, S.J., Provost, N., Marghoob, A.A., Rao, B.K., Huang, C.L., Wasti, Q., Kopf, A.W., Bart, R.S.: A study of large congenital melanocytic nevi and associated malignant melanomas: review of cases in the New York University Registry and the world literature. J. Am. Acad. Dermatol. **36**, 409–416 (1997)

19. DeDavid, M., Orlow, S.J., Provost, N., Marghoob, A.A., Rao, B.K., Wasti, Q., Huang, C.L., Kopf, A.W., Bart, R.S.: Neurocutaneous melanosis: clinical features of large congenital melanocytic nevi in patients with manifest central nervous system melanosis. J. Am. Acad. Dermatol. **35**, 529–538 (1996)

20. Duray, P.H., DerSimonian, R., Barnhill, R., Stenn, K., Ernstoff, M.S., Fine, J., Kirkwood, J.M.: An analysis of interobserver recognition of the histopathologic features of dysplastic nevi from a mixed group of nevomelanocytic lesions. J. Am. Acad. Dermatol. **27**, 741–749 (1992)

21. Garbe, C., Krüger, S., Stadler, R., Guggenmoos-Holzmann, I., Orfanos, C.E.: Markers and relative risk in a German population for developing malignant melanoma. Int. J. Dermatol. **28**, 517–523 (1989)

22. Granter, S.R., McKee, P.H., Calonje, E., Mihm Jr., M.C., Busam, K.: Melanoma associated with blue nevus and melanoma mimicking cellular blue nevus: a clinicopathologic study of 10 cases on the spectrum of so-called 'malignant blue nevus'. Am. J. Surg. Pathol. **25**, 316–323 (2001)

23. Green, A., McCredie, M., MacKie, R., Giles, G., Young, P., Morton, C., Jackman, L., Thursfield, V.: A case-control study of melanomas of the soles and palms (Australia and Scotland). Cancer Causes Control **10**, 21–25 (1999)

24. Hague, J.S., Lanigan, S.W.: Laser treatment of pigmented lesions in clinical practice: a retrospective case series and patient satisfaction survey. Clin. Exp. Dermatol. **33**, 139–141 (2008)

25. Hofmann-Wellenhof, R., Blum, A., Wolf, I.H., Piccolo, D., Kerl, H., Garbe, C., Soyer, H.P.: Dermoscopic classification of atypical melanocytic nevi (Clark nevi). Arch. Dermatol. **137**, 1575–1580 (2001)

26. Ichii-Nakato, N., Takata, M., Takayanagi, S., Takashima, S., Lin, J., Murata, H., Fujimoto, A., Hatta, N., Saida, T.: High frequency of BRAFV600E mutation in acquired nevi and small congenital nevi, but low frequency of mutation in medium-sized congenital nevi. J. Invest. Dermatol. **126**, 2111–2118 (2006)

27. Iemoto, Y., Kondo, Y.: Congenital giant cellular blue nevus resulting in dystocia. Arch. Dermatol. **120**, 798–799 (1984)

28. Kikuchi, I.: Mongolian spots remaining in schoolchildren a statistical survey in Central Okinawa. J. Dermatol. **7**, 213–216 (1980)

29. Kinsler, V.A., Chong, W.K., Aylett, S.E., Atherton, D.J.: Complications of congenital melanocytic naevi in children: analysis of 16 years' experience and clinical practice. Br. J. Dermatol. **159**, 907–914 (2008)

30. Kornberg, R., Ackerman, A.B.: Pseudomelanoma: recurrent melanocytic nevus following partial surgical removal. Arch. Dermatol. **111**, 1588–1590 (1975)

31. Krengel, S.: Nevogenesis–new thoughts regarding a classical problem. Am. J. Dermatopathol. **27**, 456–465 (2005)

32. Krengel, S., Hauschild, A., Schäfer, T.: Melanoma risk in congenital melanocytic naevi: a systematic review. Br. J. Dermatol. **155**, 1–8 (2006)

33. MacKie, R.M., English, J., Aitchison, T.C., Fitzsimons, C.P., Wilson, P.: The number and distribution of benign pigmented moles (melanocytic naevi) in a healthy British population. Br. J. Dermatol. **113**, 167–174 (1985)

34. Makkar, H.S., Frieden, I.J.: Neurocutaneous melanosis. Semin. Cutan. Med. Surg. **23**, 138–144 (2004)

35. Mooi, W.J.: Spitz nevus and its histologic simulators. Adv. Anat. Pathol. **9**, 209–221 (2002)

36. Newton, J.A.: Familial melanoma. Clin. Exp. Dermatol. **18**, 5–11 (1993)

37. Piepkorn, M.W., Barnhill, R.L., Cannon-Albright, L.A., Elder, D.E., Goldgar, D.E., Lewis, C.M., Maize, J.C., Meyer, L.J., Rabkin, M.S., Sagebiel, R.W., Skolnick, M.H., Zone, J.J.: A multiobserver, population-based analysis of histologic dysplasia in melanocytic nevi. J. Am. Acad. Dermatol. **30**, 707–714 (1994)

38. Pollock, P.M., Spurr, N., Bishop, T., Newton-Bishop, J., Gruis, N., van der Velden, P.A., Goldstein, A.M., Tucker, M.A., Foulkes, W.D., Barnhill, R., Haber, D., Fountain, J., Hayward, N.K.: Haplotype analysis of two recurrent CDKN2A mutations in 10 melanoma families: evidence for common founders and independent mutations. Hum. Mutat. **11**, 424–431 (1998)

39. Rabkin, M.S.: The limited specificity of histological examination in the diagnosis of dysplastic nevi. J. Cutan. Pathol. **35**(2), 20–23 (2008)

40. Rhodes, A.R., Harrist, T.J., Momtaz, T.K.: The PUVA-induced pigmented macule: a lentiginous proliferation of large, sometimes cytologically atypical, melanocytes. J. Am. Acad. Dermatol. **9**, 47–58 (1983)

41. Rodriguez, H.A., Ackerman, L.V.: Cellular blue nevus. Clinicopathologic study of forty-five cases. Cancer **21**, 393–405 (1968)

42. Roth, M.E., Grant-Kels, J.M., Ackerman, A.B., Elder, D.E., Friedman, R.J., Heilman, E.R., Maize, J.C., Sagebiel, R.W.: The histopathology of dysplastic nevi. Continued controversy. Am. J. Dermatopathol. **13**, 38–51 (1991)

43. Ruiz-Maldonado, R.: Measuring congenital melanocytic nevi. Pediatr. Dermatol. **21**, 178–179 (2004)

44. Ruiz-Maldonado, R., Tamayo, L., Laterza, A.M., Durán, C.: Giant pigmented nevi: clinical, histopathologic, and therapeutic considerations. J. Pediatr. **120**, 906–911 (1992)

45. Sanchez, J.L.: A unifying concept of melanotic macule. Dermatopathology **4**, 120–123 (1998)

46. Shaffer, D., Walker, K., Weiss, G.R.: Malignant melanoma in a Hispanic male with nevus of Ota. Dermatology **185**, 146–150 (1992)

47. Shapiro, P.E.: Spitz nevi. J. Am. Acad. Dermatol. **29**, 667–668 (1993)

48. Sigg, C., Pelloni, F., Schnyder, U.W.: Frequency of congenital nevi, nevi spili and café-au-lait spots and their relation to nevus count and skin complexion in 939 children. Dermatologica **180**, 118–123 (1990)

49. Stanford, D.G., Georgouras, K.E.: Dermal melanocytosis: a clinical spectrum. Australas. J. Dermatol. **37**, 19–25 (1996)

50. Steiner, A., Binder, M., Schemper, M., Wolff, K., Pehamberger, H.: Statistical evaluation of epiluminescence microscopy criteria for melanocytic pigmented skin lesions. J. Am. Acad. Dermatol. **29**, 581–588 (1993)

51. Temple-Camp, C.R., Saxe, N., King, H.: Benign and malignant cellular blue nevus. A clinicopathological study of 30 cases. Am. J. Dermatopathol. **10**, 289–296 (1988)

52. Tiede, S., Kloepper, J.E., Bodò, E., Tiwari, S., Kruse, C., Paus, R.: Hair follicle stem cells: walking the maze. Eur. J. Cell Biol. **86**, 355–376 (2007)

53. Toppe, F., Haas, N.: Blue nevus – clinical aspects and variants. Z. Hautkr. **62**, 1214–1223 (1987)

54. Tromberg, J., Bauer, B., Benvenuto-Andrade, C., Marghoob, A.A.: Congenital melanocytic nevi needing treatment. Dermatol. Ther. **18**, 136–150 (2005)

55. Tucker, M.A., Fraser, M.C., Goldstein, A.M., Struewing, J.P., King, M.A., Crawford, J.T., Chiazze, E.A., Zametkin, D.P., Fontaine, L.S., Clark Jr., W.H.: A natural history of melanomas and dysplastic nevi: an atlas of lesions in melanoma-prone families. Cancer **94**, 3192–3209 (2002)

56. Zeff, R.A., Freitag, A., Grin, C.M., Grant-Kels, J.M.: The immune response in halo nevi. J. Am. Acad. Dermatol. **37**, 620–624 (1997)

57. Zembowicz, A., Mihm, M.C.: Dermal dendritic melanocytic proliferations: an update. Histopathology **45**, 433–451 (2004)

Cutaneous Lymphoma, Leukemia and Related Disorders

3.4

Günter Burg, Werner Kempf, Reinhard Dummer, and Mirjana Urosevic-Maiwald

3.4.1 Mature T-Cell and NK-Cell Neoplasms*

Günter Burg, Werner Kempf, and Reinhard Dummer

3.4.1.1 Mycosis Fungoides

3.4.1.1.1 Definition

Mycosis fungoides (MF) is a general indolent peripheral T-cell lymphoma initially and preferentially present in the skin and showing distinct clinical, histological (except in early stages), immunophenotypical, and genotypical features. It is the most common cutaneous lymphoma [75, 100], characterized by the sequential appearance of patches, developing into plaques and finally into tumors, which tend to ulcerate.

3.4.1.1.2 ICD-O Code

9700/3

3.4.1.1.3 Synonyms

WHO/EORTC classification (2005): Mycosis fungoides
WHO classification (2001): Mycosis fungoides
REAL classification (1997): Mycosis fungoides
EORTC classification (1997): Mycosis fungoides

3.4.1.1.4 Clinical Features

Men are more frequently affected than women (male: female ratio, 2–4:1) [101, 152] showing a prevalence during the 5th–6th decades of life, although any age group may be involved. Revisions to the staging and classification of mycosis fungoides and Sezary syndrome has been elaborated by the International Society for Cutaneous Lymphomas (ISCL) and the cutaneous lymphoma task force of the European Organization of Research and Treatment of Cancer (EORTC) [125]. Mostly, the disease starts with nonspecific very unconspicuous scaly lesions resembling, chronic dermatitis, parapsoriasis, tinea corporis or other inflammatory dermatoses. Pruritus is common and often severe. Patients also may present with more distinctive irregular, well-circumscribed, scaling patches varying in size from 2–3 to 10–15 cm. The number of lesions is also variable. In some cases, the patches show a tendency to partial remission, spontaneously or due to topical treatment. This feature in combination with peripheral growth, leads to the development of lesions with unusual configurations (annular, concentric, semicircular, serpiginous) (Fig. 3.4.1). It usually takes several years until the patches progress into plaques and tumors, which may then ulcerate (Fig. 3.4.2). A subset of patients have persistent patch-stage disease without reduction of their survival time. Lymph nodes and internal organs may become involved in the later stages of MF. In the advanced stages, progression to a high-grade T-cell lymphoma is observed in approximately 25% of cases and is usually associated with an aggressive clinical course. Involvement of the mucosal tissue is rare [69].

3.4.1.1.5 Histopathology

In very early stages, there is nothing but a mild perivascular infiltrate in the upper dermis containing no atypical lymphocytes and lacking epidermotropism, rendering the histologic

G. Burg (✉)
Department of Dermatology, University Hospital of Zürich, Gloriastr. 31, 8091 Zürich, Switzerland
e-mail: g.burg@access.uzh.ch

W. Kempf
Kempf und Pfaltz, Histologische Diagnostik, Zürich, Switzerland

R. Dummer and M. Uroseric-Maiwald
Department of Dermatology, University Hospital of Zürich, Gloriastrasse 31, 8091 Zürich,
Switzerland
e-mail: reinhard.dummer@usz.ch; mirjana.urosevic@usz.ch

*all diagnostic terms follow the WHO Classification of Tumors of Haematopoietic and Lymphoid Tissues, Eds.: S. Swedlow et al., 4th Edition 2008

R. Dummer et al. (eds.), *Skin Cancer – A World-Wide Perspective*,
DOI: 10.1007/978-3-642-05072-5_3.4, © Springer-Verlag Berlin Heidelberg 2011

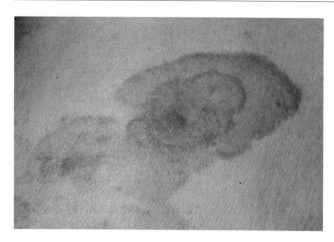

Fig. 3.4.1 Plaque stage mycosis fungoides, showing concentric features following temporary regression. Pagetoid reticulosis: sharply demarcated erythematous and scaling plaque on the foot

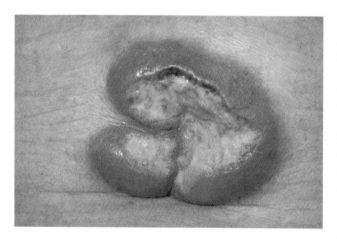

Fig. 3.4.2 Ulcerated tumorous lesion of mycosis fungoides

picture nonspecific [140, 141, 145]. Early MF can produce practically all of the patterns found in the diagnosis of inflammatory skin disease. The histological findings become diagnostic in the thin plaque stage (Fig. 3.4.3a, b). Lymphocytes are lining up in the basal layer and single-cell epidermotropism or sometimes small clusters of lymphocytes can be seen in the epidermis. The majority of cells are small, well-differentiated lymphocytes with round or only slightly cerebriform nuclei. However, there are no specific cytologic criteria discriminating tumor cells from normal lymphocytes. There can be mild acanthosis, hyperkeratosis, signs of basal layer damage (pigment incontinence), edema or fibrosis of the papillary dermis (Fig. 3.4.4a), and proliferation of postcapillary venules. The infiltrate may contain

an admixture of eosinophils, plasma cells, macrophages, and dermal dendritic cells [70].

The plaque stage is typified by a dense, subepidermal, usually band-like infiltrate containing cerebriform cells. Epidermotropism is more prominent with small intraepidermal clusters (2–3 cells) of lymphocytes (Pautrier microabscesses), which may be seen in approximately one-third of cases. Collections of atypical lymphocytes in the dermis are found in some cases.

In the tumor stage, the infiltrate is nodular or diffuse. Epidermotropism usually is lost. In addition to a predominant population of small cerebriform cells, there is a variable admixture of immunoblasts, lymphoblasts, and medium-sized or large pleomorphic or anaplastic cells (Fig. 3.4.4b).

Because MF develops slowly over several years and may have a variety of clinical presentations, it may be a diagnostic challenge, especially in the early stages which may be confused with common benign conditions such as eczema and psoriasis [136]. Therefore, clinical appraisal plus the presence of characteristic histopathologic features are needed to ensure accurate diagnosis [138].

Immunophenotypically, MF is a disease of T-helper 2 (TH2) lymphocytes expressing T-cell-associated antigens (*CD2+, CD3+, CD5+, CD4+, CD8−, CD7−, CD30−, CD45RO+, bF1+*) and clonally rearranged T-cell receptor (TCR) genes. The cytokines produced by the tumor cells (IL-4, IL-5, IL-10) [54, 165] account for the many systemic changes associated with MF, such as eosinophilia, increase of IgE or IgA, and impaired delayed-type reactivity.

3.4.1.1.6 Prognosis and Predictive Factors

The prognosis of the disease is defined by its stage. Patients with early stages have an excellent prognosis with survival similar to that of an age-, sex-, and race-matched population [51, 102, 171]. The type of skin disease present at initial diagnosis is a good prognostic indicator of survival and clinical outcome. Factors indicating poor prognosis are advanced stage and age above 60 years. When extracutaneous involvement of blood, lymph nodes or internal organs or transformation into high-grade lymphoma occurs, suspected survival is usually less than 1 year [157]. The most significant prognostic factors seem to be the patient's duration of symptoms and stage of disease at presentation [152]. It has been speculated that expression of CD44v6 may be helpful as a prognostic marker for assessing the potential for extracutaneous spread and homing behavior of the neoplastic cells.

Fig. 3.4.3 Mycosis fungoides.
(**a**) (*Upper*) nonspecific
eczematous patch stage.
H & E stain 40×. (**b**) (*Lower*)
plaque stage showing diagnostic
features like atypical cells
travelling into the epidermis
(epidermotropism). H & E
stain 10×

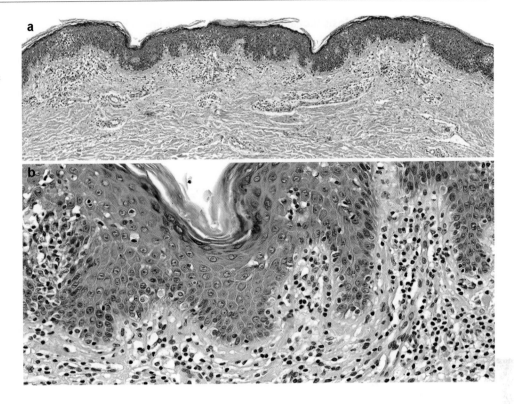

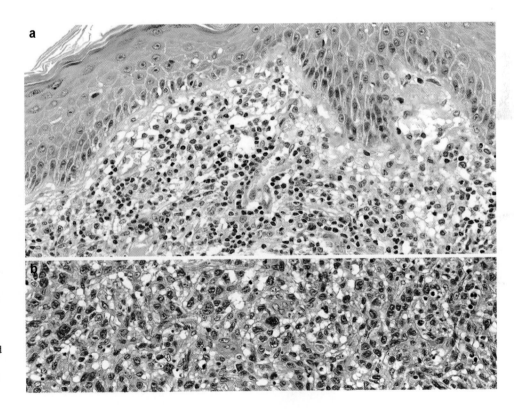

Fig. 3.4.4 Mycosis fungoides.
(**a**) (*Upper*) edema in the
papillary dermis and dilated
postcapillary venules. H & E,
40×. (**b**) (*Lower*) medium-sized
and large pleomorphic or
anaplastic cells in the tumorius
infiltrate. H & E, 63×

3.4.1.1.7 Pagetoid Reticulosis (Localized Disease)

Definition

Pagetoid reticulosis (PR) is a low grade malignant variant of mycosis fungoides (MF) with characteristic histologic features, but various phenotypes. In 1931 Ketron and Goodman described multiple lesions of the skin "apparently of epithelial origin" clinically resembling mycosis fungoides [99]. In 1939, Woringer and Kolopp reported a solitary plaque-like lesion on the arm of a 6-year old boy [168]. The term "pagetoid reticulosis" was proposed by Braun-Falco and colleagues because of the clinical and the histological appearance [23]. Most experts today consider disseminated PR a form of MF or cytotoxic epidermotropic T-cell lymphoma. The localized form of PR (Woringer Kolopp disease) is regarded as "superficial spreading" form of MF. In our opinion, only the localized form should be referred to as PR in a strict sense.

ICD-O Code

9700/3

Synonyms

WHO/EORTC (2005): Pagetoid reticulosis
WHO (2001): Not listed
REAL (1997): Not listed
EORTC (1997): Pagetoid reticulosis

Clinical Features

The localized classical Woringer-Kolopp form of PR presents as a solitary sharply demarcated psoriasiform or bowenoid erythematous, scaling or crusty plaque, exhibiting centrifugal growth [26] (Fig. 3.4.5a). The sites of predilection are the acral body areas. In contrast to MF, PR never spreads to other sites of the body, to lymph nodes, peripheral blood, internal organs or bone marrow.

Histology

The epidermis usually shows marked psoriasiform hyperplasia with para- and orthohyperkeratosis, [119] or may be atrophic in some cases. A sponge-like disaggregation of the acanthotic epidermis by medium-sized to large atypical lymphoid cells with vacuolated, abundant cytoplasm, singly or arranged in clusters, is the hallmark of PR [50] (Fig. 3.4.5b). In contrast to classical MF, more tumor cells are on the epidermis than in the dermis. The nuclei are large, hyperchromatic and sometimes convoluted resembling lymphoblasts rather than small cerebriform lymphocytes. Mitotic figures are rare. Single cells and small clusters of tumor cells can also be observed within the epithelia of adnexal structures. Towards the center of the lesion, the diffuse bandlike infiltrate increasingly involves the upper dermis. At the margins of the lesion, tumor cells are mostly found in the lower third of the epidermis.

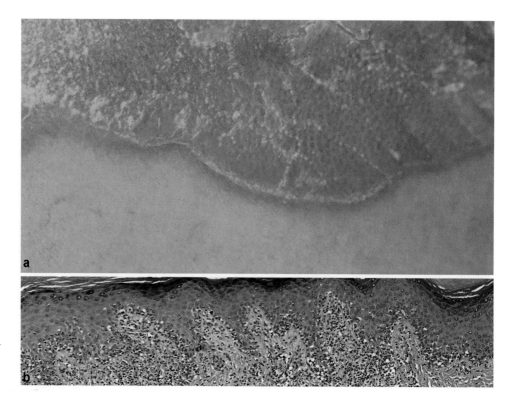

Fig. 3.4.5 Pagetoid reticulosis. (**a**) (*Upper*) solitary sharply demarcated psoriasiform plaque. (**b**) (*Lower*) pronounced epidermotropismus of lymphoid cells. H & E, 10×

Immunohistochemistry

The neoplastic cells in PR may express CD4, CD8 or be CD4/CD8 double negative. Most cases of PR express a T helper phenotype: CD3+, CD4+, CD5+, and CD8– [91]. There are reports on CD8+ cases [50, 71] or PR expressing a gamma/delta phenotype [19]. When stained for Ki67 the neoplastic cells demonstrate a higher proliferation rate in comparison to lymphocytes in the patch or plaque stage MF. The pronounced epidermotropism of neoplastic lymphocytes in PR may be explained by their strong expression of adhesion molecule alpha E beta 7 which interacts with E-cadherin on keratinocytes and the expression of cutaneous lymphocyte antigen, a skin-homing receptor interacting with E-selectin on cutaneous endothelial cells.

Prognosis and Predictive Factors

By definition, the classical localized form of PR is a solitary, locally spreading form of MF without any extracutaneous involvement. Therefore, in contrast to other CTCL, PR exhibits an excellent prognosis [108]. Recurrences after complete removal by locally aggressive procedures like surgery or X-rays seem to be rare.

3.4.1.1.8 Folliculotropic (Follicular), Syringotropic, Granulomatous Variants

Definition

Mycosis fungoides due to its variants [72, 95] may be a dermatological masquerader [123]. Follicular, syringotropic and granulomatous forms of Mycosis fungoides in the WHO/EORTC classification like Pagetoid reticulosis are referred to as variants of MF, since while exhibiting peculiar clinical and histologic features they show similar, phenotypic and genotypic profile like classical MF.

ICD-O Code

9700/3

Synonyms

WHO/EORTC classification (2005): Mycosis fungoides
WHO classification (2001): Mycosis fungoides
REAL classification (1997): Mycosis fungoides
EORTC classification (1997): Mycosis fungoides

Clinical Features and Histopathology

The clinical and histologic criteria to distinguish MF associated with follicular mucinosis from follicular MF are a matter of debate. The term "folliculotropic," which is better than "follicular" and also corresponds to the term "syringotropic," describes a particular histopathologic finding [153].

More than 80% of the patients have involvement of the face, head, and neck. The morphologic spectrum of lesions is broad and includes erythematous papules (Fig. 3.4.6a) and plaques with or without alopecia; there may be acneiform, cystic lesions or prurigo-like lesions [64, 123]. *Histologically,* folliculotropic MF may present with a broad spectrum of histopathologic changes including interstitial, granulomatous, fibrotic and acneiform reactions; there is folliculotropism of lymphocytes in the absence or presence of mild epidermotropism, with or without intrafollicular mucin [63, 153].

In *Syringotropic MF* remarkably, all patients reported to date have been men. The lesions are usually a few red–brown patches, slightly infiltrated scaling plaques or small red or skin-colored papules. Anhidrosis and hair loss in the affected areas are common.

Histologically, there is a periadnexal infiltrate composed of small cerebriform lymphocytes invading both the secretory and ductal portions of hyperplastic eccrine glands (Fig. 3.4.6b). Epidermotropism is not a prominent feature and Pautrier microabscesses are usually absent. Hair follicles may be concurrently involved resulting in alopecia. Follicular mucinosis is absent [33, 172].

Granulomatous features of various degrees are seen in about 10% of well differentiated CTCL (MF and Sézary syndrome). There are no distinct clinical features. *Histologically,* it may present as interstitial granulomatous dermatitis [49] or as sheets or clusters of giant cells. These features, which also may be seen in folliculotropic MF [123], can clearly be differentiated from the dissolute distribution of large single giant cells in granulomatous slack skin, which is a subtype of MF.

Prognosis and Predictive Factors

Folliculotropic MF seems to have a poorer prognosis than classic MF [64]. The prognosis of *syringotropic* MF due to the few cases is difficult to assess, but mostly has been reported as excellent and locally aggressive removal of single lesions using surgery or X-rays may result in complete healing. The prognostic impact of *granulomatous* features in MF remains an issue of debate [107].

Fig. 3.4.6 (**a**) Folliculotropic mycosis fungoides, showing erythematous papules. (**b**) Syringotropic mycosis fungoides with periadnexal lymphoid infiltrates. H & E, 40×

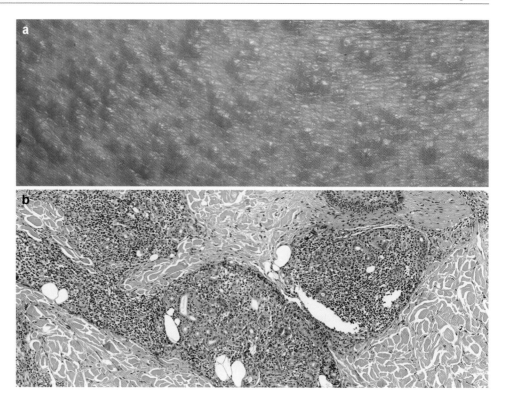

3.4.1.1.9 Granulomatous Slack Skin (GSS)

Definition

Granulomatous slack skin (GSS) is a rare granulomatous form of mycosis fungoides with pathognomonic clinical and histologic features, which has led to its designation as subtype.

ICD-O Code

9700/3

Synonyms

WHO/EORTC classification (2005): Granulomatous slack skin (subtype of mycosis fungoides)
WHO classification (2001): Not listed
REAL classification (1997): Not listed
EORTC classification (1997): Granulomatous slack skin

Clinical Features

The clinical hallmarks are the formation of skin folds, preferentially in the axillary region and the groin due to loss of elastic tissue, which is ingested by mononuclear giant cells. The clinical condition was first described in 1968 by Bazex as "Chalazodermic Besnier-Boeck-Schaumann disease" [11] and then by Convit as "progressive atrophying chronic granulomatous dermohypodermitis" [43]. A.B. Ackerman introduced the term "granulomatous slack skin" in 1978 [1]. The disease starts with slightly infiltrated, poikilodermatous plaques, preferentially in the intertriginous body areas, especially the axillary and groins. Finally, bulky pendulous skin folds develop (Fig. 3.4.7a).

GSS is seen almost exclusively in Whites and manifests usually in the third or fourth decades of life. The disease has also been reported in young children [36], finally resulting in death [121]. Men are more often affected than women.

Histopathology

Early lesions of GSS show a bandlike infiltrate of small lymphocytes without significant nuclear atypia. Numerous scattered multinucleated giant cells containing up to 40 nuclei are a hallmark (Fig. 3.4.7b, c). Elastophagocytosis and emperipolesis, i.e., phagocytosis of lymphoid cells by giant cells, are present. Elastic stains demonstrate the loss of elastic fibers within the infiltrates. More advanced lesions exhibit a dense lymphocytic infiltrate throughout the entire dermis. While some lymphoid cells may have cerebriform nuclei, nuclear atypia is less pronounced than in granulomatous MF. Histologic evidence of necrobiosis has been reported [16].

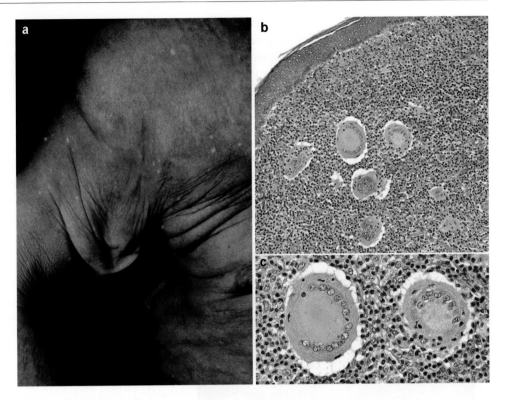

Fig. 3.4.7 Granulomatous slack skin. (**a**) Large skin folds in the axilla. (**b**, **c**) Multinucleated giant cells with nuclear dust ingested within a lymphoid infiltrate. H & E, 10× and 63×

Immunocytochemically, lymphoid tumor cells express CD4, CD45RO and show clonal T-cell receptor-gamma gene rearrangement [15]. Rarely expression of CD30 is found. The giant cells are of histiocytic origin and thus are positive for histiocytic markers such as CD68 and Mac387. The cytogenetic findings are unlike those as described for mycosis fungoides and suggest that granulomatous slack skin is a distinct primary cutaneous T-cell lymphoma [76].

Prognosis and Predictive Factors

Less than 50 patients have been reported so far. The disease usually runs an indolent, slowly progressive course over decades. Extracutaneous spread is rare. Occasionally, granulomatous lymphoadenopathy showing clonal rearrangement occurs [15]. The disease by itself does not reduce life expectancy: however other cutaneous and nodal lymphomas occur in approximately 20% of the patients, obscuring the prognosis [121, 124].

3.4.1.2 Sézary Syndrome (SS)

3.4.1.2.1 Definition

Sézary Syndrome (SS)

Sezary syndrome (SS) [75, 100] is a rare (incidence about 2% of all cutaneous lymphomas) variant of cutaneous T-cell lymphoma (CTCL), characterized by distinct clinical and hematologic features and a poor prognosis. It starts primarily as erythroderma and has to be differentiated from secondary erythroderma evolving from mycosis fungoides. Differentiation also has to be made from erythrodermas, arising from nonlymphomatous dermatologic conditions, like drug reactions, atopic dermatitis, pityriasis rubra pilaris, generalized lichen planus, and others. Coexistence with B-cell chronic lymphocytic leukemia has been reported in one case [88].

3.4.1.2.2 ICD-O Code

9701/3

3.4.1.2.3 Synonyms

WHO/EORTC classification (2005): Sézary syndrome
WHO classification (2001): Sézary syndrome
REAL classification (1997): Sézary syndrome
EORTC classification (1997): Sézary syndrome

3.4.1.2.4 Clinical Features

The typical features, described by von Zumbusch [161], later on by Sezary [161] and Baccaredda [8] have been reviewed [97]. An international working group [162, 163] has elaborated the criterias, consisting of erythroderma (Fig. 3.4.8) and circulating atypical lymphoid cells expressing the TH2-phenotype [55, 164] at a concentration of over 1,000 per mL blood. Additional symptoms are edematous swelling of the skin, itching, adenopathy of peripheral lymph nodes, hair loss, dystrophy of nails and hyperkeratosis of palms and soles and almost incurable itching. In advanced stages of the disease, tumorous transformation may occur (Fig. 3.4.8 Inset). Besides a more exfoliative type of erythroderma (Wilson-Brocq), showing dry and coarse scaling, the pityriasis rubra type of Hebra-Jadassohn has been identified, which shows brownish or dark-red discoloration of the skin with fine

scaling of the rather thin and atrophic skin, corresponding to the "homme rouge" of Hallopeau.

3.4.1.2.5 Histopathology

The epidermis is acanthotic in most cases with little or no spongiosis. In the papillary dermis, however, there is prominent edema (Fig. 3.4.9a), which helps to differentiate SS from more "dry" forms of erythroderma like in atopic dermatitis; later on fibrosis develops in the papillary dermis. Like in other CTCL, a subepidermal band-like infiltrate composed of predominantly small atypical lymphocytes, is a diagnostic hallmark. They cluster preferentially around the tips of the rete ridges. However, it is nonspecific in one third of the cases; Pautrier's microabscesses are seen only in half of the cases [158]. In advanced stages, large atypical cells occur, indicating transformation into higher malignant blast stage (Fig. 3.4.9b). There is little difference to the features of mycosis fungoides in plaque stage [87].

Immunophenotypically tumor cells in SS express a T helper phenotype (*CD2+, CD3+, CD4+ > CD8+, CD5+, CD7−, CD45RO+, CD30−*) and cutaneous lymphocyte antigen (CLA). Loss of T-cell antigens, mostly CD2, is seen in two-thirds of the cases [73]. The lack of T(reg)-cells (FOXP3) in Sézary syndrome may account for the more aggressive nature of Sezary syndrome compared with other CTCL [103].

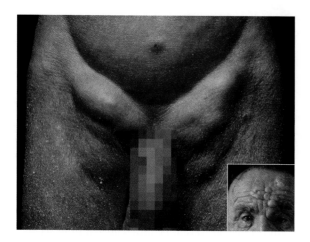

Fig. 3.4.8 Erythroderma and lymphadenopathy in a patient with Sézary syndrome

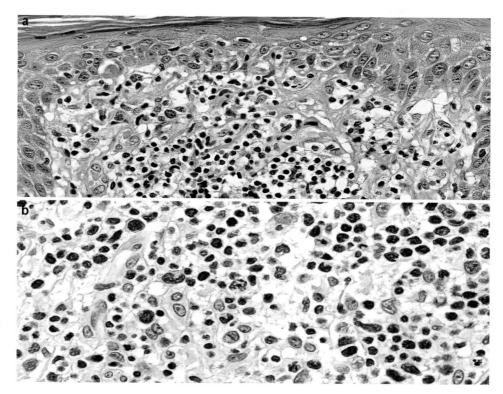

Fig. 3.4.9 Sézary syndrome. (**a**) subepidermal infiltrate and edema. H & E, 10×. (**b**) Pleomorphic infiltrate, composed of cerebriform small cells and large atypical cells, indicating transformation into higher malignancy. H & E, 63×

3.4.1.2.6 Prognosis and Predictive Factors

The prognosis of SS is worse than in mycosis fungoides showing about 20% vs. almost 90% 5-year-survival rate in SS and MF, respectively. The prognosis is worth in cases where thick plaques and tumors appear on top of the erythroderma and when blastic transformation with CD30 positive cells occurs.

3.4.1.3   Primary Cutaneous CD30+ T-Cell Lymphoproliferative Disorders

Positivity of tumor cells for CD30, a cytokine receptor belonging to the tumor necrosis factor receptor (TNFR) superfamily, is the hallmark of a clinical and morphologic spectrum of diseases including lymphomatoid papulosis (LyP), primary cutaneous CD30+ large T-cell lymphoma (CD30+ LTCL) as well as so called borderline cases [83, 92, 127]. Cutaneous neutrophil-or eosinophil-rich CD30+ anaplastic large cell lymphoma (ALCL), simulating a purulent inflammatory reaction are distinct variants of ALCL [21, 32].Future clinicopathologic classification of CD30+ cutaneous lymphoproliferative disorders should incorporate genetic and molecular criteria in order to better define the borders between benign/ malignant and aggressive/nonaggressive disorders [52, 85].

3.4.1.3.1 Lymphomatoid Papulosis (LyP)

Definition

Lymphomatoid papulosis [96] described by Macaulay [111] is a chronic recurrent, self-healing "rhythmic paradoxical" papulo-nodular skin eruption with an indolent course and histologic features of a malignant lymphoma. Verallo in 1966 has reported on Mucha-Habermann's disease (pityriasis lichenoides et varioliformis acuta PLEVA), resembling lymphoma cutis [160]. An even earlier description was given by Dupont in the German literature, reporting on a "Langsam verlaufende und klinisch gutartige Reticulopathie mit höchst maligner histologischer Struktur" [56]. Even though they share some common features, LyP and PLEVA are different nosologic entities, the latter being often infect-related and healing spontaneously and lasting no longer than 1–2 years at most, whereas the former stays for lifetime or transforms into CD30+ anaplastic large cell lymphoma or Hodgkin's disease in 5–10% of the cases [42, 94].

ICD-O Code

9718/1

Synonyms

WHO/EORTC classification (2005): CD30 lymphoproliferative disorders of the skin – lymphomatoid papulosis
WHO classification (2001): CD30 lymphoproliferative disorders of the skin – lymphomatoid papulosis
REAL classification (1997): Not listed
EORTC classification (1997): Lymphomatoid papulosis
Macauly [111] called the disease "A continuing self-healing eruption, clinically benign – histologically malignant."

Clinical Features

The overall prevalence is estimated 1–2 cases per 1,000,000 populations with a male: female ratio of 1.5:1. Usually, LyP affects people in their third or fourth decade of life (median age: 45 years), but it can be seen in patients of all ages. In children a pustular [9] and a hydroa vacciniformia-like [9] variant of LYP has been described. Mucosal involvement with oral lesions has been reported [89].

Although no definite predilection site has been identified, the face usually is spared. The individual LyP lesion starts as an erythematous, usually asymptomatic papule (initial stage) (Fig. 3.4.10a, b). Within days or few weeks, the papules become red–brown, hemorrhagic, or pustular. Some lesions undergo ulceration (ulcerative stage). This stage is followed by complete spontaneous regression of the lesion, often leaving behind hyper or hypopigmented scars with varioliform aspect. The individual lesions usually last for 2–8 weeks [24, 83].

Histopathology

The histological features of LyP are variable and considerably depend on the stage of the lesions and disease [155]. Three histologic subtypes (types A, B and C) have been delineated [166], representing a spectrum with overlapping features (Table 3.4.1). Although distinction of different histologic subtypes may be of interest, often various histologic manifestations of LyP lesions can be seen at the same time in the same patient. It makes little sense to classify LYP into types A, B and C; these letters are completely meaningless in terms of cytomorphology and may be mixed up with their usage to designate clinical tumor stages in oncology.

Fig. 3.4.10 (a, b)
Lymphomatoid papulosis.
Multiple papules in different
stages of evolution and
regression

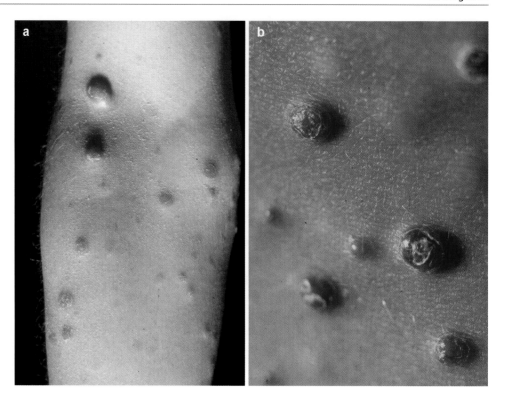

Table 3.4.1 Definition criteria for the different histologic types of LyP

Histologic type of LyP	Morphologic criteria
Classical (A) type	Scattered CD30+ blast cells in an extensive inflammatory infiltrate
MF (B) type	Mycosis fungoides-like histology with atypical CD30-negative T-cells with cerebriform nuclei
ALCL (C) type	Large clusters of CD30+ cells with few inflammatory cells, histologically suggesting a CD30+ (anaplastic) large-cell lymphoma

The predominant histological feature of a fully developed lesion is a nodular, superficial, and deep, and sometimes, wedge-shaped dermal infiltrate (Fig. 3.4.11a) that may invade the subcutaneous fat and shows epidermotropism of variable degree. The infiltrate contains medium-sized to large pleomorphic or anaplastic lymphoid cells with irregular nuclei, sparse chromatin and mitotic activity (Fig. 3.4.11b). In the classical type (A) of Lyp, CD30 positive (Fig. 3.4.11c), atypical lymphoid cells are scattered or grouped in small clusters. Epidermotropism can be present. In addition, there are numerous inflammatory cells such as neutrophils, eosinophils and histiocytes as well as few plasma cells and a prominent edema in the upper dermis [24, 34]. The MF type (B), is characterized by an epidermotropic infiltrate resembling histologic features of MF or SS and harbors atypical lymphoid cells with cerebriform nuclei but almost no CD30+ cells. The ALCL-type (C) features cohesive sheets of large atypical lymphoid cells with only a few intermingled reactive inflammatory cells, resembling anaplastic large cell lymphoma (ALCL).

Immunocytochemically, the tumor cells in LyP are activated T helper cells expressing a CD3+, CD4+, CD8−, CD30+, CD56+ (10%) phenotype, They also express activation markers such as HLA-DR and CD25 (interleukin 2-receptor) [31, 82, 93]. Characteristic markers for Reed–Sternberg cells in HD (CD15), is not expressed by tumor cells in LyP. Almost all tumor cells in LyP and CD30+ ALCL express cytotoxic molecules such as TIA-1 and granzyme B [104].

Prognosis and Predictive Factors

LyP exhibits a favorable prognosis with 5-year-survival rates of almost 100% [13, 127]. Aggressive malignant lymphoma usually with features of anaplastic large cell lymphoma occurs in about 10% of cases [68]. They can develop prior to, concurrent with, or after the manifestation of LyP and other CD30+ LPD and are usually referred to as LyP-associated malignant lymphomas [84]. They include mycosis fungoides (MF), Hodgkin's disease (HD), and systemic or cutaneous CD30+ LTCL. Fascin expression might serve as a putative prognostic marker [86].

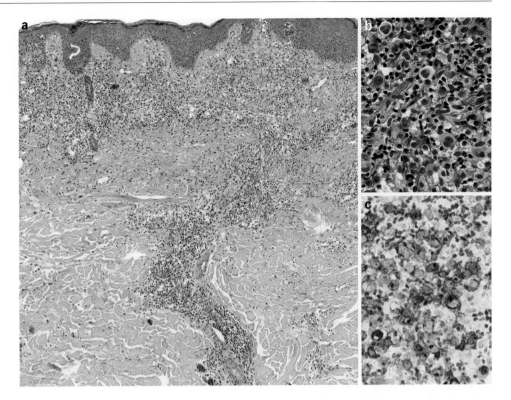

Fig. 3.4.11 Lymphomatoid papulosis. (**a**) (*Left*) wedge shaped infiltrate in the dermis. H & E, 10×. (**b**) (*Upper right*) atypical lymphoid cells. H & E, 63×. (**c**) (*Lower right*) CD30 positive activated lymphoid cells, 63×

3.4.1.3.2 Primary Cutaneous Anaplastic Large Cell Lymphoma (ALCL)

Definition

Hodgkin's disease, lymphomatoid papulosis, and cutaneous anaplastic large T-cell lymphoma are closely related [45]. Primary cutaneous and primary nodal CD30+ ALCL, however, are distinct clinical entities showing similar morphologic features, but differ in age of onset, immunophenotype, and prognosis [6]

Synonyms

WHO/EORTC classification (2005): Primary cutaneous anaplastic large-cell lymphoma
WHO classification (2001): Primary cutaneous anaplastic large cell lymphoma
REAL classification (1997): Anaplastic large cell lymphoma, CD30+
EORTC classification (1997): Primary cutaneous large cell T-cell lymphoma, CD30+
ALCL also has been referred to as "regressing atypical histiocytosis"

Clinical Features

The incidence of ALCL is 0.1 per 100,000 per year occurring mainly in people in their sixth decade with a male preponderance; however children also may be affected. The vast majority of primary cutaneous large T-cell lymphomas in HIV-infected individuals are also CD30+ [98].

Skin tumors usually are solitary or multiple confined to an extremity or a circumscribed area of the body and often undergo exulceration (Fig. 3.4.12a) followed by regression in up to 40% of the patients. Approximately 20% of the patients have multifocal disease, i.e., 2 or more lesions at multiple anatomic sites [13]. Tumors grow rapidly over a time span of 4–6 weeks without preceding patches or plaques.

Histopathology

A dense infiltrate of atypical lymphoid cells extends through all levels of the dermis into the subcutis (Fig. 3.4.12b). Epidermotropism is mostly lacking. Tumor cells grow usually in dense cohesive sheets, reminiscent of melanoma or undifferentiated carcinoma. The cytomorphologic hallmarks are large, bizarre cells with irregularly shaped nuclei and one or multiple nucleoli and an abundant, clear or eosinophilic cytoplasm (Fig. 3.4.12c). Mitoses are frequent. Within and around the tumor clusters of small reactive lymphocytes may

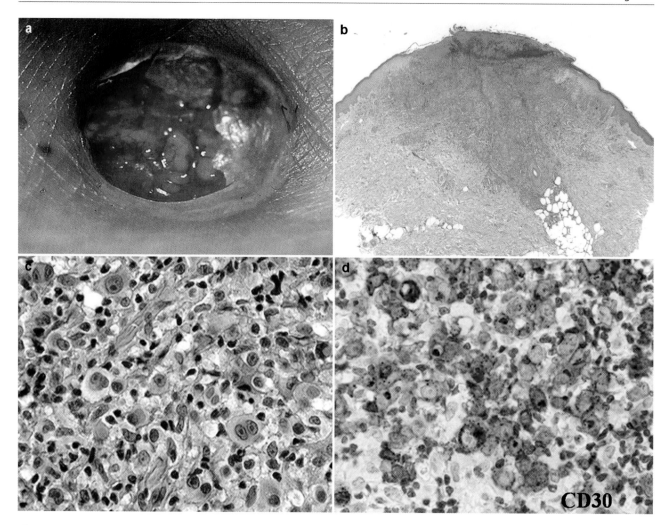

Fig. 3.4.12 Anaplastic large cell lymphoma. (**a**) (*Upper left*) solitary circumscribed tumor with ulceration. (**b**) (*Upper right*) wedge-shaped infiltrate in the dermis with some necrosis on the top. H & E, 10×. (**c**) (*Lower left*) large atypical "anaplastic" cells, 100×. (**d**) (*Lower left*) tumor cells expressing CD 30, 100×

be present. In contrast to LyP eosinophils, plasma cells, and accessory dendritic cells usually are not prominent in ALCL. *Neutrophil-rich or pyogenic CD30+ ALCL* (N-ALCL) [32, 117] is a distinct form of ALCL, which shows extensive infiltrate of neutrophils, clinically presenting with ulceration and purulent secretion.

Immunocytochemically, ALCL CD30+ have an activated T-cell phenotype with expression of T-cell associated antigens CD2, CD3, CD4, and CD45RO, and activation markers such as CD25 (IL-2R), CD30, CD71, and HLA-DR. At least 75% of the large pleomorphic or anaplastic lymphoid cells have to be CD30+ (Fig. 3.4.12d). In contrast to nodal ALCL, primary cutaneous forms do not express EMA, but may express the cutaneous lymphocyte antigen (CLA, HECA-452).

Prognosis and Predictive Factors

Primary cutaneous ALCL CD30+ shows an excellent prognosis with a 5 year-survival rate of 90% [13, 127].

Spontaneous regression, seen in almost half of the lesions and age under 60 years are associated with a better prognosis, while extracutaneous disease and age greater than 60 years have a worse outlook. Recurrences are frequent (40%). Extracutaneous spread occurs in 10% of the patients, particularly in those with multiple grouped or multifocal tumor lesions.

3.4.1.4 Subcutaneous Panniculitis-Like T-Cell Lymphoma (SPTCL)

3.4.1.4.1 Definition

Only SPTCLs which express a α/β phenotype are referred to as SPTCL sui generis according to the WHO/EORTC classification. SPTCL with a γ/δ phenotype [30] are included in the group of peripheral T-cell lymphomas, cytotoxic type.

The disorder has also been described as "hemorrhagic diathesis associated with benign histiocytic, cytophagic panniculitis and systemic histiocytosis."[167]. B-cell lymphomas that are primarily localized to the subcutaneous tissue also exist but are very rare [5].

3.4.1.4.2 ICD-O Code

9708/3

3.4.1.4.3 Synonyms

WHO/EORTC classification (2005): Subcutaneous panniculitis-like T-cell lymphoma
WHO classification (2001): Subcutaneous panniculitis-like T-cell lymphoma
REAL classification (1997): Subcutaneous panniculitis-like T-cell lymphoma
EORTC classification (1997): Subcutaneous panniculitis-like T-cell lymphoma

3.4.1.4.4 Clinical Features

Mostly patients in their fifth decade are affected without gender predilection. Multiple subcutaneous panniculitis-like tumors are found predominantly on the lower extremities, sometimes on the trunk [139]. The skin lesions may ulcerate (Fig. 3.4.13a). At the same time fever, malaise, fatigue, myalgias, chills and weight loss may be present. Some patients develop a hemophagocytic syndrome with cytopenia.

3.4.1.4.5 Histopathology

The histopathologic hallmark of this type of CTCL is the subcutaneous localization and growth pattern of focal infiltrates simulating panniculitis [120, 139] (Fig. 3.4.13b). Epidermotropism may be seen in advanced stages of the disease only. The tumor cells are lymphoid cells of varying size, often with chromatin-dense nuclei (Fig. 3.4.13c). Rimming of adipocytes by tumor cells is a common, but not specific, finding for SPCTL. Karyorrhexis with erythrophagocytosis by many histiocytes and fat necrosis are prominent features. Large and deep biopsies are mandatory to establish the diagnosis, since the lymphoproliferative process is focal.

Immunophenotypically, tumor cells express T-cell-associated antigens CD2+, CD3+, CD5+, CD4–, CD8+, CD43+ and cytotoxic proteins such as TIA-1, granzyme B and perforin [139]. A TCR α/β (βF1+) phenotype is much more frequently found than a TCR γ/δ (TCRδ-1+)

3.4.1.4.6 Prognosis and Predictive Factors

Subcutaneous panniculitic T-cell lymphoma show an indolent course with good prognosis or rapid clinical deterioration,

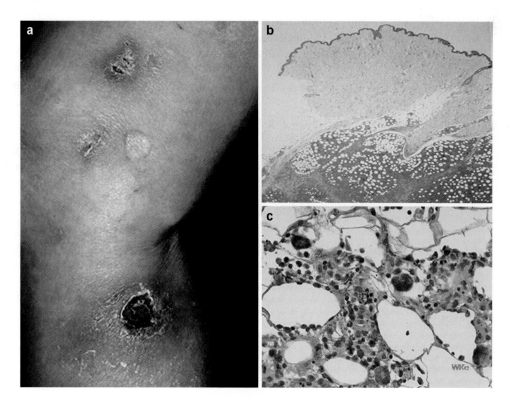

Fig. 3.4.13 Subcutaneous panniculitis-like T-cell lymphoma. (**a**) Panniculitis-like subcutaneous infiltrates with superficial ulceration and crust-formation. (**b**) Dense infiltrate in the subcutaneous tissue. H & E, 10×. (**c**) Small and medium sized lymphocytes, nuclear debris and some large atypical cells in the subcutaneous tissue. H & E, 100×

hemophagocytosis, and death. The development of hemo-phagocytic syndrome may cause rapid fatal outcome [66, 129]. A correlation exists between the course of the disease and the immunophenotype of tumor cells. A TCR α/β+/CD56- phenotype may be indicative of a more indolent course, whereas expression of TCR γ/δ+/CD56+ phenotype appears to be associated with an aggressive course and worse prognosis [80].

3.4.1.5 Primary Cutaneous Peripheral T-Cell Lymphoma (PTL)

This category constitutes a heterogeneous group of diseases, representing less than 10% of all CTCL [14]. Per definition it includes all T-cell neoplasms that do not fit into any of the other categories of T-cell lymphoma/leukemia.

3.4.1.5.1 Peripheral T-Cell Lymphoma (PTL), Unspecified

Definition

There are various subtypes of PTL, which are categorized as provisional.

Synonyms

WHO/EORTC classification (2005): Primary cutaneous peripheral T-cell lymphoma (PTL), unspecified
WHO classification (2001): Peripheral T-cell lymphoma, unspecified
REAL classification (1997): Peripheral T-cell lymphoma, unspecified
EORTC classification (1997): CTCL, pleomorphic small/medium-sized

3.4.1.6 Subtypes of PTL (Provisional)

3.4.1.6.1 Primary Cutaneous Aggressive Epidermotropic CD8-Positive Cytotoxic T-Cell Lymphoma

Definition

This Lymphoma occurs mainly in adults and is rare (less than 50 cases published Worldwide) [3, 20, 115, 143]. It shows epidermotropic infiltrates of CD8-positive, cytotoxic T-cells. However, nonepidermotropic forms exist.

Clinical Features

Lesions may be MF-like in the epidermotropic form and more nodular in the nonepidermotropic form. Lesions present as sudden eruptions of papules, nodules and tumors in a localized area or disseminated. Ulceration and necrosis may occur. Superficial, hyperkeratotic patches and plaques are seen in the MF-or pagetoid reticulosis-like form. Lesions may be hypo-or sometimes hyperpigmented. Due to the progressive course, the disease may disseminate to other visceral sites (lung, testis, central nervous system, oral mucosa), sparing lymph nodes in most of the cases [20].

Histopathology

The histopathologic feature is very variable. The epidermis may be acanthotic or atrophic, often with necrosis and ulceration [3, 20]. There may be strong epidermotropism as in pagetoid reticulosis and involvement of adnexal structures. Nodular lesions show deeper infiltrates in which epidermotropism may be lacking. The cytomorphology of tumor cells also is very variable, ranging from small to large pleomorphic cells.

Prognosis and Predictive Factors

The behavior is aggressive in most cases [143]. However CD8+ poikilodermatous mycosis fungoides with a nonaggressive clinical behavior and a good response to psoralen plus ultraviolet A treatment has been reported [2].

3.4.1.6.2 Primary Cutaneous Gamma/Delta-Positive T-Cell Lymphoma (CGD-TCL)

Definition

Cutaneous γ/δ T-cell lymphoma (CGD-TCL) is a rare (less than 50 cases reported) lymphoma composed of a clonal proliferation of mature, activated γ/δ T-cells expressing a cytotoxic phenotype. This group includes cases of subcutaneous panniculitis-like T-cell lymphoma (SPTCL) with a γ/δ phenotype. In the WHO classification 2001, these were grouped together with SPTCL of α/β origin [77]. Whether cutaneous and mucosal γ/δ TCL are all part of the same disease spectrum is unclear [7, 48].

Synonyms

WHO/EORTC classification (2005): Cutaneous γ/δ T-cell lymphoma
WHO classification (2001): Peripheral T-cell lymphoma, unspecified
REAL classification (1997): Peripheral T-cell lymphoma, unspecified
EORTC classification (1997): Not listed

Clinical Features

Nonhepatosplenic gamma/delta T-cell lymphomas have a proclivity for mucosal or cutaneous sites [7]. Primary cutaneous lymphomas expressing gamma/delta TCR are very rare. Clinically, gamma/delta lymphoma of the skin manifests with multiple plaques, tumors or subcutaneous nodules especially on the extremities, sometimes simulating subcutaneous panniculitis [30].

Histopathology

Small to intermediate-sized tumor cells and scattered large pleomorphic cells with irregular nuclei are found in the mid and deep dermis and in the subcutaneous fat tissue. Epidermotropism of reactive CD4+ T-cells, ulceration, and periadnexal infiltration are present in one-third of the biopsies [30].

Prognosis and Predictive Factors

The disease has an aggressive course with a tendency for rapid multifocal cutaneous dissemination, spread to bone marrow or lymph nodes and fatal outcome [156]. However, indolent forms also have been reported [30].

3.4.1.6.3 Primary Cutaneous Small/Medium CD4+ T-Cell Lymphoma

Definition

This is a noncytotoxic form of peripheral T-cell lymphoma, unspecified characterized by small to medium-sized pleomorphic tumor cells tumor cells, which are CD30 negative [134].

Synonyms

WHO/EORTC classification (2005): Primary cutaneous small medium CD4+ T-cell lymphoma

WHO classification (2001): Peripheral T-cell lymphoma, unspecified
REAL classification (1997): Peripheral T-cell lymphoma, unspecified
EORTC classification (1997): Not listed

Clinical Features

The mean age at diagnosis is approximately 50–60 years with a wide range. There is no gender predilection. The disease presents with localized or widespread, mostly asymptomatic and indurated papules, nodules or violaceous plaques, which appear without preceding patches as seen in MF [58].

Histopathology

The infiltrate is predominantly perivascular and periadnexal or nodular and extends to the subcutaneous tissue. Epidermotropism is absent in most cases. It consists of small to medium-sized pleomorphic lymphoid cells with irregular hyperchromatic nuclei and a pale scanty cytoplasm [58].

By definition this lymphoma has a CD3+, CD4+, CD8−, and CD30− *phenotype*. Cytotoxic proteins are not expressed [14].

Prognosis and Predictive Factors

The prognosis is favorable with an estimated 5-year survival of 60–80% [14, 58, 67].

3.4.1.7 Extranodal NK/T-Cell Lymphoma, Nasal Type

3.4.1.7.1 Hydroa Vacciniformia-Like Lymphoma (Variant) (HVLL)

Definition

Hydroa vacciniformia (HV) like T-cell lymphoma is a rare EBV-associated variant of extranodal NK/T-cell lymphoma originating from cytotoxic T-cells or NK-cells [149, 150]. It has been described in the literature as atypical HV, angiocentric cutaneous T-cell lymphoma of childhood (ACTCLC), edematous scarring vasculitic panniculitis, and EBV-associated lymphoproliferative eruption. All these disorders are not separate entities but represent a spectrum of EBV-associated lymphoproliferative diseases which affect mainly children from certain world regions where EBV infections are common, namely in Japan, Korea, Taiwan and Latin America (Mexico). The vesiculopapular skin eruption clinically resemble hydroa vacciniformie, a UV-light induced dermatosis.

ICD-O Code

9709/3

Synonyms

WHO/EORTC classification (2005): Hydroa vacciniforme-like cutaneous T-cell lymphoma
WHO classification (2001): Not listed
REAL classification (1997): Not listed
EORTC classification (1997): Not listed
It also has been referred to as angiocentric cutaneous T-cell lymphoma of childhood

Clinical Features

The disease mostly affects children or young adults of [1–5]. It is characterized by vesiculopapular eruptions, small blisters, crusts, necrotic areas and scars, occur mainly on the face, simulating Hydroa vacciniforme. The oral mucosae may be involved. UV light does not play any causative role. Additional symptoms may be present, like fever, malaise, weight loss, failure to thrive, lymphadenopathy, and hepatosplenomegaly. Laboratory tests show antibodies to EBV. There may be leukopenia, anemia, thrombocytopenia, and signs of impaired liver function.

Histopathology

Necrotic epidermis. In the dermis there is a dense perivascular/periadnexal nodular infiltrate composed of medium-sized lymphocytes with irregular, hyperchromatic nuclei, which tends to accumulate around vessels in an angiocentric/angiodestructive pattern [112]. Septal or lobular panniculitis with vasculitis involving small or larger vessels may be seen in the mid or deep dermis [126].

Immunohistochemically, the atypical cells express T-cell markers (CD3, CD45RO). B-cell-associated antigens, BCL-2 protein and CD56 are negative. CD30 antigen may be expressed on 10–40% of the atypical cells in cases showing angiocentric growth pattern [112].

Prognosis and Predictive Factors

The mortality rate is high (40–50%), due either to severe infectious complications, septicemia and/or multiorgan failure in some cases or to progression to various lymphomas or large granular lymphocyte leukemia in others. There are no clear-cut markers to predict the course of the disease. However, the prognosis is somewhat worse in the patients with angiocentric/angiodestructive features and panniculitis.

3.4.1.8 Adult T-Cell Leukemia/Lymphoma (ATLL)

3.4.1.8.1 Definition

Adult T-cell leukemia lymphoma (ATLL) is a peripheral T-cell lymphoma, etiologically associated with human T-cell leukemia virus I (HTLV-1) [147, 169]. HTLV-1 infection and ATLL is endemic in southwestern Japan and the Caribbean and rather rare in Europe and USA [109]. The disease manifests with leukemia in greater than two-thirds of patients, while the remaining patients have a lymphomatous form [116]. The spectrum of clinical manifestations and histologic features in ATLL is broad [133].

3.4.1.8.2 ICD-O Code

9827/3

3.4.1.8.3 Synonyms

WHO/EORTC classification (2005): Adult T-cell leukemia/lymphoma
WHO classification (2001): Adult T-cell leukemia/lymphoma
REAL classification (1997): Adult T-cell leukemia/lymphoma
EORTC classification (1997): Not included

3.4.1.8.4 Clinical Features

Skin involvement occurs in about 50% of the cases, presenting as purpuric papules, nodules, tumors, or as erythroderma [146]. The disease may simulate mycosis fungoides (MF) in nonendemic areas outside Japan and the Caribbean [44].

Various types can be differentiated, including an acute, a chronic, a lymphomatous and a smoldering subtype.

Peripheral blood smears show atypical lymphoid cells with convoluted nuclei (so called flower cells) and leukocytosis, sometimes in conjunction with anemia. Additional findings found in patients with acute ATLL are hypercalcemia, bone marrow involvement, lymphadenopathy, hepatosplenomegaly and pulmonary infiltrates.

3.4.1.8.5 Histopathology

Histologically, epidermotropism of lymphoid cells with formation of Pautrier microabscesses is found, simulating MF. In the upper dermis a perivascular or diffuse infiltrate of medium to large pleomorphic cells is seen. Tumor cells show pronounced nuclear pleomorphism. In chronic and smoldering variants of ATLL, small neoplastic lymphocytes show only minimal cytologic atypia. Granulomatous and angiodestructive features have been reported and some cases may present as CD30-positive anaplastic large cell lymphoma [151].

Immunocytochemically, neoplastic cells in patients with ATLL usually show a helper/inducer T-cell phenotype (CD4+, CD8−); however in some cases, CD4−, CD8+ or CD4−, CD8− phenotypes and positivity for CD30 in large atypical cells may be seen. ALK-1, TIA-1 and granzyme B are negative.

3.4.1.8.6 Prognosis and Predictive Factors

The prognosis of ATLL is generally poor especially in patients with acute or lymphomatous forms. Clinical subtype, age, increased serum calcium and LDH levels have been identified as major prognostic factors whereas, the size of tumor cells does not have prognostic implications [170]. Chronic and smoldering forms are mostly slowly progressive, but may undergo transformation into acute form of ATLL.

3.4.1.9 Angioimmunoblastic T-Cell-Lymphoma (AITL)

3.4.1.9.1 Definition

Angioimmunoblastic T-cell lymphoma (AITL) occurs mostly in middle-aged or elderly people without gender preponderance. It is a systemic malignant lymphoproliferative disorder characterized by a clonal growth of atypical lymphoid cells accompanied by the proliferation of high endothelial venules and follicular dendritic cells.

3.4.1.9.2 ICD-O Code

9766/1

3.4.1.9.3 Synonyms

WHO/EORTC classification (2005): Angioimmunoblastic T-cell lymphoma
WHO classification (2001): Angioimmunoblastic T-cell lymphoma
REAL classification (1997): Angioimmunoblastic T-cell lymphoma
EORTC classification (1997): Not included
Originally the term "angioimmunoblastic lymphadenopathy with dysproteinemia or immunoblastic lymphadenopathy" was used [59, 60].

3.4.1.9.4 Clinical Features

Skin lesions in angioimmunoblastic T-cell lymphoma (AITL) occur in half of the cases. They most commonly present as generalized erythrodermic maculopapular sometimes purpuric eruptions with a predilection for the trunk simulating viral exanthema or urticarial drug eruption [81, 113].

3.4.1.9.5 Histopathology

The histologic pattern may be variable. Usually, the skin lesions are characterized by nonspecific subtle superficial perivascular infiltrates composed of eosinophils and lymphocytes without atypia accompanied by hyperplasia of capillaries. Plasma cells and histiocytes may be present. In some cases, the disease presents as prominent vascular hyperplasia with sparse perivascular infiltrates composed of pleomorphic lymphocytes with medium-size to large reniform nuclei resembling Reed–Sternberg cells. There also may be predominance of pleomorphic cells in other cases.

Immunohistochemically, the neoplastic lymphocytes express the phenotype of mature T-helper cells (CD3+, CD4+, and CD8±). There are an increased number of dermal factor XIIIa+ dendritic cells and reactive mature B cells, plasma cells and histiocytes.

3.4.1.9.6 Prognosis and Predictive Factors

AITL exhibits an aggressive course with a mortality rate ranging from 50 to 70% and a median survival ranging from 11 to 30 months. Some patients develop secondary EBV-positive B-cell nodal lymphomas.

3.4.2 Mature Cutaneous B-Cell Neoplasms (CBCL)*

Günter Burg, Werner Kempf, and Reinhard Dummer

B-cell lymphomas are much more common in the lymph nodes. In the skin CBCL comprise 20–25% of all primary cutaneous lymphomas. Extranodal low-grade B-cell lymphoma of the mucosa-associated lymphoid tissue (MALT) type and follicle center lymphoma are the most frequent types of peripheral B-cell neoplasms seen primarily in the skin. In contrast to nodal B-cell lymphomas, CBCL have a benign overall prognosis and overtreatment must be avoided. The sub-classification and the extent of cutaneous involvement are the two most relevant prognostic factors in primary CBCL [173].

3.4.2.1 Extranodal Marginal Zone Lymphoma of the "Mucosa Associated Lymphoid Tissue" (MALT-Lymphoma)

3.4.2.1.1 Definition

Primary cutaneous marginal zone lymphoma (MZL) represents a low grade cutaneous B-cell lymphoma, composed of small B cells including marginal zone (centrocyte-like) or monocytoid cells, lymphoplasmacytoid cells and plasma cells [41]. It may develop from reactive infiltrates that represent immune responses to antigenic stimuli [53] like Borrelia burgdorferi [61] and can easily be mistaken for cutaneous lymphoid hyperplasia [106] or immunocytoma [25]. Primary cutaneous immunocytoma, primary cutaneous plasmacytoma and cutaneous follicular lymphoid hyperplasia with monotypic plasma cells are considered variants of MZL. There are still some different standpoints in the discrimination between various subtypes of FCL and MZL, which renders the subject somehow controversial.

3.4.2.1.2 ICD-O Code

9699/3

3.4.2.1.3 Synonyms

WHO/EORTC classification (2005): Cutaneous marginal zone B-cell lymphoma

WHO classification (2001): Extranodal marginal zone lymphoma of MALT type
REAL classification (1997): Extranodal marginal zone B-cell lymphoma
EORTC classification (1997): Primary cutaneous marginal zone B-cell lymphoma

3.4.2.1.4 Clinical Features

MZL affects most commonly adults over 40 years old. In contrast to follicle center cell lymphoma (FCL) which is often located on the head and neck, MZL preferentially affects the trunk (Fig. 3.4.14a) and arms, where red to violaceous infiltrated cutaneous and subcutaneous plaques or nodules with an erythematous periphery are found [144]. Biopsies should be deep in order to reflect the extent of the infiltrate.

3.4.2.1.5 Histopathology

Site-specific morphologic differences can be found in extranodal marginal zone B-cell lymphomas [135]. In the skin there is a nodular (B-cell pattern) (Fig. 3.4.14b) or diffuse infiltrate often displaying a characteristic "inverse pattern" on scanning magnification, typified by darker centers surrounded by brighter zones of pale-staining cells. Reactive follicles with distinct mantle zones are also present in the majority of cases. Occasionally, the infiltrate is arranged around adnexal structures analogous to lympho-epithelioid lesions of MALT-lymphoma of the gastrointestinal tract [144].

The infiltrate is composed of small to medium-sized lymphocytes (Fig. 3.4.14c) possessing slightly irregular nuclei with moderately dispersed chromatin, inconspicuous nucleoli and an abundant pale cytoplasm (marginal zone cells) [148, 154].

Some cells have a monocytoid appearance (reniform nuclei) or show prominent plasma cell differentiation [46]. The tumor cells proliferate mainly around the follicles and are apt to colonize them. The colonized follicles lack a distinct germinal center/mantle zone demarcation and have a more variable cellular composition, including marginal zone cells, centrocytes, and centroblasts. In the interfollicular areas small lymphocytes, lymphoplasmacytoid cells and aggregations of plasma cells are found.

The *immunophenotype* of the neoplastic cells is as follows: CD19+, CD20+, CD22+, CD79a+, CD5−, CD10−, CD23−, bcl-6−, bcl-2+. Monotypic expression of immunoglobulin light chains is seen in the majority of cases.

---

*All diagnostic terms follow the WHO Classification of Tumors of Haematopoietic and Lymphoid Tissues, Eds.: S. Swedlow et al., 4th Edition 2008

Fig. 3.4.14 Marginal zone lymphoma (MZL). (**a**) (*Left*) solitary tumor on the back, compatible with Crosti's disease. (**b**) (*Upper right*) typical B-cell pattern in MZL, (*lower right*) small to medium-sized lymphocytes (marginal zone cells)

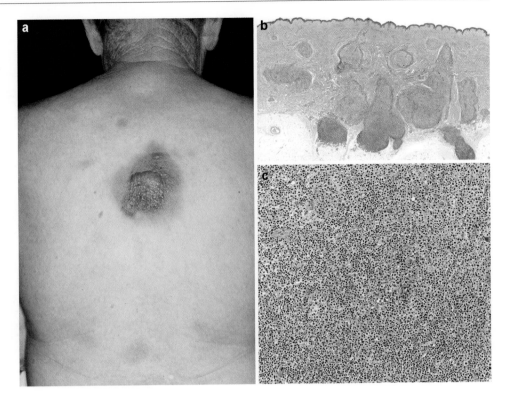

Anti-CD21 staining reveals an irregular network of follicular dendritic cells (FDC). In some cases large, expanded, diffuse FDC networks may be seen.

3.4.2.1.6 Prognosis and Predictive Factors

In general, MZL exhibits a favorable prognosis with 5-year-survival rates over 90%, however it tends to recur in more than 50% of patients. Rarely, MZL runs a fatal course.

3.4.2.2 Primary Cutaneous Follicle Center Lymphoma (FCL)

3.4.2.2.1 Definition

FCL is a common type of primary cutaneous B-cell lymphomas with differentiation of follicle center cells (centrocytes and centroblasts) [131].

3.4.2.2.2 ICD-O Code

9690/3

3.4.2.2.3 Synonyms

WHO/EORTC classification (2005): Primary cutaneous follicle center lymphoma
WHO classification (2001): Cutaneous follicle center lymphoma
REAL classification (1997): Follicle center lymphoma, follicular
EORTC classification (1997): Primary cutaneous follicle center cell lymphoma
When located on the back the disease also has been referred to as reticulohistiocytoma of the dorsum or Crosti lymphoma [18]

3.4.2.2.4 Clinical Features

Primary cutaneous follicular lymphoma usually presents with localized disease and rarely disseminates. The lesions are usually red–brown papules or nodules of very firm consistency. The preferential localizations are the scalp, forehead (Fig. 3.4.15a), neck, and trunk.

3.4.2.2.5 Histopathology

The infiltrates show a spectrum of growth patterns, with a morphologic continuum from follicular (Fig. 3.4.15b) to follicular and diffuse to diffuse. By definition, the lesions are

Fig. 3.4.15 Follicle center lymphoma (FCL). (**a**) (*Left*) firm nodules on the forehead. (**b**) (*Upper right*) nodular infiltrate, reflecting a typical B-cell pattern. H & E, 20×. (**c**) (*Lower right*) various types of follicle center cells. H & E, 40×

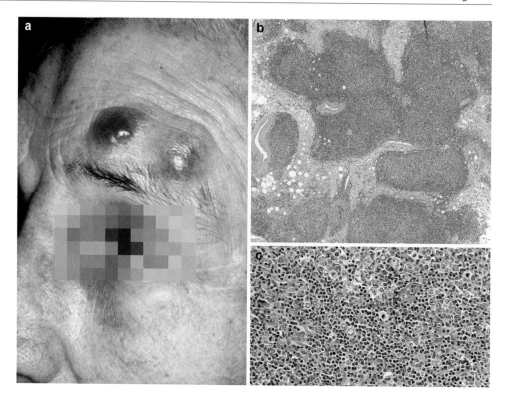

composed of centrocytes and centroblasts in varying proportions.

When morphologically identifiable, follicles are often ill-defined and show a population of small and large follicle center cells in variable mixtures (Fig. 3.4.15c), lack tingible body macrophages, and generally have an attenuated or absent mantle zone, which allows differentiation from cutaneous follicular hyperplasias (B-pseudolymphomas), which also show a higher number of mitoses. The infiltrate is button heavy reaching into the dermis, with extension into the subcutaneous tissue. The overlying epidermis is generally unaffected and a grenz zone is expressed between the epidermis and the infiltrate.

Immunophenotypically, the neoplastic B-cells express CD10+, CD19+, CD20+, CD22+, CD79a+, CD5−, CD23±, CD43− and the nuclear protein bcl-6 [57]. The bcl-2 translocation which is present in 75–95% of nodal follicular lymphomas is usually not found in primary cutaneous follicular lymphomas [39].

3.4.2.2.6 Prognosis and Predictive Factors

Primary follicular lymphoma presenting in skin has a favorable prognosis with an estimated 5-year survival of 90% [38, 132, 142].

3.4.2.3 Primary Cutaneous Diffuse Large B-Cell Lymphoma (DLBCL)

3.4.2.3.1 Definition

Diffuse large B-cell lymphoma is a heterogeneous group of non-Hodgkin lymphomas [4, 47]. Primary cutaneous diffuse large B-cell lymphomas (DLBL) comprise 1–3% of all cutaneous lymphomas and approximately 5–10% of cutaneous B-cell lymphomas. People over the age of 70 are most commonly affected. They are composed of a variety of clinical forms the most common DLBCL, leg-type usually occurs on the leg and less frequently at other sites. There also is a broad cytomorphological variation of diseases, formerly referred to as centroblastic lymphoma, immunoblastic lymphoma, anaplastic large B-cell lymphoma and multilobated large B-cell lymphoma. Other variants are referred to as DLBCL, other and comprise T-cell/histiocyte-rich LBCL, plasmablastic lymphoma and others, that do not fulfil the criteria for a DLBCL, leg type.

3.4.2.3.2 ICD-O Code

9680/3

3.4.2.3.3 Synonyms

WHO/EORTC classification (2005): Cutaneous diffuse large B-cell lymphoma DLBCL, leg-type DLBCL, other.
WHO classification (2001): Diffuse large B-cell lymphoma
REAL classification (1997): Diffuse large B-cell lymphoma
EORTC classification (1997): Primary cutaneous large B-cell lymphoma of the leg

3.4.2.3.4 Clinical Features

Usually elderly patients, women more frequently than men, are affected with a predilection of the lower leg (Fig. 3.4.16a). However, other sites of the body may be affected. Analogous to the "nasal-type" designation for a distinct extranodal variant of NK/T-cell lymphomas, the term "DLBCL, leg-type" is chosen for all cutaneous diffuse large B-cell lymphomas with the designated cytological and immunophenotypic features. Clinically, solitary or multiple disseminated or aggregated red to violaceous dome shaped tumors with a firm consistency and a shiny surface without scaling are seen. Ulceration may occur in advanced stages [74].

3.4.2.3.5 Histopathology

A diffuse destructive growth pattern is commonly found extending to all levels of the dermis and reaching into the subcutis (Fig. 3.4.16b) often obliterating adnexal structures. The epidermis is often spared, with a Grenz zone. There may be remnants of large follicle-like structures. The infiltrate is composed of medium to large sized B-cells, which are usually monomorphic in appearance. The neoplastic cells may either resemble centroblasts with large noncleaved nuclei and nucleoli attached to the nuclear membrane, or immunoblasts with a large vesicular nucleus and a prominent centrally placed nucleolus. In addition, multilobated, anaplastic or large cleaved cells can be found. Mitotic figures are frequent.

Immunocytochemically, the tumor cells express CD19, CD20, CD22 and CD79a. They are negative for CD10 and CD138, have variable Bcl-6 expression and are usually strongly positive for BCL-2 protein (Fig. 3.4.16c) and MUM-1/IRTA-4.

3.4.2.3.6 Prognosis and Predictive Factors

The 5-year survival rate is about 48%. Patients presenting with lesions confined to a circumscribed area on the trunk seem to have a better prognosis than elderly women, presenting with multiple bcl-2-positive skin tumors on the lower legs.

3.4.2.4 Intravascular Large B-Cell Lymphoma (IV-LBL)

3.4.2.4.1 Definition

Intravascular large B-cell lymphoma (IL) is a rare extranodal subtype of DLBCL characterized by the presence of large lymphoid cells within the lumina of small to medium-sized blood vessels, particularly capillaries and postcapillary venules. Rare tumors expressing a T-cell phenotype have been reported [65]. Skin is a common site of presentation, but most patients have systemic disease at time of diagnosis (Fig. 3.4.17).

Neoplastic angioendotheliomatosis has to be differentiated from reactive angioendotheliomatosis, which demonstrates a wide clinicopathologic spectrum in conjunction with a variety of underlying systemic inflammatory or neoplastic diseases [105, 118].

3.4.2.4.2 ICD-O Code

9680/3

3.4.2.4.3 Synonyms

WHO/EORTC classification (2005): Intravascular large B-cell lymphoma
WHO classification (2001): Intravascular large B-cell lymphoma
REAL classification (1997): Diffuse large B-cell lymphoma
EORTC classification (1997): Intravascular large B-cell lymphoma (provisional entity)
Other synonyms include systemic angioendotheliomatosis [130], intravascular lymphomatosis and Tappeiner–Pfleger syndrome [130].

3.4.2.4.4 Clinical Features

Skin lesions may be variable. Classical IV-LBL shows livedo-like reticulate erythema, linear erythematous streaks, and painful indurated telangiectasias; there may be also erythematous or violaceous plaques or tender indurated nodules. Lesions may imitate erythema nodosum, phlebitis,

Fig. 3.4.16 Diffuse large B-cell lymphoma (DLBCL). (**a**) (*Left*) multiple nodules, confined to one leg. (**b**) (*Upper right*) dense dermal infiltrate, sparing the epidermis. H & E, 10×. (**c**) (*Lower right*) strong expression of bcl-2

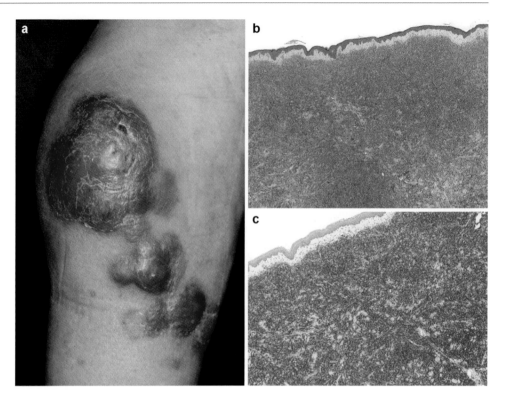

Fig. 3.4.17 Intravascular lymphoma (IVL). (**a**) (*Left*) accumulation of lymphoid cells in the dilated vascular spaces. H & E, 20×. (**b**) (*Upper right*) atypical lymphoid cells clustering in the dilated vessel. H & E, 40×. (**c**) (*Lower right*) atypical large lymphoid cells within the lumen of a small blood vessel. H & E, 100×

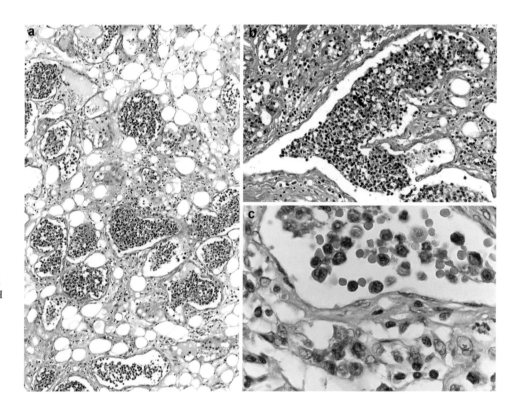

panniculitis, or vasculitis [128]. Neurologic signs and symptoms are frequent. There is a notable absence of lymphadenopathy, splenomegaly or circulating lymphoma cells in the majority of cases.

3.4.2.4.5 Histopathology

Deep biopsies are required in order to show the pathognomonic features, which are dense proliferation of atypical large lymphoid cells with vesicular nuclei, prominent nucleoli, and frequent mitoses within the lumina of small blood vessels (Fig. 3.4.17). Fibrin thrombi with partial occlusion of the vascular lumina result in reticulate and livedoid erythema. The presence of a brisk, perivascular, nonneoplastic lymphocytic infiltrate may have obscured the identification of tumor cells [10].

Immunocytology, In the more prevalent B-cell form, neoplastic cells reveal positivity of the tumor cells for CD20 and negativity for CD3, CD43, CD23 and cyclin D1 (Bcl-1) protein.

3.4.2.4.6 Prognosis and Predictive Factors

In contrast to other CBCL, the intravascular B-cell lymphoma shows a bad prognosis. The clinical course is variable, but the disease cannot be cured [22]. The involvement of the central nervous system is the most important prognostic factor.

3.4.2.5 Lymphomatoid Granulomatosis (LYG)

3.4.2.5.1 Definition

Lymphomatoid granulomatosis (LYG), originally described by Liebow et al. [110], is a rare multisystemic angiocentric and angiodestructive lymphoproliferative disease involving extranodal sites, especially the lungs, skin, and nervous system. It is composed of Epstein Barr virus (EBV)-positive B-cells admixed with T-cells and may progress to diffuse large B-cell lymphoma.

3.4.2.5.2 ICD-O Code

Not listed

3.4.2.5.3 Synonyms

WHO/EORTC classification (2005): Lymphomatoid granulomatosis
WHO classification (2001): Lymphomatoid granulomatosis

REAL classification (1997): Not listed
EORTC classification (1997): Not listed

3.4.2.5.4 Clinical Features

The skin is the most common extrapulmonary organ affected in LYG. The other commonly involved organs are brain (26%), kidney (32%), and liver (29%). Lymph nodes and spleen are spared.

The clinical features of cutaneous LYG are extremely diverse [12] and generally transient [79]. They may present as erythematous dermal papules and/or subcutaneous nodules, with or without ulceration, facial edema, and folliculitis-like eruptions [37]. Necrosis and ulceration are generally associated with larger nodules.

3.4.2.5.5 Histopathology

There is a nodular, angiocentric and angiodestructive dense, polymorphous, lymphohistiocytic infiltrate in the dermis and subcutaneous tissue leading to necrosis. Lymphocytic vasculitis with, fibrinoid necrosis may be present. Angiodestruction is less evident in the skin compared to other organs. The infiltrate surrounds and invades not only vessels but also nerves and epidermal appendages [78]. A granulomatous reaction may be seen secondary to fat necrosis.

Immunocytochemically, EBV-positive, CD20+ B-cells are frequently seen in the lung, but they are rare in the skin and may be obscured by a prominent T-cell rich infiltrate.

3.4.2.5.6 Prognosis and Predictive Factors

Almost two-thirds of patients die and the median survival is only 14 months [90]. Neurologic manifestations and presence of large numbers of atypical lymphoreticular cells within the infiltrates are unfavorable prognostic factors.

3.4.2.6 B-Cell Chronic Lymphocytic Leukemia (B-CLL)

3.4.2.6.1 Definition

B-CLL is the most common leukemia in elderly people. It is a mature B-cell neoplasm composed of small, long-lived, mature usually CD5+, CD23+, cyclin D1- B-cells. The disease affects men twice as frequently as women. Bone marrow and lymph nodes are invariably affected. Specific skin lesions occur in approximately 8% of patients. Patients with B-CLL have a greater susceptibility to infection.

3.4.2.6.2 ICD-O Code

9728/3

3.4.2.6.3 Synonyms

Chronic lymphocytic leukemia/small lymphocytic lymphoma, B-cell

3.4.2.6.4 Clinical Features

Cutaneous lesions occur in up to 25% of patients with CLL. These can be caused by either cutaneous seeding by leukemic cells or present as nonspecific lesions [137]. Specific lesions usually present as single or multiple red or violaceous macules, papules or nodules typically seen on the face (Fig. 3.4.18a) and scalp, leading to "facies leonine" [27, 159]. Nonspecific findings including purpura, ecchymoses, and maculopapular eruptions. The lesions may appear at the sites of herpes simplex and herpes zoster scars.

3.4.2.6.5 Histopathology

Cutaneous infiltrates may be superficial and deep perivascular and periadnexal, nodular-diffuse or band-like [40]. The infiltrate is typically monomorphous and consists of small- to medium-sized lymphocytes with a round nucleus, dense nuclear chromatin, small nucleoli, and scant cytoplasm (Fig. 3.4.18b). Variable numbers of eosinophils, neutrophils, and plasma cells are also present. It is typically separated from the epidermis by a narrow Grenz zone of normal collagen although isolated epidermotropic cells may be seen.

Usually the infiltrate extends through the full thickness of the dermis and into the subcutaneous fat [28]. Proliferation centers in the skin are seen only in a minority of cases.

Immunocytochemically, B-CLL cells are characterized by an aberrant immunophenotype CD20+, CD43+, CD5+ [8]. In addition they express typical B-cell markers CD19, CD23 and CD79a and show monoclonal light-chain restriction to either κ or λ.

3.4.2.6.6 Prognosis and Predictive Factors

The prognosis varies, depending upon clinical stage; the presence of specific skin lesions in patients with B-CLL does not seem to be an independent poor prognostic sign [40].

3.4.2.7 Mantle Cell Lymphoma (MCL)

3.4.2.7.1 Definition

Mantle cell lymphoma is a rare B-cell lymphoma involving the mantle cells overexpressing cyclin D1 in the mantle zone of the lymphoid follicle. MCL commonly affects extranodal sites, especially bone marrow, gastrointestinal tract and Waldeyer's ring, however, skin is rarely involved [122].

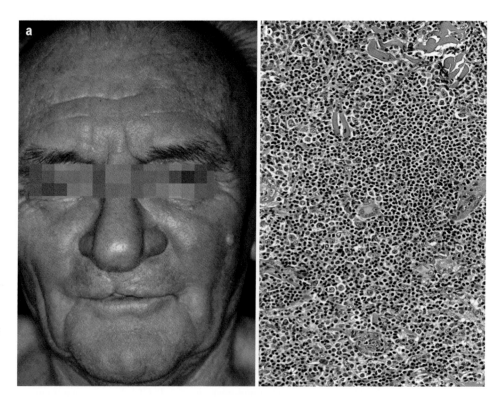

Fig. 3.4.18 Chronic lymphocytic leukemia. (**a**) (*Left*) specific skin infiltrates. (**b**) (*Right*) monomorphous infiltrate consisting of small- to medium-sized lymphocytes. H & E, 40×

3.4.2.7.2 ICD-O Code

9673/3

3.4.2.7.3 Synonyms

WHO/EORTC classification (2005): Mantle cell lymphoma
WHO classification (2001): Mantle cell lymphoma
REAL classification (1997): Mantle cell lymphoma
EORTC classification (1997): Not listed

3.4.2.7.4 Clinical Features

Approximately 4–6% of non-Hodgkin lymphomas are mantle cell lymphomas. Mantle cell lymphoma presenting in skin is seen mostly in cases with stage IV disease. Only a few cases have been reported in the literature [17, 62, 114]. Clinically multiple erythematous plaques or nodules are found.

3.4.2.7.5 Histopathology

Skin infiltrates in MCL occur in the dermis sometimes with extension to the subcutaneous tissue. A grenz-zone is present. The infiltrate may be relatively scanty and perivascular, form nodules or be very dense and diffuse.

Cytologically, the lymphoid cells are small to medium sized, usually slightly larger than normal lymphocytes, with dispersed chromatin, scant pale cytoplasm, and inconspicuous nucleoli. The nuclei have an irregular or cleaved configuration in most cases. In the blastoid variant, which may be more common in cutaneous lesions, the cells resemble lymphoblasts or large and pleomorphic cells of a diffuse large B-cell lymphoma.

Immunocytochemically, the most specific marker for MCL is the expression of cyclin D1. Additionally, the lymphoid cells are CD20+, CD79a, CD43+, IgM+, IgD+, CD10–, CD23–, bcl-2+, bcl-6–.

3.4.2.7.6 Prognosis and Predictive Factors

The prognosis of primary cutaneous MCL is controversial in the literature. Survival times between 18 months after diagnosis [92] and 17 years [17] have been reported.

3.4.2.8 Burkitt Lymphoma (BL)

3.4.2.8.1 Definition

Burkitt lymphoma is an aggressive B-cell lymphoma-associated with Epstein–Barr virus infection (EBV) in most cases and featuring translocation of the *c-myc* gene [35]. BL occurs endemically in children under 10 years in the so-called lymphoma belt of Central Africa. However, sporadic cases are seen in children and young adults throughout the world.

3.4.2.8.2 ICD-O Code

9680/3

3.4.2.8.3 Synonyms

WHO/EORTC classification (2005): Burkitt lymphoma
WHO classification (2001): Burkitt lymphoma / leukemia
REAL classification (1997): Burkitt lymphoma
EORTC classification (1997): Not listed

3.4.2.8.4 Clinical Features

Patients with BL present with large tumors due to the high proliferation rate and rapid growth of tumor cells. The most frequently involved sites are tissues that are comparatively poor in lymphoreticular elements like the jaws, ovaries, testes, thyroid, adrenals, and breasts. The skin may show secondary involvement.

3.4.2.8.5 Histopathology

The infiltrate is monotonous and shows a cohesive proliferation of medium-sized cells with many mitotic figures and a high rate of spontaneous cell death. The cytoplasm is deeply basophilic and usually contains lipid vacuoles. Their nuclei are round or ovoid and have fine or coarse granular chromatin. The apoptotic tumor cells are ingested by macrophages whose scattered distribution creates the typical "starry sky" pattern [29].

Immunocytochemically, the tumor cells express B-cell associated antigens (CD19, CD20, CD22), are positive for CD10, Bcl-6 (pointing to a germinal center origin), and are negative for CD5, CD23, Bcl-2 and TdT.

3.4.2.8.6 Prognosis and Predictive Factors

The prognosis depends on the degree of systemic spread of the disease. If properly treated, the outlook for patients with BL is favorable.

3.4.3 Immature Hematopoietic Malignancies

Mirjana Urosevic-Maiwald

3.4.3.1 *Blasti Plasmacytoid Dendritic Cell Neoplasm*

3.4.3.1.1 Definition

Blastic NK cell lymphoma is a rare and clinically aggressive neoplasm with a high incidence of skin involvement and risk of leukemic dissemination [17, 30, 41]. Recent evidence implies in most of the cases a close histogenetic relationship to plasmacytoid dendritic cell or its putative precursor [17]. Due to unclear precursor cells, the term CD4+CD56+ hematodermic neoplasm is preferred [39].

3.4.3.1.2 ICD-O Code

Blastic NK-cell lymphoma [9727/3] [1]

3.4.3.1.3 Synonyms

WHO-EORTC classification (2005): CD4+CD56+ hematodermic neoplasm [39]
WHO classification of tumors (2001): Blastic NK-cell lymphoma [20]

REAL classification (1997): Not listed
EORTC classification (1997): Not listed

- Dendritic cell 2 related CD4+/CD56+ blastic tumor of the skin
- Early plasmacytoid dendritic cell leukemia/lymphoma
- Agranular CD4+/CD56+ hematodermic tumor
- CD4+/CD56+ acute leukemia
- CD56+ TdT+ blastic NK cell tumor of skin
- Dendritic cell 2 precursor acute leukemia
- (Lympho) blastoid NK-leukemia/lymphoma
- Agranular CD4+/CD56+ blastic NK leukemia/lymphoma
- Primary cutaneous CD4+/CD56+ hematolymphoid neoplasm
- Myelomonocytic precursor cell-related lymphoma
- Cutaneous agranular CD2−/CD4+/CD56+ lymphoma
- Acute agranular CD4+ NK-cell leukemia
- CD4+/CD56+ acute monoblastic leukemia
- Histiocyte-associated hematologic malignancy

3.4.3.1.4 Clinical Features

Blastic NK-cell lymphoma/CD4+CD56+ hematodermic neoplasm (HN) primarily affects elderly patients, even though 30% of the cases are presented in patients younger than 50 years [39]. Pediatric cases are rare, but described [17]. Skin involvement occurs in up to 90% and manifests as asymptomatic solitary or multifocal skin lesions. Skin lesions are typically nodules, patch-plaques or bruise-like areas that measure from a few millimeters up to 10 cm (Fig. 3.4.19a).

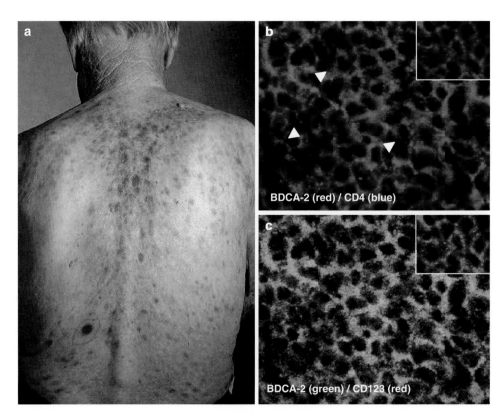

Fig. 3.4.19 CD4+ CD56+ hematodermic neoplasm. (**a**) Clinical manifestation. (**b**, **c**) Immunophenotype of tumor cells shown with confocal microscopy. Costaining of tumor cells with BDCA-2 (*red*) and CD4 (*blue*) is shown in magenta color (**b**). Costaining of tumor cells with BDCA-2 (*green*) and CD123 (*blue*) is shown in *yellow* color (**c**)

BDCA-2 (red) / CD4 (blue)

BDCA-2 (green) / CD123 (red)

Associated erythema, hyperpigmentation and ulceration can be seen. In almost 50% of the cases, the skin lesions represent the only detectable extramedullary tumor manifestation. Concomitant lymph node involvement is common (40–50%), but splenomegaly (~20%) or involvement of other mucosal sites (~10%) is relatively infrequent [17, 30, 41]. Systemic B symptoms are rare at diagnosis. Most cases display low-level blood marrow and peripheral blood involvement (60–90%). However, initial fulminant leukemia, even in the absence of the skin lesions, is rare (5–25%) [17]. Another common finding at the diagnosis is the presence of cytopenias, which are sometimes so severe that the patients are diagnosed to have a coincident myelodysplastic syndrome. This finding may be strengthened by the presence of megaloblastoid erythroid maturation and tumor-associated monocytosis. The disease progresses quickly with development of true lymph node, bone marrow and central nervous system involvement. Development of fulminant leukemia is a feature of HN progression or relapse, and is nearly always present at terminal stage. Relapse as myelomonocytic leukemia can also occur [23]. Thus, CD4+CD56+ HN should be principally differentiated from myelomonocytic leukemia cutis, and conceptually relates to so-called "aleukemic leukemia cutis" [41].

3.4.3.1.5 Histopathology and Immunophenotype

Skin involvement in CD4+CD56+ HN is diffusely dermal. Early-stage lesions may show predominantly perivascular or periadnexal patterns [17]. Histologically, nonepidermotropic monotonous dense infiltrates of medium-to-large sized cells with sparse cytoplasm, nuclear polymorphism, finely clumped chromatin and absent or indistinct nucleoli, resembling large lymphoblasts or myeloblasts are seen in the dermis [7, 17]. The epidermis is spared and separated from the dermis by a distinct grenz zone. Mitotic figures are frequent. Inflammatory cells are rare. There is generally no necrosis or angioinvasion. Inflammatory cells are absent. Erythrocyte extravasation is a characteristic feature, explaining the bruise-like appearance of the skin lesions [7]. Extensive involvement of the subcutis is only seen in large tumor lesions.

Immunophenotypically, tumor cells in HN express CD4 and CD56 in the absence of common linage-specific markers for lymphoid or myelomonocytic cells [7, 17, 41]. The blastic morphology, CD56 expression and lack of definitive myeloid or T-cell markers initially resulted in assignment of this tumor to the NK-cell lineage. Chaperot et al. showed that leukemic CD4+CD56+ cells express a constellation of markers very similar to the one present on the plasmacytoid dendritic cells (pDCs), i.e., lack of common lineage markers with concomitant expression of CD123/interleukin-3 receptor α chain, HLA-DR and CD45RA [10]. Indeed, the expression of CD43, HLA-DR and CD45RA, also expressed by B-cells and naïve T-cells, can be detected in tumor cells in most of the cases [8, 17, 36, 41]. The selectin ligand,

cutaneous lymphocyte antigen (CLA, HECA-452) is usually highly expressed in skin lesions [31]. Terminal deoxynucleotidyl transferase (TdT), a lymphoblastic marker, is expressed in up to 50% of HN [8, 17, 41]. As already mentioned, tumor cells in HN also express the markers associated with pDCs. CD123 (interleukin-3 receptor α chain) is sensitive and largely specific marker for pDCs and can be demonstrated in more than 90% of HN cases. Occasionally, dim CD123 can be found in some myelomonocytic leukemias, but the staining does not show the strong and uniform pattern seen in HN [17]. T-cell leukemia 1 (TCL1) is an Akt kinase regulator and lymphoid protooncogene, with expression restricted to nonneoplastic pDCs and B-cells [27, 31, 38]. TCL1 is expressed in 90% of HN [18], a feature that can help discriminate from CD123^weak myelomonocytic leukemias, which are nearly always negative for TCL1 [18, 31]. Variable expression of CD7, CD33, CD68, CD94 and CD99, as seen in pDC subsets, was also described in HN [17]. Whereas TCL1, CD68, CD123 and HLA-DR can also be expressed on other lymphoid or myeloid cells, blood DC antigen 2 (BDCA-2) was until recently the only specific marker expressed on human pDCs [13]. BDCA-2 expression has been reported in a subset of HN, and may identify a more mature differentiation state of the tumor cells [21]. The expression of BDCA-2 and CD123 on tumor cells of HN is shown in (Fig. 3.4.19b, c). Conversely, TdT expression shows an inverse correlation with BDCA-2 and seems to define a less mature, precursor pDC leukemia/lymphoma [21]. Furthermore, these tumor cells also express MxA protein, which is indicative of the pDC function to produce interferons [32, 36]. A new pDC-specific marker has been introduced recently – CD2AP adaptor protein, which was absent in almost all leukemia cutis [26]. Finally, the expression of EBV antigens, myeloperoxidase (MPO), lysosyme, PAX-5, CD20, CD22, T-cell receptor protein (TCR) should exclude the diagnosis of HN.

3.4.3.1.6 Prognosis and Predictive Factors

The clinical course is aggressive. The patients with CD4+CD56+ HN have an overall dismal prognosis, with a median overall survival between 12 and 14 months, irrespective of the initial pattern of the disease [17, 41]. Most patients have shown an initial response to multiagent chemotherapy (80–90%), but relapses with subsequent drug resistance occurring in the vast majority of cases after a median of 9–11 months. Long-lasting remissions or sporadic cures were featured in rare reports, usually in younger patients who received acute leukemia-induction therapy followed by an allogeneic stem cell transplantation in first complete remission [6, 15, 17, 30, 33, 34].

Immunoreactivity of tumor cells for BDCA-2 was shown to significantly reduce the overall and disease-specific survival in a small group of patients [21]. On the contrary, expression of TdT was identified as an independent positive prognostic in a larger series of patients [6, 35].

3.4.3.2 Precursor Lymphoblastic Leukemia/ Lymphoma

3.4.3.2.1 Definition

Lymphoblastic leukemias/lymphomas are neoplasms of immature lymphoid cells. Depending on the involved lineage, T-cell and B-cell lymphoblastic leukemia/lymphoma are recognized [20]. When the process of precursor B-cell neoplasm is confined to a solid tissue mass without evidence of blood and marrow involvement, the disorder is referred to as lymphoma. When the process includes extensive blood and marrow involvement, lymphoblastic leukemia is the appropriate term. Lymphoblastic leukemia/lymphoma is rare, accounting for 3.5–7% of all cutaneous lymphomas.

3.4.3.2.2 ICD-O Code

T-cell lymphoblastic leukemia [9837/3], lymphoma [9729/3]
B-cell lymphoblastic leukemia [9835/3], lymphoma [9728/3]

3.4.3.2.3 Precursor T-Cell Lymphoblastic Leukemia/ Lymphoblastic Lymphoma (T-ALL/T-LBL)

T-ALL constitutes 15% of childhood acute lymphoblastic leukemias (ALL) and 25% of adult ALL [5, 16]. Precursor T-LBL comprises about 85–90% of lymphoblastic lymphoma. T-ALL patients present with a high leukocytosis and often a large mediastinal mass, in contrast to B-ALL, which has variable leukocyte counts and only rarely a mass. T-ALL and presumably T-LBL is thought to result from malignant thymocytes that arise at defined stages of intrathymic T-cell differentiation [2]. An abnormal karyotype is found in approximately 50% of T-ALL cases [16]. T-cell receptor genes from chromosomes 7 and 14 are often involved in translocations with different transcription factor, such as TAL1, LYL1 and HOX11. In addition, fusion genes are generated that encode for chimeric proteins with oncogenic properties, such as SIL-TAL1 and MLL-partner gene fusions. Cryptic deletions leading to the loss of tumor suppressor genes also occur in T-ALL, the most common of which are the deletion at chromosome 6q and the deletion of CDKN2A^{INK4} at chromosome 9p21. Recently, it has also been found that T-ALL cases involve mutations in the key regulator of T-cell fate, the NOTCH1 molecule [40]. Although current treatment protocols have improved the overall outcome for patients with T-ALL, a significant number of patients remain at high risk of relapse, and only a few survive when the disease reoccurs. The existence and frequency of NOTCH1 mutations in T-ALL provides a compelling possibility for the use of either inhibitors of the Notch pathway, such as γ-secretase antagonists, or inhibitors of NF-κB pathway, such as bortezomib, in the treatment of T-ALL [2].

3.4.3.2.4 Precursor B-Cell Lymphoblastic Leukemia/ Lymphoblastic Lymphoma (B-ALL/B-LBL)

B-ALL is primarily a disease of children, accounting for 80–85% of childhood ALL. B-LBL is a rare type of lymphoma that preferentially affects young people, accounting for approximately 10% of lymphoblastic lymphomas. Precursor B-ALL always involves blood and bone marrow with frequent extramedullary involvement of central nervous system, lymph nodes, spleen and gonads. Leukocyte counts vary and may be decreased, normal or increased at presentation. Different genetic abnormalities have been described in B-ALL, some of which also have prognostic implications [24]. Over 50% of the children with B-ALL have the good hyperploid karyotype or the t(12, 21), which predicts 85–90% long-term survival. Almost three-fourths of the patients with B-LBL reported in the literature seem to have skin lesions (with or without adjacent nodal involvement) [25]. B-LBL has a high remission rate despite aggressive multiagent chemotherapy in combination with or without radiotherapy [24, 25].

3.4.3.2.5 Skin Manifestations and Histopathology of Precursor Lymphoblastic Leukemia/ Lymphoma

The skin is relatively rarely affected by the precursor lymphoblastic leukemias/lymphomas (1% of all leukemia/lymphoma cases) [9, 11]. Precursor B-cell malignancies occur more frequently in the skin than those of precursor T-cell origin. The most common clinical presentation in cutaneous and extranodal sites is a single nodule or a tumor. In the skin, there are typically one or multiple erythematous papules and nodules, often encountered in the head and neck region, especially in patients with B-ALL/B-PBL. The high likelihood to develop bone marrow involvement is an important consideration for therapy, as these patients are considered to have systemic disease.

The cytomorphologic features of precursor lymphoblastic leukemia/lymphoma are almost identical [11, 39]. Typically, the infiltrates are deep seated in the dermis and lack epidermotropism. The pattern of infiltration can be perivascular or even diffuse. The cells are interspersed among dermal collagen fibers, without a stromal inflammatory response. Morphologically, the cells have usually a uniform appearance giving rise to monotonous infiltrate, composed of intermediate (small- to medium-) sized cells with round scarce perinuclear contours and blastic chromatin resembling lymphoblasts. Numerous mitotic and apoptotic figures can be often observed. Stromal fibrosis is frequently seen.

3.4.3.2.6 Immunophentype of Precursor Lymphoblastic Leukemia/Lymphoma

T-ALL/T-LBL: These tumors are positive for CD1a, CD3, CD10 and TdT. CD99 is usually positive. CD3 in combination with TdT and/or CD1a is the most specific marker for the identification of this type of precursor neoplasms. Other useful T-cell lineage markers are CD2, CD4, CD5 and CD8. A subset of cases expresses CD4 and CD8. It is of note that CD99 (surface antigen MIC2) can be expressed in nonhematopoietic tumors and should not be considered as a specific marker for precursor leukemia/lymphoma [3, 4, 19, 29].

B-ALL/B-LBL: Tumor cells express CD10, CD19 and CD79a in most of the cases. CD20, CD22 and CD24 are variably expressed. Pax5 (B-cell lineage specific activator protein, BSAP) is a B-cell specific transcription factor that is essential for commitment of lymphoid precursors to the B-cell lineage [12]. Pax5 is detectable in pro-B-cell stage and subsequently in all further stages of B-cell lymphopoiesis, except in plasma cells, where it is down-regulated. The combination of Pax5 and TdT is very useful to identify this type of precursor neoplasms. However, Pax5 can also be found in AML, for example in conjunction with t(8, 21) translocation [14, 37].

3.4.3.3 Myeloid and Monocytic Leukemias

Leukemia cutis represents a secondary infiltration of the skin by malignant leukocytes (either of myeloid or lymphoid origin), which results in clinically identifiable cutaneous lesions. Leukemia cutis composed of neoplastic granulocytic precursors has also been designated as myeloid sarcoma, granulocytic sarcoma, primary extramedullary leukemia, or chloroma [20, 39]. When composed of neoplastic monocytic precursors (monoblasts and promonocytes), leukemia cutis was also termed monoblastic sarcoma. Myeloid sarcoma and extramedullary myeloid cell tumor often encompass both granulocytic and monocytic tumors. Involvement of the skin occurs in 10–15% of patients with acute myeloid leukemia

(AML) and less frequently in chronic myeloproliferative diseases [11, 39]. Various types of AML are responsible for different frequencies of leukemia cutis. Up to 50% of patients with acute myelomonocytic (AMMoL) and monocytic leukemia (AMoL) present with leukemia cutis. On the other hand, skin involvement in patients with chronic myelomonocytic leukemia (CML) is less common. Children seem to be more affected than adults by leukemia cutis; as many as 30% of infants with congenital leukemia, most frequently of AML type, show skin involvement.

Clinical manifestations of leukemia cutis range from solitary to multiple violaceous, red–brown or hemorrhagic papules/plaques and nodules of varying sizes [11, 20, 28, 39]. Different leukemia cutis lesions can be present in the same patient. Lower extremities are most commonly affected, followed by arms, trunk, scalp, and face. Leukemic infiltration tends to prefer the sites of previous or concomitant inflammation. Unusual clinical presentations of leukemia include pronounced gingival hyperplasia and oral petechiae AMoL, leonine faces in AMMoL, eczematous lesions, penile and scrotal ulcers, and erythema nodosum-like panniculitis. Almost 90% of the patients with leukemia cutis show attendant involvement of other extramedullary sites, in particular meninges. Most cases of leukemia cutis are diagnosed after the discovery of systemic leukemia. Coexistence of skin and systemic leukemia was observed in up to one-third of the cases. Occasionally, skin infiltration may precede bone marrow and peripheral blood involvement and is termed "aleukemic leukemia cutis" or "primary extramedullary leukemia." This uncommon event occurs predominantly in patient with AML and is usually manifested in wide-spread and papulo-nodular lesions.

Histologically, the infiltrate in leukemia cutis can be nodular with perivascular or periadnexal distribution or interstitial and/or diffuse [11]. A characteristic feature is the presence of rows of atypical cells between collagen bundles. Tumor cells in AMoL and AMMoL are medium- to large-sized and show round, oval or folded nuclei, small nucleoli, and amphophilic cytoplasm reminiscent of promonocytes. Mitotic figures are usually present. Extension into subcutaneous fat can also be seen. Epidermotropism is rare. Skin involvement in CML reveals more pleomorphic infiltrate, dominated by variably mature cells of granulocytic lineage. The majority of tumor cells show reactivity for myeloperoxidase, lysozyme and CD68. CD56, a neural cell adhesion molecule N-CAM, can also be expressed in some cases of AML. CD117, a c-lit product, is present in AML, including the myeloblastic component of AMMoL. Conversely, the majority of AMoL cases are negative. CD117 is not specific, due to its expression on mast cell and other lymphoid cell infiltrates.

The presence of leukemia cutis in AML or CML patients implies an aggressive course and portends poor prognosis [11, 39]. In one series, all patients died within 24 months after appearance of specific skin manifestations [22].

References

Mature T-Cell and NK-Cell Neoplasms

1. Ackerman, A.: Granulomatous slack skin. Histologic diagnosis of inflammatory skin diseases, pp. 483–485. Lea and Febiger, Philadelphia (1978)

2. Ada, S., Gulec, A.T.: CD8+ poikilodermatous mycosis fungoides with a nonaggressive clinical behaviour and a good response to psoralen plus ultraviolet A treatment. Br. J. Dermatol. **157**(5), 1064–1066 (2007)

3. Agnarsson, B.A., Vonderheid, E.C., et al.: Cutaneous T cell lymphoma with suppressor/cytotoxic (CD8) phenotype: identification of rapidly progressive and chronic subtypes. J. Am. Acad. Dermatol. **22**(4), 569–577 (1990)

4. Akinyemi, E., Mai, L., et al.: Diffuse large B-cell lymphoma mimicking advanced basal cell carcinoma. J. Natl. Med. Assoc. **99**(8), 948–950 (2007)

5. Alaibac, M., Bordignon, M., et al.: Primary subcutaneous B-cell lymphoma: case report and literature review. Acta Derm. Venereol. **88**(2), 151–154 (2008)

6. Amagai, M., Kawakubo, Y., et al.: Lymphomatoid papulosis followed by Ki-1 positive anaplastic large cell lymphoma: proliferation of a common T-cell clone. J. Dermatol. **22**(10), 743–746 (1995)

7. Arnulf, B., Copie-Bergman, C., et al.: Nonhepatosplenic gammadelta T-cell lymphoma: a subset of cytotoxic lymphomas with mucosal or skin localization. Blood **91**(5), 1723–1731 (1998)

8. Baccaredda, A.: Reticulohistiocytosis cutanea hyperplastica benigna cum melanodermia. Arch. Dermatol. Syphilol. **179**, 209–256 (1939)

9. Barnadas, M.A., Lopez, D., et al.: Pustular lymphomatoid papulosis in childhood. J. Am. Acad. Dermatol. **27**(4), 627–628 (1992)

10. Barnett, C.R., Seo, S., et al.: Intravascular B-cell lymphoma: the role of skin biopsy. Am. J. Dermatopathol. **30**(3), 295–299 (2008)

11. Bazex, A., Dupre, A., et al.: Chalazodermic Besnier-Boeck-Schaumann disease? Bull. Soc. Fr. Dermatol. Syphiligr. **75**(4), 448–449 (1968)

12. Beaty, M.W., Toro, J., et al.: Cutaneous lymphomatoid granulomatosis: correlation of clinical and biologic features. Am. J. Surg. Pathol. **25**(9), 1111–1120 (2001)

13. Bekkenk, M.W., Geelen, F.A., et al.: Primary and secondary cutaneous CD30(+) lymphoproliferative disorders: a report from the Dutch Cutaneous Lymphoma Group on the long-term follow-up data of 219 patients and guidelines for diagnosis and treatment. Blood **95**(12), 3653–3661 (2000)

14. Bekkenk, M.W., Vermeer, M.H., et al.: Peripheral T-cell lymphomas unspecified presenting in the skin: analysis of prognostic factors in a group of 82 patients. Blood **102**(6), 2213–2219 (2003)

15. Belousova, I.E., Nikonova, S.M., et al.: Granulomatous slack skin with clonal T-cell receptor-gamma gene rearrangement in skin and lymph node. Br. J. Dermatol. **157**(2), 405–407 (2007)

16. Benton, E.C., Morris, S.L., et al.: An unusual case of granulomatous slack skin disease with necrobiosis. Am. J. Dermatopathol. **30**(5), 462–465 (2008)

17. Bertero, M., Novelli, M., et al.: Mantle zone lymphoma: an immunohistologic study of skin lesions. J. Am. Acad. Dermatol. **30**(1), 23–30 (1994)

18. Berti, E., Alessi, E., et al.: Reticulohistiocytoma of the dorsum. J. Am. Acad. Dermatol. **19**, 259–272 (1988)

19. Berti, E., Cerri, A., et al.: Primary cutaneous gamma/delta T-cell lymphoma presenting as disseminated pagetoid reticulosis. J. Invest. Dermatol. **96**, 718–723 (1991)

20. Berti, E., Tomasini, D., et al.: Primary cutaneous CD8-positive epidermotropic cytotoxic T cell lymphomas. A distinct clinicopathological entity with an aggressive clinical behavior. Am. J. Pathol. **155**(2), 483–492 (1999)

21. Bittencourt, A.L., Rothers, S., et al.: Primary cutaneous eosinophil-rich anaplastic large cell lymphoma: report of an unusual case and literature review. J. Cutan. Med. Surg. **12**(2), 88–92 (2008)

22. Bogomolski-Yahalom, V., Lossos, I.S., et al.: Intravascular lymphomatosis–an indolent or aggressive entity? Leuk. Lymphoma **29**(5–6), 585–593 (1998)

23. Braun-Falco, O., Marghescu, S., et al.: Pagetoide reticulosis–Woringer-Kolopp's disease. Hautarzt **24**(1), 11–21 (1973)

24. Braun-Falco, O., Nikolowski, J., et al.: Lymphomatoid papulosis. Review and personal observation of 4 patients. Hautarzt **34**(2), 59–65 (1983)

25. Braun-Falco, O., Guggenberger, K., et al.: Immunozytom unter dem Bild einer Acrodermatitis chronica atrophicans. Hautarzt **29**, 644–647 (1978)

26. Braun, F.O., Schmoeckel, C., et al.: Pagetoid reticulosis. A further case report with a review of the literature. Acta Derm. Venereol. Suppl. (Stockh). **59**(85), 11–21 (1979)

27. Buechner, S., Su, W.: Leukemia cutis. In: Arndt, K.A., Robinson, J.K., Leboit, P.E., Wintroub, B.U. (eds.) Cutaneous Medicine and Surgery, p. 1670. W.B.Saunders, Philadelphia (1996)

28. Buechner, S.A., Li, C.Y., et al.: Leukemia cutis. A histopathologic study of 42 cases. Am. J. Dermatopathol. **7**(2), 109–119 (1985)

29. Burg, G., Braun-Falco, O.: Cutaneous lymphomas, pseudolymphomas and related disorders. Springer, Berlin (1983)

30. Burg, G., Dummer, R., et al.: A subcutaneous delta positive T-cell lymphoma that produces interferon gamma. N. Engl. J. Med. **325**, 1078–1081 (1991)

31. Burg, G., Hoffmann, F.G., et al.: Lymphomatoid papulosis: a cutaneous T-cell pseudolymphoma. Acta Derm. Venereol. **61**(6), 491–496 (1981)

32. Burg, G., Kempf, W., et al.: Pyogenic lymphoma of the skin: a peculiar variant of primary cutaneous neutrophil-rich CD30+ anaplastic large-cell lymphoma. Clinicopathological study of four cases and review of the literature. Br. J. Dermatol. **148**(3), 580–586 (2003)

33. Burg, G., Schmockel, C.: Syringolymphoid hyperplasia with alopecia–a syringotropic cutaneous T-cell lymphoma? Dermatology **184**(4), 306–307 (1992)

34. Burg, G., Ziffer, S., et al.: Light and electron microscopy findings in lymphomatoid papulosis. In: Muller, S. (ed.) Parapsoriasis, pp. 78–81. Mayo Foundation, Rochester (1990)

35. Burkitt, D.: A sarcoma involving the jaws in African children. Br. J. Surg. **46**, 218–223 (1958)

36. Camacho, F.M., Burg, G., et al.: Granulomatous slack skin in childhood. Pediatr. Dermatol. **14**(3), 204–208 (1997)

37. Carlson, K.C., Gibson, L.E.: Cutaneous signs of lymphomatoid granulomatosis. Arch. Dermatol. **127**(11), 1693–1698 (1991)

38. Cerroni, L., Arzberger, E., et al.: Primary cutaneous follicle center cell lymphoma with follicular growth pattern. Blood **95**(12), 3922–3928 (2000)

39. Cerroni, L., Volkenandt, M., et al.: bcl-2 Protein expression and correlation with the interchromosomal 14;18 translocation in cutaneous lymphomas and pseudolymphomas. J. Invest. Dermatol. **102**(2), 231–235 (1994)

40. Cerroni, L., Zenahlik, P., et al.: Specific cutaneous infiltrates of B-cell chronic lymphocytic leukemia: a clinicopathologic and prognostic study of 42 patients. Am. J. Surg. Pathol. **20**(8), 1000–1010 (1996)

41. Cho-Vega, J.H., Vega, F., et al.: Primary cutaneous marginal zone B-cell lymphoma. Am. J. Clin. Pathol. **125**(suppl), S38–S49 (2006)

42. Christensen, H.K., Thomsen, K., et al.: Lymphomatoid papulosis: a follow-up study of 41 patients. Semin. Dermatol. **13**(3), 197–201 (1994)

43. Convit, J., Kerdel, F., et al.: Progressive, atrophing, chronic granulomatous dermohypodermitis. Autimmune disease? Arch. Dermatol. **107**, 271 (1973)

44. D'Incan, M., Antoniotti, O., et al.: HTLV-I-associated lymphoma presenting as mycosis fungoides in an HTLV-I non-endemic area: a viro-molecular study. Br. J. Dermatol. **132**(6), 983–988 (1995)

45. Davis, T.H., Morton, C.C., et al.: Hodgkin's disease, lymphomatoid papulosis, and cutaneous T-cell lymphoma derived from a common T-cell clone. N. Engl. J. Med. **326**(17), 1115–1122 (1992)

46. de la Fouchardiere, A., Balme, B., et al.: Primary cutaneous marginal zone B-cell lymphoma: a report of 9 cases. J. Am. Acad. Dermatol. **41**(2 pt 1), 181–188 (1999)

47. De Paepe, P., De Wolf-Peeters, C.: Diffuse large B-cell lymphoma: a heterogeneous group of non-Hodgkin lymphomas comprising several distinct clinicopathological entities. Leukemia **21**(1), 37–43 (2007)

48. de Wolf-Peeters, C., Achten, R.: gammadelta T-cell lymphomas: a homogeneous entity? Histopathology **36**(4), 294–305 (2000)

49. Debarbieux, S., Balme, B., et al.: Interstitial granulomatous dermatitis. Ann. Dermatol. Vénéréol. **134**(11), 889–891 (2007)

50. Deneau, D.G., Wood, G.S., et al.: Woringer-Kolopp disease (pagetoid reticulosis). Four cases with histopathologic, ultrastructural, and immunohistologic observations. Arch. Dermatol. **120**(8), 1045–1051 (1984)

51. van Doorn, R., Van Haselen, C.W., et al.: Mycosis fungoides: disease evolution and prognosis of 309 Dutch patients. Arch. Dermatol. **136**, 504–510 (2000)

52. Droc, C., Cualing, H.D., et al.: Need for an improved molecular/genetic classification for CD30+ lymphomas involving the skin. Cancer Control **14**(2), 124–132 (2007)

53. Du, M.Q.: MALT lymphoma: recent advances in aetiology and molecular genetics. J. Clin. Exp. Hematop. **47**(2), 31–42 (2007)

54. Dummer, R., Kohl, O., et al.: Peripheral blood mononuclear cells in patients with nonleukemic cutaneous T-cell lymphoma. Reduced proliferation and preferential secretion of a T helper-2-like cytokine pattern on stimulation. Arch. Dermatol. **129**(4), 433–436 (1993)

55. Dummer, R., Posseckert, G., et al.: Soluble interleukin-2 receptors inhibit interleukin 2-dependent proliferation and cytotoxicity: explanation for diminished natural killer cell activity in cutaneous T-cell lymphomas in vivo? J. Invest. Dermatol. **98**(1), 50–54 (1992)

56. Dupont, A.: Langsam verlaufende und klinisch gutartige Reticulopathie mit höchst maligner histologischer Struktur. Hautarzt **16**, 284–286 (1965)

57. Falini, B., Fizzotti, M., et al.: Bcl-6 protein expression in normal and neoplastic lymphoid tissues. Ann. Oncol. **8**(suppl 2), 101–104 (1997)

58. Friedmann, D., Wechsler, J., et al.: Primary cutaneous pleomorphic small T-cell lymphoma. A review of 11 cases. The French Study Group on Cutaneous Lymphomas. Arch. Dermatol. **131**(9), 1009–1015 (1995)

59. Frizzera, G., Kaneko, Y., et al.: Angioimmunoblastic lymphadenopathy and related disorders: a retrospective look in search of definitions. Leukemia **3**(1), 1–5 (1989)

60. Frizzera, G., Moran, E.M., et al.: Angio-immunoblastic lymphadenopathy. Diagnosis and clinical course. Am. J. Med. **59**(6), 803–818 (1975)

61. Garbe, C., Stein, H., et al.: Borrelia burgdorferi-associated cutaneous B cell lymphoma: clinical and immunohistologic characterization of four cases. J. Am. Acad. Dermatol. **24**(4), 584–590 (1991)

62. Geerts, M.L., Busschots, A.M.: Mantle-cell lymphomas of the skin. Dermatol. Clin. **12**(2), 409–417 (1994)

63. Gerami, P., Guitart, J.: The spectrum of histopathologic and immunohistochemical findings in folliculotropic mycosis fungoides. Am. J. Surg. Pathol. **31**(9), 1430–1438 (2007)

64. Gerami, P., Rosen, S., et al.: Folliculotropic mycosis fungoides: an aggressive variant of cutaneous T-cell lymphoma. Arch. Dermatol. **144**(6), 738–746 (2008)

65. Gleason, B.C., Brinster, N.K., et al.: Intravascular cytotoxic T-cell lymphoma: a case report and review of the literature. J. Am. Acad. Dermatol. **58**(2), 290–294 (2008)

66. Gonzalez, C.L., Medeiros, L.J., et al.: T-cell lymphoma involving subcutaneous tissue. A clinicopathologic entity commonly associated with hemophagocytic syndrome. Am. J. Surg. Pathol. **15**(1), 17–27 (1991)

67. Grange, F., Hedelin, G., et al.: Prognostic factors in primary cutaneous lymphomas other than mycosis fungoides and the Sezary syndrome. The French Study Group on Cutaneous Lymphomas. Blood **93**(11), 3637–3642 (1999)

68. Gruber, R., Sepp, N.T., et al.: Prognosis of lymphomatoid papulosis. Oncologist **11**(8), 955–957 (2006). author reply 957

69. Gruson, L.M., Heller, P., et al.: Mycosis fungoides involving the nasal mucosa. J. Am. Acad. Dermatol. **56**(5 suppl), S112–S114 (2007)

70. Guitart, J., Kennedy, J., et al.: Histologic criteria for the diagnosis of mycosis fungoides: proposal for a grading system to standardize pathology reporting. J. Cutan. Pathol. **28**(4), 174–183 (2001)

71. Haghighi, B., Smoller, B.R., et al.: Pagetoid reticulosis (Woringer-Kolopp disease): an immunophenotypic, molecular, and clinicopathologic study. Mod. Pathol. **13**(5), 502–510 (2000)

72. Hanna, S., Walsh, N., et al.: Mycosis fungoides presenting as pigmented purpuric dermatitis. Pediatr. Dermatol. **23**(4), 350–354 (2006)

73. Harmon, C.B., Witzig, T.E., et al.: Detection of circulating T cells with Cd4(+)Cd7(−) immunophenotype in patients with benign and malignant lymphoproliferative dermatoses. J. Am. Acad. Dermatol. **35**(3 pt 1), 404–410 (1996)

74. Hembury, T.A., Lee, B., et al.: Primary cutaneous diffuse large B-cell lymphoma: a clinicopathologic study of 15 cases. Am. J. Clin. Pathol. **117**(4), 574–580 (2002)

75. Hwang, S.T., Janik, J.E., et al.: Mycosis fungoides and Sezary syndrome. Lancet **371**(9616), 945–957 (2008)

76. Ikonomou, I.M., Aamot, H.V., et al.: Granulomatous slack skin with a translocation t(3;9)(q12;p24). Am. J. Surg. Pathol. **31**(5), 803–806 (2007)

77. Jaffe, E.: Subcutaneous panniculitis-like T-cell lymphoma. WHO classification of tumors. In: Jaffe ES, H.N., Stein, H., Vardiman, J.W. (eds.) Pathology and Genetics of Tumors of Haematopoietic and Lymphoid Tissues, pp. 212–213. IARC, Lyon (2001)

78. Jambrosic, J., From, L., et al.: Lymphomatoid granulomatosis. J. Am. Acad. Dermatol. **17**(4), 621–631 (1987)

79. James, W.D., Odom, R.B., et al.: Cutaneous manifestations of lymphomatoid granulomatosis. Report of 44 cases and a review of the literature. Arch. Dermatol. **117**(4), 196–202 (1981)

80. Jang, K.A., Choi, J.H., et al.: Primary CD56 + nasal-type T/natural killer-cell subcutaneous panniculitic lymphoma: presentation as haemophagocytic syndrome. Br. J. Dermatol. **141**(4), 706–709 (1999)

81. Jayaraman, A.G., Cassarino, D., et al.: Cutaneous involvement by angioimmunoblastic T-cell lymphoma: a unique histologic presentation, mimicking an infectious etiology. J. Cutan. Pathol. **33**(suppl 2), 6–11 (2006)

82. Kadin, M.E.: Common activated helper-T-cell origin for lymphomatoid papulosis, mycosis fungoides, and some types of Hodgkin's disease. Lancet **2**(8460), 864–865 (1985)

83. Kadin, M.E.: The spectrum of Ki-1+ cutaneous lymphomas. Curr. Probl. Dermatol. **19**(132), 132–143 (1990)

84. Kadin, M.E.: Lymphomatoid papulosis and associated lymphomas. How are they related? Arch. Dermatol. **129**(3), 351–353 (1993)

85. Kadin, M.E.: Pathobiology of CD30+ cutaneous T-cell lymphomas. J. Cutan. Pathol. **33**(suppl 1), 10–17 (2006)

86. Kadin, M.E., Levi, E., et al.: Progression of lymphomatoid papulosis to systemic lymphoma is associated with escape from growth inhibition by transforming growth factor-beta and CD30 ligand. Ann. N. Y. Acad. Sci. **941**, 59–68 (2001)

87. Kamarashev, J., Burg, G., et al.: Comparative analysis of histological and immunohistological features in mycosis fungoides and Sezary syndrome. J. Cutan. Pathol. **25**(8), 407–412 (1998)

88. Karsai, S., Hou, J.S., et al.: Sezary syndrome coexisting with B-cell chronic lymphocytic leukemia: case report and review of the literature. Dermatology 216(1), 68–75 (2008)

89. Kato, N., Tomita, Y., et al.: Involvement of the tongue by lymphomatoid papulosis. Am. J. Dermatopathol. 20(5), 522–526 (1998)

90. Katzenstein, A.L., Carrington, C.B., et al.: Lymphomatoid granulomatosis: a clinicopathologic study of 152 cases. Cancer 43(1), 360–373 (1979)

91. Kaudewitz, P., Burg, G., Stein, H., Klepzig, K., Mason, D.Y., Braun-Falco, O.: Monoclonal antibody patterns in lymphomatoid papulosis. Dermatol. Clin. 3, 749–757 (1985)

92. Kaudewitz, P., Burg, G.: Lymphomatoid papulosis and Ki-1 (CD30)-positive cutaneous large cell lymphomas. Semin. Diagn. Pathol. 8(2), 117–124 (1991)

93. Kaudewitz, P., Stein, H., et al.: Detection of Sternberg-Reed- and Hodgkin cell specific antigen on atypical cells in lymphomatoid papulosis. In: Second International Conference on Malignant Lymphoma, Lugano (1984)

94. Kaudewitz, P., Stein, H., et al.: Hodgkin's disease followed by lymphomatoid papulosis. Immunophenotypic evidence for a close relationship between lymphomatoid papulosis and Hodgkin's disease. J. Am. Acad. Dermatol. 22, 999–1006 (1990)

95. Kazakov, D.V., Burg, G., et al.: Clinicopathological spectrum of mycosis fungoides. J. Eur. Acad. Dermatol. Venereol. 18(4), 397–415 (2004)

96. Kempf, W.: CD30+ lymphoproliferative disorders: histopathology, differential diagnosis, new variants, and simulators. J. Cutan. Pathol. 33(suppl 1), 58–70 (2006)

97. Kerl, H.: Das Sézary-Syndrom. Zentralbl. Haut Geschlechtskr. 144, 359–446 (1981)

98. Kerschmann, R.L., Berger, T.G., et al.: Cutaneous presentations of lymphoma in human immunodeficiency virus disease. Predominance of T cell lineage. Arch. Dermatol. 131(11), 1281–1288 (1995)

99. Ketron, L.W., Goodman, M.H.: Multiple lesions of the skin apparently of epithelial origin resembling clinically mycosis fungoides. Arch. Dermatol. 24, 758–777 (1931)

100. Kim, E.J., Lin, J., et al.: Mycosis fungoides and sezary syndrome: an update. Curr. Oncol. Rep. 8(5), 376–386 (2006)

101. Kim, Y.H., Hoppe, R.T.: Mycosis fungoides and the Sezary syndrome. Semin. Oncol. 26(3), 276–289 (1999)

102. Kim, Y.H., Liu, H.L., et al.: Long-term outcome of 525 patients with mycosis fungoides and Sezary syndrome: clinical prognostic factors and risk for disease progression. Arch. Dermatol. 139(7), 857–866 (2003)

103. Klemke, C.D., Fritzsching, B., et al.: Paucity of FOXP3+ cells in skin and peripheral blood distinguishes Sezary syndrome from other cutaneous T-cell lymphomas. Leukemia 20(6), 1123–1129 (2006)

104. Kummer, J.A., Vermeer, M.H., et al.: Most primary cutaneous CD30-positive lymphoproliferative disorders have a CD4-positive cytotoxic T-cell phenotype. J. Invest. Dermatol. 109(5), 636–640 (1997)

105. Lazova, R., Slater, C., et al.: Reactive angioendotheliomatosis. Case report and review of the literature. Am. J. Dermatopathol. 18(1), 63–69 (1996)

106. LeBoit, P.E., McNutt, N.S., et al.: Primary cutaneous immunocytoma. A B-cell lymphoma that can easily be mistaken for cutaneous lymphoid hyperplasia. Am. J. Surg. Pathol. 18(10), 969–978 (1994)

107. LeBoit, P.E., Zackheim, H.S., et al.: Granulomatous variants of cutaneous T-cell lymphoma. The histopathology of granulomatous mycosis fungoides and granulomatous slack skin. Am. J. Surg. Pathol. 12(2), 83–95 (1988)

108. Lee, J., Viakhireva, N., et al.: Clinicopathologic features and treatment outcomes in Woringer-Kolopp disease. J. Am. Acad. Dermatol. 59(4), 706–712 (2008)

109. Levine, P.H., Jaffe, E.S., et al.: Human T-cell lymphotropic virus type I and adult T-cell leukemia/lymphoma outside Japan and the Caribbean Basin. Yale J. Biol. Med. 61(3), 215–222 (1988)

110. Liebow, A.A., Carrington, C.R., et al.: Lymphomatoid granulomatosis. Hum. Pathol. 3(4), 457–558 (1972)

111. Macaulay, W.L.: Lymphomatoid papulosis. A continuing self-healing eruption, clinically benign–histologically malignant. Arch. Dermatol. 97(1), 23–30 (1968)

112. Magana, M., Sangueza, P., et al.: Angiocentric cutaneous T-cell lymphoma of childhood (hydroa-like lymphoma): a distinctive type of cutaneous T-cell lymphoma. J. Am. Acad. Dermatol. 38(4), 574–579 (1998)

113. Martel, P., Laroche, L., et al.: Cutaneous involvement in patients with angioimmunoblastic lymphadenopathy with dysproteinemia: a clinical, immunohistological, and molecular analysis. Arch. Dermatol. 136(7), 881–886 (2000)

114. Marti, R.M., Campo, E., et al.: Cutaneous lymphocyte-associated antigen (CLA) expression in a lymphoblastoid mantle cell lymphoma presenting with skin lesions. Comparison with other clinicopathologic presentations of mantle cell lymphoma. J. Cutan. Pathol. 28(5), 256–264 (2001)

115. Massone, C., Chott, A., et al.: Subcutaneous, blastic natural killer (NK), NK/T-cell, and other cytotoxic lymphomas of the skin: a morphologic, immunophenotypic, and molecular study of 50 patients. Am. J. Surg. Pathol. 28(6), 719–735 (2004)

116. Matutes, E.: Adult T-cell leukaemia/lymphoma. J. Clin. Pathol. 60(12), 1373–1377 (2007)

117. McCluggage, W.G., Walsh, M.Y., et al.: Anaplastic large cell malignant lymphoma with extensive eosinophilic or neutrophilic infiltration. Histopathology 32(2), 110–115 (1998)

118. McMenamin, M.E., Fletcher, C.D.: Reactive angioendotheliomatosis: a study of 15 cases demonstrating a wide clinicopathologic spectrum. Am. J. Surg. Pathol. 26(6), 685–697 (2002)

119. Medenica, M., Lorincz, A.L.: Pagetoid reticulosis (Woringer-Kolopp disease). Histopathologic and ultrastructural observations. Arch. Dermatol. 114(2), 262–268 (1978)

120. Mehregan, D.A., Su, W.P., et al.: Subcutaneous T-cell lymphoma: a clinical, histopathologic, and immunohistochemical study of six cases. J. Cutan. Pathol. 21(2), 110–117 (1994)

121. Moreno-Gimenez, J.C., Jimenez-Puya, R., et al.: Granulomatous slack skin disease in a child: the outcome. Pediatr. Dermatol. 24(6), 640–645 (2007)

122. Motegi, S., Okada, E., et al.: Skin manifestation of mantle cell lymphoma. Eur. J. Dermatol. 16(4), 435–438 (2006)

123. Nashan, D., Faulhaber, D., et al.: Mycosis fungoides: a dermatological masquerader. Br. J. Dermatol. 156(1), 1–10 (2007)

124. Noto, G., Pravata, G., et al.: Granulomatous slack skin: report of a case associated with Hodgkin's disease and a review of the literature. Br. J. Dermatol. 131(2), 275–279 (1994)

125. Olsen, E., Vonderheid, E., et al.: Revisions to the staging and classification of mycosis fungoides and Sezary syndrome: a proposal of the International Society for Cutaneous Lymphomas (ISCL) and the cutaneous lymphoma task force of the European Organization of Research and Treatment of Cancer (EORTC). Blood 110(6), 1713–1722 (2007)

126. Oono, T., Arata, J., et al.: Coexistence of hydroa vacciniforme and malignant lymphoma. Arch. Dermatol. 122(11), 1306–1309 (1986)

127. Paulli, M., Berti, E., et al.: CD30/Ki-1-positive lymphoproliferative disorders of the skin–clinicopathologic correlation and statistical analysis of 86 cases: a multicentric study from the European Organization for Research and Treatment of Cancer Cutaneous Lymphoma Project Group. J. Clin. Oncol. 13(6), 1343–1354 (1995)

128. Perniciaro, C., Winkelmann, R.K., et al.: Malignant angioendotheliomatosis is an angiotropic intravascular lymphoma. Immunohistochemical, ultrastructural, and molecular genetics studies. Am. J. Dermatopathol. 17(3), 242–248 (1995)

129. Perniciaro, C., Zalla, M.J., et al.: Subcutaneous T-cell lymphoma. Report of two additional cases and further observations [see comments]. Arch. Dermatol. 129(9), 1171–1176 (1993)

130. Pfleger, L., Tappeiner, J.: Zur Kenntnis der systemisierten Endotheliomatose der cutanen Blutgefaesse (Reticuloendotheliomatose?). Hautarzt **10**, 359–363 (1959)

131. Pimpinelli, N.: New aspects in the biology of cutaneous B-cell lymphomas. J. Cutan. Pathol. **33**(suppl 1), 6–9 (2006)

132. Pimpinelli, N., Santucci, M., et al.: Primary cutaneous follicular centre-cell lymphoma–a lymphoproliferative disease with favourable prognosis. Clin. Exp. Dermatol. **14**(1), 12–19 (1989)

133. Plumelle, Y., Pascaline, N., et al.: Adult T-cell leukemia-lymphoma: a clinico-pathologic study of twenty-six patients from Martinique. Hematol. Pathol. **7**(4), 251–262 (1993)

134. Ralfkiaer, E., Willemze, R., et al.: Primary cutaneous peripheral T-cell lymphoma, unspecified. In: LeBoit, G.B.P., Weedon, D., Sarasin, A. (eds.) WHO Books: Tumors of the Skin, pp. 184–188. IARC, Lyon (2006)

135. Rawal, A., Finn, W.G., et al.: Site-specific morphologic differences in extranodal marginal zone B-cell lymphomas. Arch. Pathol. Lab. Med. **131**(11), 1673–1678 (2007)

136. Reddy, K., Bhawan, J.: Histologic mimickers of mycosis fungoides: a review. J. Cutan. Pathol. **34**(7), 519–525 (2007)

137. Robak, E., Robak, T.: Skin lesions in chronic lymphocytic leukemia. Leuk. Lymphoma **48**(5), 855–865 (2007)

138. Robson, A.: The pathology of cutaneous T-cell lymphoma. Oncology (Williston Park) **21**(2 suppl 1), 9–12 (2007)

139. Salhany, K.E., Macon, W.R., et al.: Subcutaneous panniculitis-like T-cell lymphoma: clinicopathologic, immunophenotypic, and genotypic analysis of alpha/beta and gamma/delta subtypes. Am. J. Surg. Pathol. **22**(7), 881–893 (1998)

140. Santucci, M., Biggeri, A., et al.: Efficacy of histologic criteria for diagnosing early mycosis fungoides: an EORTC cutaneous lymphoma study group investigation. European Organization for Research and Treatment of Cancer. Am. J. Surg. Pathol. **24**(1), 40–50 (2000)

141. Santucci, M., Burg, G., et al.: Interrater and intrarater reliability of histologic criteria in early cutaneous T-cell lymphoma. An EORTC Cutaneous Lymphoma Project Group study. Dermatol. Clin. **12**(2), 323–327 (1994)

142. Santucci, M., Pimpinelli, N., et al.: Primary cutaneous B-cell lymphoma: a unique type of low-grade lymphoma. Clinicopathologic and immunologic study of 83 cases. Cancer **67**(9), 2311–2326 (1991)

143. Santucci, M., Pimpinelli, N., et al.: Cytotoxic/natural killer cell cutaneous lymphomas. Report of EORTC Cutaneous Lymphoma Task Force Workshop. Cancer **97**(3), 610–627 (2003)

144. Servitje, O., Estrach, T., et al.: Primary cutaneous marginal zone B-cell lymphoma: a clinical, histopathological, immunophenotypic and molecular genetic study of 22 cases. Br. J. Dermatol. **147**(6), 1147–1158 (2002)

145. Shapiro, P.E., Pinto, F.J.: The histologic spectrum of mycosis fungoides/Sezary syndrome (cutaneous T-cell lymphoma). A review of 222 biopsies, including newly described patterns and the earliest pathologic changes. Am. J. Surg. Pathol. **18**(7), 645–667 (1994)

146. Shimizu, S., Yasui, C., et al.: Cutaneous-type adult T-cell leukemia/lymphoma presenting as a solitary large skin nodule: a review of the literature. J. Am. Acad. Dermatol. **57**(5 suppl), S115–S117 (2007)

147. Siegel, R., Gartenhaus, R., et al.: HTLV-I associated leukemia/lymphoma: epidemiology, biology, and treatment. Cancer Treat. Res. **104**, 75–88 (2001)

148. Spencer, J., Perry, M.E., et al.: Human marginal-zone B cells. Immunol. Today **19**(9), 421–426 (1998)

149. Stokkermans-Dubois, J., Jouary, T., et al.: A case of primary cutaneous nasal type NK/T-cell lymphoma and review of the literature. Dermatology **213**(4), 345–349 (2006)

150. Suzuki, R., Takeuchi, K., et al.: Extranodal NK/T-cell lymphoma: diagnosis and treatment cues. Hematol. Oncol. **26**(2), 66–72 (2008)

151. Takahara, T., Masutani, K., et al.: Adult T-cell leukemia/lymphoma in which the pathohistological diagnosis was identical to that of Ki-1 positive anaplastic large cell lymphoma. Intern. Med. **38**(10), 824–828 (1999)

152. Tan, E.S., Tang, M.B., et al.: Retrospective 5-year review of 131 patients with mycosis fungoides and Sezary syndrome seen at the National Skin Centre, Singapore. Australas. J. Dermatol. **47**(4), 248–252 (2006)

153. Tan, S.H., Sim, C.S., et al.: Follicular mycosis fungoides mimicking a cutaneous B-cell lymphoproliferative disorder. Australas. J. Dermatol. **45**(3), 188–191 (2004)

154. Tomaszewski, M.M., Abbondanzo, S.L., et al.: Extranodal marginal zone B-cell lymphoma of the skin: a morphologic and immunophenotypic study of 11 cases. Am. J. Dermatopathol. **22**(3), 205–211 (2000)

155. Tomaszewski, M.M., Lupton, G.P., et al.: A comparison of clinical, morphological and immunohistochemical features of lymphomatoid papulosis and primary cutaneous CD30(Ki-1)-positive anaplastic large cell lymphoma. J. Cutan. Pathol. **22**(4), 310–318 (1995)

156. Toro, J.R., Liewehr, D.J., et al.: Gamma-delta T-cell phenotype is associated with significantly decreased survival in cutaneous T-cell lymphoma. Blood **101**(9), 3407–3412 (2003)

157. Toro, J.R., Stoll Jr., H.L., et al.: Prognostic factors and evaluation of mycosis fungoides and Sezary syndrome. J. Am. Acad. Dermatol. **37**(1), 58–67 (1997)

158. Trotter, M.J., Whittaker, S.J., et al.: Cutaneous histopathology of Sezary syndrome: a study of 41 cases with a proven circulating T-cell clone. J. Cutan. Pathol. **24**(5), 286–291 (1997)

159. Varkonyi, J., Zalatnai, A., et al.: Secondary cutaneous infiltration in B cell chronic lymphocytic leukemia. Acta Haematol. **103**(2), 116–121 (2000)

160. Verallo, V.M., Haserick, J.R.: Mucha-Habermann's disease simulating lymphoma cutis. Report of two cases. Arch. Dermatol. **94**(3), 295–299 (1966)

161. Von Zumbusch, L.: Fallbericht. Arch. Dermatol. Syphilol. **51**, 119 (1915)

162. Vonderheid, E.C., Bernengo, M.G., et al.: Update on erythrodermic cutaneous T-cell lymphoma: report of the International Society for Cutaneous Lymphomas. J. Am. Acad. Dermatol. **46**(1), 95–106 (2002)

163. Vonderheid, E.C., Pena, J., et al.: Sezary cell counts in erythrodermic cutaneous T-cell lymphoma: Implications for prognosis and staging. Leuk. Lymphoma **47**(9), 1841–1856 (2006)

164. Vowels, B., Cassin, M., et al.: Aberrant cytokine production by Sezary syndrome patients: cytokine secretion pattern resembles murine Th2 cells. J. Invest. Dermatol. **99**, 90–94 (1992)

165. Vowels, B.R., Lessin, S.R., et al.: Th2 cytokine mRNA expression in skin in cutaneous T-cell lymphoma. J. Invest. Dermatol. **103**(5), 669–673 (1994)

166. Willemze, R., Meyer, C.J., et al.: The clinical and histological spectrum of lymphomatoid papulosis. Br. J. Dermatol. **107**(2), 131–144 (1982)

167. Winkelmann, R.K., Bowie, E.J.W.: Hemorrhagic diathesis associated with benign histiocytic, cytophagic panniculitis and systemic histiocytosis. Arch. Intern. Med. **140**, 1460–1463 (1980)

168. Woringer, F., Kolopp, P.: Lesion erythemato-squameuse polycyclique de l'avant-bras evoluant depuis 6 ans chez un garconnet de 13 ans. Ann. Dermatol. Syphil. **10**, 945–958 (1939)

169. Yamaguchi, K., Takatsuki, K.: Adult T cell leukaemia-lymphoma. Baillières Clin. Haematol. **6**(4), 899–915 (1993)

170. Yamamura, M., Yamada, Y., et al.: Circulating interleukin-6 levels are elevated in adult T-cell leukaemia/lymphoma patients and correlate with adverse clinical features and survival. Br. J. Haematol. **100**(1), 129–134 (1998)

171. Zackheim, H.S., Amin, S. Kashani-Sabet, M. McMillan, A.: "Prognosis in cutaneous T-cell lymphoma by skin stage: long-term

survival in 489 patients." J Am Acad Dermatol. **40**(3), 418–425 (1999)

172. Zelger, B., Sepp, N., et al.: Syringotropic cutaneous T-cell lymphoma: a variant of mycosis fungoides? Br. J. Dermatol. **130**(6), 765–769 (1994)

173. Zinzani, P.L., Quaglino, P., et al.: Prognostic factors in primary cutaneous B-cell lymphoma: the Italian Study Group for Cutaneous Lymphomas. J. Clin. Oncol. **24**(9), 1376–1382 (2006)

Immature Hematopoietic Malignancies

1. ICD-O-3 Coding materials. (2001) http://seer.cancer.gov/icd-o-3/

2. Aifantis, I., Raetz, E., Buonamici, S.: Molecular pathogenesis of T-cell leukaemia and lymphoma. Nat. Rev. Immunol. **8**, 380–390 (2008)

3. Ali, A., Serra, S., Asa, S.L., et al.: The predictive value of CK19 and CD99 in pancreatic endocrine tumors. Am. J. Surg. Pathol. **30**, 1588–1594 (2006)

4. Alsaad, K.O., Serra, S., Perren, A., et al.: CK19 and CD99 immunoexpression profile in goblet cell (mucin-producing neuroendocrine tumors) and classical carcinoids of the vermiform appendix. Int. J. Surg. Pathol. **15**, 252–257 (2007)

5. Bassan, R., Gatta, G., Tondini, C., et al.: Adult acute lymphoblastic leukaemia. Crit. Rev. Oncol. Hematol. **50**, 223–261 (2004)

6. Bekkenk, M.W., Jansen, P.M., Meijer, C.J.L.M., et al.: CD56+ hematological neoplasms presenting in the skin: a retrospective analysis of 23 new cases and 130 cases from the literature. Ann. Oncol. **15**, 1097–1108 (2004)

7. Burg, G., Kempf, W., Cozzio, A., et al.: WHO/EORTC classification of cutaneous lymphomas 2005: histological and molecular aspects. J. Cutan. Pathol. **32**, 647–674 (2005)

8. Burg, G., Kempf, W., Cozzio, A., et al.: Cutaneous malignant lymphomas: update 2006. J. Dtsch Dermatol. Ges. **4**, 914–933 (2006)

9. Büchner, S.A.: Specific and nonspecific skin manifestations in leukemia. Praxis (Bern 1994) **91**, 1071–1077 (2002)

10. Chaperot, L., Bendriss, N., Manches, O., et al.: Identification of a leukemic counterpart of the plasmacytoid dendritic cells. Blood **97**, 3210–3217 (2001)

11. Cho-Vega, J.H., Medeiros, L.J., Prieto, V.G., et al.: Leukemia cutis. Am. J. Clin. Pathol. **129**, 130–142 (2008)

12. Cobaleda, C., Schebesta, A., Delogu, A., et al.: Pax5: the guardian of B cell identity and function. Nat. Immunol. **8**, 463–470 (2007)

13. Dzionek, A., Sohma, Y., Nagafune, J., et al.: BDCA-2, a novel plasmacytoid dendritic cell-specific type II C-type lectin, mediates antigen capture and is a potent inhibitor of interferon alpha/beta induction. J. Exp. Med. **194**, 1823–1834 (2001)

14. Feldman, A.L., Dogan, A.: Diagnostic uses of Pax5 immunohistochemistry. Adv. Anat. Pathol. **14**, 323–334 (2007)

15. Feuillard, J., Jacob, M., Valensi, F., et al.: Clinical and biologic features of CD4(+)CD56(+) malignancies. Blood **99**, 1556–1563 (2002)

16. Graux, C., Cools, J., Michaux, L., et al.: Cytogenetics and molecular genetics of T-cell acute lymphoblastic leukemia: from thymocyte to lymphoblast. Leukemia **20**, 1496–1510 (2006)

17. Herling, M., Jones, D.: CD4+/CD56+ hematodermic tumor: the features of an evolving entity and its relationship to dendritic cells. Am. J. Clin. Pathol. **127**, 687–700 (2007)

18. Herling, M., Teitell, M.A., Shen, R.R., et al.: TCL1 expression in plasmacytoid dendritic cells (DC2s) and the related CD4+ CD56+ blastic tumors of skin. Blood **101**, 5007–5009 (2003)

19. Ishizawa, K., Komori, T., Shimada, S., et al.: Olig2 and CD99 are useful negative markers for the diagnosis of brain tumors. Clin. Neuropathol. **27**, 118–128 (2008)

20. Jaffe, E.S., Harris, N.L., Stein, H., Vardiman, J.W. (eds.): WHO classification of tumors: pathology and genetics of tumors of haematopoietic and lymphoid tissues. International Agency for Research on Cancer (IARC), Lyon (2001)

21. Jaye, D.L., Geigerman, C.M., Herling, M., et al.: Expression of the plasmacytoid dendritic cell marker BDCA-2 supports a spectrum of maturation among CD4+ CD56+ hematodermic neoplasms. Mod. Pathol. **19**, 1555–1562 (2006)

22. Kaddu, S., Zenahlik, P., Beham-Schmid, C., et al.: Specific cutaneous infiltrates in patients with myelogenous leukemia: a clinicopathologic study of 26 patients with assessment of diagnostic criteria. J. Am. Acad. Dermatol. **40**, 966–978 (1999)

23. Khoury, J.D., Medeiros, L.J., Manning, J.T., et al.: CD56(+) TdT(+) blastic natural killer cell tumor of the skin: a primitive systemic malignancy related to myelomonocytic leukemia. Cancer **94**, 2401–2408 (2002)

24. Leclair, S.J., Rodak, B.F.: The new WHO nomenclature: lymphoid neoplasms. Clin. Lab. Sci. **15**, 55–59 (2002)

25. Maitra, A., McKenna, R.W., Weinberg, A.G., et al.: Precursor B-cell lymphoblastic lymphoma. A study of nine cases lacking blood and bone marrow involvement and review of the literature. Am. J. Clin. Pathol. **115**, 868–875 (2001)

26. Marafioti, T., Paterson, J.C., Ballabio, E., et al.: Novel markers of normal and neoplastic human plasmacytoid dendritic cells. Blood **111**, 3778–3792 (2008)

27. Narducci, M.G., Pescarmona, E., Lazzeri, C., et al.: Regulation of TCL1 expression in B- and T-cell lymphomas and reactive lymphoid tissues. Cancer Res. **60**, 2095–2100 (2000)

28. Paydaè, S., Zorludemir, S.: Leukaemia cutis and leukaemic vasculitis. Br. J. Dermatol. **143**, 773–779 (2000)

29. Pelosi, G., Leon, M.E., Veronesi, G., et al.: Decreased immunoreactivity of CD99 is an independent predictor of regional lymph node metastases in pulmonary carcinoid tumors. J. Thorac. Oncol. **1**, 468–477 (2006)

30. Petrella, T., Bagot, M., Willemze, R., et al.: Blastic NK-cell lymphomas (agranular CD4+CD56+ hematodermic neoplasms): a review. Am. J. Clin. Pathol. **123**, 662–675 (2005)

31. Petrella, T., Meijer, C.J.L.M., Dalac, S., et al.: TCL1 and CLA expression in agranular CD4/CD56 hematodermic neoplasms (blastic NK-cell lymphomas) and leukemia cutis. Am. J. Clin. Pathol. **122**, 307–313 (2004)

32. Pilichowska, M.E., Fleming, M.D., Pinkus, J.L., et al.: CD4+/CD56+ hematodermic neoplasm ("blastic natural killer cell lymphoma"): neoplastic cells express the immature dendritic cell marker BDCA-2 and produce interferon. Am. J. Clin. Pathol. **128**, 445–453 (2007)

33. Reichard, K.K., Burks, E.J., Foucar, M.K., et al.: CD4(+) CD56(+) lineage-negative malignancies are rare tumors of plasmacytoid dendritic cells. Am. J. Surg. Pathol. **29**, 1274–1283 (2005)

34. Reimer, P., Rüdiger, T., Kraemer, D., et al.: What is CD4+CD56+ malignancy and how should it be treated? Bone Marrow Transplant. **32**, 637–646 (2003)

35. Suzuki, R., Nakamura, S., Suzumiya, J., et al.: Blastic natural killer cell lymphoma/leukemia (CD56-positive blastic tumor): prognostication and categorization according to anatomic sites of involvement. Cancer **104**, 1022–1031 (2005)

36. Urosevic, M., Conrad, C., Kamarashev, J., et al.: CD4+CD56+ hematodermic neoplasms bear a plasmacytoid dendritic cell phenotype. Hum. Pathol. **36**, 1020–1024 (2005)

37. Valbuena, J.R., Medeiros, L.J., Rassidakis, G.Z., et al.: Expression of B cell-specific activator protein/PAX5 in acute myeloid leuke-

mia with t(8;21)(q22;q22). Am. J. Clin. Pathol. **126**, 235–240 (2006)

38. Virgilio, L., Narducci, M.G., Isobe, M., et al.: Identification of the TCL1 gene involved in T-cell malignancies. Proc. Natl. Acad. Sci. U. S. A. **91**, 12530–12534 (1994)

39. Weedon, D., LeBoit, P., Burg, G., Sarasin, A. (eds.): WHO classification of tumors: pathology and genetics of tumors of the skin. International Agency for Research on Cancer (IARC), Lyon (2005)

40. Weng, A.P., Ferrando, A.A., Lee, W., et al.: Activating mutations of NOTCH1 in human T cell acute lymphoblastic leukemia. Science **306**, 269–271 (2004)

41. Willemze, R., Jaffe, E.S., Burg, G., et al.: WHO-EORTC classification for cutaneous lymphomas. Blood **105**, 3768–3785 (2005)

Histiocytoses

3.5

Keiji Iwatsuki

Core Messages

> Histiocytoses are a group of disorders encompassing reactive and neoplastic conditions derived from macrophages, dendritic cells, and histiocytes. The terminology and categorization of histiocytic disorders have been a controversial issue because of the vague definition of histiocytes. Recently, however, the cell lineage of myeloid-derived macrophages and dendritic cells is becoming clear through immunophenotypic analysis. The classification based on cell lineage provides us new insight into histiocytoses, although there are still some controversies between clinical and pathological entities. This chapter reviews the current definition, etiology, clinicopathologic features, and cell lineage of histiocytic disorders involving the skin, with special attention to the representative entities: Langerhans cell histiocytosis (LCH), Rosai–Dorfman disease, juvenile xanthogranuloma, and reticulohistiocytosis

3.5.1 Introduction

Histiocytoses are classified into two major categories: Langerhans cell histiocytosis (LCH) and non-LC histiocytosis (non-LCH). The latter may include the xanthogranuloma family and other histiocytic disorders. In 1987, the Histiocyte Society proposed a classification of histiocytic syndromes: (1) class I histiocytosis (LCH), (2) class II histiocytosis (non-LCH), and (3) class III histiocytosis

(malignant histiocytosis) [17]. Recently, the revised classification of histiocytic disorders, including hematological disorders, was proposed based on cell lineage and biological behaviors: (1) dendritic cell-related, (2) macrophage-related, and (3) malignant disorders [4, 11]. According to this immunophenotypic classification, the dendritic cell group may include both LCH and the juvenile xanthogranuloma family, in which the proliferative histiocytoid cells share dermal/interstitial dendritic cells markers such as factor XIII and fascin. In order to avoid controversy in classification, this chapter describes the representative histiocytic disorders involving the skin, using dermatological diagnoses (Table 3.5.1).

3.5.1.1 Langerhans Cell Histiocytosis

Synonyms: Histiocytosis X, Langerhans cell disease (LCD), class I histiocytosis (by Histiocyte Society), Letterer–Siwe disease (acute disseminated LCD), Hand–Schüller–Christian disease (chronic multifocal LCD), eosinophilic granuloma (chronic focal LCD), congenital self-healing reticulohistiocytosis (Hashimoto–Pritzker disease)

3.5.1.1.1 Definition

LCH is defined as a proliferative disorder of LC type dendritic cells characterized by expression of S100 protein, CD1a and Langerin (CD207), and by racquet-shaped Birbeck granules in the cytoplasm. LCH may include four clinical subtypes previously used: (1) Letterer–Siwe disease for the acute, disseminated, or visceral LCH, (2) Hand–Schüller–Christian disease for the chronic but progressive, multifocal form, (3) eosinophilic granuloma for chronic, localized LCH, and (4) Hashimoto–Pritzker disease for the benign, self-healing variant. Langerhans cell sarcoma, or malignant LCH is a rare, high-grade malignant neoplasm with a LC-like phenotype and overt nuclear pleomorphism.

K. Iwatsuki
Department of Dermatology, Okayama University Graduate School of Medicine, Dentistry and Pharmaceutical Sciences,
2-5-1 Shikata-cho, Okayama 700-8558, Japan
e-mail: keijiiwa@cc.okayama-u.ac.jp

R. Dummer et al. (eds.), *Skin Cancer – A World-Wide Perspective*,
DOI: 10.1007/978-3-642-05072-5_3.5, © Springer-Verlag Berlin Heidelberg 2011

Table 3.5.1 Histiocytic disorders involving the skin [3, 4, 7, 9, 11, 17]

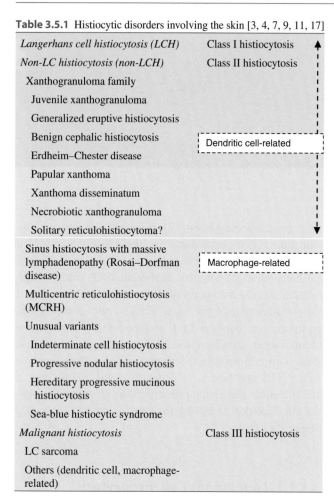

Langerhans cell histiocytosis (LCH)	Class I histiocytosis
Non-LC histiocytosis (non-LCH)	Class II histiocytosis
Xanthogranuloma family	
Juvenile xanthogranuloma	
Generalized eruptive histiocytosis	
Benign cephalic histiocytosis	Dendritic cell-related
Erdheim–Chester disease	
Papular xanthoma	
Xanthoma disseminatum	
Necrobiotic xanthogranuloma	
Solitary reticulohistiocytoma?	
Sinus histiocytosis with massive lymphadenopathy (Rosai–Dorfman disease)	Macrophage-related
Multicentric reticulohistiocytosis (MCRH)	
Unusual variants	
Indeterminate cell histiocytosis	
Progressive nodular histiocytosis	
Hereditary progressive mucinous histiocytosis	
Sea-blue histiocytic syndrome	
Malignant histiocytosis	Class III histiocytosis
LC sarcoma	
Others (dendritic cell, macrophage-related)	

3.5.1.1.2 Etiology

A clonal proliferation of LC type dendritic cells has been demonstrated by X-linked polymorphic DNA probes including HUMARA [16]. In contrast, primary pulmonary LCH arising in cigarette smokers might be both clonal and non-clonal [18] and may have allelic loss of tumor suppressor genes [13]. Bombesin-like peptides in cigarettes may stimulate alveolar macrophages, leading to the proliferation of Langerhans cells [14]. A subset of LCH is hereditary, especially in monozygotic twins [1].

3.5.1.1.3 Clinical Manifestations

LCH shows a broad spectrum of symptoms, severity, organ involvement, and prognosis. The localized form of LCH, formerly designated as eosinophilic granuloma commonly occurs in the bones and skin, and lymph node or lung involvement is occasionally seen. The clinical course is usually indolent, and spontaneous regression may occur.

Hashimoto–Pritzker disease has been designated as congenital self-healing reticulohistiocytosis, because the lesions are usually present at birth and composed of a few to several nodules or multiple, disseminated cutaneous papules. Spontaneous clearance occurs by 2–3 months of age.

Hand–Schüller–Christian disease is a subtype of LCH characterized by multiple cutaneous lesions associated with systemic symptoms such as diabetes insipidus, exophthalmos, and multiple osteolytic lesions, although other visceral organs and lymph nodes may be affected. The disease is usually progressive, and needs systemic treatments.

Letterer–Siwe disease is the most aggressive form of LCH associated with multisystem involvement. Lesions on the skin and mucosa consist of multiple, disseminated papules, coalescent plaques, and ulcerative nodules (Fig. 3.5.1a, b). Hemorrhagic papules and vesicles may occur in aggressive cases. Systemic symptoms include fever, lymphadenopathy, anemia, thrombocytopenia, hepatosplenomegaly, pulmonary infiltration, and hemophagocytic syndrome.

3.5.1.1.4 Histopathology

LCH cells have a characteristic lobulated, folded, or kidney-shaped nucleus and consistently express S100 protein, CD1a, and Langerin (CD207) (Fig. 3.5.1c, d; Table 3.5.2). Ultrastructually, tennis racquet-shaped Birbeck granules are observed in cytoplasm and very rarely in the nucleus (Fig. 3.5.1e, f). Three histologic reactions have been reported in LCH: proliferative, granulomatous and xanthomatous type. The proliferative type presents with acute, disseminated papules, in which LCH cells are infiltrating beneath or within the epidermis, associated with T-cell infiltration (Fig. 3.5.1d). The granulomatous type is usually associated with the chronic stage of the disease and composed of multinucleated giant cells, eosinophils, and other cell types. The xanthomatous type may be seen in the bone lesions of Hand–Schüller–Christian type LCH with foam cells, eosinophils, and other reactive cells, the feature of which is similar to xanthogranuloma. In Hashimoto–Pritzker disease, the infiltrate is composed of LCH cells with abundant cytoplasm and giant cells showing a "ground glass" appearance.

3.5.1.1.5 Differential Diagnosis

Letterer–Siwe type LCH should be differentiated clinically from seborrheic dermatitis, Darier's disease, pityriasis lichenoides, prurigo, and non-LC histiocytoses. Some cases of Hashimoto–Pritzker disease may be confused with blueberry muffin baby. Immunological phenotyping differentiates LCH from other non-LCH and class II histiocytosis (by Histiocyte Society) by expressing CD68 but not CD1a or Langerin (CD207).

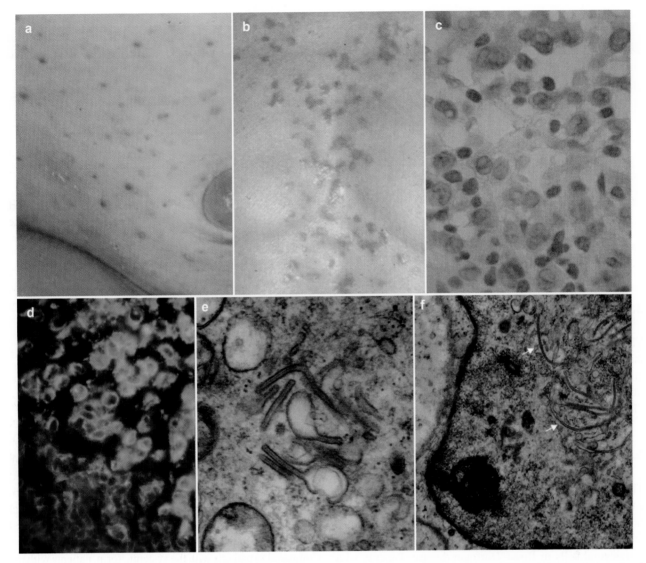

Fig. 3.5.1 Langerhans cell histiocytosis (LCH): Discrete, reddish or purpuric papules on the abdomen of an infant (**a**), and grouping, reddish papules on the anterior chest of an elderly individual, mimicking Darier's disease (**b**). Histiocytoid cells with a bilobulated nucleus express Langerin (CD207) (**c**). LCH cells expressing CD1a (*green*) and CD3-positive T lymphocytes (**d**). Racquet-shaped Birbeck granules in the cytoplasm (**e**) and very rarely in the nucleus (**f**; *arrows*)

3.5.1.1.6 Therapy and Prognosis

See Chap. 4.4

3.5.1.2 *Indeterminate Cell Histiocytosis*

Synonyms: Indeterminate dendritic cell tumor

3.5.1.2.1 Definition

A group of histiocytic lesions composed of possible indeterminate dendritic cells expressing S100 proteins and CD1a

without Langerin (CD207) or Birbeck granules [10] and not consistent with other histiocitoses.

3.5.1.2.2 Etiology

Indeterminate cell histiocytosis can occur de novo or in association with a B-cell lymphoma, possibly as a result of B-cell dedifferentiation [7].

3.5.1.2.3 Clinical Features

Patients with indeterminate cell histiocytosis have a wide age range, from infants to the elderly, and may present with a

Table 3.5.2 Immunophenotypes of LCH cells and related cell lineage [4, 7, 11]

	Immunophenotype						
	S100	CD1a	Langerin	XIIIa	Fascin	CD68	MHC II
LCH	+	+	+	−	−	±	+cytoplasm
Interdigitating DC	+	+	−	−	+	±	+surface
Dermal/interstitial DC	±	−	−	+	+	+	±
Indeterminate DC	+	+	−	−	−		
Rosai–Dorfman	+	−	−	−	−	+	
Xanthogranuloma cells	−	−	−	+	+	+	
Veil cell/migrating LC	+	+	±	−	−		
Macrophage	±	−	−	−	±	+	+

variety of cutaneous manifestations: one or a few nodules to multiple papulonodules mimicking LCH.

3.5.1.2.4 Histopathology

The lesion is composed of mononuclear cell infiltrate containing foam cells and giant cells. The infiltrating histiocytes are similar to LCH cells in phenotype except for the absence of Langerin (CD207) reactivity and Birbeck granules (Table 3.5.2) [1].

3.5.1.2.5 Differential Diagnosis

The diagnosis can be made possible by exclusion of LCH and other histiocytic diseases by immunophenotyping. Indeterminate cells should be distinguished from LCH cells, interdigitating cells, dermal/interstitial dendritic cells, and histiocytoid cells in Rosai–Dorfman disease. Patients with nodular scabies and pityriasis rosea may contain similar cell types. It is difficult to exclude the lesions composed of accumulation of veil cells/migrating LC (if present).

3.5.1.2.6 Treatment and Prognosis

No clear data available.

3.5.1.3 *Sinus Histiocytosis With Massive Lymphadenopathy (Rosai–Dorfman Disease)*

3.5.1.3.1 Definition

A benign nodal or extranodal disease characterized by infiltration of histiocytoid cells harboring mononuclear cells in the cytoplasm (emperipolesis) and an immunophenotype of CD68+, S100+ without CD1a and Langerin (CD207).

3.5.1.3.2 Etiology

Unknown. EB virus or HHV-6 infection has been postulated.

3.5.1.3.3 Clinical Features

Rosai–Dorfman disease primarily involves cervical lymph nodes and is frequently associated with cutaneous lesions [15]. Cervical lymphadenopathy presents with fever, elevated ESR, leukocytosis or leukopenia, and polyclonal hypergammaglobulinemia. Cutaneous Rosai–Dorfman disease without nodal involvement occurs less commonly. Brownish, indurated plaques and nodules may occur in the skin solely (Fig. 3.5.2a). Compared to patients with the systemic form, patients with the cutaneous form are older and most commonly women [2, 5].

3.5.1.3.4 Histopathology

The cutaneous lesion is composed of a mixture of infiltrates: lymphocytes, plasma cells, neutrophils, macrophages, and histiocytoid cells harboring lymphocytes in pale abundant cytoplasm (emperipolesis) (Fig. 3.5.2b, c). The histiocytoid cells are positive for CD68 and S100 protein (Fig. 3.5.2d) and negative for CD1a and Langerin (CD207).

3.5.1.3.5 Differential Diagnosis

The clinical differential diagnoses may include abscesses, scrofuloderma, lupus vulgaris, cutaneous lymphoma, and sarcoidosis. Histologically, foreign body granuloma, reticulohistiocytoma, xanthogranuloma, LCH, and Malakoplakia (Michaelis–Gutmann bodies) should be differentiated.

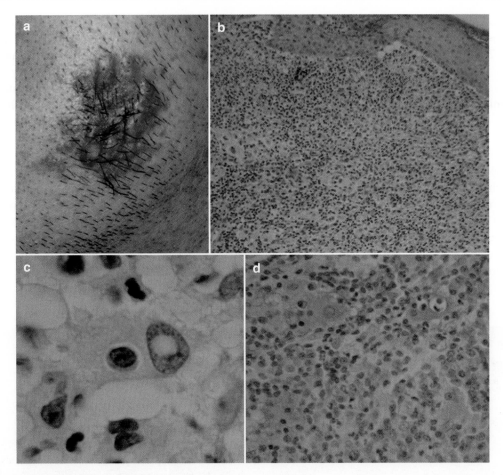

Fig. 3.5.2 Cutaneous Rosai–Dorfman disease: A reddish, indurated plaque with nodules (**a**) is composed of an admixture of histiocytoid cells, mononuclear cells, plasma cells and neutrophils (**b**). The histio-cytoid cells contain lymphocytes in the cytoplasm (emperipolesis) (**c**), and express S100 protein (**d**). (Courtesy of Dr. N. Takiyoshi, Hirosaki University)

3.5.1.3.6 Treatment and Prognosis

Most cases with Rosai–Dorfman disease resolve spontaneously in months to years [2, 5, 15] but may recur in some cases. Surgical removal of the solitary skin lesion is an option for treatment.

3.5.1.4 Juvenile Xanthogranuloma

Synonyms: Xanthogranuloma (XG), non-X histiocytosis, class II histiocytosis (by Histiocyte Society)

3.5.1.4.1 Variants

Disseminated juvenile XG (JXG), deep JXG, generalized eruptive histiocytosis, benign cephalic histiocytosis, mononuclear xanthogranuloma, xanthoma disseminatum, papular xanthoma, scalloped cell xanthogranuloma, spindle cell xanthogranuloma, reticulohistiocytoma, Erdheim–Chester disease, necrobiotic xanthogranuloma.

3.5.1.4.2 Definition

A group of non-LCH (CD68+, CD1a−, Langerin−) associated with xanthomatous tissue reaction, but no clear consensus classification exists for this category. The infantile forms are usually benign and self-healing, with some cases presenting with organ involvement. The adult-onset, systemic diseases include Erdheim–Chester and necrobiotic XG.

3.5.1.4.3 Etiology

A triple association between JXG, NF-1 and myelomonocytic leukemia occurs [19], and LCH may also be associated [12]. The cell lineage of JXG has been postulated to be dermal/interstitial dendritic cells because of the expression of factor XIII and fascin, but its specificity is still controversial (Table 3.5.2) [4, 11].

3.5.1.4.4 Clinical Features

The cutaneous lesions vary from one or several papules to numerous, disseminated papules and preferentially occur on the head, neck and trunk shortly after birth (Fig. 3.5.3a, b). No lipid abnormality is found. According to the Kiel Pediatric Tumor Registration [8], 34.5% of JXG were congenital, and 71.0% were diagnosed within the first year of life. Most cases of cutaneous JXG were solitary (81.0%), and 3.9% presented with visceral (systemic) involvement which may not be related to the dissemination of the cutaneous lesions. The early lesions are reddish and become brownish yellow because of the accumulation of foam cells. JXG with systemic involvement is rare, but significant morbidity and occasional deaths may occur. Of 34 children with systemic JXG [6], the extracutaneous site of disease was the subcutaneous soft tissue in 12 patients, central nervous system in 8 (Fig. 3.5.3c), liver/spleen in 8, lung in 6, and eye/orbit, oropharynx, and muscle in 4 patients each.

Solitary XG and reticulohistiocytoma are both self-limiting diseases that may occur in adults. Erdheim–Chester disease is an adult-onset, disseminated histiocytosis which predominantly affects the bones, lungs and kidneys, with a high mortality rate [3]. Necrobiotic XG may be associated with paraproteinemia or hematological malignancies such as plasma cell dyscrasia and multiple myeloma.

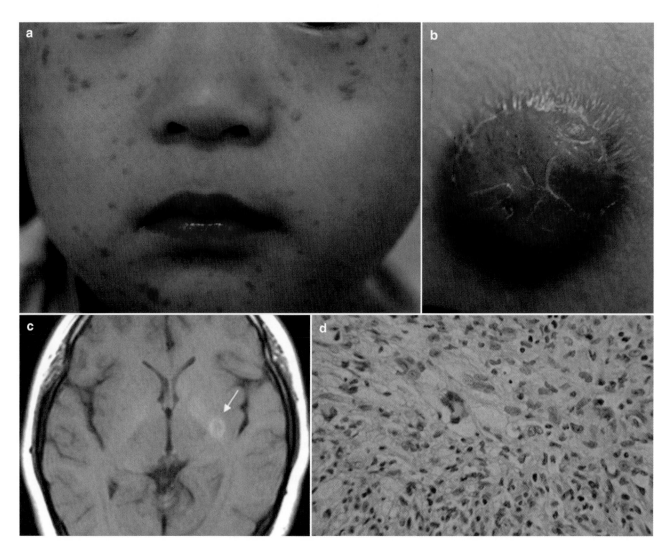

Fig. 3.5.3 Juvenile xanthogranuloma: Similarly-sized, reddish papules scattered on the face (**a**). A yellowish brown nodule on the chest in a 14 year-old girl (**b**) who presented with a solitary tumor in the brain (**c**; *arrow*). A mixed infiltrate of mononuclear cells, neutrophils and multinucleated giant cells containing lipid (**d**)

3.5.1.4.5 Histopathology

Infiltrates contain mononuclear cells and an admixture of other inflammatory cells such as lymphocytes and neutrophils (Fig. 3.5.3d). The early lesions are composed of mainly mononuclear cells, and the mature lesions contain a variable number of foam cells, characteristically Touton cells. Proliferating histiocytoid cells may express both macrophage and dermal/interstitial dendritic cell markers, including CD68, α1-antitrypsin, chymotrypsin, lysozyme, factor XIIIa, and fascin, and consistently negative for LCH markers such as S100 protein and CD1a (Table 3.5.2) [3, 4, 9, 11]. Based on these phenotypes, the JXG family has been classified as a group of dentritic cell tumors, but this has been a controversial issue. Solitary reticulohistiocytoma, a possible variant of XG, may contain many oncocytic macrophages and multinucleated histiocytes characterized by abundant, eosinophilic, finely granular cytoplasm, the feature of which is a so-called "ground glass" appearance.

3.5.1.4.6 Differential Diagnosis

Nodular JXG must be distinguished from Hashimoto–Pritzker disease, mastocytoma, and Spitz nevus. The multiple papules should be differentiated from LCH and early onset sarcoidosis. Patients with numerous papulonodules may be classified into the variants of JXG histopathologically, including xanthoma disseminatum, generalized eruptive histiocytosis, and benign cephalic histiocytosis.

3.5.1.4.7 Treatment and Prognosis

Both mucocutaneous lesions and organ involvement of JXG show spontaneous regression in most patients. Solitary or few lesions are successfully treated with excision. Patients with systemic JXG have been treated with radiation or systemic chemotherapy (see detail in Chap. 4.4).

3.5.1.5 Reticulohistiocytosis

3.5.1.5.1 Definition

Reticulohistiocytosis is divided into two categories: solitary reticulohistiocytoma and multicentric reticulohistiocytosis (MCRH). The solitary form, a possible variant of xanthogranuloma (see Chap. 3.4.1.4), generally occurs as a brownish yellow nodule on the head. MCRH is characterized by multiple, glossy, cutaneous lesions and is very frequently associated with fever, weight loss, and systemic symptoms such as symmetric erosive arthritis, various malignancies, and systemic inflammatory diseases [9].

3.5.1.5.2 Variant

Diffuse cutaneous reticulohistiocytosis (purely cutaneous from)

3.5.1.5.3 Etiology

Unknown, but immunologic responses to underlying autoimmune diseases or neoplasms have been postulated.

3.5.1.5.4 Clinical Features

MCRH preferentially occurs in females of the fifth or sixth decade, and presents with multiple, small papules or nodules on the extremities and face (Fig. 3.5.4a). Grouped papules around the periungal areas are called "coral beads." Oral or nasal mucosa may also be affected. Multiple papules and nodules on the mutilating fingers, due to erosive arthritis, suggest MCRH. Most patients with MCRH have polyarthritis, and some may have underlying disorders such as tuberculosis, hypothyroidism, diabetes mellitus, or internal malignancies, including carcinomas of cervix, ovary, breast, stomach and colon, melanoma, and hematological disorders [9].

3.5.1.5.5 Histopathology

The cutaneous lesion is composed of histiocytic infiltrates and multinucleated, eosinophilic giant cells with "ground glass" cytoplasm (Fig. 3.5.4b). The cells are positive for CD68 and negative for S100 protein, CD1a, and factor XIIIa. Similar histiocytoid cells are present in the synovium.

3.5.1.5.6 Differential Diagnosis

The differential diagnoses for MCRH are rheumatoid arthritis, sarcoidosis, Gottron's papules in dermatomyositis, and tophi.

3.5.1.5.7 Treatments and Prognosis

See Chap. 4.4

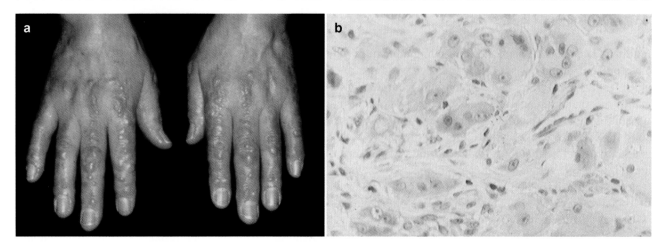

Fig. 3.5.4 Multicentric reticulohistiocytosis (MCRH): Skin-colored, glossy nodules on the dorsal surfaces of hands (**a**). Multinucleated giant cells with abundant, eosinophilic cytoplasm ("ground glass appearance") (**b**)

References

1. Arico, M., Nichol, K., Whitlock, J.A., Arceci, R., Haupt, R., Mittler, U., Kuhne, T., Lombardi, A., Ishii, E., Egeler, R.M., Danesino, C.: Familical clustering of Langerhans cell histiocytosis. Br. J. Haematol. **107**, 883–888 (1999)
2. Brenn, T., Calonje, E., Granter, S.R., Leonard, N., Grayson, W., Fletcher, C.D., McKee, P.H.: Cutaneous Rosai-Dorfman disease is a distinct clinical entity. Am. J. Dermatopathol. **24**, 385–391 (2002)
3. Caputo, R., Marzano, A.V., Passoni, E., Berti, E.: Unsual varinats of non-Langerhans cell histiocytosis. J. Am. Acad. Dermatol. **57**, 1031–1045 (2007)
4. Favara, B.E., Feller, A.C.; WHO Committee, the Histiocyte Society: Contemporary classification of histiocytic disorders. Med. Pediatr. Oncol. **29**, 157–166 (1997)
5. Frater, J.L., Maddox, J.S., Obadiah, J.M., Hurley, M.Y.: Cutaneous Rosai-Dorfman disease: comprehensive review of cases reported in the medical literature since 1990 and presentation of an illustrative case. J. Cutan. Med. Surg. **10**, 281–290 (2006)
6. Freyer, D.R., Kennedy, R., Bostrom, B.C., Kohut, G., Dehner, L.P.: Juvenile xanthogranuloma: forms of systemic disease and their clinical implications. J. Pediatr. **129**, 227–237 (1996)
7. Jaffe, R., Pileri, S.A., Facchetti, F., Jones, D.M., Jaffe, E.S.: Histiocytic and dendritic cell neoplasms, introduction. In: Swerdlow, S., et al. (eds.) WHO Classification of Tumors of Haematopoietic and Lymphoid Tissues, pp. 354–355. IARC, Lyon (2008)
8. Janssen, D., Harms, D.: Juvenile xanthogranuloma in childhood and adolescence: a clinicopathologic study of 129 patients from the Kiel pediatric tumor registry. Am. J. Surg. Pathol. **29**, 21–28 (2005)
9. Newman, B., Hu, W., Nigro, K., Gilliam, A.C.: Aggressive histiocytic disorders that can involve the skin. J. Am. Acad. Dermatol. **56**, 302–316 (2007)
10. Rezk, S.A., Spagnolo, D.V., Brynes, R.K., Weiss, L.M.: Indeterminate cell tumor: a rare dendritic neoplasm. Am. J. Surg. Pathol. **32**, 1868–1876 (2008)
11. Satter, E.K., High, W.A.: Langerhans cell histiocytosis: a review of the current recommendations of the Histiocyte Society. Pediatr. Dermatol. **3**, 291–295 (2008)
12. Tran, D.T., Wolgamot, G.M., Olerud, J., Hurst, S., Argenyi, Z.: An 'eruptive' variant of juvenile xanthogranuloma associated with Langerhans cell histiocytosis. J. Cutan. Pathol. **35**(suppl 1), 5054 (2008)
13. Dacic, S., Trusky, C., Bakker, A., Finkelstein, S.D., Yousem, S.A.: Genotypic analysis of pulmonary Langerhans cell histiocytosis. Hum. Pathol. **34**, 1345–1349 (2003)
14. Vassallo, R., Ryu, J.H., Colby, T.V., Hartman, T., Limper, A.H.: Pulmonary Langerhaqns'-cell histiocytosis. N. Engl. J. Med. **342**, 1969–1978 (2000)
15. Wang, K.H., Chen, W.Y., Liu, H.N., Huang, C.C., Lee, W.R., Hu, C.H.: Cutaneous Rosa-Dorfman disease: clinicopathological profiles, spectrum and evolution of 21 lesions in six patients. Br. J. Dermatol. **154**, 277–286 (2006)
16. Willman, C.L., Busque, L., Griffith, B.B., Favara, B.E., McClain, K.L., Duncan, M.H., Gilliland, D.G.: Langerhans'-cell histiocytosis (histiocytosis X): a clonal proliferative disease. N. Engl. J. Med. **331**, 154–160 (1994)
17. Writing Group of the Histiocyte Society: Histiocytosis syndromes in children. Lancet **1**, 208–209 (1987)
18. Yousem, S.A., Colby, T.V., Chen, Y.Y., Chen, W.G., Weiss, L.M.: Pulmonary Langerhans' cell histiocytosis: molecular analysis of clonality. Am. J. Surg. Pathol. **25**, 630–636 (2001)
19. Zvulunov, A., Barak, Y., Metzker, A.: Juvenile xanthogranuloma, neurofibroma, and juvenile chronic myelogenous leukemia. World statistical analysis. Arch. Dermatol. **132**, 1390–1391 (1995)

Mastocytosis, Vascular, Muscular and Fibrohistiocytic Tumors

3.6

Naohito Hatta, Nagwa M. Elwan, L. Weibel, Luis Requena, Davide Donghi, Jürg Hafner, Beata Bode-Lesniewska, and Kenji Asagoe

N. Hatta (✉)
Division of Dermatology, Toyama Prefectural Central Hospital,
2-2-78 Nishinagae, Toyama, 930-8550, Japan
e-mail: hattanao@tch.pref.toyama.jp

N.M. Elwan
Department of Medicine, Tanta University, Tanta-Egypt
e-mail: elwan2egy@yahoo.com

L. Weibel
Department of Dermatology, University Hospital Zurich,
Gloriastrasse 31, 8091 Zurich, Switzerland

L. Requena
Department of Dermatology, Fundación Jiménez Díaz,
Universidad Autónoma, Madrid, Spain
e-mail: lrequena@fjd.es

D. Donghi
Department of Dermatology, University Hospital Zurich,
Gloriastrasse 31, 8091 Zurich, Switzerland
e-mail: davide.donghi@usz.ch

J. Hafner
Department of Dermatology, University Hospital Zurich,
Gloriastrasse 31, 8091 Zurich, Switzerland
e-mail: juerg.hafner@usz.ch

B. Bode-Lesniewska
Institut für klinische Pathologie, Universitätsspital Zürich,
Schmelzbergstrasse, 128091 Zurich, Switzerland
e-mail: beata.bode@usz.ch

K. Asagoe
Department of Dermatology, Okayama University
Graduate School of Medicine, Dentistry and
Pharmaceutical Sciences, 2-5-1 Shikata-cho, Okayama,
700-8558, Japan
e-mail: asakoshi@cc.okayama-u.ac.jp

3.6.1 Mastocytosis

Naohito Hatta

3.6.1.1 Definition

Mastocytosis is a very heterogeneous disease. In cutaneous mastocytosis, the abnormal growth of mast cells is limited to a cutaneous lesion while in systemic mastocytosis at least one extracutaneous organ is involved. An updated consensus classification for mastocytosis was proposed in 2001 (Table 3.6.1) [4]. In cutaneous mastocytosis, normal-appearing mast cells are increased predominantly around blood vessels and skin appendages in the papillary dermis. The diagnosis of systemic mastocytosis is made by multifocal compact mast cell infiltrations consisting at least 15 cells that are detected in bone marrow or other extracutaneous organs [4].

3.6.1.2 Molecular Abnormality

Mast cells are derived from CD34+ multipotent hematopoietic progenitor cells. During the maturation process, interaction of the Kit proto-oncogene and stem cell factor (SCF) play an important role. Gain of functional mutations in Kit, such as D816V result in ligand-independent constitutive activation of Kit signaling and uncontrolled mast cell proliferation and resistance to apoptosis [1]. This somatic mutation is found in the vast majority of patients with systemic mastocytosis, and can be used as a minor diagnostic criterion [3].

R. Dummer et al. (eds.), *Skin Cancer – A World-Wide Perspective*,
DOI: 10.1007/978-3-642-05072-5_3.6, © Springer-Verlag Berlin Heidelberg 2011

Table 3.6.1 WHO classification of mastocytosis

Cutaneous mastosytosis (CM)
Maculopapular CM=urticaria pigmentosa (UP)
Diffuse CM
Solitary mastocytoma of skin
Systemic mastocytosis (SM)
Indolent SM (ISM)
SM with an associated clonal hematologic non-mast cell lineage disease (SM-AHNMD)
Aggressive SM (ASM)
Mast cell leukemia (MCL)
Mast cell sarcoma (MCS)
Extracutaneous mastocytoma

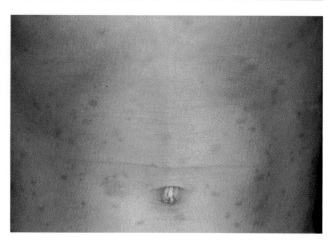

Fig. 3.6.1 Urticaria pigmentosa. Numerous typical reddish-brown maculopapules and pigmentations in a young child

3.6.1.3 Clinical Examination

A biopsy of cutaneous lesions is desirable to confirm the diagnosis. A full blood count should be performed; however, unless systemic mastocytosis is suspected, routine bone marrow examination is not required. As tryptase is stored within the secretary granules of mast cells, serum tryptase levels >20 ng/mL suggest the presence of systemic mastocytosis. Abdominal ultrasound and bone scans can be considered to evaluate liver, spleen, and bone involvement.

3.6.1.4 Cutaneous Mastocytosis

Cutaneous mastocytosis (CM) without systemic involvement that develops in childhood has a favorable prognosis. CM should be diagnosed when the patient shows typical clinical aspects of skin lesions, typical focal infiltrate of mast cells in the dermis, and the absence of systemic mastocytosis criteria. Mechanical irritation such as physical exercise, hot baths, and scratching causes the release of mast cell mediators and symptoms of flushing, itching, and gastrointestinal disturbance.

3.6.1.4.1 Urticaria Pigmentosa

Urticaria pigmentosa (UP) is equivalent to maculopapular cutaneous mastosytosis, and the commonest pattern in this category. Although UP occurs in both children and adults, most patients are children. Numerous reddish-brown maculopapules, plaques, and nodules appear on the body except on the face, head, palms, and soles of the feet (Fig. 3.6.1). Cases with a few nodules similar to mastocytoma may also be regarded as multiple mastocytoma of the skin [5]. In

patients with childhood onset, spontaneous clearance or fading of the disease is frequently observed during puberty.

3.6.1.4.2 Diffuse Cutaneous Mastocytosis

Diffuse cutaneous mastocytosis (DCM) is characterized by diffuse erythrodermic rash rather than the typical maculaopapular lesions typically seen in UP. DCM appears to be a less frequent form of CM than UP. Due to the extensive infiltration of mast cells, some patients show diffusely thickened skin or nodules.

3.6.1.4.3 Mastocytoma

Cutaneous mastocytomas present as solitary red, pink, or yellowish nodules or plaques in infancy or early childhood. These plaques are usually solitary and tend to blister with friction. Histologically, the lesion consists of dense, mature-appearing mast cells without atypia. Usually, the lesion disappears spontaneously in adolescence.

3.6.1.5 Indolent Systemic Mastocytosis

Indolent systemic mastocytosis (ISM) is defined by the presence of skin lesions and an absence of clinical or laboratory signs of (1) smoldering disease, (2) aggressive disease, (3) mast cell leukemia (MCL), and (4) an associated clonal hematological non-mast cell lineage disease (AHNMD). ISM is the most common variant of SM and usually involves both the skin and the bone marrow. Typical ISM presents with UP-like skin lesions and shows mediator-related symptoms. The bone marrow contains multifocal, dense infiltrates of mast cells. Although most ISM has a prolonged clinical course, transformation into a more aggressive form of SM has been reported.

Smoldering systemic mastocytosis (SSM) exhibits at least two of the following criteria; (1) a bone marrow infiltration grade of >30% and serum tryptase >200 ng/mL, (2) discrete signs of myelodysplasia or myeloproliferation, and (3) palpable organomegaly or visceral lymphadenopathy detected by US or CT without impairment of organ function due to MC infiltration (C-findings).

3.6.1.6 Aggressive Systemic Mastocytosis

Aggressive systemic mastocytosis (ASM) is much less common than ISM and lacks typical skin lesions. ASM is defined by hepatosplenomegaly and generalized lymphadenopathy with the presence of <20% bone marrow mast cells in bone marrow smears and no signs of an associated MCL and SM-AHNMD. Clinical symptoms of ASM include impaired organ function such as severe cytopenias, malabsorption, bone fractures, and liver dysfunction.

Lymphadenopathic mastocytosis with eosinophilia is a rare variant of ASM and characterized by prominent eosinophilia of blood and tissues and generalized lymphadenopathy [2].

3.6.1.7 Systemic Mastocytosis with an Associated Clonal Hematologic Non-Mast Cell Lineage Disease

Systemic mastocytosis with an associated clonal hematologic non-mast cell lineage disease (SM-AHNMD) is the second most frequent subtype of systemic mastocytosis. Most SM-AHNMDs are accompanied myeloid disorders such as myelodysplastic syndrome, myeloproliferative syndrome, acute myeloid leukemia, chronic myeloid leukemia and chronic myelomonocytic leukemia. The prognosis of SM-AHNMD is mainly determined by the severity of "AHNMD."

3.6.1.8 Mast Cell Leukemia

Mast cell leukemia (MCL) is characterized by leukemic infiltration of various organs by immature neoplastic mast cells. The diagnosis is made by the presence of circulating mast cells and more than 20% of mast cells in the bone marrow smear.

3.6.2 Disease Entities of Kaposi Sarcoma

Nagwa M. Elwan

Kaposi sarcoma (KS) is a multifocal neoplasm of the endothelium. KS has been classified into four clinical-epidemiological variants including the original classic KS, African or endemic KS, epidemic or AIDS-associated KS, and iatrogenic or immunosuppression-related KS.

3.6.2.1 Clinical Features

The clinical course varies from indolent cutaneous lesions often limited to the lower extremities to rapidly progressive disease with extensive coetaneous and visceral disease. Clinical features of KS can be classified into cutaneous and extacutaneous KS.

3.6.2.2 Cutaneous KS

Classic KS occurs mainly in older men, in whom KS tumors usually occur on the lower legs and feet. Typical lesions are initially solitary or few, asymptomatic erythematous or violaceous macules or nodules. Disease progression is variable; macules or tumors can remain unchanged for months to years or grow rapidly within few weeks and disseminate. Rapid growth can lead to localized pain and a yellow–green discoloration of the area around the tumor as a result of hemorrhage. Further progression can lead to central necrosis and ulceration of KS lesions. Plaque-like and nodular KS lesions often become confluent and can be accompanied by massive edema [4].

Commonly, KS-AIDS first presents with multiple nodules on the upper body, head and neck, and tends to evolve swiftly on the skin, mucous membranes, and in viscera with dissemination leading to organ dysfunction and mortality [16].

3.6.2.3 Clinical Variants of Cutaneous KS

KS has many, and sometimes coexisting, morphological variants including: (1) patch stage, (2) localized (nondestructive) plaque, (3) exophytic KS, (4) infiltrative KS, (5) generalized lymphadenopathic KS with widespread cutaneous lesions, (6) disseminated cutaneous and visceral KS, (7) telangiectatic, (8) keloidal, (9), ecchymotic, and (10) lymphangioma-like or cavernous KS [27]. The common forms include localized nodular, locally aggressive, and generalized lymphadenopathic. Lymphadenopathic KS is a clinically aggressive form often associated with widespread lymph node and cutaneous involvement. Mucous membranes and viscera are also affected. It is the predominant form in African children [9, 32].

Post traumatic KS and post irradiation primary KS are reported. KS can occur at the site of other unrelated skin diseases or trauma, what is termed "isotopic response" [3, 31]. Conjunctival, oral and penile KS are also reported [5, 13, 17].

3.6.2.4 Extracutaneous KS

Systemic or extracutaneous KS have been linked to significant mortality and morbidity. The most evident visceral KS is reported in gut and lymph nodes [20, 22]. In AIDS-associated KS, the most common visceral involvement sites were the lungs, gastrointestinal tract, and lymph nodes [15]. The liver and heart are also common extracutaneous involvement sites [20]. Other organs which may be involved include the kidneys, adrenals, pancreas, brain, testes, urinary bladder, and thyroid [29, 30].

3.6.2.5 Staging of KS

1. The AIDS clinical trials group classification by Krown et al. [12] uses the following three categories, with a tumor/immune system/systemic illness (TIS) grading method: *Tumor (T)*: high or low risk signs (good when KS is confined to skin and/or lymph nodes and/or demonstrates minimal oral disease). *Immune system (I)*: CD4 cell level ≥150/mm^3 (low risk) vs. <150/mm^3 (high risk). *Systemic illness (S)*: low or high risk.

2. Another classification by Mitsuyasu [18] divides KS into four stages. *Stage I*: localized nodular KS in elderly men in North America and Europe. *Stage II*: localized, invasive and aggressive KS (mostly seen in Africa). *Stage III*: disseminated mucocutaneous KS in African children and homosexual patients. *Stage IV*: stage III with visceral involvement.

3. Schwartz et al. [26, 27] prefer the following classification. *Stage I*: localized nodular KS, with ≤15 cutaneous lesions or involvement restricted to one bilateral anatomic site, and few, if any, gut nodules. *Stage II*: includes both exophytic destructive KS and locally infiltrative cutaneous lesions and locally aggressive KS or nodular KS, or >15 cutaneous lesions or involvement of more than one bilateral anatomic site, and few or many gut nodules. *Stage III*: generalized lymphadenopathic KS with widespread lymph node involvement, with or without cutaneous KS, but with limited if any visceral involvement. *Stage IV*: (disseminated visceral KS): widespread KS, usually progressing from stage II or III, with involvement of multiple visceral organs with or without cutaneous KS. Although other staging ideas are reported, staging of KS remains a challenge.

3.6.2.6 Histopathology of KS

Unlike most cancers, which arise from the clonal outgrowth of a single cell type, KS lesions are histologically complex [8]. The principal proliferating cell in KS lesions is the spindle cell. Pathologists have argued about the origin of KS spindle cells. Many suggestions are reported, including ideas that spindle cell are of endothelial lineage, bearing many endothelial markers including CD31, CD 34 and CD36 [21]. Confusion has accompanied the finding that KS spindle cells display significant heterogeneity in marker expression, e.g., some spindle cells stain for muscle alpha-actin, leading some researchers to speculate that spindle cells may arise from biopotential mesenchymal precursors of vascular cells [11]. Another view is that the spindle cells arise from lymphatic endothelium [1]. Irrespective of their precise origin, spindle cells clearly represent the main proliferative element in KS. From a pathogenetic point of view, KS is composed of three parallel processes: a proliferative component involving mainly spindle cells), an inflammatory component, and an angiogenic component [7].

KS histology is not static, but varies considerably with the evolutionary state of the lesion. KS tends to evolve from the early inflammatory or patch stage to the nodular/plaque stage. *Patch stage* KS shows glomerulus-like vascular formations and an angioendotheliomatous pattern. Angioneoplasia may occur in clinically uninvolved perilesional KS skin [23]. In *nodular stage* KS, endothelialized vessels and non-endothelialized slit-like spaces may become evident in addition to spindle cells infiltrating dermal collagen bundles. The slit-like spaces often contain erythrocytes which may extravasate. The inflammatory cell component is unaltered. The plaque stage shows the same histologic features seen in the nodular stage, with diffuse dermal involvement [25].

Immunohistochemical evaluation of immune cell infiltrate in cutaneous KS revealed increased density of immune cells (CD68, CD3) in the nodular lesions, reflecting increased antigenicity of these lesions [10]. Immunohistochemical testing favors the endothelial cell, probably of lymphoid type, as the cell of origin for KS. The presence of factor VIII-related antigen, the lectin *Ulex eurpeaus* agglutinin 1, and reactivity with two monoclonal antibodies (EN4 and PALE) suggest that KS is derived from endothelium of lymphatic origin. On the other hand, KS spindle cells express CD34 which is expressed by endothelial cells of small blood vessels but not those of lymphatic origin [19]. Expression of a monoclonal antibody to vascular endothelial growth factor receptor-3 (VEGFR-3) is a sensitive marker for KS, but does not reliably distinguish KS from other angiosarcomas [6].

3.6.2.7 Prognosis

Prognosis of KS depends on the clinical manifestations and staging of the disease. Prognosis appears to correlate with the degree of immunosuppression and older age in classic KS patients [24]. The prognosis is excellent in cases of localized nodular KS and iatrogenic KS, while locally aggressive KS has an intermediate prognosis. Patients with AIDS-KS usually develop disseminated KS or severe opportunistic infection within 3 years of diagnosis, with a 3-year survival rate closer to 0% without therapy [2, 28]. Protease inhibitor-based HAART was associated with a median survival of 31 months in HIV associated advanced KS patients treated with chemotherapy, compared to only 7 months without HAART [14]. The mean survival rate of patients with AIDS-KS has been 15–24 months approximately. Patients may die from associated opportunistic infections or from gastrointestinal KS with hemorrhage [14].

3.6.3 Hemangiomas of Infancy

Nagwa M. Elwan and L. Weibel

Vascular birthmarks can be classified into hemangiomas and vascular malformations. Hemangiomas are common benign tumors of early infancy, characterized by endothelial hyperplasia and proliferation, rapid neonatal growth, and slow involution during childhood. Vascular malformations show a normal endothelial turnover, they are usually present at birth and grow in proportion with the child [38]. It is important to distinguish between hemangiomas (vascular tumors) and vascular malformation (static lesion), although this differentiation may occasionally be difficult on clinical grounds alone [1].

Several types of hemangiomas have been described including: (a) hemangiomas of infancy (HOI), (b) Congenital hemangiomas (rapidly involuting and non-involuting), (c) miliary hemangiomas (benign neonatal; cutaneous-limited, and disseminated neonatal) [1].

3.6.3.1 Hemangiomas of Infancy

This is the most common type of hemangiomas. The true incidence of infantile hemangiomas is difficult to determine due to the methodologic limitations of the few relevant studies, but some reports suggest that the incidence is about 4–5% [7]. Other reports showed that the incidence of infantile hemangiomas is 10–12% in Caucasian infants and lower in dark-skinned infants [8].

3.6.3.2 Clinical Features

Hemangiomas of infancy (HOI) are more common in females than males (3:1–5:1 ratio). They appear during the neonatal period, usually within 2 weeks [13]. Their size varies from a few millimeters to large plaques of more than 10 cm. Most hemangiomas are solitary, but some infants show multiple lesions. Superficial hemangiomas are recognized by their bright strawberry-red color, while deep lesions can present with a normal to bluish skin hue related to their location [12]. The growth of HOI is often divided into phases: *(a) The initial nascent phase*: in 50% hemangioma precursor lesions are visible on the first day of life in the form of a telangiectatic macule surrounded by a pale halo, an erythematous macule, or a pinhead sized cherry red papule. *(b) The proliferative phase*: starts within weeks of the appearance of the hemangioma, and is most pronounced during the first 3–6 months of life, often showing rapid growth. *(c) The stationary phase (plateau)*: static size after 6–10 months. *(d) The involuting phase*: usually starts during the second year of life. Initially the color fades and then the tumor slowly shrinks in size. The skin usually lightens completely and normal skin is restored, however in approximately one-third of the children residual telangiectasia and textural changes of the skin persist [2, 14]. HOI are most commonly located on the head and neck (60%), followed by the trunk and extremities [14]. They may occur at extracutaneous sites including the liver, gastrointestinal tract, central nervous system, and pancreas.

3.6.3.3 Classification

HOI are classified as superficial (strawberry or capillary) Fig. 3.6.2a, deep (cavernous), or mixed. Recently, hemangiomas were further classified as follows [3]: *(a) Localized*: those that seem to grow from a single focal point, *(b) Segmental*: plaque-type hemangiomas demonstrating linear and/or geographic distribution, *(c) Indeterminate*: not readily classified as either localized or segmental, and *(d) Multifocal*: 10 or more cutaneous hemangiomas. HOI should be differentiated from other infantile vascular tumors including rapidly involuting congenital hemangiomas (RICH), non-involuting congenital hemangiomas (NICH), kaposiform hemangioendotheliomas and tufted angiomas [12], and from non-vascular benign or malignant lesions such as nasal glioma, infantile fibrosarcoma, angiosarcoma, and dermatofibrosarcoma protuberans.

3.6.3.4 Histopathology

Proliferating hemangiomas are composed of nearly solid masses of small capillaries with plump, rapidly dividing endothelial cells with or without lumens. They are grouped in delicately defined lobules separated by fine strands of connective tissue. None of the lobules are encapsulated [10]. During the involution process, the vascular lumens dilate, endothelial cells flatten, and progressive deposition of fibrous

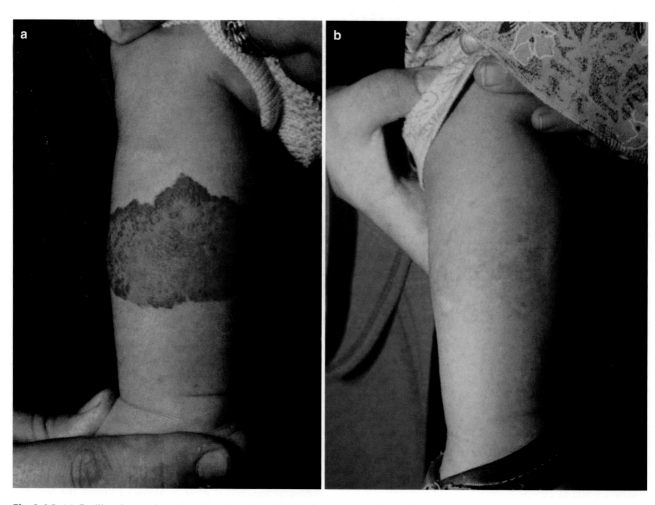

Fig. 3.6.2 (**a**) Capillary hemangioma in an Egyptian infant. (**b**) Capillary hemanangioma after treatment with pulsed dye laser (PDL)

tissue occurs, giving the hemangioma a lobular architecture. Fully involuted lesions contain few tiny vessels and draining veins, with flattened endothelium in a surrounding stroma of fibrofatty tissue, collagen, and reticulin fibers [7].

Stimulators of angiogenesis such as vascular endothelial growth factor (VEGF), basic fibroblast growth factor (bFGF), monocytochrome attractant protein-1, insulin-like growth factor-2 (IGF-2), and allograft inflammatory factor-1 are upregulated in proliferating hemangiomas [4–6]. Common expression of immunohistochemical markers such as glucose uptake transporter-1, Glut-1, merosin, FcRII, and Lewis Y antigen may suggest that hemangiomas either derived from or share a common precursor to the placenta [11]. Glut-1 expression is positive in HOI, while it is negative in congenital hemangiomas and all cases of vascular malformations [5, 9]. Also, infantile hemangioma cells are VEGF-receptor, CD31, and CD34 positive, similar to the embryonal cardinal vein, suggesting that these cells are arrested in an immature stage of vascular development, leading to their rapid proliferation [4].

3.6.3.5 Prognosis and Management

The majority of infantile hemangiomas are uncomplicated and involute spontaneously with a good cosmetic result. Approximately 10% of all infantile hemangiomas require treatment, usually due to their location (periocular area, nose, lips, airways, perianal area), large size or ulceration. Until recently systemic corticosteroids have been the mainstay of treatment for complicated hemangiomas, apart from other treatment options such as intralesional corticosteroids, laser therapy (Fig. 3.6.2b), interferon-alpha, vincristine and surgery. However, betablockers such as propranolol have now been discovered to be highly effective for the treatment of proliferating infantile hemangiomas [16]. Potential explanations for the therapeutic effect of propranolol – a nonselective beta-adrenergic receptor blocker – on infantile hemangiomas include vasoconstriction, which is immediately visible as a change in color, associated with a palpable softening of the hemangioma; decreased expression of vascular endothelial growth factor (*VEGF*) and basic fibroblast growth factor (*bFGF*) genes through the down-regulation of the RAF – mitogen-activated protein kinase pathway; and the triggering of apoptosis of capillary endothelial cells [16].

This novel treatment option has been adapted worldwide with great success and follow-up studies confirm the consistent rapid therapeutic effect of propranolol, leading to considerable shortening of the natural course of HOI with good clinical tolerance [17].

Betablockers will probably shortly replace most previous therapies and represent the treatment of choice for complicated infantile hemangiomas.

3.6.4 Disease Entities of Cherry Hemangioma

Nagwa M. Elwan

Cherry hemangiomas (cherry angiomas or senile angiomas) are very common single or multiple bright red papules, up to a few millimeters in diameter, occurring predominantly on the trunk and proximal parts of the limbs. Cherry angiomas are rare before puberty, but the incidence rises sharply in the fourth decade [1].

3.6.4.1 Histopathology

In small early lesions, one or more dilated interconnecting thin-walled vascular channels are present in the dermal papillae. In older lesions, there is loss of rete ridges and atrophy of the superficial epidermis, with formation of a polypoid lesion composed of a network of dilated communicating channels with scant intervening connective tissue. These lesions appear to be the dilated and interconnected segments of venous capillaries and post capillary venules in the dermal papillae. The vessels of the upper horizontal plexus are not involved [2].

3.6.5 Disease Entities of Sinusoidal Hemangioma

Nagwa M. Elwan

Sinusoidal hemangioma (SH) was described by two pathologists, Calonje and Fletcher, in 1991 [1]. They described twelve cases of sinusoidal hemangioma (SH), a distinctive subset of the group of lesions known as cavernous hemangioma. Clinically, SH presented as solitary subcutaneous, deep dermal lesions in adults, predominantly females; the trunk (including the breast) and limbs were the most commonly affected sites [1]. It is an acquired lesion and has therefore not been included with the "hamartomas or malformations."

3.6.5.1 Histopathology

SH are characterized by dilated, interconnecting, thin-walled vascular channels that frequently show a pseudopapillary pattern. These vessels have a predominantly lobular architecture but peripherally show focally ill-defined spread into subcutaneous tissue. The lining endothelium is single-layered but may show focal pleomorphism and hyperchromasia; mitotic figures, however, are not seen. Follow up of those cases has revealed no tendency for either local recurrence or metastasis [1, 2].

3.6.6 Disease Entities of Glomeruloid Hemangioma

Nagwa M. Elwan

Chan and colleagues coined the term "glomeruloid hemangioma" (GH) for a characteristic benign vascular tumor which they considered a cutaneous marker for POEMS syndrome [1]. POEMS syndrome is a multisystem disorder characterized by polyneuropathy, organomegaly, endocrinopathy, M-protein, and skin changes [5, 9]. Multicentric Castleman's disease and POEMS syndrome are overlapping conditions [4, 8]. On the other hand, solitary or localized cutaneous glomeruloid hemangiomas have been reported to occur outside of POEMS syndrome [3, 6, 7]. Clinically, GH are multiple or single dome-shaped red papules affecting the trunk and limbs [9]. GH in the form of hemangioma with cerebriform morphology have been reported [2].

3.6.6.1 Histopathology

In the characteristic GH described by Chan et al. 1990 [1], there are dilated dermal vascular spaces filled with grape-like aggregates of small capillary vessels, resulting in structures resembling renal glomeruli. Cells within the capillary loops are lined by endothelial cells with scant cytoplasm; (CD3 + CD34+, CD68−, CD105 + UEA-1+), while the outer surfaces of the loops were covered with either swollen endothelial cells containing PAS (−) and immunoglobulin-positive eosinophilic hyaline globules (CD31+, CD34−, CD68±, CD105−, UEA-1−) or cells without globules. These two phenotypically different endothelial cells are separated by alpha-smooth muscle actin-positive pericytes. Pericytes and endothelial cells covering the outer surface of the loops are bordered by basement membrane [9].

3.6.7 Hobnail Hemangioma (Targetoid Hemosiderotic Hemangioma)

Luis Requena

Hobnail hemangiomas are benign cutaneous vascular proliferations characterized by irregular vascular channels lined with endothelial cells with a hobnail appearance [1–20]. Targetoid hemosiderotic hemangioma [1] and hobnail hemangioma [15] are currently considered the same entity by most authors.

3.6.7.1 Clinical Features

Most hobnail hemangiomas appear as a solitary brown to violaceous central papule, surrounded by a thin, pale area and a peripheral ecchymotic ring (Fig. 3.6.3). The ecchymotic halo ultimately disappears, whereas the central papule persists. However, there are also hobnail hemangiomas without targetoid appearance. The lower limbs, specifically the thighs, are the most frequently involved sites. Trauma may play a pathogenic role in the development of hobnail hemangioma, and some authors believe that this lesion results from trauma in a preexisting lymphangioma or angiokeratoma [14, 18].

3.6.7.2 Histopathologic Features

Hobnail hemangioma consists of a wedge-shaped dermal vascular proliferation with a distinctive biphasic appearance [15]. The center and the superficial areas of the lesion are composed of dilated, irregular, thin-walled ectatic

vascular spaces involving the superficial dermis (Fig. 3.6.4a). These vascular spaces sometimes exhibit intraluminal papillary projections and fibrin thrombi at different stages of organization. Prominent, plump, endothelial cells with a hobnail appearance line both the vessel lumina and the papillary projections (Fig. 3.6.4b). As the vascular structures descend into the reticular dermis, they become smaller and appear as irregular, angulated, thin-walled slit-shaped channels that dissect between collagen bundles of the dermis [15]. In these deep areas, dermal fibrosis, hemosiderin, extravasated red blood cells, and a mild mononuclear inflammatory infiltrate are common histopathologic findings.

Immunohistochemical studies have demonstrated that the endothelial cells lining the vascular spaces of hobnail hemangioma stain weakly for factor VIII-related antigen and strongly for *Ulex europaeus* I lectin and CD31 [1–3, 16]. The lack of actin labeled pericytes, the CD34 negativity of endothelial cells lining the vascular structures, and the immunoreactivity of these endothelial cells for D2-40 support lymphatic differentiation in hobnail hemangioma [19].

The histopathologic differential diagnosis from the patch-stage of Kaposi's sarcoma may be difficult. However, the superficial and central areas of hobnail hemangioma show dilated vessels with intraluminal papillary projections lined by prominent endothelial cells, a feature that is absent in Kaposi's sarcoma. In hobnail hemangioma the vascular channels at the periphery of the lesion do not surround preexisting vascular and adnexal structures in the dermis, as is the case in the patch-stage of Kaposi's sarcoma. Immunohistochemical investigations of human herpes virus 8 (HHV-8) has proven consistently negative in hobnail hemangiomas [20].

3.6.7.3 Treatment

The lesion is entirely benign, and surgical excision is curative. No recurrences have been reported after excision.

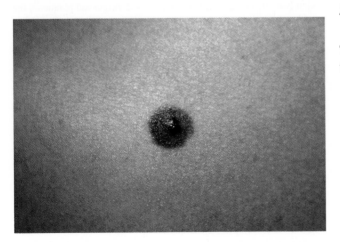

Fig. 3.6.3 Clinical appearance of hobnail hemangioma. Some lesions, such as the one shown in this case, show a targetoid morphology, with a central papule of angiomatous appearance and an ecchymotic halo

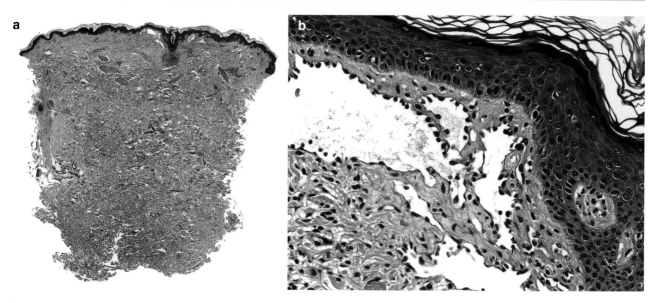

Fig. 3.6.4 (**a**) Scanning power showing dilated irregular thin-walled vascular structures in the superficial dermis. (**b**) The dilated vascular structures are lined by prominent, plump, endothelial cells with a hobnail appearance

3.6.8 Microvenular Hemangioma

Luis Requena

Microvenular hemangioma is a benign, acquired, slowly growing cutaneous asymptomatic lesion with angiomatous appearance [1–12].

3.6.8.1 Clinical Features

Microvenular hemangioma appears as a solitary, well circumscribed, bright red papule or small plaque (Fig. 3.6.5). It most commonly affects the upper limbs, particularly the forearms, varying in size from 0.5 to 2 cm. Examples of microvenular hemangioma have been also described on the trunk, face, and lower limbs [3, 4, 9]. A histogenetic relationship between microvenular hemangioma and hormonal factors such as pregnancy and hormonal contraceptives was originally postulated [2, 4], but this feature has not been corroborated by other authors. An example of microvenular hemangioma developed in a patient with Wiskott–Aldrich syndrome [9], and hemangiomas identical to microvenular hemangioma have been also described in patients with POEMS syndrome [10, 12]

3.6.8.2 Histopathologic Features

Histopathologically, microvenular hemangioma appears as a poorly circumscribed proliferation of irregularly branched,

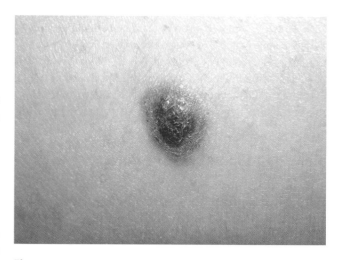

Fig. 3.6.5 Clinical appearance of microvenular hemangioma. The lesion consisted of a sharply circumscribed, bright red plaque on the anterior trunk

round to oval, thin-walled blood vessels lined with a single layer of monomorphous endothelial cells (Fig. 3.6.6). They involve the entire reticular dermis, and slightly sclerotic collagen bundles are seen between the neoformed vascular structures. The lumina of the neoplastic blood vessels are inconspicuous and often collapse with only a few red cells within them. Immunohistochemically, endothelial cells lining the vascular lumina express positivity for factor VIII-related antigen and *Ulex europaeus* I lectin [1–3]. Some smooth muscle actin positive pericytes have also been described surrounding the vascular spaces [3, 5].

The main differential diagnosis of microvenular hemangioma is the patch stage lesions of Kaposi's sarcoma. Kaposi's sarcoma shows irregular anastomosing vascular spaces, newly

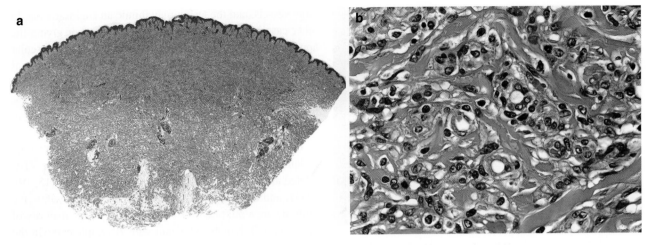

Fig. 3.6.6 (**a**) Scanning magnification showing the involvement of the upper half of the reticular dermis. (**b**) Higher magnification demonstrated that the lesion was composed of round to oval thin walled blood vessels lined by a single layer of endothelial cells, some of them containing erythrocytes within their small lumina

formed ectatic vascular channels surrounding preexisting normal blood vessels and adnexa (promontory sign), plasma cells, hyaline (eosinophilic) globules, and small interstitial fascicles of spindle cells. All of these features are absent in microvenular hemangioma, which is characterized by the presence of monomorphous, small, elongated blood vessels with inconspicuous lumina involving the full thickness of the reticular dermis. Furthermore, immunohistochemical investigations of human herpes virus 8 (HHV-8) has proven negative in microvenular hemangiomas [11], with the exception of an African patient with POEMS syndrome and Castleman's disease who showed immunoexpression of HHV-8 in the endothelial cells of a microvenular hemangioma, probably as a result of immunosuppression [12].

3.6.8.3 *Treatment*

Microvenular hemagioma is a benign lesion which is cured with simple excision.

3.6.9 Angiolymphoid Hyperplasia with Eosinophilia

Luis Requena

Angiolymphoid hyperplasia with eosinophilia (ALHE) is a benign cutaneous or subcutaneous vascular proliferation composed of immature blood vessels lined with epithelioid endothelial cells and variable proportions of chronic inflammatory infiltrate containing lymphocytes and eosinophils. ALHE was originally considered a late stage of Kimura disease [1, 2], but currently, most authors believe that ALHE and Kimura's disease are two separate entities [3–8].

3.6.9.1 *Clinical Features*

Clinically, ALHE is characterized by erythematous or violaceous papules or nodules of angiomatoid appearance with a predilection for the head (Fig. 3.6.7), especially around the ears, forehead, and scalp. Less commonly reported sites include the oral mucosa [9, 10], trunk, extremities [11, 12], vulva [13, 14], penis [15], and inner canthus of the eye [16]. In cases of multiple lesions, they tend to be grouped or confluent. Symptomatic lesions may be pruritic, painful, or pulsatile. Lesions do not involute spontaneously and often recur after excision [17]. Some patients have peripheral eosinophilia, but this feature is less frequent and less marked than in Kimura's disease, and lymphadenopathy, asthma, increased serum IgE, and proteinuria are not seen in patients with ALHE.

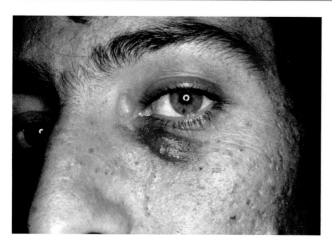

Fig. 3.6.7 Angiolymphoid hyperplasia with eosinophilia involving the lower eyelid

3.6.9.2 Histopathologic Features

Histopathologically, ALHE consists of well-circumscribed nodules (Fig. 3.6.8a) involving the dermis and/or the subcutaneous fat that at scanning magnification may show a lobular configuration. There are two distinct components in ALHE, namely irregular blood vessels and dense inflammatory infiltrate. The vascular component comprises irregular thick walled blood vessels lined with epithelioid endothelial cells, which protrude into the lumen. The walls of the vessels often reveal thickened bundles of smooth muscle and abundant mucin. The endothelial cells show large round to oval nuclei and abundant eosinophilic cytoplasm, which often contains prominent vacuoles as a sign of primitive vascular differentiation (Fig. 3.6.8b). These endothelial cells may also form solid sheets, and the angiomatous nature of the lesion then becomes less evident. Sometimes the proliferation of the endothelial cells is especially prominent within the lumina of

large vessels, and the lesion may mimic an angiosarcoma. In other cases, the endothelial cells group together giving the appearance of multinucleated cells with immature vascular lumina [18]. The stroma of ALHE consists of fibrovascular tissue that invariably contains lymphocytes, eosinophils, mast cells, and, sometimes, mucin deposits. In some cases, lymphoid follicles with germinal centers are present, but usually they are not as prominent as in Kimura's disease.

Immunohistochemical studies have demonstrated that the endothelial cells express immunoreactivity for factor VIII-related antigen [9, 19–22], *Ulex europaeus* I lectin [15, 19], CD31, and CD34 [23]. The lymphocytes present within the infiltrate are a mixture of T and B cells, with the majority of them being T lymphocytes and with B lymphocytes in the germinal centers [20]. In one series, T-cell monoclonality was detected in the infiltrate of ALHE, which may define a subgroup of ALHE with a higher tendency to recurrences [20]. Ultrastructurally, the characteristic endothelial cells contain Weibel–Palade bodies [9, 19–21, 24, 25].

The true nature of ALHE is uncertain. Human herpes virus 8 (HHV8) has been detected in some lesions of ALHE [26, 27], but these findings could be not confirmed by other authors [12, 28, 29]. In some cases there is an antecedent of trauma [30]. When the biopsy is large and deep enough, an arteriovenous shunt is found in a significant percentage of cases [31]. These features suggest that ALHE is not a true neoplasm, but a reactive hyperplastic process which probably occurs secondary to damage and repair of an artery or vein [30].

The differential diagnosis with Kimura's disease can be established on the basis of both the clinical and histopathological features [3–8]. Clinically, Kimura's disease consists of skin-colored subcutaneous masses that, in extreme cases, distort the outline of the face dramatically as a consequence of the presence of large infiltrates of inflammatory cells within the dermis and subcutaneous tissues. Usually patients

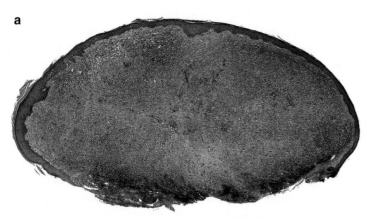

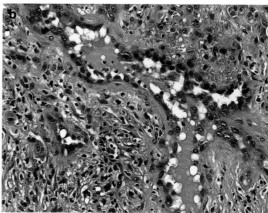

Fig. 3.6.8 (**a**) Scanning power of angiolymphoid hyperplasia with eosinophilia showing a dome shaped papule. (**b**) Higher magnification showing irregular vascular structures lined with prominent endothelial cells with epithelioid appearance. Some of the endothelial cells show cytoplasmic vacuolization as sign of primitive vascular differentiation. Note also the presence of eosinophils in the stroma

also show intense peripheral eosinophilia and lymphadenopathy. Histopathologically, Kimura's disease is devoid of the vascular abnormalities seen in ALHE, and when plump endothelial cells are present in the blood vessels, they are a focal finding. The main finding is the presence of numerous, closely packed lymphoid follicles that extend throughout the dermis and subcutaneous fat and sometimes into the lymph nodes and internal organs. Within these infiltrates, there are numerous eosinophils. In brief, Kimura's disease is not a disorder of blood vessels but an inflammatory systemic process of unknown etiology.

3.6.9.3 Treatment

Lesions of ALHE can be adequately managed with surgery, cryotherapy, or laser therapy [32–37], but larger lesions show a tendency to persist unless the arteriovenous shunt is excised.

3.6.10 Spindle-Cell Hemangioma

Luis Requena

This lesion was originally described as spindle cell hemangioendothelioma, because it was considered as a low grade malignant vascular proliferation [1]. Subsequently, more than 200 cases have reported in the literature, and all of them showed benign biological behavior [2–39]. Accordingly, the lesion was renamed spindle cell hemangioma [28, 39–42].

3.6.10.1 Clinical Features

Spindle cell hemangioma is preferentially located in the distal regions of the extremities (Fig. 3.6.9) of children and young adults [3], although examples of this lesion have been reported in several areas including the buttock [16], oral cavity [23], spinal cord [26], and penis [32]. It affects both sexes equally. Several cases of spindle cell hemangioma have been described in patients with Maffucci syndrome [1, 3, 7, 18, 21, 22, 24, 25, 28, 29, 31, 34]. Interestingly, three of the patients with co-existence of spindle cell hemangioma and Maffucci's syndrome developed angiosarcomas in other regions of the body, separate from those affected by the

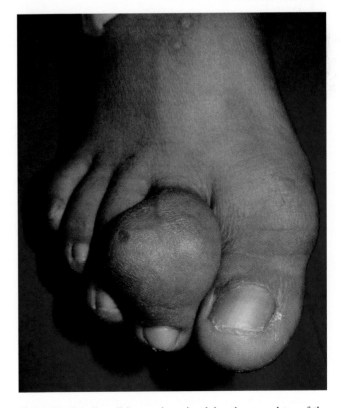

Fig. 3.6.9 Spindle cell hemangioma involving the second toe of the right foot

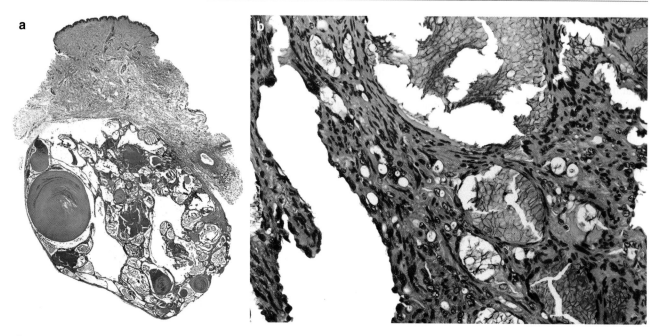

Fig. 3.6.10 (a) At scanning magnification spindle cell hemangioma appears as a well-circumscribed nodule composed of dilated vascular structures, some of them with their lumina occupied by organized thrombi and phleboliths. (b) At higher magnification there are short fascicles of spindle cells, some of them showing prominent cytoplasmic vacuolization

spindle cell hemangioma [11, 24, 28]. Although many lesions present initially as a single nodule, most become multifocal within an anatomical region acquiring the characteristics of firm, bluish nodules.

3.6.10.2 Histopathologic Features

At low power, spindle cell hemangioma consists of well circumscribed but not encapsulated nodules (Fig. 3.6.10a). The nodules are composed of dilated, thin walled blood vessels, sometimes occupied by organized thrombi and phleboliths. A stroma of spindle cells arranged in fascicles and closely resembling Kaposi's sarcoma is interspersed between the blood vessels. The fascicles often also contain round cells with vacuolated cytoplasm (Fig. 3.6.10b), which sometimes may be misinterpreted as entrapped adipose tissue [28, 37]. Immunohistochemical studies have demonstrated that the endothelial cells that line the blood vessels and the plump rounded cells with vacuolated cytoplasm express immunoreactivity for factor VIII-related antigen, *Ulex europaeus* I lectin, and CD34 [1, 3, 10, 11, 14, 18, 22]. In contrast, the spindle cells are negative for these markers but express immunoreactivity for smooth muscle markers, including HHF35, alpha-smooth muscle actin, desmin, and collagen type IV thus providing evidence that they are immature pericytes [22]. Immunohistochemical studies with proliferating markers regularly disclose low proliferative activity [25]. Electron microscopic studies have demonstrated that the round cells show ultrastructural characteristics of endothelial cells, whereas the spindle cells were less differentiated mesenchymal cells showing features of fibroblasts [3, 10, 11, 14, 15].

Histopathologic differential diagnosis with nodular lesions of Kaposi's sarcoma may be challenging, but immunohistochemical studies for the presence of the human herpesvirus 8 in spindle cell hemangioma are consistently negative [30].

3.6.10.3 Treatment

Spindle cell hemangioma may be approached surgically, but the lesion often recurs [28]. Although the clinical course of spindle cell hemangioma is benign, a close follow-up is needed in patients with spindle cell hemangioma and Maffucci syndrome to aid in early detection of chondrosarcoma in these patients.

3.6.11 Tufted Angioma

Luis Requena

Tufted angioma is an unusual, acquired, benign vascular neoplasm [1] that has also been described under the names of progressive capillary hemangioma [2] and angioblastoma [3–5].

3.6.11.1 Clinical Features

Lesions of tufted angioma mostly involve children and young adults, but both congenital and very late onset examples have been also described [6–10]. Most cases are sporadic, but there are also reports of tufted angioma effecting several members of a family with an autosomal dominant transmission [11]. The lesions have a predilection for the neck, upper chest, back, and shoulders (Fig. 3.6.11) [4, 12, 13], although examples of tufted angioma have also been reported on the head, extremities, and oral mucosa [14–17]. The neoplasm grows slowly and insidiously, and may eventually come to cover a large area of the trunk or neck. Spontaneous regression is rare [18].

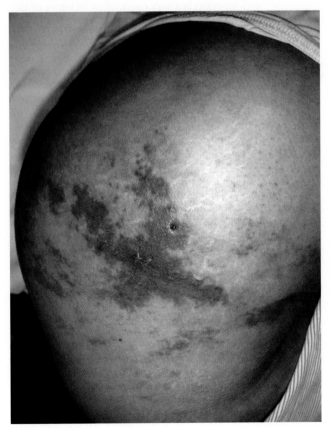

Fig. 3.6.11 Tufted hemangioma involving the shoulder of an obese woman

The clinical appearance of tufted angioma is variable. The most common presentations are enlarging erythematous or brown macules or plaques with an angiomatous appearance. In other cases, the lesions may resemble granulomas or a connective tissue nevus. Pain [19, 20] and hyperhidrosis [20, 21] have been described in some cases of tufted angioma. Dome-shaped papules on the surface of the lesion resembling pyogenic granulomas [22], sometimes arranged in a linear fashion [23], have also been reported [23]. Several disorders have been described in association with tufted angioma, including nevus flammeus [24, 25] and other vascular malformations [26], pregnancy [27], non-regressing lipodystrophy centrifugalis abdominalis [28], and liver transplantation [29]. Many cases of Kasabach–Merritt syndrome are associated with tufted angioma or with kaposiform hemangioendothelioma, and these two neoplasms are now considered closely related vascular proliferations by most authors [30–36].

3.6.11.2 Histopathologic Features

Tufted angioma appears histopatologically composed of multiple individual capillary lobules scattered within the dermis and subcutaneous fat (Fig. 3.6.12a), which are more prominent in the middle and lower part of the dermis. Each lobule is composed of aggregates of endothelial cells that whorl concentrically around a preexisting vascular structure. Some lobules bulge into the walls of dilated thin-walled vascular structures, giving these vessels a slit-like or semilunar appearance [22, 27, 37] (Fig. 3.6.12b). Small capillary lumina are identified within the aggregations of endothelial cells. Uncommon histopathologic features of tufted angioma lesions include mucinous stroma [21], numerous eccrine units [38], and intravenous location [39].

Immunohistochemically, neoplastic endothelial cells of the capillary lobules weakly express immunoreactivity for factor VIII related antigen, but they exhibit strong positivity for *Ulex europaeus* I lectin, EN4, CD31, CD34, and alpha-smooth muscle actin [4, 40]. Cells expressing reactivity for smooth muscle actin most likely represent pericytes rather than endothelial cells [2]. Ultrastructural studies have demonstrated characteristic crystalloid inclusions and Weibel–Palade bodies within proliferating endothelial cells [1].

3.6.11.3 Treatment

Spontaneous regression is rare in tufted angioma [23, 39, 41–43]. Satisfactory responses have been reported with surgery [44], soft radiation [12], pulse dye laser [10, 45], high-dose of systemic steroids [46], interferon-alpha [47–51], and intralesional injections of alpha-interferon [52].

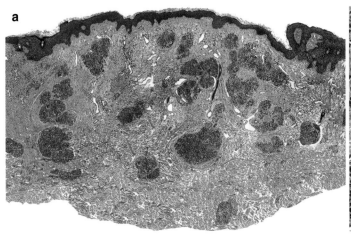

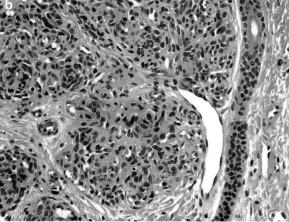

Fig. 3.6.12 (**a**) At scanning magnification there are several lobules of capillary hemangioma scattered in the dermis. (**b**) Higher magnification showing one of the lobules of capillary hemangioma and a vascular lumen with semi-lunar appearance at the periphery

3.6.12 Disease Entities of Arteriovenous Hemangioma

Nagwa M. Elwan

Arteriovenous hemangioma (acral arteriovenous tumor) presents as a solitary, red or purple papule with a predilection for the lips, perioral skin, nose, and eyelids of middle aged to elderly men [3]. It is usually asymptomatic and appears to have an association with chronic liver disease [1].

Arteriovenous malformations (AVMs) seems to be a distinct entity. AVMs are fast-flow vascular lesions composed of dysmorphic arterial and venous vessels connected directly to one another, without an intervening capillary bed [2]. AVMs occur with equal frequency in males and females. Forty to sixty percent of lesions are visible at birth, and 30% become clinically apparent during childhood. They are more common in the head and neck area [4]. AVMs may progress through four different stages: stage I (the quiescent phase), stage II (the progressive phase), stage III (deep destruction with chronic ulceration, pain, and hemorrhage), stage IV (cardiac decompensation) [4].

3.6.12.1 Histopahtology of Arteriovenous Hemangioma

There is a collection of large, thick-walled vessels in the upper and mid dermis, which is well-circumscribed but non-encapsulated. These vessels, lined with endothelium, reveal a fibromuscular wall containing elastic fibers but no definite elastic laminae. Most vessels have the characteristics of veins. In about one-third of cases, there are thin-walled dilated angiomatous capillaries superficial to the large tumor vessels. The stroma is often myxoid [5].

3.6.13 Disease Entities of Cutaneous Angiosarcoma

Davide Donghi

3.6.13.1 Definition

Cutaneous angiosarcoma is a very rare malignant tumor of vascular endothelial origin, which often presents diagnostic and therapeutic challenges, resulting in an unfavorable outcome.

3.6.13.2 Epidemiology

The overall incidence of this tumor is approximately 0.01/100,000. Less than 1% of all malignant tumors are soft tissue sarcomas, 2% of which are angiosarcomas. About 60% of all angiosarcomas are primarily located in the skin or subcutaneous tissue. Cutaneous angiosarcoma shows a slight male preponderance (1.6–3:1) and almost exclusively affects patients over 50 years of age, with a peak incidence in the eighth decade.

3.6.13.3 Etiopathogenesis

In most cases unknown, although an elevated incidence in post-radiation areas and chronic lymphedematous limbs (see below) has been proven. Different factors promoting vascular proliferation (serum VEGF-D and angiopoietin) or inducing T-lymphocyte apoptosis (Fas-ligand) were found to be highly expressed in cutaneous angiosarcomas, while vascular endothelial cadherine (VE-cadherin) was absent in most tumors thus diminishing cell–cell-cohesion. In contrast with other malignant vascular tumors like Kaposi-sarcoma, no HHV-8-DNA was found in neoplastic tissue.

3.6.13.4 Clinical Appearance

Unfortunately, clinical suspicion of angiosarcoma is frequently evoked too late, because the tumor is almost always asymptomatic and can mimic many inflammatory dermatoses and other benign/less malignant tumors, especially when located on the face or scalp.

Mainly, three clinical types of cutaneous angiosarcoma have been identified:

- *Classical, "head-and-neck"-type angiosarcoma* accounts for 50–60% of all cases, particularly in elderly patients. It mostly appears as a bruise-like red-violaceous patch (Fig. 3.6.13), which shows no tendency to heal and becomes larger and ill-defined with progression. In later stages, the tumor can show pink-reddish nodes, which later ulcerate and bleed. Noteworthy is that histologically documented tumor extension often exceeds clinical evidence, thus making an in sano surgical treatment even more difficult. A highly malignant histologically defined form, the epithelioid angiosarcoma, is considered a subtype of this group.
- *Post-radiation angiosarcoma*: once concentrated in women post radiation for breast cancer, the incidence of radiation-induced angiosarcomas is decreasing with the diminished use of extramammary full-dose radiation therapy in oncological practice. Post-radiation angiosarcoma can appear as late as 30 years after the conclusion of treatment.
- *Lymphedema-associated angiosarcoma*: this form was first described by *Stewart and Treves* in 1948, who reported six cases of tumor development after mastectomy and axillary

lymph node dissection, resulting in chronic lymphedema of the arm. About 10% of all cutaneous angiosarcomas belong to this group, with time to diagnosis ranging from 4 to 30 years after the first manifestation of lymphedema.

3.6.13.5 Histopathology

The histologic diagnosis of a cutaneous angiosarcoma can be a real challenge even to an experienced dermatopathologist. Distinctive features of these tumors include:

- Bizarre vascular configuration in the upper dermis
- Dissecting vascular growth with "lightning"-like vascular slits
- Atypical endothelial lining and/or pseudopapillae protruding into the lumen
- Endothelial pleomorphism with atypical mitoses
- Clusters of epithelioid-like tumor cells

Different immunohistochemical assays have proven helpful in the diagnosis of angiosarcoma. The vascular markers CD31 and CD34 are almost always positive, whereas in later stages and with progressing tumor cell dedifferentiation CD34 can become negative. HHV-8-DNA is invariably negative. VEGFR-3, a tyrosine kinase receptor expressed by lymphatic endothelium, is positive in about 50% of all angiosarcomas; although it can't be used to discriminate between this tumor and Kaposi's sarcoma, it could play a predicting role when a therapy with tyrosine kinase inhibitors like Imatinib is planned. Ki-67, a cell proliferation marker, can be of prognostic value in differentiating between low and high malignant evolution.

3.6.13.6 Differential Diagnosis

Clinical differential diagnoses include hematomas, inflammatory diseases like rosacea (Fig. 3.6.14), eczema (seborrheic, contact or atopic), cellulitis, lupus erythematosus, eosinophilic granuloma, sarcoidosis and many others, as well as other tumors such as malignant melanomas (especially amelanotic), metastases, and cutaneous lymphomas.

3.6.13.7 Clinical Course and Prognosis

Angiosarcoma is believed to have the worst prognosis among malignant skin tumors. It is likely to produce distant metastasis, most commonly in the lung, liver, lymph nodes, and spleen, while the central nervous system and heart are rarely affected. Local recurrence was reported in about 50%

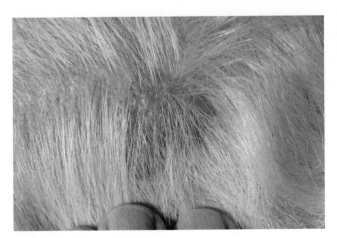

Fig. 3.6.13 Classical, "head-and-neck"-type angiosarcoma

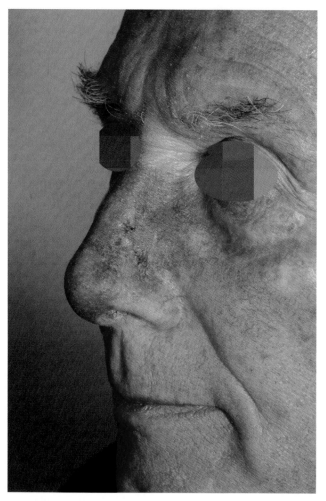

Fig. 3.6.14 Cutaneous angiosarcoma mimicking rosacea

3.6.14 Lymphatic Tumors

Jürg Hafner

3.6.14.1 Lymphangioma Circumscriptum

Lymphangioma circumscriptum (LC) and hematolymphangioma circumscriptum (HLC) are vascular malformations, according to the Hamburg Classification of Belov and Weber [1, 3, 6, 7, 9]. They represent malformations of small, extratruncular vessels, lymphatic (LC) or complex lymphatic-venous (HLC).

Clinically, they form grouped subepidermal vesicles resembling frogspawn. The most typical localizations are the proximal extremities, perineum, axillary folds, neck, buccal mucosa and tongue. Based on the work of Whimster et al., it was found that the subepidermal vesicles communicate with large lymphatic cisterns deep in the subcutis or muscle. Whimster supposed that the subepidermal vesicles formed from the pressure transmitted by the pulsatile deep lymphatic cisterns [2, 10].

LC is usually present at birth or becomes apparent within the first 2 years of life. Quite often, such lesions are best left untreated. Aesthetic considerations, persistent lymphatic drainage and recurrent infection (erysipelas) are the three major indications for interventional treatment. When surgical treatment may be considered, thorough imaging with ultrasound or, preferably, magnetic resonance imaging should be recommended. Incomplete excision of the interconnected subcutaneous lymphatic cysts is regularly followed by recurrences. Sclerotherapy can, therefore, be an adjunct or a true alternative to surgical treatment, for removal of the majority of the malformation. Otherwise, ablative laser surgery or semiselective photothermolysis can be used to vaporize the subepidermal vesicles and "seal" the lesional skin area by means of a superficial dermal scar (Fig. 3.6.15a, b). This procedure effectively stops lymphatic leakage and recurrent infection.

Acquired progressive lymphangiectasias, e.g., of the vulva, can be most frequently seen after treatment for cervical or endometrial cancer with lymphadenectomy or radiotherapy but also in hereditary syndromes including vascular malformations, e.g., proteus syndrome. Their origin of elevated lymphatic pressure, extending into the subpapillary lymphatics, is different, but the resulting skin lesions are undistinguishable from LC [8].

of patients with histologically tumor-free resection margins and occurred mostly within the first 2 years of initial diagnosis. Likeliness of local recurrence was mainly influenced by initial tumor size.

The prognosis quoad vitam is poor, with an overall 5-year survival rate ranging from 12 to 20% (median survival 18–28 months). The most important prognostic feature is tumor size. Patients with an external tumor diameter >5 cm at diagnosis have a definitively worse prognosis than patients with tumor diameter <5 cm. Recently, Deyrup et al. proposed a method for risk stratification for tumors <5 cm using a combination of histologic features: high-risk tumors presented necrosis and/or epithelioid cell morphology, while low-risk tumors did not show necrosis or epithelioid cell morphology. In fact, 3-year survival rates differed substantially (24% for high-risk and 77% for low-risk); 5-year survival for high-risk patients was 0%.

Other significant factors in terms of prognosis include depth of invasion greater than 3 mm, mitotic count over 3/mm^2, and, of course, metastases, local recurrence, and positive surgical margins.

3.6.14.2 Progressive Lymphangioma

Progressive lymphangioma is a congenital cavernous lymphatic malformation. More often in pediatrics, but also in

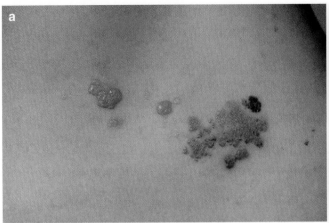

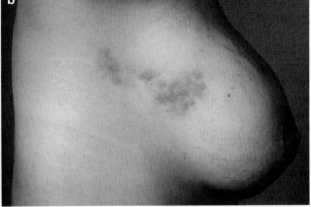

Fig. 3.6.15 (**a**) Lymphangioma circumscriptum of the breast. Subepidermal vesicles resembling frog spawn. Demand for treatment for aesthetical considerations and two epi. (**b**) Same patient after one session with the CO_2-laser, defocused technique. Aesthetic improvement and cessation of erysipelas

adult medicine, extensive lymphangiomatosis of the chest with chylothorax [11], mesenterial lymphangioma, or retroperitoneal lymphangioma can represent a major therapeutic challenge, that is currently, when feasible, often treated by laparascopic extirpation. Progressive lymphangiomas of the head and neck (e.g., cystic hygroma of the face) can represent a major challenge in ENT surgery and dermatology [4, 5]. In recent years, sclerotherapy of head- and neck lymphangiomas with OK-432 (picibanil) has added substantially to the therapeutic armamentarium of these difficult to treat malformations [12].

3.6.15   Smooth and Skeletal Muscle Tumors

Nagwa M. Elwan

3.6.15.1   Disease Entities of Pilar Leiomyoma

Pilar leiomyoma is a benign smooth muscle tumor leiomyoma is arising from the arrector pili muscle. The tumor is often multiple than solitary (Fig. 3.6.16). Multiple lesions usually have their onset in the late second or third decade of life, presenting as multiple, firm, painful reddish-brown papulonodules with a predilection for the face, back and the extensor aspects of the extremities [1, 3]. Rarely, leiomyomas are distributed in a linear fashion or seem to follow a dermatome, giving the presentation of painful unilateral, zosteriform cutaneous leiomyoma [6]. Multiple leiomyomas have been associated with uterine leiomyomas in some females [2]. Some cases of cutaneous leiomyoma with cytologic atypia were reported and it was suggested that cutaneous leiomyomas may exhibit bizarre or "symplastic" patterns analogous to their uterine counterparts [4]. Minor trauma or exposure to cold temperatures may lead to severe pain in the tumors [7]. There are only sparse reports of leiomyoma of the nipple [5]. Leiomyomas of genital skin is quite uncommon, with only few reported cases of scrotal and vulval lesions [5].

3.6.15.1.1   Histopathology

Pilar leiomyomas are circumscribed non-encapsulated tumors, centered in the dermis, with an overlying uninvolved subepidermal zone (Grenz zone). The tumor is composed of bundles of smooth muscles, arising from arrector pili muscle

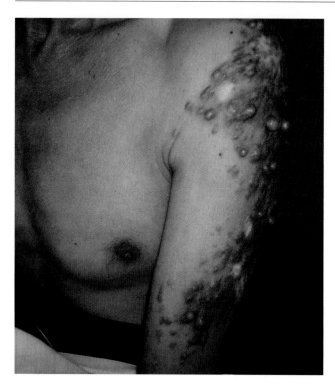

Fig. 3.6.16 Multiple pilor leiomyomes of the arm of an Egyptian patient

3.6.16 Smooth and Skeletal Muscle Tumors

Beata Bode-Lesniewska

3.6.16.1 Cutaneous Leiomyosarcoma

Cutaneous leiomyosarcoma is a malignant soft tissue tumor showing smooth muscle differentiation and originating in the dermis [1, 2]. The subcutaneous tissue is involved only in advanced, long standing or recurrent lesions. The tumor affects both genders with a male predilection and occurs mainly in elderly adults on extremities, mostly on hair covered extensor surfaces, scalp and trunk. Due to its superficial localization, the lesion is usually diagnosed before it grows beyond 2–3 cm in size. Microscopically, ill defined, sometimes nodular proliferation of elongated spindle cells with abundant eosinophilic cytoplasm is found (Fig. 3.6.17a). They form interlacing fascicles that infiltrate the collagen framework of the dermis, intermingling with local pilar erector muscles. The nuclei show mild to moderate atypia with hyperchromasia and variation in size and shape. Mitotic figures, both typical and atypical can easily be found. Primary cutaneous leiomyosarcomas are mainly well to moderately differentiated tumors, with high grade pleomorphic lesions being exceptional; in these cases, metastases from distant sites must be ruled out. Due to the early stage and a relatively small size at first diagnosis, secondary changes such as necrosis or hemorrhage are rare. In many cases, the tumors are confined to the dermis and thus have a favorable prognosis with virtually no risk of metastases. Spread to subcutaneous tissue is associated with a 30–40% risk of metastases, similar to the clinical course of non-cutaneous soft tissue leiomyosarcomas [3–5].

Immunohistochemically, virtually all leiomyosarcomas express smooth muscle actin (Fig. 3.6.17b). Desmin is found less commonly. Some tumors may show focal weak cytokeratin positivity.

Cutaneous leiomyosarcoma, similar to their soft tissue counterparts, does not show consistent reproducible genetic alterations.

Local excision with clear margins is the treatment of choice, offering a good chance of a cure [6].

and arranged in an interlacing or a whorled pattern. The cells are well-differentiated, having abundant eosinophilic cytoplasm and elongated nuclei with blunt ends (cigar-shaped nuclei). There are usually no mitoses in the pilar variant. Long standing tumors may show fibrous tissue in the stroma with occasional focal hyalinization. Focal stromal myxoid changes may be noted, and hair follicles are sometimes found within the tumor. The smooth muscle nature of the cells can be confirmed with the Masson trichrome stain and desmin; the immunoperoxidase marker for smooth muscles [5, 8].

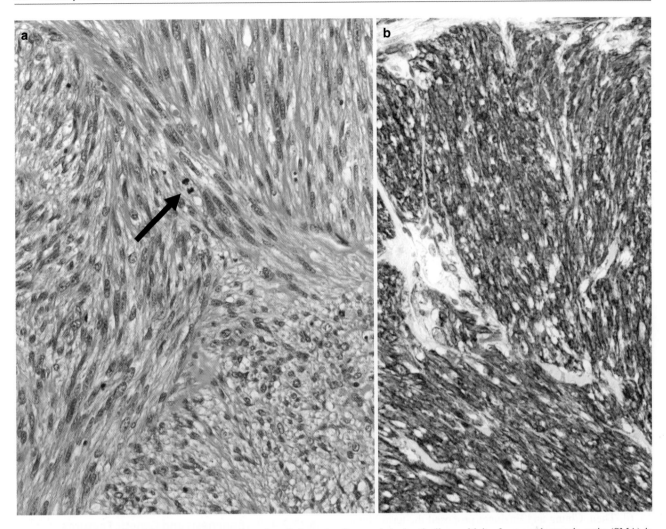

Fig. 3.6.17 (**a**) Cutaneous leiomyosarcoma consists of well formed bundles of spindle, elongated cells with eosinophilic cytoplasm. Mitotic figures (*arrow*) and mild to moderate atypia are easily found. (**b**) Immunohstochemically, positivity for smooth muscle actin (SMA) is found in virtually all cases

3.6.17   Fibrous, Fibrohistiocytic, and Histiocytic Tumors

Kenji Asagoe and Beata Bode-Lesniewska

3.6.17.1   *Dermatomyofibroma*

3.6.17.1.1   Definition

Dermatomyofibroma, first described by Kamino et al. in 1992 [4], is a benign soft tissue tumor of the skin characterized by the proliferation of fibroblasts and myofibroblasts.

3.6.17.1.2   Clinical Features

Dermatomyofibroma is a slowly growing tumor, localized mostly on the shoulder or trunk, with a predilection for young females. It presents as a solitary, asymptomatic, oval- or annular-shaped, skin-colored or brownish red plaque/nodule measuring 1–2 cm in diameter [4].

3.6.17.1.3   Histopathology

Dermatomyofibroma (synonym: plaque-like dermal fibromatosis) is a rare, dermal, benign, myo-fibroblastic proliferation, occurring mainly, but not exclusively, in young women in the shoulder/axilla region [2].

Histologically, a poorly defined, cutaneous proliferation of bland spindle cells, characteristically showing parallel alignment to the skin surface, is found. The cells contain scant, pale cytoplasm. The collagen rich extracellular matrix shows a slightly increased number of elastic fibers, enabling the distinction of dermatomyofibroma from scars. Immunohistochemistry demonstrates variable positivity for alpha-smooth muscle actin in about half of the tumors and negativity for S100, CD34, desmin and caldesmone.

3.6.17.1.4 Pathogenesis and Genetic Features

No pathogenetic factors or genetic abnormalities have been indicated.

3.6.17.1.5 Therapy

Simple excision is usually curative.

3.6.17.1.6 Prognosis

The tumor does not show infiltrative growth. Local recurrence is rare.

3.6.17.2 Infantile Myofibromatosis

3.6.17.2.1 Definition

Infantile myofibromatosis was previously described by Williams and Schurm in 1951 as "congenital fibrosarcoma" and by Stout in 1954 as "congenital generalized fibromatosis" [5, 6]. Then, Chung and Enzinger proposed the term "infantile myofibromatosis" [7]. This disorder is a rare fibromatosis characterized by the proliferation of myofibroblasts, occurring mainly during the neonatal period. The lesion can be solitary or multiple. If multiple lesions develop, the lesions are described as "myofibromatosis."

3.6.17.2.2 Clinical Features

The disorder mostly presents congenitally or in infancy, but may also develop in children and adults with a male predilection. The head, neck and trunk are commonly affected. Two thirds to one half of patients have a solitary lesion [8, 9]. Solitary lesion usually involves dermis, subcutaneous fat and, less commonly, skeletal muscles. The superficial lesions present as movable, grayish-white or purplish nodules that measure several centimeters in diameter. In contrast with solitary lesion, multiple lesions more frequently accompany lesions in the bone, lung, heart, gastrointestinal tract and/or other internal organs (multicentric form).

3.6.17.2.3 Histopathology

One third of the patients diagnosed with a myofibroma have multiple tumors, a condition which is defined as myofibromatosis. In most cases of myofibromatosis, the tumors are present at birth or appear within the first 2 years of life (congenital generalized fibromatosis, infantile myofibromatosis), but adult onset also occurs. One-third to one half of the lesions are located in deep soft tissues, with the remainder located in the skin and/or subcutaneous tissue, mostly in the head and neck region or on the trunk. Myofibromatosis is more common in male patients [2, 10, 11].

Histologically, myofibroma/myofibromatosis is a solitary or multicentric, benign, nodular, moderately cellular proliferation, consisting of myoid perivascular cells. The cells are elongated and spindle-shaped, with some eosinophilic cytoplasm and are oriented in short fascicles. The lesions are well circumscribed and display, particularly in the center of the nodules, a characteristic, prominent, vascular, hemangiopericytoma-like pattern, giving the lesion a biphasic aspect. Focal necrosis with areas of hemorrhage and hyalinization may be observed. Mitoses are variable in number but not atypical. Immunohistochemically, there is positivity for alpha-smooth muscle actin, with variable positivity for desmin. S100 and cytokeratins are negative.

Local excision of dermal myofibromas/myofibromatosis is curative, and recurrence is unlikely. Visceral presentation, however, may prove fatal.

3.6.17.2.4 Pathogenesis and Genetic Features

Myopericytic origin of the tumors has been suggested [12]. Most of the patients do not have a familial history, although some cases suggesting autosomal dominant or recessive inheritance have been reported [13]. No definite cytogenetic alteration has been identified.

3.6.17.2.5 Therapy

Lesions without visceral involvement tend to regress spontaneously. Solitary lesions can be treated by simple excision without recurrence [7, 9].

3.6.17.2.6 Prognosis

Lesions of the skin, soft tissues and bone follow a benign course and often regress spontaneously, while internal involvement often causes fatal symptoms that do not respond to treatment [7, 9].

3.6.17.3 Sclerotic Fibroma

3.6.17.3.1 Definition

Sclerotic fibroma, also known as "storiform collagenoma," is a benign fibrotic tumor composed of hyalinized collagen bundles with sparse cellular components [14]. Multiple lesions are associated with Cowden's disease (multiple hamartoma syndrome).

3.6.17.3.2 Clinical Features

Sclerotic fibroma presents as a solitary, asymptomatic, dome-shaped, whitish and waxy nodule up to 1–2 cm in diameter, which develops on any anatomical site.

3.6.17.3.3 Histopathology

Sclerotic fibroma (synonym: (circumscribed) storiform collagenoma) is a benign, rare, dermal, paucicellular, soft tissue tumor occurring in both sexes, at any age, in various locations but particularly on the face [2, 15]. It is sharply delineated and consists of thick collagen bundles arranged in a storiform pattern with only few bland fibroblasts. No immunohistochemical expression of actin, desmin or S100 is found. Interestingly, multiple tumors are typical of Cowden disease [16].

3.6.17.3.4 Pathogenesis and Genetic Features

Although some authors suggest a close relation to dermatofibroma [17], this is not yet confirmed. No genetic background has been documented in solitary lesions, whereas multiple tumors develop in patients with a rare genodermatosis, Cowden's disease.

3.6.17.3.5 Therapy

Simple excision is usually curative.

3.6.17.3.6 Prognosis

Malignant transformation has not been reported. Some tumors become large if they remain untreated.

3.6.17.4 Pleomorphic Fibroma

3.6.17.4.1 Definition

Pleomorphic fibroma is a rare, benign tumor with a polypoid shape and is histologically characterized by the appearance of abnormal stromal cells [18].

3.6.17.4.2 Clinical Features

Pleomorphic fibroma develops on the extremities, trunk, head, and neck of adults, as a slowly growing, asymptomatic, skin-colored, polypoid or dome-shaped nodule between 0.5 and 2 cm in diameter. Females are affected slightly more often than males. Clinical differential diagnoses include skin tags, neurofibroma, nevus cell nevus, and hemangioma.

3.6.17.4.3 Histopathology

Pleomorphic fibroma is a well demarcated, dermal, polypoid or dome-shaped, skin-colored solitary nodule, which occurs in adult patients, on the trunk or extremities, and may reach 2 cm in size [2, 15]. It is asymptomatic and slowly growing.

Histologically, the polypoid lesion consists of a subepidermal, collagen rich, hypocellular nodule, with a varying number of scattered spindle or stellate cells showing conspicuous variations in the size and form of the nuclei as well as hyperchromatic chromatin and small nucleoli. Some multinucleated cells can also be observed. Rare mitoses may occur; however no atypical mitosis or tumor necrosis is found. The etiology of the cellular atypia remains unsettled, however ischemia or paracrine influence is thought to be causative. Focal immunohistochemical positivity for smooth muscle actin or CD34 may occasionally be seen. Cytokeratin, S100 and desmin are negative.

3.6.17.4.4 Pathogenesis and Genetic Features

Degeneration or ischemia may be causative factors in the development of cytologic atypia. Myofibroblastic differentiation of tumor cells has also been suggested [19].

3.6.17.4.5 Therapy

Simple excision is usually curative with rare local recurrence.

3.6.17.4.6 Prognosis

Despite the presence of cytologically atypical fibrohistio-cytic cells, the tumor shows benign clinical behavior.

3.6.17.5 Dermatofibrosarcoma Protuberans

3.6.17.5.1 Definition

Dermatofibrosarcoma protuberans (DFSP) is a locally aggressive tumor arising in the dermis and subcutis, histologically showing a storiform growth pattern with fibroblastic differentiation.

3.6.17.5.2 Clinical Features

DFSP often develops in young and middle-aged adults, and males are more frequently affected than females. It presents as a cutaneous nodule or, less frequently, a subcutaneous mass with a slight predilection for the trunk and proximal extremities. The tumor starts as an asymptomatic, small, firm, skin-colored to reddish nodule/plaque. Progression is usually slow but persistent, forming a large, coalescent, irregular, infiltrative nodule. Rarely, an atrophic lesion also develops (Fig. 3.6.18a). Advanced lesions grow rapidly and may cause multinodular lesion and ulceration. Pigmented DFSP (Bedner tumor), which was previously reported as a type of neurofibroma, is a rare variant of DFSP.

3.6.17.5.3 Histopathology

Dermatofibrosarcoma protuberans (DFSP) is a nodular, mesenchymal cutaneous and subcutaneous tumor, occurring in young adults of both genders with a male predominance [2, 20]. It affects mainly the trunk and, less commonly, proximal extremities. It shows slow but persistent growth, sometimes with a history of a nodule growing over several years.

Histologically, an extensive, poorly demarcated infiltration of subcutaneous tissue by spindle cells is found, with infiltration of the dermis and diffuse spread among adipocytes (Fig. 3.6.19a). The cells are fairly monomorph, with a prominent storiform growth pattern. Some tumors may show extensive myxoid change or contain foci of cells with more abundant eosinophilic cytoplasm (myoid nodules). Scattered melanin containing cells may be present in some tumors, called Bednar tumors or pigmented DFSP. Mitotic activity can regularly be observed and is generally lower than 5/10

HPF. Isolated cases may contain areas identical to giant cell fibroblastoma. As described above, both tumors exhibit the same genetic aberration (translocation t(17;22)(q22;q13)), leading to overexpression of PDGFB, stimulating an autocrine loop which affects the growth of tumor cells. This event can be disrupted by specific tyrosine kinase inhibitors. These inhibitors can thus be applied clinically in locally incurable tumors.

Diffuse positivity for CD34 (Fig. 3.6.19c) is characteristic immunohistochemical finding, allowing for discrimination from a dermatofibroma. Other markers (S100, SMA, desmin, keratins, EMA) remain negative discriminating DFSP from epithelial, myogenic and neural neoplasms.

DFSPs carry a high risk of local recurrence if not treated with adequate resection with 2–3 cm clear surgical margin. The tumor does not metastasize, however in rare cases areas resembling fibrosarcoma with increased mitotic activity and atypia may be found. Tumors containing sarcomatous foci may give rise to metatstatic disease [21, 22].

3.6.17.5.4 Differential Diagnoses

Clinical differential diagnoses include dermatofibroma (fibrous histiocytoma), keloid/hypertrophic scar and malignant melanoma. Atrophic DFSP mimics morphea and lichen sclerosis et atrophicus.

3.6.17.5.5 Pathogenesis and Genetic Features

Association with a previous burn or trauma has been referred, but not confirmed.

Cytogenetically, it has been shown that DFSP exhibits t(17;22) (q22;q13) translocation [23]. The translocation fuses the various exons of the collagen type 1 alpha1 (COL1A1) gene with the exon 2 of the platelet-derived growth factor beta (PDGFB) gene (Fig. 3.6.18b, c), resulting in the generation of COL1A1-PDGFB fusion protein, which stimulates tumor cells by binding to the PDGFB receptor [24, 25].

3.6.17.5.6 Therapy

The preferred treatment for patients with DFSP is a wide local excision with 2–3 cm margin. A wider excision might be needed for large, ill-defined tumors. Radiotherapy has been recommended for unresectable tumors, especially on the head and neck, or for tumors with incomplete excision [26]. Imatinib mesylate, a tyrosine kinase inhibitor

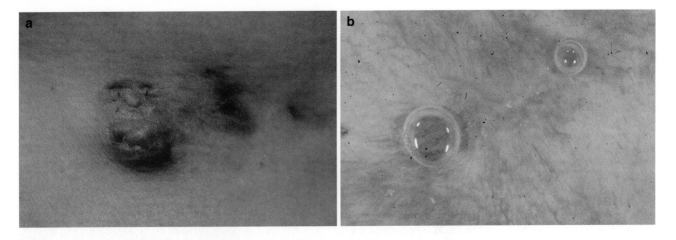

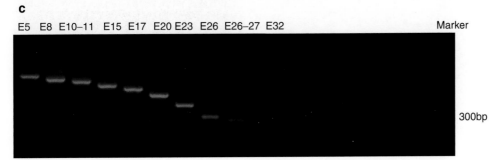

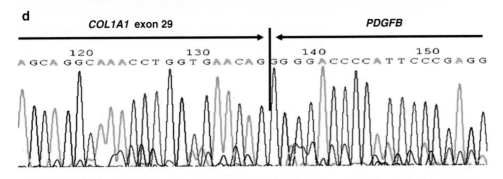

COL1A1 exon 29   **PDGFB**

Fig. 3.6.18 Dermatofibrosarcoma protuberans. Clinical appearance (**a**). Dermoscopic findings (**b**). The *COL1A1-PDGFB* fusion transcript in RT-PCR assay (**c, d**; courtesy of Gen Nakanishi MD). Amplified products are detected using the exon 5, 8, 10–11, 15, 17, 20, 23, 26 or 26–27 primer of the *COL1A1* gene and the primer of the *PDGFB* gene (E5 lane to E26-27 lane), but no amplified products are detected when exon 32 primer of the *COL1A1* gene is used, indicating that there is a breakpoint located downstream of *COL1A1* exon 27 (**c**). Partial nucleotide sequence of the *COL1A1-PDGFB* fusion transcripts shows fusion of *COL1A1* exon 29 with *PDGFB* exon 2 (**d**)

that inhibits signal transduction from PDGF receptors, has recently been applied in the treatment of advanced tumors [27].

3.6.17.5.7 Prognosis

The recurrence rate in DFSP patients treated with wide local excision has been reported to be 10–20% [28]. Despite its locally aggressive behavior, DFSP without fibrosarcomatous transformation metastasizes quite rarely. However, the fibrosarcomatous variant more frequently recurs locally and develops metastatic diseases [22].

3.6.17.6 Dermatofibroma (Fibrous Histiocytoma)

3.6.17.6.1 Definition

Dermatofibroma (fibrous histiocytoma) is a benign, dermal or superficial subcutaneous proliferation of oval- to spindle-shaped cells resembling histiocytes or fibroblasts, accompanied by an increase in collagen bundles and inflammatory cells. Recent studies suggest the neoplastic nature of this tumor but it is still controversial whether dermatofibroma is a neoplastic disease or an inflammatory disease [29, 30].

Fig. 3.6.19 Giant cell fibroblastoma and dermatofibrosarcoma protuberans: (**a**) Spindle cells of both lesions diffusely infiltrate subcutaneous fatty tissue spreading along the collagen septa (hematoxylin and eosin staining; original magnification 100×). (**b**) Giant cell fibroblastoma consists of spindle cells and characteristic multinucleated giant cells (*arrow*). Pseudovascular clefts (*star*) may be lined by both spindle and/or giant cells (hematoxylin and eosin staining; original magnification 200×). (**c**) Diffuse strong positivity for CD34 is observed in cells of both tumors (original magnification 100×)

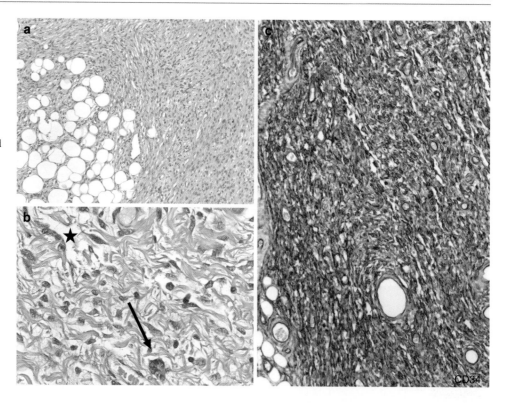

3.6.17.6.2 Clinical Features

Dermatofibroma commonly localizes on the extremities of young or middle-aged adults with a slight predilection for females. The tumor usually presents as a solitary, slowly growing, round to oval, slightly elevated to hemispheric nodule or plaque. The tumor is usually less than 2 cm in diameter, but larger lesions can grow up to 5 cm. The color of the tumors is erythematous in early lesions but becomes brownish or skin-colored over time (Fig. 3.6.20a). Multiple dermatofibromas may occur particularly in immunosuppressed patients with systemic lupus erythematosus [31], Sjogren syndrome, pemphigus vulgaris or other autoimmune diseases.

There are some variants of dermatofibroma such as cellular, aneurysmal, atypical and epithelioid. Among these variants, aneurysmal and epithelioid variants reveal characteristic clinical features. The aneurysmal variant (benign aneurysmal histiocytoma) usually displays a rapidly growing, violaceous to blackish nodule mimicking vascular or melanocytic lesions (Fig. 3.6.20c). The epithelioid variant presents as a solitary, reddish, polypoid or papillomatous nodule resembling pyogenic granuloma.

Dermoscopic findings in common types of dermatofibroma frequently include central whitish patches and a delicate pigment network at the periphery [32] (Fig. 3.6.20b). The aneurysmal variant exhibits similar dermoscopic findings to vascular lesions (red–blue lacunas, red-bluish to

red–black homogeneous areas) in the center, but usually shows the same features as common dermatofibromas at the periphery (delicate pigment network) [33] (Fig. 3.6.20d).

3.6.17.6.3 Histopathology

Dermatofibroma (synonyms: dermal benign fibrous histiocytoma, fibroma durum, subepidermal nodular fibrosis or sclerosis, sclerotic or sclerosing fibroma, sclerosing hemangioma) is the most common tumor in this category [2, 34]. It occurs mainly during early or middle adulthood and can localize on various areas, although it is most commonly seen in the extremities. An association with insect bites or other forms of minor trauma has been reported, however the findings of clonal chromosomal changes support the neoplastic nature of this tumor [35–37]. In 30% of cases multiple tumors may occur. Synchronous appearance has been reported in the setting of immunosppression.

Histologically, several morphological variants may be discerned, but all dermatofibromas share some general features. The tumors usually consist of predominantly dermal, unencapsulated, poorly defined spindle and/or rounded mesenchymal cells, exhibiting variable levels of cellular proliferation (Fig. 3.6.21b). The cells are fairly monomorph, with few mitotic figures. The lesions contain haphazardly arranged, thick collagen bundles, which are particularly prominent in the periphery, leading to the "trapping" aspect

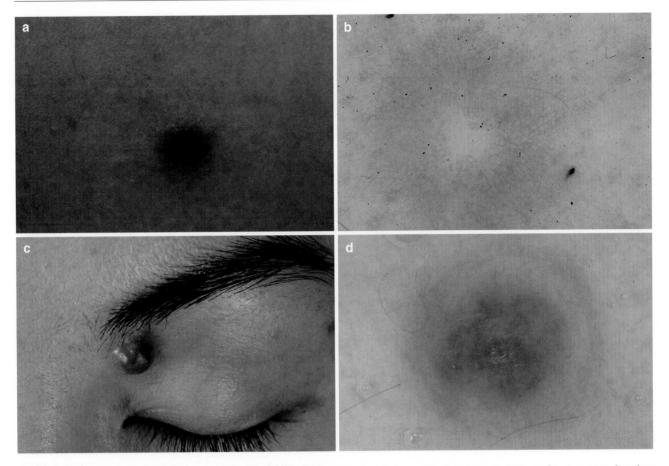

Fig. 3.6.20 Dermatofibroma (fibrous histiocytoma), common type. Clinical appearance (**a**). Dermoscopic findings (**b**). Aneurysmal variant (benign aneurysmal histiocytoma). Clinical appearance (**c**). Dermoscopic findings (**d**)

(Fig. 3.6.21a). Admixture of a variable number of inflammatory and hemosiderin loaded histiocytic cells as well as the accompanying hyperplasia of the overlying epidermis (Fig. 3.6.21a), including the melanocytes (causing hyperpigmentation of the overlying skin), are characteristic in these tumors. Numerous subtypes of dermatofibroma are described according to their divergence from the general cytological presentation of lesional cells, cellular density or secondary stromal changes (morphological variants include the following subtypes: cellular, atypical, aneurysmal, epitheloid, hemosiderotic, atrophic, clear cell, myxoid, lipidized, lichenoid, ossifying, granular, with osteoclast-like giant cells, with eosionophilic infiltrate, etc.).

Immunohistochemistry is usually not contributory, showing positivity for factor XIII and variable, mostly focal and weak expression of smooth muscle actin an/or CD34, other markers are negative. The main differential diagnosis of dermatofibroma, particularly of its cellular variant, is dermatofibrosarcoma protuberans (DFSP). In contrast to dermatofibroma, DFSP presents with slender cells in a prominent storiform pattern, wide infiltration of the dermis and subcutaneous adipose tissue, and distinctly diffuse expression of CD34.

The standard treatment for dermatofibroma is local excision with clear margins. The local recurrence rate may be high in inadequately treated tumors, especially in some of the histologic variants (e.g., cellular, aneurysmal). Isolated, histologically otherwise typical cases with dissemination to the local lymph nodes or lungs have been reported [38].

3.6.17.6.4 Differential Diagnoses

Clinical differential diagnoses include dermatofibrosarcoma protuberans, keloid/hypertrophic scar, nodular prurigo, malignant melanoma, epidermal cyst. The aneurysmal variant is similar to vascular tumors and melanocytic nevi.

3.6.17.6.5 Pathogenesis and Genetic Features

Previous histories of minor trauma or arthropod bites have been suggested as causative factors [39]. On the contrary, some authors demonstrated clonality in some cases of dermatofibromas using cytogenetic analysis, thus indicating the

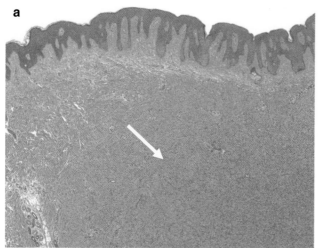

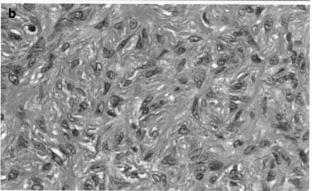

Fig. 3.6.21 Dermatofibroma. (**a**) General architecture of the tumor with hyperplasia of the overlaying epidermis and collagen "trapping" at the periphery of the nodule (*arrow*) (hematoxylin and eosin staining; original magnification 25×). (**b**) Typical cell type of dermatofibroma (hematoxylin and eosin staining; original magnification 400×)

neoplastic nature of this disease [37]. Whether dermatofibromas are reactive or neoplastic is still debated.

3.6.17.6.6 Therapy

Simple excision is usually curative with rare local recurrence. However, no treatment is necessary, with the exception of lesions that are cosmetically troubling. For the cellular, aneurysmal or atypical variants, complete excision has been recommended because local recurrences and occasional metastases have been reported [38].

3.6.17.6.7 Prognosis

Dermatofibromas are essentially benign tumors, but recurrence may rarely occur after the incomplete excision. It has been noted that the cellular, aneurysmal and atypical variants may recur more frequently. Furthermore, the cellular

variant has been reported to show aggressive growth and metastasis [38].

3.6.17.7 Giant Cell Fibroblastoma

3.6.17.7.1 Definition

Giant cell fibroblastoma, first described by Shmookler and Enzinger [40], is a clinicopathological variant of dermatofibrosarcoma protuberans (DFSP), which predominantly affects infants and children.

3.6.17.7.2 Clinical Features

Giant cell fibroblastoma presents as an intradermal or subcutaneous, ill-demarcated tumor localized most often on the trunk and, next frequently, proximal extremities. Children are mainly affected. The tumor tends to be asymptomatic and grows slowly, up to several centimeters (0.8–8 cm) in diameter [41, 42].

3.6.17.7.3 Histopathology

Giant cell fibroblastoma is a histologic variant of dermatofibrosarcoma protuberans (DFSP) (described below), occurring in children within the first decade of life [20]. It generally affects males and has a predilection for the skin of the trunk, shoulder and groin, a distribution which is very similar to that of DFSP. Microscopically, the tumor consists of a mostly subcutaneous, poorly circumscribed mass, with variable cellularity and extension into the dermis. Slender spindle cells are found loosely arranged against a background of thick collagen fibers with some myxoid areas. Typical, mainly multinucleated giant cells are found as a characteristic feature (Fig. 3.6.19b). Irregularly branching, pseudovascular spaces or clefts, lined with spindle and giant cells, are seen in the extracellular matrix. More cellular areas resembling typical DFSP may focally be present. Immunohistochemically, diffuse positivity for CD34 is seen without expression of other markers (Fig. 3.6.19c).

Both giant cell fibroblastoma and DFSP exhibit the same translocation, t(17;22)(q22;q13), between the collagen type 1 alpha1 gene and PDGFB gene. The fusion product has biologic effects similar to normal PDGFB [24, 43].

3.6.17.7.4 Pathogenesis and Genetic Features

Giant cell fibroblastoma has been shown to have the same genetic alteration as DFSP, t(17;22) (q22;q13) translocation.

The minor difference is that the linear chromosome occurs in giant cell fibroblastoma as well as DFSP developed in children, whereas the ring chromosome occurs more frequently in DFSP of the adults [44].

3.6.17.7.5 Therapy

Wide local excision is required, as is done in DFSP.

3.6.17.7.6 Prognosis

About half of the patients experience local recurrence [41]. However, metastasis has not been reported.

References

Mastocytosis

1. Furitsu, T., Tsujimura, T., Tono, T., et al.: Identification of mutations in the coding sequence of the proto-oncogene c-kit in a human mast cell leukemia cell line causing ligand-independent activation of c-kit product. J. Clin. Invest. **92**, 1736–1744 (1993)
2. Hauswirth, A.W., Sperr, W.R., Ghannadan, M., et al.: A case of smouldering mastocytosis with peripheral blood eosinophilia and lymphadenopathy. Leuk. Res. **26**, 601–606 (2002)
3. Horny, H.P., Sotlar, K., Valent, P.: Mastocytosis: state of the art. Pathobiology **74**, 121–132 (2007)
4. Valent, P., Horny, H.P., Li, C.Y., et al.: Mastocytosis (mast cell disease). In: Jaffe, E.S., Harris, N.L., Stein, H., et al. (eds.) World Health Organization Classification of Tumors. Pathology and genetics of Tumors of Haematopoietic and Lymphoid Tissues., pp. 291–302. IARC, Geneva (2001)
5. Wolff, K., Komar, M., Petzelbauer, P.: Clinical and histopathological aspects of cutaneous mastocytosis. Leuk. Res. **25**, 519–528 (2001)

Disease Entities of Kaposi Sarcoma

1. Beckstead, J.H., Wood, G.S., Fletcher, V.: Evidence for the origin of Kaposi's sarcoma from lymphatic endothelium. Am. J. Pathol. **119**, 294–300 (1995)
2. Brenner, B., Weissmann-Brenner, A., Rakowsky, E., et al.: Classical Kaposi sarcoma: prognostic factor analysis of 248 patients. Cancer **95**, 1982–1987 (2002)
3. De Pasquale, R., Nasca, M.R., Micali, G.: Postirradiation primary Kaposi's sarcoma of the head and neck. J. Am. Acad. Dermatol. **40**, 312–314 (1999)
4. Di Lorenzo, G., Konstantinopoulos, P.A., Pantanowitz, L., et al.: Management of AIDS-related Kaposi's sarcoma. Lancet Oncol. **8**, 167–176 (2007)
5. Feller, L., Lemmer, J., Wood, N.H., et al.: Necrotizing gingivitis of Kaposi sarcoma affected gingivae. SADJ. **61**, 314–317 (2006)
6. Folpe, A.L., Veikkola, T., Valtola, R., et al.: Vascular endothelial growth factor receptor-3 (VEGFR-3): a marker of vascular tumors with presumed lymphatic differentiation, including Kaposi's sar-

coma, kaposiform and Dabska-type hemangioendotheliomas, and a subset of angiosarcomas. Mod. Pathol. **13**, 180–185 (2000)
7. Ganem, D.: KSHV infection and the pathogenesis of Kaposi's sarcoma. Annu. Rev. Pathol. **1**, 273–296 (2006)
8. Herndier, B., Ganem, D.: The biology of Kaposi's sarcoma. Cancer Treat. Res. **104**, 89–126 (2001)
9. Hussein, M.R.: Cutaneous and lymphadenopathic Kaposi's sarcoma: a case report and review of literature. J. Cutan. Pathol. **35**, 575–578 (2008)
10. Hussein, M.R.: Immunohistological evaluation of immune cell infiltrate in cutaneous Kaposi's sarcoma. Cell Biol. Int. **32**, 157–162 (2008)
11. Kaaya, E.E., Parravicini, C., Ordonez, C., et al.: Heterogeneity of spindle cells in Kaposi's sarcoma: comparison of cells in lesions and in culture. J. Acquir. Immune Defic. Syndr. Hum. Retrovirol. **10**, 295–305 (1995)
12. Krown, S.E., Metroka, C., Wernz, J.C.: Kaposi's sarcoma in the acquired immune deficiency syndrome: a proposal for uniform evaluation, response, and staging criteria. AIDS Clinical Trials Group Oncology Committee. J. Clin. Oncol. **7**, 1201–1207 (1989)
13. Kua, H.W., Merchant, W., Waugh, M.A.: Oral Kaposi's sarcoma in a non-HIV homosexual White male. Int. J. STD AIDS **15**, 775–777 (2004)
14. Leitch, H., Trudeau, M., Routy, J.P.: Effect of protease inhibitor-based highly active antiretroviral therapy on survival in HIV-associated advanced Kaposi's sarcoma patients treated with chemotherapy. HIV Clin. Trials **4**, 107–114 (2003)
15. Lemlich, G., Schwam, L., Lebwohl, M.: Kaposi's sarcoma and acquired immunodeficiency syndrome. Postmortem findings in twenty-four cases. J. Am. Acad. Dermatol. **16**, 319–325 (1987)
16. Levine, A.M., Tulpule, A.: Clinical aspects and management of AIDS-related Kaposi's sarcoma. Eur. J. Cancer **37**, 1288–1295 (2001)
17. Micali, G., Nasca, M.R., De Pasquale, R., et al.: Primary classic Kaposi's sarcoma of the penis: report of a case and review. J. Eur. Acad. Dermatol. Venereol. **17**, 320–323 (2003)
18. Mitsuyasu, R.T.: Clinical variants and staging of Kaposi's sarcoma. Semin. Oncol. **14**, 13–18 (1987)
19. Pyakurel, P., Pak, F., Mwakigonja, A.R., et al.: Lymphatic and vascular origin of Kaposi's sarcoma spindle cells during tumor development. Int. J. Cancer **119**, 1262–1267 (2006)
20. Reed, W.B., Kamath, M., Weiss, L.: Kaposi sarcoma, with emphasis on the internal manifestations. Arch. Dermatol. **110**, 115–118 (1974)
21. Regezi, J.A., MacPhail, L.A., Daniels, T.E., et al.: Oral Kaposi's sarcoma: a 10-year retrospective histopathologic study. J. Oral Pathol. Med. **22**, 292–297 (1993)
22. Rosella, M., Masotti, A., Cottoni, F.: Endoscopic examination in Kaposi's sarcoma. J. Eur. Acad. Dermatol. Venereol. **14**, 225–226 (2000)
23. Ruszczak, Z., Mayer-Da Silva, A., Orfanos, C.E.: Kaposi's sarcoma in AIDS. Multicentric angioneoplasia in early skin lesions. Am. J. Dermatopathol. **9**, 388–398 (1987)
24. Sapienza, G., Nasca, M.R., Dinotta, F., et al.: Guess what. Classic Kaposi's sarcoma. Eur. J. Dermatol. **11**, 157–158 (2001)
25. Satta, R., Cossu, S., Massarelli, G., et al.: Anaplastic transformation of classic Kaposi's sarcoma: clinicopathological study of five cases. Br. J. Dermatol. **145**, 847–849 (2001)
26. Schwartz, R.A., Volpe, J.A., Lambert, M.W., et al.: Kaposi's sarcoma. Semin. Dermatol. **3**, 303–315 (1984)
27. Schwartz, R.A., Micali, G., Nasca, M.R., et al.: Kaposi sarcoma: a continuing conundrum. Am. Acad. Dermatol. **S9**, 179–206 (2008)
28. Spano, J.P., Salhi, Y., Costagliola, D., et al.: Factors predictive of disease progression and death in AIDS-related Kaposi's sarcoma. HIV Med. **1**, 232–237 (2000)

29. Templeton, A.C.: Studies in Kaposi's sarcoma. Postmortem findings and disease patterns in women. Cancer **30**, 854–867 (1972)
30. Templeton, A.C.: Kaposi's sarcoma. Pathol. Annu. **16**, 315–336 (1981)
31. Wolf, R., Brenner, S., Ruocco, V., et al.: Isotopic response. Int. J. Dermatol. **34**, 341–348 (1995)
32. Ziegler, J.L., Katongole-Mbidde, E.: Kaposi's sarcoma in childhood: an analysis of 100 cases from Uganda and relationship to HIV infection. Int. J. Cancer **65**, 200–203 (1996)

Hemangiomas of Infancy

1. Bruckner, A.L., Frieden, I.J.: Hemangiomas of infancy. J. Am. Acad. Dermatol. **48**, 477–493 (2003)
2. Chan, Y.C., Giam, Y.C.: Guidelines of care for cutaneous haemangiomas. Ann. Acad. Med. Singapore **34**, 117–123 (2005)
3. Chiller, K.G., Passaro, D., Frieden, I.J.: Hemangiomas of infancy: clinical characteristics, morphologic subtypes, and their relationship to race, ethnicity, and sex. Arch. Dermatol. **138**, 1567–1576 (2002)
4. Dadras, S.S., North, P.E., Bertoncini, J., et al.: Infantile hemangiomas are arrested in an early developmental vascular differentiation state. Mod. Pathol. **17**, 1068–1079 (2004)
5. Elwan, N.M., Soliman, M.M., Hassan, A.M., et al.: CD34, VEGF and Glut-1 in some congenital vascular lesions before and after PDL and KTP laser therapy. Egypt J. Derm. Androl. **27**, 19–32 (2006)
6. Jia, J., Zhao, Y.F., Zhao, J.H.: Potential roles of allograft inflammatory factor-1 in the pathogenesis of hemangiomas. Med. Hypotheses **68**, 288–290 (2007)
7. Kilcline, C., Frieden, I.J.: Infantile hemangiomas: how common are they? A systematic review of the medical literature. Pediatr. Dermatol. **25**, 168–173 (2008)
8. Klement, G., Fishman, S.J.: Vascualr anomalies: hemangiomas and malformations. In: Grosfeld, J.L., O'Neill Jr., J.A., Fonkalsrud, E.W., Coran, A.G. (eds.) Pediatric Surgery, 6th edn, p. 2094. Mosby El-Sevier, Phialdelphia (2006)
9. Leon-Villapalos, J., Wolfe, K., Kangesu, L., et al.: GLUT-1: an extra diagnostic tool to differentiate between haemangiomas and vascular malformations. Br. J. Plast. Surg. **58**, 348–352 (2005)
10. North, P.E., Waner, M., James, C.A., et al.: Congenital nonprogressive hemangioma: a distinct clinicopathologic entity unlike infantile hemangioma. Arch. Dermatol. **137**, 1607–1620 (2001)
11. North, P.E., Waner, M., Mizeracki, A., et al.: A unique microvascular phenotype shared by juvenile hemangiomas and human placenta. Arch. Dermatol. **137**, 559–570 (2001)
12. Pandey, A., Gangopadhyay, A.N., Upadhyay, V.D.: Evaluation and management of infantile hemangioma: an overview. Ostomy Wound Manage. **54**, 16–18 (2008). 20, 22–26, 28–9
13. Phung, T.L., Hochman, M., Mihm, M.C.: Current knowledge of the pathogenesis of infantile hemangiomas. Arch. Facial Plast. Surg. **7**, 319–321 (2005)
14. Tanner, J.L., Dechert, M.P., Frieden, I.J.: Growing up with a facial hemangioma: parent and child coping and adaptation. Pediatrics **101**, 446–452 (1998)
15. Willenberg, T., Baumgartner, I.: Vascular birthmarks. Vasa. **37**, 5–17 (2008)
16. Léauté-Labrèze, C., Dumas de la Roque, E., Hubiche, T., Boralevi, F., Thambo, J.-B., Taïeb: Propranolol for severe hemangiomas of infancy. N. Engl. J. Med. **358**, 2649–2651 (2008)
17. Sans V, Dumas de la Roque E, Berge J., et al.: Propranolol for severe infantile hemangiomas: follow-up report. Pediatrics. (2009) Aug 10 (Epub ahead of print)

Disease Entities of Cherry Hemangioma

1. Bean, W.B.: Vascular Spiders and Related Lesions of the Skin, p. 228. Blackwell Scientific Publications, Oxford (1958)
2. Weedon, D.: Vascular tumors. In: Weedon, D. (ed.) Skin pathology, 2nd edn, p. 1001. Churchill Livingstone, London (2002)

Disease Entities of Sinusoidal Hemangioma

1. Calonje, E., Fletcher, C.D.: Sinusoidal hemangioma. A distinctive benign vascular neoplasm within the group of cavernous hemangiomas. Am. J. Surg. Pathol. **15**, 1130–1135 (1991)
2. Enjolras, O., Wassef, M., Brocheriou-Spelle, I., et al.: Sinusoidal hemangioma. Ann. Dermatol. Venereol. **125**, 575–580 (1998)

Disease Entities of Glomeruloid Hemangioma

1. Chan, J.K., Fletcher, C.D., Hicklin, G.A., et al.: Glomeruloid hemangioma. A distinctive cutaneous lesion of multicentric Castleman's disease associated with POEMS syndrome. Am. J. Surg. Pathol. **14**, 1036–1046 (1990)
2. Chan, P.T., Lee, K.C., Chong, L.Y., et al.: Glomeruloid haemangioma with cerebriform morphology in a patient with POEMS syndrome. Clin. Exp. Dermatol. **31**, 775–777 (2006)
3. Forman, S.B., Tyler, W.B., Ferringer, T.C., et al.: Glomeruloid hemangiomas without POEMS syndrome: series of three cases. J. Cutan. Pathol. **34**, 956–957 (2007)
4. Perdaens, C., De Raeve, H., Goossens, A., et al.: POEMS syndrome characterized by glomeruloid angioma, osteosclerosis and multicentric Castleman disease. J. Eur. Acad. Dermatol. Venereol. **20**, 480–481 (2006)
5. Phillips, J.A., Dixon, J.E., Richardson, J.B., et al.: Glomeruloid hemangioma leading to a diagnosis of POEMS syndrome. J. Am. Acad. Dermatol. **55**, 149–152 (2006)
6. Piña-Oviedo, S., López-Patiño, S., Ortiz-Hidalgo, C.: Glomeruloid hemangiomas localized to the skin of the trunk with no clinical features of POEMS syndrome. Int. J. Dermatol. **45**, 1449–1450 (2006)
7. Vélez, D., Delgado-Jiménez, Y., Fraga, J.: Solitary glomeruloid haemangioma without POEMS syndrome. J. Cutan. Pathol. **32**, 449–452 (2005)
8. Yang, S.G., Cho, K.H., Bang, Y.J., et al.: A case of glomeruloid hemangioma associated with multicentric Castleman's disease. Am. J. Dermatopathol. **20**, 266–270 (1998)
9. Yuri, T., Yamazaki, F., Takasu, K., et al.: Glomeruloid hemangioma. Pathol. Int. **58**, 390–395 (2008)

Hobnail Hemangioma (Targetoid Hemosiderotic Hemangioma)

1. Santa Cruz, D.J., Aronberg, J.: Targetoid hemosiderotic hemangioma. J. Am. Acad. Dermatol. **19**, 550–558 (1988)
2. Rapini, R.P., Golitz, L.E.: Targetoid hemosiderotic hemangioma. J. Cutan. Pathol. **17**, 233–235 (1990)
3. Vion, B., Frenk, E.: Targetoid hemosiderotic hemangioma. Dermatology **184**, 300–302 (1992)

4. Benes, P., Douglass, M., Lowe, L.: Targetoid hemosiderotic hemangioma; a series of four cases [Abstract]. J. Cutan. Pathol. **20**, 533 (1993)
5. Krahl, D., Petzoldt, D.: Targetoides hämosiderotisches Hämangiom. Eine weitere Differentialdiagnose des Kaposi-Sarkoms. Hautarzt **45**, 34–37 (1994)
6. Lowe, L.: Self assessment-1993. Targetoid hemosiderotic hemangioma. J. Cutan. Pathol. **21**, 568–569 (1994)
7. Perrin, C., Rodot, S., Ortonne, J.P., Michiels, J.F.: L'hémangiome en cible hémosidérinique. Ann. Dermatol. Venereol. **122**, 111–114 (1995)
8. Margaroth, G.S., Tigelaar, R.E., Longley, J., Luck, L.E., Leffell, D.J.: Targetoid hemangioma associated with pregnancy and the menstrual cycle. J. Am. Acad. Dermatol. **32**, 282–284 (1995)
9. Held, J.L., Malhotra, R.: Targetoid hemosiderotic hemangioma. Fitzpatrick's J. Clin. Dermatol. **3**, 70 (1995)
10. Fariña, M.C., Montalvo, N., Piqué, E., Escalonilla, P., Olivares, M., Barat, A., Martín, L., Requena, L.: Hemangioma hemosiderótico en diana: un nuevo caso y revisión de la literatura. Actas Dermosifiliogr. **86**, 383–387 (1995)
11. Ho, C., McCalmont, T.H.: Targetoid hemosiderotic hemangioma: report of 24 cases, with emphasis on unusual features and comparison to early Kaposi's sarcoma [Abstract]. J. Cutan. Pathol. **22**, 67 (1995)
12. Ly, S., Versapuech, J., Vergier, B., Beylot-Barry, M., Beylot, C.: Guess what? Targetoid hemosiderotic hemangioma. Eur. J. Dermatol. **8**, 583–585 (1998)
13. Avci, O., Soyal, M.C., Sagol, O., Gunes, A.T.: Targetoid hemosiderotic hemangioma [Letter]. J. Eur. Acad. Dermatol. Venereol. **11**, 186–187 (1998)
14. Carlson, J.A., Daulat, S., Goodheart, H.P.: Targetoid hemosiderotic hemangioma – a dynamic vascular tumor: report of 3 cases with episodic and cyclic changes and comparison with solitary angiokeratomas. J. Am. Acad. Dermatol. **41**, 215–224 (1999)
15. Guillou, L., Calonje, E., Speight, P., Rosai, J., Fletcher, C.D.: Hobnail hemangioma: a pseudomalignant vascular lesion with a reappraisal of targetoid hemosiderotic hemangioma. Am. J. Surg. Pathol. **23**, 97–105 (1999)
16. Santonja, C., Torrelo, A.: Hobnail hemangioma. Dermatology **191**, 154–156 (1995)
17. Mentzel, T., Partanen, T.A., Kutzner, H.: Hobnail hemangioma ("targetoid hemosiderotic hemangioma"): clinicopathologic and immunohistochemical analysis of 62 cases. J. Cutan. Pathol. **26**, 279–286 (1999)
18. Christenson, L.J., Seabury Stone, M.: Trauma-induced simulator of targetoid hemosiderotic hemangioma. Am. J. Dermatopathol. **23**, 221–223 (2001)
19. Franke, F.E., Steger, K., Marks, A., Kutzner, H., Mentzel, T.: Hobnail hemangiomas (targetoid hemosiderotic hemangiomas) are true lymphangiomas. J. Cutan. Pathol. **31**, 362–367 (2004)
20. Gutzner, R., Kaspari, M., Herbst, R.A., Kapp, A., Kiehl, P.: Absence of HHV-8 DNA in hobnail hemangiomas. J. Cutan. Pathol. **29**, 154–158 (2002)

Microvenular Hemangioma

1. Hunt, S.J., Santa Cruz, D.J., Barr, R.J.: Microvenular hemangioma. J. Cutan. Pathol. **18**, 235–240 (1991)
2. Bantel, E., Grosshans, E., Ortonne, J.P.: Zuz Kenntnis mickrokapillärer angiome, beobachtungen bei schwangeren bzw. Unter hormoneller antikonzeption stehenden Frauen. Z. Hautkr. **64**, 1071–1074 (1989)
3. Aloi, F., Tomasini, C., Pippione, M.: Microvenular hemangioma. Am. J. Dermatopathol. **15**, 534–538 (1993)
4. Satge, D., Grande-Goburdhun, J., Grosshans, E.: Hemangiome microcapillaire. Ann. Dermatol. Venereol. **120**, 297–298 (1993)
5. Horn, M.S., Stern, J.B.: Small red nodule on the leg of a young woman. Microvenular hemangioma. Arch. Dermatol. **131**, 483 (1995)
6. Black, R.J., McCusker, G.M., Eedy, D.J.: Microvenular haemangioma. Clin. Exp. Dermatol. **20**, 260–262 (1995)
7. Sanz Trelles, A., Ojeda Martos, A., Jiménez Fernández, A., VeraCastaño, A.: Microvenular hemangioma: a new case in a child. Histopathology **32**, 89–90 (1998)
8. Fukunaga, M., Ushigome, S.: Microvenular hemangioma. Pathol. Int. **48**, 237–239 (1998)
9. Rikihisa, W., Yamamoto, O., Kohda, F., Hamada, M., Yasumoto, S., Kiryu, H., Asahi, M.: Microvenular haemangioma in a patient with Wiskott-Aldrich syndrome. Br. J. Dermatol. **141**, 752–754 (1999)
10. Ackerman, A.B., Guo, Y., Vitale, P.: Clues to Diagnosis in Dermatopathology II, pp. 285–288. ASCP, Chicago (1992)
11. Ben-Dor, D., Chan, J.K.: Immunostaining for human herpes virus 8 latent nuclear antigen-1 helps distinguish Kaposi sarcoma from its mimickers. Am. J. Clin. Pathol. **121**, 335–342 (2004)
12. Hudnall, S.D., Chen, T., Brown, T., Angel, T., Schwartz, M.R., Tyring, S.K.: Human herpes virus-8-positive microvenular hemangioma in POEMS syndrome. Arch. Pathol. Lab. Med. **127**, 1034–1036 (2003)

Angiolymphoid Hyperplasia with Eosinophilia

1. Wells, G.C., Whimster, I.W.: Subcutaneous angiolymphoid hyperplasia with eosinophilia. Br. J. Dermatol. **81**, 1–15 (1969)
2. Kimura, T., Yoshimura, S., Ishikawa, E.: Abnormal granuloma with proliferation of lymphoid tissue. Trans. Soc. Pathol. Jpn. **37**, 179–180 (1948)
3. Chan, J.K.C., Hui, P.K., Ng, C.S., Yuen, N.W.F., Kung, I.T.M., Gwi, E.: Epithelioid hemangioma (angiolymphoid hyperplasia with eosinophilia) and Kimura's disease in Chinese. Histopathology **15**, 557–574 (1989)
4. Googe, P.B., Harris, N.L., Mihm Jr., M.C.: Kimura's disease and angiolymphoid hyperplasia with eosinophilia: two distinct histopathological entities. J. Cutan. Pathol. **14**, 263–271 (1987)
5. Kung, I.T.M., Gibson, J.B., Bannatyne, P.M.: Kimura's disease: a clinico-pathological study of 21 cases and its distinction from angiolymphoid hyperplasia with eosinophilia. Pathology **16**, 39–44 (1984)
6. Kuo, T.T., Shih, L.Y., Chan, H.L.: Kimura's disease. Involvement of regional lymph nodes and distinction from angiolymphoid hyperplasia with eosinophilia. Am. J. Surg. Pathol. **12**, 843–854 (1988)
7. Rosai, J.: Angiolymphoid hyperplasia with eosinophilia of the skin. Its nosological position in the spectrum of the histiocytoid hemangioma. Am. J. Dermatopathol. **4**, 175–184 (1982)
8. Urabe, A., Tsuneyoshi, M., Enjoji, M.: Epithelioid hemangioma versus Kimura's disease. A comparative clinicopathologic study. Am. J. Surg. Pathol. **11**, 758–766 (1987)
9. Masa, F.C., Fretzin, D.F., Chowdhury, L., et al.: Angiolymphoid hyperplasia demonstrating extensive skin and mucosal lesions controlled with vinblastine therapy. J. Am. Acad. Dermatol. **11**, 333–339 (1984)
10. Tsuboi, H., Fujimura, T., Katsuoka, K.: Angiolymphoid hyperplasia with eosinophilia in the oral mucosa. Br. J. Dermatol. **145**, 365–366 (2001)

11. Imbling Jr., F.D., Viegas, S.F., Sanchez, R.L.: Multiple angiolymphoid hyperplasia with eosinophilia of the hand: report of a case and review of the literature. Cutis **58**, 345–348 (1996)

12. Arnold, M., Geilen, C.C., Coupland, S.E., Krengel, S., Dippel, E., Sproder, J., Goerdt, S., Orfanos, C.E.: Unilateral angiolymphoid hyperplasia with eosinophilia involving the left arm and hand. J. Cutan. Pathol. **26**, 436–440 (1999)

13. Aguilar, A., Ambrojo, P., Requena, L., Olmos, L., Sanchez Yus, E.: Angiolymphoid hyperplasia with eosinophilia limited to the vulva. Clin. Exp. Dermatol. **15**, 65–67 (1990)

14. Scurry, J., Dennerstein, G., Brenan, J.: Angiolymphoid hyperplasia with eosinophilia of the vulva. Aust. N. Z. Obstet. Gynaecol. **35**, 347–348 (1995)

15. Srigley, J.R., Ayala, A.G., Ordoñez, N.G., et al.: Epithelioid hemangioma of the penis: a rare and distinctive vascular lesion. Arch. Pathol. Lab. Med. **109**, 51–54 (1985)

16. Mariatos, G., Gorgoulis, V.G., Laskaris, G., Kittas, C.: Epithelioid hemangioma (angiolymphoid hyperplasia with eosinophilia) in the inner canthus. J. Eur. Acad. Dermatol. Venereol. **15**, 90–91 (2001)

17. Bendl, B.J., Asano, K., Lewis, R.J.: Nodular angioblastic hyperplasia with eosinophilia and lymphofolliculosis. Cutis **19**, 327–329 (1977)

18. Sakamoto, F., Hashimoto, T., Takenouchi, T., Ito, M., Nitto, H.: Angiolymphoid hyperplasia with eosinophilia presenting multinucleated cells in histology: an ultrastructural study. J. Cutan. Pathol. **25**, 322–326 (1998)

19. Angervall, L., Kindblom, L.G., Karlsson, K., et al.: Atypical hemangioendothelioma of venous origin: a clinicopathologic angiographic immunohistochemical, and ultrastructural study of two endothelial tumors within the concept of histiocytoid hemangioma. Am. J. Surg. Pathol. **9**, 504–516 (1985)

20. Kempf, W., Haeffner, A.C., Zepter, K., Sander, C.A., Flaig, M.J., et al.: Angiolymphoid hyperplasia with eosinophilia: evidence for a T-cell lymphoproliferative origin. Hum. Pathol. **33**, 1023–1029 (2002)

21. Ose, D., Vollmer, R., Shelburne, J., et al.: Histiocytoid hemangioma of the skin and scapula: a case report with electron microscopy and immunohistochemistry. Cancer **51**, 1656–1662 (1983)

22. Burgdorf, W.H.C., Mukai, K., Rosai, J.: Immunohistochemical identification of factor VIII related antigen in endothelial cells of cutaneous lesions of alleged vascular nature. Am. J. Clin. Pathol. **75**, 167–171 (1981)

23. Macarenco, R.S., Leite do Canto, A., Gonzalez, S.: Angiolymphoid hyperplasia with eosinophilia showing prominent granulomatous and fibrotic reaction: a morphological and immunohistochemical study. Am. J. Dermatopathol. **28**, 514–517 (2006)

24. Daniels, D.G., Schrodt, G.R., Fliegelman, M.T., et al.: Ultrastructural study of a case of angiolymphoid hyperplasia with eosinophilia. Arch. Dermatol. **109**, 870–872 (1974)

25. Eady, R.A.J., Wilson Jones, E.: Pseudopyogenic granuloma: enzyme histochemical and ultrastructural study. Hum. Pathol. **8**, 653–668 (1977)

26. Gyulai, R., Kemeny, L., Adam, E., Nagy, F., Dobozy, A.: HHV8 DNA in angiolymphoid hyperplasia of the skin. Lancet **347**, 1837 (1996)

27. Oksenhendler, E., Cazals-Hatem, D., Schulz, T.F., Barateau, V., Grollet, L., Sheldon, J., Clauvel, J.P., Sigaux, F., Agbalika, F.: Transient angiolymphoid hyperplasia and Kaposi's sarcoma after primary infection with human herpesvirus 8 in a patient with human immunodeficiency virus infection. N. Engl. J. Med. **338**, 1585–1590 (1998)

28. Lebbe, C., Pellet, C., Flageul, B., Sastre, X., Avril, M.F., Bonvalet, D., Morel, P., Calvo, F.: Sequences of human herpesvirus 8 are not detected in various non-Kaposi sarcoma vascular lesions. Arch. Dermatol. **133**, 919–920 (1997)

29. Jang, K.A., Ahn, S.J., Choi, J.H., Sung, K.J., Moon, K.C., Koh, J.K., Shim, Y.H.: Polymerase chain reaction (PCR) for human herpesvirus 8 and heteroduplex PCR for clonality assessment in angiolymphoid hyperplasia with eosinophilia and Kimura's disease. J. Cutan. Pathol. **28**, 363–367 (2001)

30. Vadlamudi, G., Schinella, R.: Traumatic pseudoaneurism: a possible early lesion in the spectrum of epithelioid hemangioma/angiolymphoid hyperplasia with eosinophilia. Am. J. Dermatopathol. **20**, 113–117 (1998)

31. Onishi, Y., Ohara, K.: Angiolymphoid hyperplasia with eosinophilia associated with arteriovenous malformation: a clinicopathological correlation with angiography and serial estimation of serum levels or renin, eosinophil cationic protein and interleukin 5. Br. J. Dermatol. **140**, 1153–1156 (1999)

32. Hobbs, E.R., Bailin, P.L., Ratz, J.L., Yarbrough, C.L.: Treatment of angiolymphoid hyperplasia of the external ear with carbon dioxide laser. J. Am. Acad. Dermatol. **19**, 345–349 (1988)

33. Letzman, B.H., McMeekin, T., Gaspari, A.A.: Pulsed dye laser treatment of angiolymphoid hyperplasia with eosinophilia lesions. Arch. Dermatol. **133**, 920–921 (1997)

34. Rohrer, T.E., Allan, A.E.: Angiolymphoid hyperplasia with eosinophilia successfully treated with a long-pulsed tunable dye laser. Dermatol. Surg. **26**, 211–214 (2000)

35. Papadavid, E., Krausz, T., Chu, A.C., Walker, N.P.: Angiolymphoid hyperplasia with eosinophilia successfully treated with the flashlamp pulsed-dye laser. Br. J. Dermatol. **142**, 192–194 (2000)

36. Gupta, G., Munro, C.S.: Angiolymphoid hyperplasia with eosinophilia: successful treatment with pulsed dye laser using the double pulse technique. Br. J. Dermatol. **143**, 214–215 (2000)

37. Fosko, S.W., Glaser, D.A., Rogers, C.J.: Eradication of angiolymphoid hyperplasia with eosinophilia by copper vapor laser. Arch. Dermatol. **137**, 863–865 (2001)

Spindle-Cell Hemangioma

1. Weiss, S.W., Enzinger, F.M.: Spindle cell hemangioendothelioma: a low grade angiosarcoma resembling cavernous hemangioma and Kaposi's sarcoma. Am. J. Surg. Pathol. **10**, 521–530 (1986)

2. Lessard, M., Barnhill, R.L.: Spindle cell hemangioendothelioma. J. Am. Acad. Dermatol. **18**, 393–395 (1988)

3. Scott, G.A., Rosai, J.: Spindle cell hemangioendothelioma. Report of seven additional cases of a recently described neoplasm. Am. J. Dermatopathol. **10**, 281–288 (1988)

4. Wu, K.K.: Spindle cell hemangioendothelioma of the foot. J. Foot Surg. **28**, 475–478 (1989)

5. Zoltie, N., Roberts, P.F.: Spindle cell haemangioendothelioma in association with epithelioid haemangioendothelioma. Histopathology **15**, 544–546 (1989)

6. Rios Martín, J.J., Gonzalez Campora, R., Armas Padron, J.R., Moreno Jimenez, J.C., Camacho Martínez, F.: Hemangioendotelioma de células fusiformes. Actas Dermosifiliogr. **80**, 481–484 (1989)

7. Lawson, J.P., Scott, G.: Case report 602: spindle cell hemangioendothelioma (SCH) and enchondromatosis (a form of Maffuci syndrome) in a patient with acute myelocytic leukemia (AML). Skeletal Radiol. **19**, 158–162 (1990)

8. Habeck, J.O.: Das spindelzellhamangioendotheliom-ein niedrig malignes Angiosarkom. Pathologe **11**, 94–96 (1990)

9. Steinbach, L.S., Ominsky, S.H., Shpall, S., Perkocha, L.A.: MR imaging of spindle cell hemangioendothelioma. J. Comput. Assist. Tomogr. **15**, 155–157 (1991)

10. Terashi, H., Itami, S., Kurata, S., Sonoda, T., Takayasu, S., Yokoyama, S.: Spindle cell hemangioendothelioma. Report of three cases. J. Dermatol. **18**, 104–111 (1991)

11. Fletcher, C.D.M., Beham, A., Schmid, C.: Spindle cell haemangioendothelioma: a clinicopathological and immunohistochemical study indicative of a non-neoplastic lesion. Histopathology **18**, 291–301 (1991)

12. Nikorowitsch, R., Kindermann, D.: Zum Spindelzellhamangioendotheliom. Histomorphologische, immunohistochemische und DNA zytometrische Befunde. Pathologe **12**, 327–330 (1991)

13. Marcoval Caus, J., Pagerols Bonilla, X., Iñiguez Navarro, D., Sais Puigdemont, G., Moreno Carazo, A., Peyri Rey, J.: Hemangioendotelioma de células fusiformes. Estudio de dos casos y revisión de la literatura. Actas Dermosifiliogr. **32**, 449–451 (1991)

14. Ding, J., Hashimoto, H., Imayama, S., Tsuneyoshi, M., Enjoji, M.: Spindle cell haemangioendothelioma: probably a benign vascular lesion not a low-grade angiosarcoma. A clinicopathological, ultrastructural and immunohistochemical study. Virchows Arch Pathol. Anat. **420**, 77–85 (1992)

15. Imayama, S., Murakamai, Y., Hashimoto, H., Hori, Y.: Spindle cell hemangioendothelioma exhibits the ultrastructural features of reactive vascular proliferation rather than of angiosarcoma. Am. J. Clin. Pathol. **97**, 279–287 (1992)

16. Ono, C.M., Mitsunaga, M.M., Lockett, L.J.: Intragluteal spindle cell hemangioendothelioma. An unusual presentation of a recently described vascular neoplasm. Clin Orthop **281**, 224–228 (1992)

17. Battocchio, S., Facchetti, F., Brisigotti, M.: Spindle cell hemangioendothelioma: further evidence against its proposed neoplastic nature. Histopathology **22**, 296–298 (1993)

18. Murakami, J., Sarker, A.B., Teramoto, N., Horie, Y., Taguchi, K., Akagi, T.: Spindle cell hemangioendothelioma: a report of two cases. Acta Pathol. Jpn **43**, 529–534 (1993)

19. Eltorky, M., Chesney, T., Sebes, J., Hall, J.C.: Spindle cell hemangioendothelioma. Report of three cases and review of the literature. J. Dermatol. Surg. Oncol. **20**, 196–202 (1994)

20. Azadeh, B., Attallach, M.F., Ejeckam, G.C.: Spindle cell hemangioendothelioma in association with epithelioid hemangioendothelioma. Cutis **53**, 134–136 (1994)

21. Pellegrini, A.E., Drake, R.D., Qualman, S.J.: Spindle cell hemangioendothelioma: a neoplasm associated with Maffuci's syndrome. J. Cutan. Pathol. **22**, 173–176 (1995)

22. Fukunaga, M., Ushigome, S., Nikaido, T., Ishikawa, E., Nakamori, K.: Spindle cell hemangioendothelioma: an immunohistochemical and flow cytometric study of six cases. Pathol. Int. **45**, 589–595 (1995)

23. Tosios, K., Koutlas, I.G., Kapranos, N., Papanicolau, S.I.: Spindlecell hemangioendothelioma of the oral cavity. A case report. J. Oral Pathol. Med. **24**, 379–382 (1995)

24. Fanburg, J.C., Meis-Kindblom, J.M., Rosemberg, A.E.: Multiple enchondromas associated with spindle-cell hemagioendotheliomas. An overlooked variant of Maffucci's syndrome. Am. J. Surg. Pathol. **19**, 1029–1038 (1995)

25. Hisaoka, M., Kouho, H., Aoki, T., Hashimoto, H.: DNA cytometric and immunohistochemical analysis of proliferative activity in spindle cell haemangioendothelioma. Histopathology **27**, 451–456 (1995)

26. Mahdavi, Z., Grafe, M.R., Ostrup, R., Kormanik, P., Chamberlain, M.C.: Spindle cell hemangioendothelioma of the spinal cord. J. Neurooncol. **27**, 231–234 (1996)

27. Patel, S.V., Bass, F.D., Niemi, W.J., Pressman, M.M.: Spindle cell hemangioendothelioma: a case presentation and literature review of a rare lower extremity tumor. J. Foot Ankle Surg. **35**, 309–311 (1996)

28. Perkins, P., Weiss, S.W.: Spindle cell hemangioendothelioma. An analysis of 78 cases with reassessment of its pathogenesis and biologic behavior. Am. J. Surg. Pathol. **20**, 1196–1204 (1996)

29. Hisaoka, M., Aoki, T., Kouho, H., Chosa, H., Hashimoto, H.: Maffucci's syndrome associated with spindle cell hemangioendothelioma. Skeletal Radiol. **26**, 191–194 (1997)

30. Hisaoka, M., Hashimoto, H., Iwamasa, T.: Diagnostic implication of Kaposi's sarcoma-associated herpesvirus with special reference to the distinction between spindle cell hemangioendothelioma and Kaposi's sarcoma. Arch. Pathol. Lab. Med. **122**, 72–76 (1998)

31. Yañez, S., Val-Bernal, J.F., Mira, C., Echevarria, M.A., González-Vela, M.C., Arce, F.: Spindle cell hemangioendothelioma associated with multiple skeletal enchondromas: a variant of Maffucci's syndrome. Gen. Diagn. Pathol. **143**, 331–335 (1998)

32. Gradner, T.L., Elston, D.M.: Multiple lower extremity and penile spindle cell hemangioendotheliomas. Cutis **62**, 23–26 (1998)

33. Bodemer, C., Fraitag, S., Amoric, J.C., Benaceur, S., Brunelle, F., De Prost, Y.: Hemangioendotheliome a cellules fusiformes dans une variete monomelique et multinodulaire chez l'enfant. Ann. Dermatol. Venereol. **124**, 857–860 (1997)

34. Enjolras, O., Wassef, M., Merland, J.J.: Syndrome de Maffucci: une fausse malformation veineuse? Un cas avec hemangioendothelioma a cellules fusiformes. Ann. Dermatol. Venereol. **125**, 512–515 (1998)

35. Keel, S.B., Rosemberg, A.E.: Hemorrhagic epithelioid and spindle cell hemangioma: a newly recognized, unique vascular tumor of bone. Cancer **85**, 1966–1972 (1999)

36. Isayama, T., Iwasaki, H., Ogata, K., Naito, M.: Intramuscular spindle cell hemangioendothelioma. Skeletal Radiol. **28**, 477–480 (1999)

37. Tomasini, C., Aloi, F., Soro, E., Elia, V.: Spindle cell hemangioma. Dermatology **199**, 274–276 (1999)

38. Setoyama, M., Shimada, H., Miyazono, N., Baba, Y., Kanzaki, T.: Spindle cell hemangioendothelioma: successful treatment with recombinant interleukin-2. Br. J. Dermatol. **142**, 1238–1239 (2000)

39. Weiss, S.W., Goldblum, J.R.: Enzinger and Weiss's Soft Tissue Tumors, 4th edn, pp. 853–856. Mosby, St. Louis (2001)

40. Mentzel, T., Kutzner, H.: Hemangioendotheliomas: heterogeneous vascular neoplasms. Dermatopathol. Pract. Concept **5**, 102–109 (1999)

41. Requena, L., Ackerman, A.B.: Hemangioendothelioma? Dermatopathol. Pract. Concept **5**, 110–112 (1999)

42. Fletcher, C.D.M.: The non-neoplastic nature of spindle cell hemangioendothelioma. Am. J. Clin. Pathol. **98**, 545–546 (1992)

Tufted Angioma

1. Wilson Jones, E.: Malignant vascular tumors. Clin. Exp. Dermatol. **1**, 287–312 (1976)

2. MacMillan, A., Champion, R.H.: Progressive capillary haemangioma. Br. J. Dermatol. **85**, 492–493 (1971)

3. Nakagawa, K.: Case report of angioblastoma of the skin. Nippon Hifuka Gakkai Zasshi **59**, 92–94 (1949)

4. Wilson Jones, E., Orkin, M.: Tufted angioma (angioblastoma). A benign progressive angioma not to be confused with Kaposi's sarcoma or low-grade angiosarcoma. J. Am. Acad. Dermatol. **20**, 214–225 (1989)

5. Igarashi, M., Oh-i, T., Koga, M.: The relationship between angioblastoma (Nakagawa) and tufted angioma: report of four cases with angioblastoma and a literature-based comparison of the two conditions. J. Dermatol. **27**, 537–542 (2000)

6. Satomi, I., Tanaka, Y., Murata, J., Fujisawa, R.: A case of angioblastoma (Nakagawa). Rinsho Dermatol (Tokyo) **23**, 703–709 (1981)

7. Kim, K.J., Lee, M.W., Choi, J.H., Sung, K.J., Moon, K.C., Koh, J.K.: A case of congenital tufted angioma mimicking cavernous hemangioma. J. Dermatol. **28**, 514–515 (2001)

8. Hebeda, C.L., Scheffer, E., Starink, T.M.: Tufted angioma of late onset. Histopathology **23**, 191–193 (1993)
9. Descours, H., Grezard, P., Chouvet, B., Labeille, B.: Angiome en touffes acquis de l'adulte. Ann. Dermatol. Venereol. **125**, 44–46 (1998)
10. Dewerdt, S., Callens, A., Machet, L., Grangeponte, M.C., Vaillant, L., Lorette, G.: Angiome en touffes acquis de l'adulte: echec du traitement par laser a colorant pulse. Ann. Dermatol. Venereol. **125**, 47–49 (1998)
11. Heagerty, A.H.M., Rubin, A., Robinson, T.W.E.: Familial tufted angioma. Clin. Exp. Dermatol. **17**, 344–345 (1992)
12. Kumakiri, M., Muramoto, F., Tsukinaga, I., Yoshida, T., Ohura, T., Miura, Y.: Crystalline lamellae in the endothelial cells of a type of hemangioma characterized by the proliferation of immature endothelial cells and pericytes-angioblastoma (Nakagawa). J. Am. Acad. Dermatol. **8**, 68–75 (1983)
13. Okada, E., Tamura, A., Ishikawa, O., Miyachi, Y.: Tufted angioma (angioblastoma): case report and review of 41 cases in the Japanese literature. Clin. Exp. Dermatol. **25**, 627–630 (2000)
14. Ward, K.A., Kennedy, C.T., Ashworth, M.T.: Acquired tufted angioma frequently develops at sites other than the neck and upper trunk. Clin. Exp. Dermatol. **21**, 80 (1996)
15. Kleinegger, C.L., Hammond, H.L., Vincent, S.D., Finkelstein, M.W.: Acquired tufted angioma: a unique vascular lesion not previously reported in the oral mucosa. Br. J. Dermatol. **142**, 794–799 (2000)
16. Daley, T.: Acquired tufted angioma of the lower lip mucosa. J. Can. Dent. Assoc. **66**, 137 (2000)
17. Michel, S., Hohenleutner, U., Stolz, W., Knuchel-Clarke, R., Helmig, M., Landthaler, M.: Buschelartiges angiom ("tufted angioma"). Klin. Pädiatr. **213**, 39–42 (2001)
18. Allen, P.W.: Three new vascular tumors – tufted angioma, kaposiform infantile hemangioendothelioma, and proliferative cutaneous angiomatosis. Int. J. Surg. Pathol. **2**, 63–72 (1994)
19. Sumitra, S., Yesudian, P.: Painful tufted angioma precipitated by trauma. Int. J. Dermatol. **33**, 675–676 (1994)
20. Bernstein, E.F., Kantor, G., Howe, N., Savit, R.M., Koblenzer, P., Uitto, J.: Tufted angioma of the thigh. J. Am. Acad. Dermatol. **31**, 307–311 (1994)
21. Cho, K.H., Kim, S.H., Park, K.C., Lee, A.Y., Song, K.Y., Chi, J.G., Lee, Y.S., Kim, K.J.: Angioblastoma (Nakagawa) – is it the same as tufted angioma? Clin. Exp. Dermatol. **16**, 110–113 (1991)
22. Padilla, R.S., Orkin, M., Rosai, J.: Acquired "tufted" angioma (progressive capillary hemangioma). A distinctive clinicopathologic entity related to lobular capillary hemangioma. Am. J. Dermatopathol. **9**, 292–300 (1987)
23. Jang, K.A., Choi, J.H., Sung, K.J., Moon, K.C., Koh, J.K.: Congenital linear tufted angioma with spontaneous regression. Br. J. Dermatol. **138**, 912–913 (1998)
24. Alessi, E., Bertani, E., Sala, F.: Acquired tufted angioma. Am. J. Dermatopathol. **8**, 426–429 (1986)
25. Kim, T.H., Choi, E.H., Ahn, S.K., Lee, S.H.: Vascular tumors arising in port-wine stains: two cases of pyogenic granuloma and a case of acquired tufted angioma. J. Dermatol. **26**, 813–816 (1999)
26. Michel, S., Hohenleutner, U., Stolz, W., Landthaler, M.: Acquired tufted angioma in association with a complex cutaneous vascular malformation. Br. J. Dermatol. **141**, 1142–1144 (1999)
27. Kim, Y.K., Kim, H.J., Lee, K.G.: Acquired tufted angioma associated with pregnancy. Clin. Exp. Dermatol. **7**, 458–459 (1992)
28. Hiraiwa, A., Takai, K., Fukui, Y., Adachi, A., Fujii, H.: Non-regressing lipodystrophia centrifugalis abdominalis with angioblastoma (Nakagawa). Arch. Dermatol. **126**, 206–209 (1990)
29. Chu, P., LeBoit, P.E.: An eruptive vascular proliferation resembling acquired tufted angioma in the recipient of a liver transplant. J. Am. Acad. Dermatol. **26**, 322–325 (1992)
30. Enjolras, O., Wassef, M., Mazoyer, E., Frieden, I.J., Rieu, P.N., Drouet, L., Taieb, A., Stalder, J.F., Escande, J.P.: Infant with

Kasabach-Merritt syndrome do not have "true" hemangiomas. J. Pediatr. **130**, 631–640 (1997)
31. Leaute-Labreze, C., Bioulac-Sage, P., Labbe, L., Meraud, J.P., Taieb, A.: Tufted angioma associated with platelet trapping syndrome: response to aspirin. Arch. Dermatol. **133**, 1077–1079 (1997)
32. Enjolras, O., Wassef, M., Dosquet, C., Drouet, L., Fortier, G., Josset, P., Merland, J.J., Escande, J.P.: Syndrome de Kasabach-Merritt sur angiome en touffes congenital. Ann. Dermatol. Venereol. **125**, 257–260 (1998)
33. Nakamura, E., Ohnishi, T., Watanabe, S., Takahashi, H.: Kasabach-Merritt syndrome associated with angioblastoma. Br. J. Dermatol. **139**, 164–166 (1998)
34. Seo, S.K., Suh, J.C., Na, G.Y., Kim, I.S., Sohn, K.R.: Kasabach-Merritt syndrome: identification of platelet trapping in a tufted angioma by immunohistochemistry technique using monoclonal antibody to CD61. Pediatr. Dermatol. **16**, 392–394 (1999)
35. Enjolras, O., Mulliken, J.B., Wassef, M., Frieden, I.J., Rieu, P.N., Burrows, P.E., Salhi, A., Leaute-Labreze, C., Kozakewich, H.P.: Residual lesions after Kasabach-Merritt phenomenon in 41 patients. J. Am. Acad. Dermatol. **42**, 225–235 (2000)
36. Alvarez-Mendoza, A., Lourdes, T.S., Ridaura-Sanz, C., Ruiz-Maldonado, R.: Histopathology of vascular lesions found in Kasabach-Merritt syndrome: review based on 13 cases. Pediatr. Dev. Pathol. **3**, 556–560 (2000)
37. Croue, A., Habersetzer, M., Leclech, C., Forest, J.L., Saint-Andre, J.P., Verret, J.L.: Le "tufted angioma" (angiome en touffes). Une tumeur vasculaire benigne a differencier du sarcome de Kaposi. Arch. Anat. Cytol. Pathol. **41**, 159–163 (1993)
38. Ban, M., Kamiya, H., Kitajima, Y.: Tufted angioma of adult onset, revealing abundant eccrine glands and central regression. Dermatology **201**, 68–70 (2000)
39. Fukunaga, M.: Intravenous tufted angioma. APMIS **108**, 287–292 (2000)
40. Mentzel, T., Wollina, U., Castelli, E., Kutzner, H.: Buschelartiges Hamangiom ("tufted angioma"). Klinisch-pathologische und immunohistologische Analyse von funf Fallen einer distinkten Entitat im Spektrum der kapillaren Hamangiome. Hautarzt **47**, 369–375 (1996)
41. Miyamoto, T., Mihara, M., Mishima, E., et al.: Acquired tufted angioma showing spontaneous regression. Br. J. Dermatol. **127**, 645–648 (1992)
42. Lam, W.Y., Mac-Moune Lai, F., Look, C.N., Choi, P.C., Allen, P.W.: Tufted angioma with complete regression. J. Cutan. Pathol. **21**, 461–466 (1994)
43. McKenna, K.E., McCusker, G.: Spontaneous regression of a tufted angioma. Clin. Exp. Dermatol. **25**, 656–658 (2000)
44. Verret, J.L., Leclech, C., Croue, A., Forest, J.L., Peria, P.H., Matard, B.: Tufted angioma (angioblastome). Ann. Dermatol. Venereol. **121**, 140 (1994)
45. Frenk, E., Vion, B., Merot, Y., Ruffieux, C.: Tufted angioma. Dermatologica **181**, 242–243 (1990)
46. Munn, S.E., Jackson, J.E., Russell Jones, R.: Tufted haemangioma responding to high-dose systemic steroids: a case report and review of the literature. Clin. Exp. Dermatol. **19**, 511–514 (1994)
47. Suarez, S.M., Pensler, J.M., Paller, A.S.: Response of deep tufted angioma to interferon alpha. J. Am. Acad. Dermatol. **33**, 124–126 (1995)
48. Park, K.C., Ahn, P.S., Lee, Y.S., Kim, K.H., Cho, K.H.: Treatment of angioblastoma with recombinant interferon-alpha 2. Pediatr. Dermatol. **12**, 184–186 (1995)
49. Robenzadeh, A., Don, P.C., Weinberg, J.M.: Treatment of tufted angioma with interferon alfa: role of bFDG. Pediatr. Dermatol. **15**, 482 (1998)
50. Wilmer, A., Kaatz, M., Bocker, T., Wollina, U.: Tufted angioma. Eur. J. Dermatol. **9**, 51–53 (1999)

51. Wollina, U.: Interferon for tufted angioma. Pediatr. Dermatol. **16**, 338 (1999)
52. Fariña, M.C., Torrelo, A., Mediero, I.G., Zambrano, A.: Angioma en penacho. Actas Dermosifiliogr. **87**, 563–567 (1996)

Disease Entities of Arteriovenous Hemangioma

1. Akiyama, M., Inamoto, N.: Arteriovenous haemangioma in chronic liver disease: clinical and histopathological features of four cases. Br. J. Dermatol. **144**, 604–609 (2001)
2. Garzon, M.C., Huang, J.T., Enjolras, O., et al.: Vascular malformations. J. Am. Acad. Dermatol. **56**, 353–370 (2007)
3. Girard, C., Graham, J.H., Johnson, W.C.: Arteriovenous hemangioma (arteriovenous shunt). A clinicopathological and histochemical study. J. Cutan. Pathol. **1**, 73–87 (1974)
4. Kohout, M.P., Hansen, M., Pribaz, J.J., et al.: Arteriovenous malformations of the head and neck: natural history and management. Plast. Reconstr. Surg. **102**, 643–654 (1998)
5. Koutlas, I.G., Jessurun, J.: Arteriovenous hemangioma: a clinicopathological and immunohistochemical study. J. Cutan. Pathol. **21**, 343–349 (1994)

Disease Entities of Cutaneous Angiosarcoma

1. Maddox, J.C., Evans, H.L.: Angiosarcoma of skin and soft tissue: a study of forty-four cases. Cancer **48**(8), 1907–1921 (1981)
2. Shin, S.J., Lesser, M., Rosen, P.P.: Hemangiomas and angiosarcomas of the breast. Arch. Pathol. Lab. Med. **131**, 538–544 (2007)
3. Brown, L.F., Dezube, B.J., Tognazzi, K., Dvorak, H.F., Yancopoulos, G.D.: Expression of Tie 1, Tie2, and angiopoietins 1, 2, and 4 in Kaposi's sarcoma and cutaneous angiosarcoma. Am. J. Pathol. **156**, 2179–2183 (2000)
4. Rao, J., DeKoven, J.G., Beatty, J.D., Jones, G.: Cutaneous angiosarcoma as a delayed complication of radiation therapy for carcinoma of the breast. J. Am. Acad. Dermatol. **49**, 532–538 (2003)
5. Brown, L.F., Tognazzi, K., Dvorak, H.F., Harrist, T.J.: Strong expression of kinase insert domain-containing receptor, a vascular permeability factor/vascular endothelial growth factor receptor in AIDS-associated Kaposi's sarcoma and cutaneous angiosarcoma. Am. J. Pathol. **148**, 1065–1074 (1996)
6. Aguila, L.I., Sanchez, J.L.: Angiosarcoma of the face resembling rhinophyma. J. Am. Acad. Dermatol. **49**, 530–531 (2003)
7. Folpe, A.L., Johnston, C.A., Weiss, S.W.: Cutaneous angiosarcoma arising in a gouty tophus. Am. J. Dermatopathol. **22**(5), 418–421 (2000)
8. Cannavò, S.P., Lentini, M., Magliolo, E., Guarneri, C.: Cutaneous angiosarcoma of the face. J. Eur. Acad. Dermatol. Venereol. **17**, 594–595 (2003)
9. Murray, S., Simmons, I., James, C.: Cutaneous angiosarcoma of the face and scalp presenting as alopecia. Australas. J. Dermatol. **44**, 273–276 (2003)
10. Sinclair, S.A., Sviland, L., Natarajan, S.: Angiosarcoma arising in a chronically lymphoedematous leg. Br. J. Dermatol. **138**, 692–694 (1998)
11. Folpe, A.L., Veikkola, T., Valtola, R., Weiss, S.W.: Vascular endothelial growth factor receptor-3 (VEGFR-3): a marker of vascular tumors with presumed lymphatic differentiation, including Kaposi's

sarcoma, kaposiform and Dabska-type hemangioendotheliomas, and a subset of angiosarcomas. Mod. Pathol. **13**(2), 180–185 (2000)
12. Neisius, U.W., Schuler, G., Lüftl, M.: Lividfarbener tumor am capillitium. Hautarzt **56**, 778–782 (2005)
13. Pawlik, T.M., Paulino, A.F., Mcginn, C.J., Baker, L.H., Cohen, D.S., Morris, J.S., Rees, R., Sondak, V.K.: Cutaneous angiosarcoma of the scalp. Cancer **98**, 1716–1726 (2003)
14. Rich, A.L., Berman, P.: Cutaneous angiosarcoma presenting as an unusual facial bruise. Age Ageing **33**, 512–514 (2004)
15. Den Bakker, M.A., Flood, S.J., Kliffen, M.: CD31 staining in epithelioid sarcoma. Virchows Arch. **443**, 93–97 (2003)
16. Pestoni, C., Paredes-Suarez, C., Peteiro, C., Toribio, J.: Early detection of cutaneous angiosarcoma of the face and scalp and treatment with paclitaxel. J. Eur. Acad. Dermatol. Venereol. **19**, 357–359 (2005)
17. Morgan, M.B., Swann, M., Somach, S., Eng, W., Smoller, B.: Cutaneous angiosarcoma: a case series with prognostic correlation. J. Am. Acad. Dermatol. **50**, 867–874 (2004)
18. Mendenhall, W.M., Mendenhall, C.M., Werning, J.W., Reith, J.D., Mendenhall, N.P.: Cutaneous angiosarcoma. Am. J. Clin. Oncol. **29**, 524–528 (2006)
19. Fink-Puches, R., Smolle, J., Beham, A., Kerl, H., Soyer, H.P.: Kutane Angiosarkome. Hautarzt **51**, 479–485 (2000)
20. Fayette, J., et al.: Angiosarcomas, a heterogeneous group of sarcomas with specific behavior depending on primary site: a retrospective study of 161 cases. Ann. Oncol. **18**(12), 2030–2036 (2007)
30. Vogt, T.: Angiosarkom. Hautarzt **59**, 237–251 (2008)
31. DeMartelaere, S.L., Roberts, D., Burgess, M.A., et al.: Neoadjuvant chemotherapy-specific and overall treatment outcomes in patients with cutaneous angiosarcoma of the face with periorbital involvement. Head Neck **30**(5), 639–646 (2008)
32. Abraham, J.A., Hornicek, F.J., Kaufman, A.M., Harmon, D.C., et al.: Treatment and outcome of 82 patients with angiosarcoma. Ann. Surg. Oncol. **14**(6), 1953–1967 (2007)
33. Mark, R.J., Poen, J.C., Tran, L.M., et al.: Angiosarcoma: a report of sixty-seven patients and a review of the literature. Cancer **77**, 2400–2406 (1996)
34. Stewart, F.W., Treves, N.: Classics in oncology: lymphangiosarcoma in postmastectomy lymphedema: a report of six cases in elephantiasis chirurgica. CA Cancer J. Clin. **31**(5), 284–299 (1981)
35. Braun-Falco, O., Plewig, G., Wolff, H.H., Burgdorf, W.H.C., Landthaler, M.: Dermatologie und Venerologie, 5th edn. Springer, Berlin (2005)

Lymphatic Tumors

1. Belov, S.: Classification of congenital vascular defects. Int. Angiol. **9**, 141–146 (1990)
2. Browse, N.L., Whimster, I., Stewart, G., Helm, C.W., Wood, J.J.: Surgical management of "lymphangioma circumscriptum. Br. J. Surg. **73**, 585–588 (1986)
3. Enjolras, O., Mulliken, J.B.: The current management of vascular birthmarks. Pediatr. Dermatol. **10**, 311–313 (1993)
4. Greinwald Jr., J., Cohen, A.P., Hemanackah, S., Azizkhan, R.G.: Massive lymphatic malformations of the head, neck and chest. J. Otolyryngol. Head Neck Surg. **37**, 169–173 (2008)
5. Khanna, G., Sato, Y., Smith, R.J., Bauman, N.M., Nerad, J.: Causes of facial swelling in pediatric patients: correlation of clinical and radiologic findings. Radiographics **26**, 157–171 (2006)
6. Landthaler, M., Hohenleutner, U.: Classifications of vascular abnormalities and neoplasms. Hautarzt **48**, 622–628 (1997)
7. Mulliken, J.B., Glowacki, J.: Hemangiomas and vascular malformations in infants and children: a classification based on endothelial characteristics. Plast. Reconstr. Surg. **69**, 412–422 (1982)

8. Stewart, C.J., Chan, T., Platten, M.: Acquired lymphangiectasia ("lymphangioma circumscriptum") of the vulva: a report of eight cases. Pathology **26**, 1–6 (2009)
9. Weber, J.: Invasive radiological diagnostic of congenital vascular malformations (CVM). Int. Angiol. **9**, 168–174 (1990)
10. Whimster, I.: The pathology of lymphangioma circumscriptum. Br. J. Dermatol. **94**, 473–486 (1976)
11. Yeager, N.D., Hammond, S., Mahan, J., Davis, J.T., Adler, B.: Unique diagnostic features and successful management of a patient with disseminated lymphangiomatosis and chylothorax. J. Pediatr. Hematol. Oncol. **30**, 66–69 (2009)
12. Yoo, J.C., Ahn, Y., Lim, Y.S., Hah, J.H., Kwon, T.K., Sung, M.W., Kim, K.H.: OK-432 sclerotherapy in head and neck lymphangiomas: long-term follow-up result. Otolaryngol. Head Neck Surg. **140**, 120–123 (2009)

Smooth and Skeletal Muscle Tumors

1. Gökdemir, G., Altunay, I.K., Köslü, A., et al.: A case of multiple facial painless leiomyomata. J. Eur. Acad. Dermatol. Venereol. **14**, 144–145 (2000)
2. Jolliffe, D.S.: Multiple cutaneous leiomyomata. Clin. Exp. Dermatol. **3**, 89–92 (1978)
3. Latoni, J.D., Neuburg, M., Matloub, H.S.: Pilar leiomyoma: a case report and review of the literature. Ann. Plast. Surg. **45**, 662–664 (2000)
4. Mahalingam, M., Goldberg, L.J.: Atypical pilar leiomyoma: cutaneous counterpart of uterine symplastic leiomyoma? Am. J. Dermatopathol. **23**, 299–303 (2001)
5. Newman, P.L., Fletcher, C.D.: Smooth muscle tumors of the external genitalia: clinicopathological analysis of a series. Histopathology **18**, 523–529 (1991)
6. Sahoo, B., Radotra, B.D., Kaur, I., et al.: Zosteriform pilar leiomyoma. J. Dermatol. **28**, 759–761 (2001)
7. Spencer, J.M., Amonette, R.A.: Tumors with smooth muscle differentiation. Dermatol. Surg. **22**, 761–768 (1996)
8. Thyresson, H.N., Su, W.P.: Familial cutaneous leiomyomatosis. J. Am. Acad. Dermatol. **4**, 430–434 (1981)

Smooth and Skeletal Muscle Tumors

1. Weedon, D., Williamson, R.M., Patterson, J.W.: Smooth and skeletal muscle tumors. In: LeBoit, P.E., Burg, G., Sarasin, A. (eds.) World Health Organization Classification of Tumors Skin Tumors, pp. 250–253. IARC, Lyon (2006)
2. Weiss, S.W., Goldblum, J.R.: Leiomyosarcoma. In: Weiss, S.W., Goldblum, J.R. (eds.) Enzinger and Weiss's Soft Tissue Tumors, 5th edn, pp. 545–564. Mosby Elsevier, St. Louis (2008)
3. Bellezza, G., Sidoni, A., Cavaliere, A., Scheibel, M., Bucciarelli, E.: Primary cutaneous leiomyosarcoma: a clinicopathological and immunohistochemical study of 7 cases. Int. J. Surg. Pathol. **12**(1), 39–44 (2004)
4. Jensen, M.L., Jensen, O.M., Michalski, W., Nielsen, O.S., Keller, J.: Intradermal and subcutaneous leiomyosarcoma: a clinicopathological and immunohistochemical study of 41 cases. J. Cutan. Pathol. **23**(5), 458–463 (1996)
5. Kaddu, S., Beham, A., Cerroni, L., Humer-Fuchs, U., Salmhofer, W., Kerl, H., et al.: Cutaneous leiomyosarcoma. Am. J. Surg. Pathol. **21**(9), 979–987 (1997)

6. Humphreys, T.R., Finkelstein, D.H., Lee, J.B.: Superficial leiomyosarcoma treated with Mohs micrographic surgery. Dermatol. Surg. **30**(1), 108–112 (2004)

Fibrous, Fibrohistiocytic and Histiocytic Tumors

1. LeBoit, P.E., Burg, G., Weedon, D., Sarasin, A. (eds.): Pathology and Genetics of Skin Tumors. IARC, Lyon (2006)
2. Weyers, W., Mentzel, T., Kasper, R.C., et al.: Fibrous, fibrohistiocytic and histiocytic tumors. In: LeBoit, P.E., Burg, G., Sarasin, A. (eds.) World Health Organization Classification of Tumors. Skin Tumors, pp. 254–262. IARC Press, Lyon (2006)
3. Fletcher CDM, Unni KK, Mertens F (eds.) So-called fibrohistiocytic tumors. In: World Health Organization Classification of Tumors. Tumors of Soft Tissue and Bone, pp. 109–26. IARC, Lyon (2002)
4. Kamino, H., Reddy, V.B., Gero, M., et al.: Dermatomyofibroma. A benign cutaneous, plaque-like proliferation of fibroblasts and myofibroblasts in young adults. J. Cutan. Pathol. **19**, 85–93 (1992)
5. Williams, J.O., Schrum, D.: Congenital fibrosarcoma; report of a case in a newborn infant. AMA Arch. Pathol. **51**, 548–552 (1951)
6. Stout, A.P.: Juvenile fibromatoses. Cancer **7**, 953–978 (1954)
7. Chung, E.B., Enzinger, F.M.: Infantile myofibromatosis. Cancer **48**, 1807–1818 (1981)
8. Dimson, O.G., Drolet, B.A., Southern, J.F., et al.: Congenital generalized myofibromatosis in a neonate. Arch. Dermatol. **136**, 597–600 (2000)
9. Wiswell, T.E., Davis, J., Cunningham, B.E., et al.: Infantile myofibromatosis: the most common fibrous tumor of infancy. J. Pediatr. Surg. **23**, 315–318 (1988)
10. Rubin, B.P., Brodge, J.A.: Myofibroma/Myofibromatosis. In: Fletcher, C.D.M., Unni, K.K., Mertens, F. (eds.) World Health Organization Classification of Tumors. Tumors of Soft Tissue and Bone, pp. 59–61. IARC Press, Lyon (2002)
11. Weiss SW, Goldblum JR (eds.) Fibrous tumors of infancy and childhood. In: Enzinger and Weiss's Soft Tissue Tumors, 5th edn, pp. 257–302. Mosby Elsevier, St. Louis (2008)
12. Granter, S.R., Badizadegan, K., Fletcher, C.D.: Myofibromatosis in adults, glomangiopericytoma, and myopericytoma: a spectrum of tumors showing perivascular myoid differentiation. Am. J. Surg. Pathol. **22**, 513–525 (1998)
13. Zand, D.J., Huff, D., Everman, D., et al.: Autosomal dominant inheritance of infantile myofibromatosis. Am. J. Med. Genet. A **126A**, 261–266 (2004)
14. Rapini, R.P., Golitz, L.E.: Sclerotic fibromas of the skin. J. Am. Acad. Dermatol. **20**, 266–271 (1989)
15. Weiss SW, Goldblum JR (eds.) Benign fibroblastic/myofibroblastic proliferations. In: Enzinger and Weiss's Soft Tissue Tumors, 5th edn, pp. 175–225. Mosby Elsevier, St. Louis (2008)
16. Al-Daraji, W.I., Ramsay, H.M., Ali, R.B.: Storiform collagenoma as a clue for Cowden disease or PTEN hamartoma tumor syndrome. J. Clin. Pathol. **60**, 840–842 (2007)
17. Pujol, R.M., de Castro, F., Schroeter, A.L., et al.: Solitary sclerotic fibroma of the skin: a sclerotic dermatofibroma? Am. J. Dermatopathol. **18**, 620–624 (1996)
18. Kamino, H., Lee, J.Y., Berke, A.: Pleomorphic fibroma of the skin: a benign neoplasm with cytologic atypia. A clinicopathologic study of eight cases. Am. J. Surg. Pathol. **13**, 107–113 (1989)
19. Garcia-Doval, I., Casas, L., Toribio, J.: Pleomorphic fibroma of the skin, a form of sclerotic fibroma: an immunohistochemical study. Clin. Exp. Dermatol. **23**, 22–24 (1998)

20. Weiss SW, Goldblum JR (eds.) Fibrohistiocytic tumors of intermediate malignancy. In: Enzinger and Weiss's Soft Tissue Tumors, 5th edn, pp. 371–402. Mosby Elsevier, St. Louis (2008).

21. Abbott, J.J., Oliveira, A.M., Nascimento, A.G.: The prognostic significance of fibrosarcomatous transformation in dermatofibrosarcoma protuberans. Am. J. Surg. Pathol. 30, 436–443 (2006)

22. Mentzel, T., Beham, A., Katenkamp, D., et al.: Fibrosarcomatous ("high-grade") dermatofibrosarcoma protuberans: clinicopathologic and immunohistochemical study of a series of 41 cases with emphasis on prognostic significance. Am. J. Surg. Pathol. 22, 576–587 (1998)

23. Pedeutour, F., Simon, M.P., Minoletti, F., et al.: Translocation, t(17;22)(q22;q13), in dermatofibrosarcoma protuberans: a new tumor-associated chromosome rearrangement. Cytogenet. Cell Genet. 72, 171–174 (1996)

24. O'Brien, K.P., Seroussi, E., Dal Cin, P., et al.: Various regions within the alpha-helical domain of the COL1A1 gene are fused to the second exon of the PDGFB gene in dermatofibrosarcomas and giant-cell fibroblastomas. Genes Chromosomomes Cancer 23, 187–193 (1998)

25. Nakanishi, G., Lin, S.N., Asagoe, K., et al.: A novel fusion gene of collagen type I alpha 1 (exon 31) and platelet-derived growth factor B-chain (exon 2) in dermatofibrosarcoma protuberans. Eur. J. Dermatol. 17, 217–219 (2007)

26. Suit, H., Spiro, I., Mankin, H.J., et al.: Radiation in management of patients with dermatofibrosarcoma protuberans. J. Clin. Oncol. 14, 2365–2369 (1996)

27. McArthur, G.A., Demetri, G.D., van Oosterom, A., et al.: Molecular and clinical analysis of locally advanced dermatofibrosarcoma protuberans treated with imatinib: Imatinib Target Exploration Consortium Study B2225. J. Clin. Oncol. 23, 866–873 (2005)

28. Gloster Jr., H.M., Harris, K.R., Roenigk, R.K.: A comparison between Mohs micrographic surgery and wide surgical excision for the treatment of dermatofibrosarcoma protuberans. J. Am. Acad. Dermatol. 35, 82–87 (1996)

29. Zelger, B.G., Zelger, B.: Dermatofibroma (fibrous histiocytoma): an inflammatory or neoplastic disorder? Histopathology 38, 379–381 (2001)

30. Calonje, E.: Is cutaneous benign fibrous histiocytoma (dermatofibroma) a reactive inflammatory process or a neoplasm? Histopathology 37, 278–280 (2000)

31. Newman, D.M., Walter, J.B.: Multiple dermatofibromas in patients with systemic lupus erythematosus on immunosuppressive therapy. N Engl J. Med. 289, 842–843 (1973)

32. Zaballos, P., Puig, S., Llambrich, A., et al.: Dermoscopy of dermatofibromas: a prospective morphological study of 412 cases. Arch. Dermatol. 144, 75–83 (2008)

33. Zaballos, P., Llambrich, A., Ara, M., et al.: Dermoscopic findings of haemosiderotic and aneurysmal dermatofibroma: report of six patients. Br. J. Dermatol. 154, 244–250 (2006)

34. Weiss, S.W., Goldblum, J.R.: Benign fibrohistiocytic tumors. In: Weiss, S.W., Goldblum, J.R. (eds.) Enzinger and Weiss`s Soft Tissue Tumors, 5th edn, pp. 331–370. Mosby Elsevier, Philadelphia (2008)

35. Chen, T.C., Kuo, T., Chan, H.L.: Dermatofibroma is a clonal proliferative disease. J. Cutan. Pathol. 27, 36–39 (2000)

36. Hui, P., Glusac, E.J., Sinard, J.H., et al.: Clonal analysis of cutaneous fibrous histiocytoma (dermatofibroma). J. Cutan. Pathol. 29, 385–389 (2002)

37. Vanni, R., Fletcher, C.D., Sciot, R., et al.: Cytogenetic evidence of clonality in cutaneous benign fibrous histiocytomas: a report of the CHAMP study group. Histopathology 37, 212–217 (2000)

38. Guillou, L., Gebhard, S., Salmeron, M., et al.: Metastasizing fibrous histiocytoma of the skin: a clinicopathologic and immunohistochemical analysis of three cases. Mod. Pathol. 13, 654–660 (2000)

39. Evans, J., Clarke, T., Mattacks, C.A., et al.: Dermatofibromas and arthropod bites: is there any evidence to link the two? Lancet 2, 36–37 (1989)

40. Shmookler, B.M., Enzinger, F.M., Weiss, S.W.: Giant cell fibroblastoma. A juvenile form of dermatofibrosarcoma protuberans. Cancer 64, 2154–2161 (1989)

41. Fletcher, C.D.: Giant cell fibroblastoma of soft tissue: a clinicopathological and immunohistochemical study. Histopathology 13, 499–508 (1988)

42. Maeda, T., Hirose, T., Furuya, K., et al.: Giant cell fibroblastoma associated with dermatofibrosarcoma protuberans: a case report. Mod. Pathol. 11, 491–495 (1998)

43. Shimizu, A., O'Brien, K.P., Sjoblom, T., et al.: The dermatofibrosarcoma protuberans-associated collagen type I alpha1/platelet-derived growth factor (PDGF) B-chain fusion gene generates a transforming protein that is processed to functional PDGF-BB. Cancer Res. 59, 3719–3723 (1999)

44. Sirvent, N., Maire, G., Pedeutour, F.: Genetics of dermatofibrosarcoma protuberans family of tumors: from ring chromosomes to tyrosine kinase inhibitor treatment. Genes Chromosomes Cancer 37, 1–19 (2003)

Neural Tumors

Jürgen C. Becker and Herman Kneitz

3.7.1 Merkel Cell Carcinoma

Merkel cell carcinoma (MCC) is a very aggressive neuroendocrine carcinoma of the skin [1]. In 1972 Toker described five patients with unusual skin tumors where histologically anastomosing trabeculae and cell nests in the dermis dominated, so that he used the name "trabecular carcinoma of the skin" [2].

3.7.1.1 Clinical Features

MCC characteristically develops rapidly over weeks to months on chronic sun-damaged skin as an asymptomatic, firm-elastic hemispherical tumor with a smooth, shiny surface [3]. The majority of patients state in their case history a rapid growth of the tumor within 3 months. The most common color of the primary lesion is red/pink, seen in more than half of the patients; a blue/violaceous color of the tumors is noted in a quarter of the patients. The typical clinical features of MCC can be explained by the fact that the tumor usually grows in a hemispherical fashion to the outside and in an iceberg-like fashion into the deep, so that the intact epidermis is stretched. In addition to the frequent hemispherical or nodular forms, more rarely plaque-like variants occur, especially on the trunk. Most primary tumors are located on sun-exposed skin, i.e., head and neck, lower limbs, and upper extremities; however, the tumors may also be present on the buttock or other minimally sun-exposed areas [1]. Moreover, nodal disease in the setting of no identified primary tumor may be the first presentation of disease in more than 10% of the patients. Even initially MCC grows in an infiltrating manner, but ulcerations are very rare and are observed only in very advanced tumors. Satellite metastases can occur quite early.

Recently, Heath et al. reported the presumed clinical diagnosis of subsequently confirmed series of 106 patients with MCC [4]. The majority (56%) of clinical impressions were benign: A cyst or acneiform lesion was the single most common presumptive diagnosis (32%), followed by lipoma (6%), dermatofibroma or fibroma (4%), and vascular lesion (4%). Malignant diagnoses comprised an additional 36% of presumptive diagnoses, e.g., nonmelanoma skin cancer lymphoma, metastatic carcinoma, and sarcoma. Notably, the correct clinical diagnosis of MCC was made presumptively in only two cases. Prompted by this disturbing observation, Heath et al. proposed five clinical features that may serve as clues for the diagnosis of MCC: asymptomatic/lack of tenderness, expanding rapidly, immunosuppression, older than 50 years, and location on an ultraviolet-exposed site. At least three of these features, which can be memorized by the acronym AEIOU, were present in almost 90% of their series of MCC cases [4].

3.7.1.2 Histopathology

Due to the relatively uncharacteristic features of MCC, the diagnosis in most cases is first made on the basis of histopathology [5]. Histologically, MCC appears as an asymmetric dermal tumor with irregular margins composed of tumor cells arranged in strands or nests [6]. The tumor spreads into the reticular dermis and subcutis; the papillary dermis, epidermis, and adnexa are usually spared. In the hematoxylin-eosin stain the cells are monomorphous and display a typical nuclear chromatin pattern (Fig. 3.7.1). The tumor cells are characterized by a large, relatively pale nucleus. The cytoplasm is scant and contains argyrophil granules and often displays thread-like extensions. A further criterion is paranuclear plaques consisting of whorls of intermediate filaments [7]. The mitotic index is very high and many atypical mitoses are seen. According to the arrangement and appearance of the tumor cells three histologic patterns are

J.C. Becker (✉) and H. Kneitz
J.C. Becker (✉) and H. Kneitz
Dept. General Dermatology, Medical University of Graz,
Auenbruggerplatz 8, A-8010 Graz, Austria
e-mail: juergen.becker@medunigraz.at

R. Dummer et al. (eds.), *Skin Cancer – A World-Wide Perspective*,
DOI: 10.1007/978-3-642-05072-5_3.7, © Springer-Verlag Berlin Heidelberg 2011

differentiated: the trabecular, the intermediate, and the small cell type. The trabecular type originally described by Toker is relatively rare with about 10%; the tumor cells are somewhat larger than in the other types and grow in a distinct trabecular fashion in the dermis [8]. The intermediate type is the most frequent (about 80%); the tumor cells are medium-sized and possess large, lobed nuclei and scant, pale stained cytoplasm. The tumor cells of small cell MCC are small and possess a hyperchromatic nucleus; the small cell type occurs in about 10% of cases. Mixed and transitional forms between the three types are very frequent. The tumor cell formations, especially in the trabecular type, but

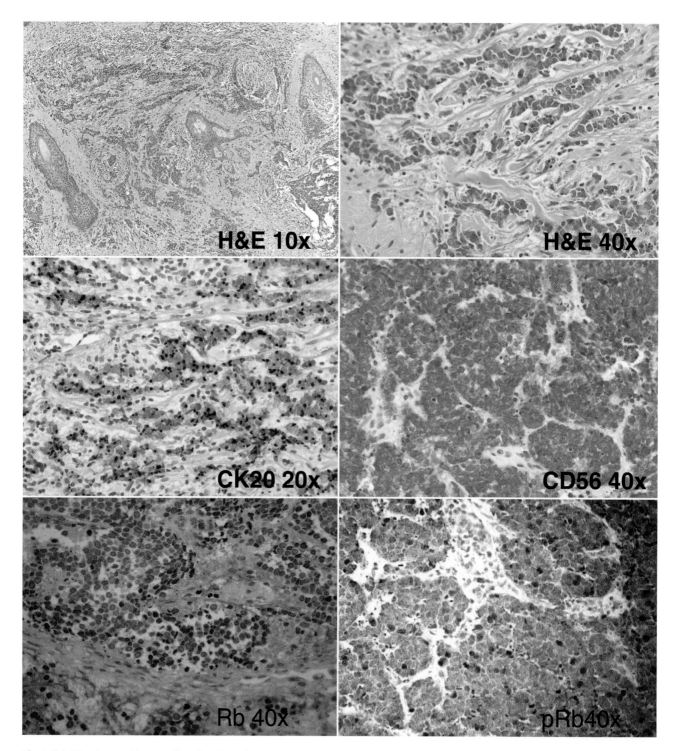

Fig. 3.7.1 Histology and immunohistochemistry of Merkel cell carcinoma

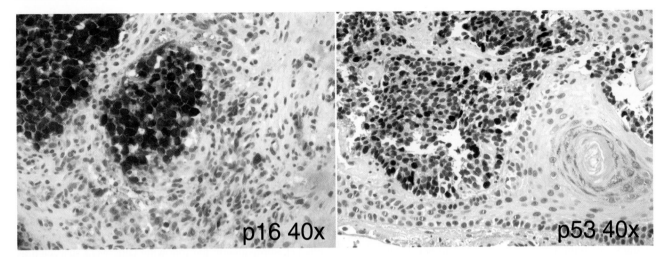

Fig. 3.7.1 (continued)

also in the intermediate type, are interrupted by connective tissue septa.

Due to the uncharacteristic histomorphologic cellular features of MCC, immunohistochemistry is required for definitive diagnosis (Fig. 3.7.1) [5]. This is especially necessary to differentiate histologic differential diagnoses such as small cell lung cancer, small B-cell lymphomas, or anaplastic small cell melanomas. In general, the immunohistochemical identification of cytokeratin (CK) 20 and neuron-specific enolase (NSE) is performed, with the former being quite specific but not always positive and the latter usually positive but relatively unspecific. These tests are combined with stains for leukocyte common antigen (LCA), thyroid transcription factor 1 (TTF-1), and vimentin, which are usually negative (Table 3.7.1) [8]. CK20 is found in the tumor cells in a remarkable paranuclear plaque (dot-like pattern) as well as to a significantly less extent along the cytoskeleton. Further, the tumor cells of MCC display additional antigens in varying frequency and intensity; these include, among others, chromogranin A, synaptophysin, tenascin-C, CD56, as well as various neurofilaments and neuropeptides. Expression of the inhibitor of apoptosis (IAP) survivin and the member of the p53 family, p63, appears to be associated with a poorer prognosis [9–11]. Transmission electron microscopy reveals characteristic electron-dense cytoplasmic granules (diameter about 100 nm) as well as intermediate filaments [8].

3.7.1.3 Staging

MCC prognosis is highly associated with the stage of disease at presentation. The stage classification for MCC is not uniformly defined. Usually the stage classification shown in Table 3.7.2 is employed [5]. Disease-specific survival for local disease (stage I) is greater than 90%, decreasing to 52% with nodal involvement (stage II). In stage III, i.e., presence of distant metastases, expected survival is typically less than 10% at 3 years [12].

Table 3.7.1 Immunohistochemistry of Merkel cell carcinoma (MCC)

	MCC	B-cell lymphoma	Melanoma	Small cell lung cancer
CK 20	+[a]	–	–	–
Vimentin	–	+	+	–
Neurofilaments	+[b]	–	–	–
Chromogranin A (CgA)	±	–	–	(±)[c]
Neuron-specific enolase (NSE)	+	–	+	±
S100	–	(±)[c]	+	–
Leukocyte common antigen (LCA)	–	+	–	–
Thyroid transcription factor 1 (TTF-1)	–	–	–	+

[a]Plaques; [b]in the majority of cases; [c]in rare cases

Table 3.7.2 Stage classification of MCC

Stage	Primary tumor
Ia	Diameter <2 cm
Ib	Diameter >2 cm
II	Locoregional metastases
III	Distant metastases

For initial staging the current guidelines recommend ultrasonography of the draining lymph nodes and the abdomen as well as a chest X-ray [5]. Further imaging should be considered for unclear findings. Due to the high frequency of lymphatic metastases, sentinel lymph node biopsy is generally performed and reveals micrometastatic involvement in about 25% of cases [13, 14]. The presence of micrometastases in the sentinel lymph nodes appears to denote poorer prognosis. When distant metastases are expected, appropriate imaging of the various organs should be performed [15]. Somatostatin receptor scintigraphy does not appear very suited to determine tumor spread. The value of the recently introduced ^{68}Gallium-DOTATOC PET is currently being investigated [16].

Most recurrences occur within 2 years after the diagnosis of the primary tumor [1, 17]. Retrospective studies on over 400 patients reported in the literature reveal the following unfavorable prognostic factors: advanced tumor stage (locoregional metastases or distant metastases), male gender, location of the primary tumor in the head and neck region or on the trunk, and presence of immunosuppression. Prognostic significance is also assigned to the histological type: the trabecular type is the best differentiated, while the small cell type is least differentiated; measuring tumor thickness also appears to allow for prognostic classification [8]. Further histologic characteristics of prognostic significance are the presence or absence of tumor-infiltrating lymphocytes as well as the overexpression of p63 or survivin [7, 9–11].

To date no scientifically founded studies on follow-up of MCC exist. In most German departments of dermatology in the first year tight control in short intervals of 6 weeks is done due to the risk of local recurrences and regional lymph node metastases [1]. After this, in the following year, follow-up is done quarterly and later in half-year intervals. In the course of follow-up, in addition to clinical examination with lymph node, palpation lymph node sonography, especially of the regional lymph node basins, is performed. Once-yearly abdominal sonography and a chest X-ray or perhaps other forms of imaging are performed. The role of determining serum markers such as, for example, chromogranin A or NSE, to improve evaluation of prognosis or early detection of metastases is unclear [5].

3.7.2 Granular Cell Tumor

Granular cell tumor (GCT) was originally described as granular cell myoblastoma and was believed to be of myogenic origin [1]; thus, GCT is also known as myoblastoma or Abrikossoff's tumor. GCT is a very rare disease. In general, it appears as a singular benign lesion; however, anecdotal cases of malignant multicentric forms have been reported [2]. Whether true GCT may be indeed malignant is somewhat controversial. In any case, GCT may be multicentric, occasionally shows pleomorphism and mitotic activity, or recurs, thereby causing concern for malignancy.

The genesis of the GCT is uncertain. In the beginning, Abrikossoff considered myoblastic stem cells as originating cells [1]; subsequently the following cells were suspected as precursory in the histogenesis of GCT: neural cells, fibroblasts, undifferentiated mesenchymal cells, and Schwann cells [3, 4]. It was suggested that the GCT could develop from a variety of cells that have the ability to take the form of the histiocytes and the phagocytes. The most substantiated hypothesis, however, is that GCT is a consequence of altered cellular metabolism of the Schwann cells or of their precursors. This notion is supported by the constant presence of the protein S-100.

GCT typically occurs in the skin and the subcutis, along mucosal surfaces, and occasionally within the skeletal muscle [2, 4, 5]. Clinically, it appears as a firm solitary nodular lesion, with a 5–20 mm diameter that slowly grows. It is generally asymptomatic, but in rare cases some pruritic, painful, and/or tender tumors have been found, mainly on the hands and fingers. The age range most commonly affected by GCT is from the second to sixth decades of life, with an average age of 50 years. However, GCT may also appear in children: in a series of 95 cases, 12 patients (12.6%) were younger than 19 years old [6>]. It occurs twice as often in women than in men [2, 4, 5]. The lesion generally appears in solitary form. Still, the incidence of multiple GCT occurring either synchronously or metachronously, compared to the total number of GCTs, is 4–30% [7, 8]. Notably, more than 30 cases of multiple GCT in children have been described; interestingly in about one third of these the GCT was in association with somatic defects, which could involve various organs, e.g., the skin, the cardiovascular system, the musculoskeletal tissues, and the nerve tissues [9–11]. Moreover, multiple GCT in pediatric patients may be associated with genetic syndromes, such as neurofibromatosis type I or Noonan syndrome, and familial cases have been described [12, 13].

In the first description of GCT, Abrikossoff reported a lesion of the tongue [1]; subsequently other authors reported cases with tumors located in different sites, including nose, oral cavity, breast, respiratory system, gastrointestinal system, urinary system, female genitals, uvea, neurohypophysis, and central and peripheral nervous systems [14–19]. Thus, the clinical differential diagnoses are manifold.

Indeed, in a comprehensive review of historic cases filed in the Departments of Pathology at the National Naval Medical and Dental Centers and the Georgetown University Hospital over a period spanning more than 30 years, Lack et al. noted that the correct preoperative diagnosis was made in only three patients, and in each, the tumor was located on the dorsum of the tongue [5]. The clinical diagnosis most frequently made was fibroma or sebaceous cyst; fibroadenoma was suspected in half of the women with GCT arising in breast parenchyma; in three cases a clinical diagnosis of carcinoma was made.

Histologically, GCT consists of polymorphous polygonal cells with a small round nucleus or oval hyperchromatic with one or two nuclei [4]. The tumor cells have a low mitotic index. Their cytoplasm contains an abundant granular eosinophilic substance. The cells usually are periodic acid-Schiff (PAS)-positive. Immunhistochemistry in virtually all cases reveals a constant diffuse positivity for S-100 protein, CD68, and Galectin-3 [3, 20] (Fig. 3.7.2). HBME-1 is positive in about 95% of cases. Distinction from several other benign and malignant neoplasms that may show granular cell features, such as smooth muscle, vascular, fibrohistiocytic, true histiocytic, and melanocytic proliferations, is extremely important with regard to treatment and prognosis [3, 20].

Malignancy of GCT should be clinically suspected if rapid growth, broad dimensions (>4 cm), and necrotic/hemorrhagic areas are present [2, 21, 22]. Histological suspicious facts are a high mitotic index, as well as cellular and nuclear pleomorphism. In the cases of malignant GCT, the organs most affected by metastasis are the local lymph nodes, the bony tissue, the peripheral nerves, the peritoneal cavity, and the lungs. Notably, cases of metastasis have also been discovered 14 years after identification of the primary lesion [3, 20].

The treatment of choice for GCT is surgical; it consists of local excision of the tumor with the adjacent mucosa/skin and periosteum [23]. A reliable preoperative estimate of the features suggestive of malignancy would be important for surgical planning. Tumor size, patient age at presentation,

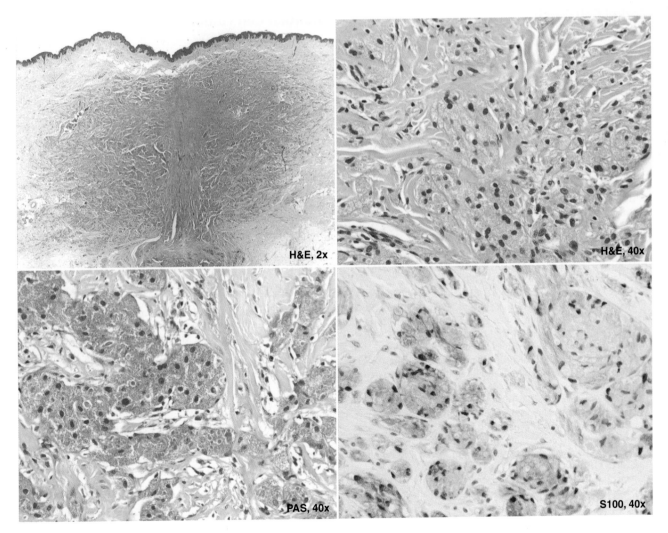

Fig. 3.7.2 Histological and Immunhistological Morphology of Granular Cell Tumor

and tumor location may provide some indication of behavior. Diagnosis and prognostication based on findings from preoperative fine-needle aspiration biopsy are hampered by the fact that the cytologic features of malignant GCT have not been well defined yet [24]. If the preoperative histological diagnosis suggests a malignant transformation, a local lymphadenoidectomy may be considered. Local reappearance after incomplete excision occurs in 15% of cases, whereas true relapse occurs only in 1–3% of cases. Mohs micrographic surgery as a highly effective treatment for cutaneous neoplasms when tissue conservation is crucial may be considered for GCT in particular locations where only limited safety margins are possible [25, 26]. Whether radio- or chemotherapy is advisable in treating malignant and metastatic forms of GCT remains an unsolved issue.

References

Merkel Cell Carcinoma

1. Weller, K., Vetter-Kauzcok, C., Kähler, K., Hauschild, A., Eigentler, T., Pföhler, C., Neuber, K., Moll, I., Krause, M., Kneisel, L., Nashan, D., Thoelke, A., Letsch, B., Näher, H., Becker, J.C.: Umsetzung von Leitlinien bei seltenen Erkrankungen am Beispiel des Merkelzellkarzinoms. Guideline implementation in Merkel cell carcinoma: an example of a rare disease. Dtsch. Arztebl. 103, 2791–2796 (2006)
2. Toker, C.: Trabecular carcinoma of the skin. Arch. Dermatol. 105, 107–110 (1972)
3. Poulsen, M.: Merkel-cell carcinoma of the skin. Lancet Oncol. 5, 593–599 (2004)
4. Heath, M., Jaimes, N., Lemos, B., Mostaghimi, A., Wang, L.C., Penas, P.F., Nghiem, P.: Clinical characteristics of Merkel cell carcinoma at diagnosis in 195 patients: the AEIOU features. J. Am. Acad. Dermatol. 58, 375–381 (2008)
5. Becker, J.C., Mauch, C., Kortmann, R.D., keilholz, U., Bootz, F., Garbe, C., Hauschild, A., Moll, I.: Short German guidelines: Merkel cell carcinoma. JDDG 6(S1), 15–16 (2008)
6. Bickle, K., Glass, L.F., Messina, J.L., Fenske, N.A., Siegrist, K.: Merkel cell carcinoma: a clinical, histopathologic, and immunohistochemical review. Semin. Cutan. Med. Surg. 23, 46–53 (2004)
7. Llombart, B., Monteagudo, C., Lopez-Guerrero, J.A., Carda, C., Jorda, E., Sanmartin, O., Almenar, S., Molina, I., Martin, J.M., Llombart-Bosch, A.: Clinicopathological and immunohistochemical analysis of 20 cases of Merkel cell carcinoma in search of prognostic markers. Histopathology 46, 622–634 (2005)
8. Plaza, J.A., Suster, S.: The Toker tumor: spectrum of morphologic features in primary neuroendocrine carcinomas of the skin (Merkel cell carcinoma). Ann. Diagn. Pathol. 10, 376–385 (2006)
9. Asioli, S., Righi, A., Volante, M., Eusebi, V., Bussolati, G.: p63 expression as a new prognostic marker in Merkel cell carcinoma. Cancer 110, 640–647 (2007)
10. Kim, J., McNiff, J.M.: Nuclear expression of survivin portends a poor prognosis in Merkel cell carcinoma. Mod. Pathol. 21, 764–769 (2008)
11. Tucci, M.G., Lucarini, G., Giangiacomi, M., Zizzi, A., Criante, P., Ricotti, G., Biagini, G.: Immunohistochemical study of apoptosis

markers and involvement of chemokine CXCR4 in skin Merkel cell carcinoma. J. Eur. Acad. Dermatol. Venereol. 20, 1220–1225 (2006)
12. Agelli, M., Clegg, L.X.: Epidemiology of primary Merkel cell carcinoma in the United States. J. Am. Acad. Dermatol. 49, 832–841 (2003)
13. Civantos, F.J., Moffat, F.L., Goodwin, W.J.: Lymphatic mapping and sentinel lymphadenectomy for 106 head and neck lesions: contrasts between oral cavity and cutaneous malignancy. Laryngoscope 112, 1–15 (2006)
14. Ortin-Perez, J., van Rijk, M.C., Valdes-Olmos, R.A., Vidal-Sicart, S., Nieweg, O.E., Vilalta, A., Kroon, B.B., Pons, F.: Lymphatic mapping and sentinel node biopsy in Merkel's cell carcinoma. Eur. J. Surg. Oncol. 33, 119–122 (2007)
15. Nguyen, B.D., McCullough, A.E.: Imaging of Merkel cell carcinoma. Radiographics 22, 367–376 (2002)
16. Gabriel, M., Decristoforo, C., Kendler, D., Dobrozemsky, G., Heute, D., Uprimny, C., Kovacs, P., Von Guggenberg, E., Bale, R., Virgolini, I.J.: 68Ga-DOTA-Tyr3-octreotide PET in neuroendocrine tumors: comparison with somatostatin receptor scintigraphy and CT. J. Nucl. Med. 48, 508–518 (2007)
17. Hodgson, N.C.: Merkel cell carcinoma: changing incidence trends. J. Surg. Oncol. 89, 1–4 (2005)

Granular Cell Tumor

1. Abrikossoff, A.: Über myome, ausgehened von der quergestreiften willkürlichen muskulatur. Virchows Arch. 260, 215–223 (1926)
2. Khansur, T., Balducci, L., Tavassoli, M.: Granular cell tumor. Clinical spectrum of the benign and malignant entity. Cancer 60, 220–222 (1987)
3. Le, B.H., Boyer, P.J., Lewis, J.E., Kapadia, S.B.: Granular cell tumor: immunohistochemical assessment of inhibin-alpha, protein gene product 9.5, S100 protein, CD68, and Ki-67 proliferative index with clinical correlation. Arch. Pathol. Lab. Med. 128, 771–775 (2004)
4. Ordonez, N.G.: Granular cell tumor: a review and update. Adv. Anat. Pathol. 6, 186–203 (1999)
5. Lack, E.E., Worsham, G.F., Callihan, M.D., Crawford, B.E., Klappenbach, S., Rowden, G., Chun, B.: Granular cell tumor: a clinicopathologic study of 110 patients. J. Surg. Oncol. 13, 301–316 (1980)
6. Strong, E.W., McDivitt, R.W., Brasfield, R.D.: Granular cell myoblastoma. Cancer 25, 415–422 (1970)
7. Curtis, B.V., Calcaterra, T.C., Coulson, W.F.: Multiple granular cell tumor: a case report and review of the literature. Head Neck 19, 634–637 (1997)
8. Gross, V.L., Lynfield, Y.: Multiple cutaneous granular cell tumors: a case report and review of the literature. Cutis 69, 343–346 (2002)
9. Muscardin, L.M., Paradisi, M., Provini, A., Cota, C., Marzetti, G.: Multiple cutaneous granular cell tumors, joint hypermobility and mild facial dysmorphism in a child. Int. J. Dermatol. 45, 847–850 (2006)
10. Seiter, S., Ugurel, S., Tilgen, W., Reinhold, U.: Multiple granular cell tumors and growth hormone deficiency in a child. Pediatr. Dermatol. 16, 308–310 (1999)
11. Tomson, N., Abdullah, A., Tan, C.Y.: Multiple granular cell tumors in a child with growth retardation. Report of a case and review of the literature. Int. J. Dermatol. 45, 1358–1361 (2006)
12. Bakos, L.: Multiple cutaneous granular cell tumors with systemic defects: a distinct entity? Int. J. Dermatol. 32, 432–435 (1993)
13. Martin III, R.W., Neldner, K.H., Boyd, A.S., Coates, P.W.: Multiple cutaneous granular cell tumors and neurofibromatosis in childhood. A case report and review of the literature. Arch. Dermatol. 126, 1051–1056 (1990)

14. D'Andrea, V., Ambrogi, V., Biancari, F., De Antoni, E., Di Matteo, G.: Granular cell myoblastoma (Abrikossoff tumor) of the chest wall: a never described site of a rare tumor. J. Thorac. Cardiovasc. Surg. **108**, 792–793 (1994)
15. Enoz, M., Kiyak, E., Katircioglu, S., Gulluoglu, M.: Abrikossoff tumor of the larynx. Acta Medica (Hradec. Kralove). **50**, 157–158 (2007)
16. Lowe, D.L., Chaudhary, A.J., Lee, J.R., Chamberlain, S.M., Schade, R.R., Cuartas-Hoyos, U.: Four cases of patients with gastrointestinal granular cell tumors. South. Med. J. **100**, 298–300 (2007)
17. Narra, S.L., Tombazzi, C., Datta, V., Ismail, M.K.: Granular cell tumor of the esophagus: report of five cases and review of the literature. Am. J. Med. Sci. **335**, 338–341 (2008)
18. Ortiz-Hidalgo, C., de, l V., Moreno-Collado, C.: Granular cell tumor (Abrikossoff tumor) of the clitoris. Int. J. Dermatol. **36**, 935–937 (1997)
19. Yang, J.H., Mitchell, K.B., Poppas, D.P.: Granular cell tumor of the glans penis in a 9-year-old boy. Urology **71**, 546–552 (2008)
20. Bellezza, G., Colella, R., Sidoni, A., Del Sordo, R., Ferri, I., Cioccoloni, C., Cavaliere, A.: Immunohistochemical expression of Galectin-3 and HBME-1 in granular cell tumors: a new finding. Histol. Histopathol. **23**, 1127–1130 (2008)
21. Fanburg-Smith, J.C., Meis-Kindblom, J.M., Fante, R., Kindblom, L.G.: Malignant granular cell tumor of soft tissue: diagnostic criteria and clinicopathologic correlation. Am. J. Surg. Pathol. **22**, 779–794 (1998)
22. Gartmann, H.: Malignant granular cell tumor. Hautarzt **28**, 40–44 (1977)
23. Becelli, R., Perugini, M., Gasparini, G., Cassoni, A., Fabiani, F.: Abrikossoff's tumor. J. Craniofac. Surg. **12**, 78–81 (2001)
24. Wieczorek, T.J., Krane, J.F., Domanski, H.A., Akerman, M., Carlen, B., Misdraji, J., Granter, S.R.: Cytologic findings in granular cell tumors, with emphasis on the diagnosis of malignant granular cell tumor by fine-needle aspiration biopsy. Cancer **93**, 398–408 (2001)
25. Abraham, T., Jackson, B., Davis, L., Yu, J., Peterson, C.: Mohs surgical treatment of a granular cell tumor on the toe of a child. Pediatr. Dermatol. **24**, 235–237 (2007)
26. Smith, S.B., Farley, M.F., Albertini, J.G., Elston, D.M.: Mohs micrographic surgery for granular cell tumor using S-100 immunostain. Dermatol. Surg. **28**, 1076–1078 (2002)

Non-Melanoma Skin Cancer

4.1

Severin Läuchli, Jürg Hafner, Günther F.L. Hofbauer,
Antonio Cozzio, and Mirjana Urosevic-Maiwald

4.1.1 Surgery

Severin Läuchli and Jürg Hafner

4.1.1.1 *Indication*

The aim of any skin cancer treatment is to eliminate all tumor cells. This can be achieved by excision of the tumor with a certain margin, physical destruction of tumor cells by various means such as cryosurgery, electrodessication or irradiation, or pharmacological destruction of tumor cells. For the vast majority of non-melanoma skin cancer, surgery is the curative treatment of choice as it provides the best means of controlling that the entire tumor is removed and thus the cancer is eradicated [6, 34, 49].

The type of treatment chosen depends on patient factors as well as the tumor's risk of local recurrence and metastasis. Amongst patient factors to be considered are age, concomitant medications, and comorbidities. As most skin cancer surgery can be performed under local anesthesia with minimal pain and discomfort to the patient, the procedure carries a low treatment-associated morbidity and can be performed in almost all patients with very few contraindications. Only patients with numerous or severe comorbidities, i.e., severe heart disease or bone marrow aplasia, may pose a risk for surgical treatment under local anesthesia. Immunosuppression per se is not a contraindication for surgical treatment but requires more generous use of perioperative antibiotic prophylaxis. Medication with anticoagulants or platelet aggregation inhibitors is only a relative contraindication. If extensive repairs are required or the procedure site cannot compressed, this medication should be discontinued prior to the operation. Otherwise, it is sufficient to make sure that anticoagulation is at an INR below 2.5, whereas antiplatelet medications can be continued [1, 24, 38]. Very large tumors or those with invasion of underlying tissues (muscle, bone, tendons) usually require a multidisciplinary surgical approach and general anesthesia [25].

Factors influencing the risk of recurrence are: location of the tumor (Mid-face, temples, ear > cheeks, forehead, scalp > trunk, extremities), size (>2 cm), definition of borders, immunosuppression, history of recurrence, tumor histology, and perineural invasion [30]. Low-risk tumors can be treated with standard excision or an ablative modality such as curettage and electrodessication or cryosurgery. For high-risk tumors, standard excision should only be performed in select cases, if the tumor can be excised with a large margin and the defect can be closed directly [3, 48]. Many high-risk non-melanoma skin cancers show a growth pattern with subclinical extension into surrounding tissue, which cannot be clinically recognized and is often missed with simple excision; this residual tissue in turn leads to recurrences. It is, therefore, preferred to excise the tumor using a step-by-step procedure with examination of the specimen's entire surgical margin (micrographically controlled surgery or Mohs surgery) (Fig. 4.1.1) [31]. Most high-risk tumors should be excised using micrographically controlled surgery. Besides having a lower recurrence rate, this method allows for narrower margins, and therefore, facilitates an esthetically and functionally pleasing reconstruction.

S. Läuchli (✉) and J. Hafner
Department of Dermatology, University Hospital,
Zürich, Switzerland
e-mail: severin.laeuchli@usz.ch; juerg.hafner@usz.ch

G.F.L. Hofbauer
Dermatologische Klinik, Universitätsspital Zürich,
Gloriastrasse 31, Zürich, Switzerland
e-mail: hofbauer@usz.ch

A. Cozzio
Department of Dermatology,
University Hospital of Zurich,
Zurich, Switzerland
e-mail: antonio.cozzio@usz.ch

M. Urosevic-Maiwald
Department of Dermatology, University Hospital Zurich,
Gloriastrasse 31, Zürich, Switzerland
e-mail: mirjana.urosevic@usz.ch

R. Dummer et al. (eds.), *Skin Cancer – A World-Wide Perspective*,
DOI: 10.1007/978-3-642-05072-5_4.1, © Springer-Verlag Berlin Heidelberg 2011

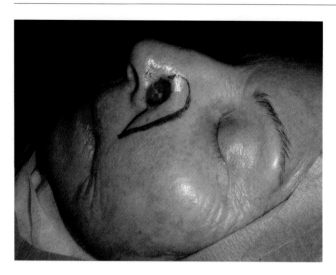

Fig. 4.1.1 Defect after Mohs surgery of a basal cell carcinoma, involving the paranasal sulcus

Table 4.1.1 Indications for micrographically controlled surgery

Tumor- related indications
Aggressive histological growth pattern (e.g., infiltrating/sclerosing BCC)
Recurrent tumors
Ill-defined clinical margins
Tumor size (>2 cm)
Perineural or perivascular invasion
Location-related indications
Locations that require complex reconstructions and maximal tissue sparing (e.g., nose, lips, eyelids)
Locations with high rates of recurrence (mid-face, eyelids, ears)

Thus, indications for micrographically controlled surgery are, on one hand, tumors that have a strong tendency to recur or display an infiltrative growth pattern (e.g., infiltrative BCC, tumors with perineural invasion) or, on the other hand, tumors in a location where minimal excision defects and saving as much tissue as possible is of the utmost importance (e.g., tumors on the nose) (cf. Table 4.1.1) [33, 52].

4.1.1.2 Technique

4.1.1.2.1 Standard Excision

For most low-risk non-melanoma skin cancers, standard excision with a margin is the easiest and most straightforward approach [14, 50]. The border of the tumor is clinically delineated, and a margin, depending on the tumor type, is

chosen. There are no universally agreed-upon margins. For primary nodular basal cell carcinomas (BCC), a margin of 3–5 mm is usually chosen [54], whereas wider margins are needed for recurrent tumors [7]. For tumors with a more infiltrative growth pattern, e.g., sclerodermiform BCCs, the margin should be 6–15 mm [5]. For squamous cell carcinomas, wider security margins (of 5–7 mm) are generally chosen, due to their high recurrence rates and metastatic potential [42]. Curettage of the tumor prior to its excision is preferred by some surgeons as it may allow better delineation of the tumor borders [8, 16]. After infiltration of the tissue underneath and surrounding the tumor with local anesthesia, a vertical incision is performed along a previously marked line. The specimen is then detached by dissecting along the mid subcutis or, preferably, along the next underlying anatomical structure. Excessive bleeding can be stopped with electrocoagulation. After undermining along the anatomical plane chosen for the depth of the excision, the wound margins can be adapted, usually with a side-to-side closure. The direction of the resulting scar should be along the relaxed skin tension lines (or perpendicular to the direction of lowest resistance, which can be determined by pinching the skin with two fingers).

4.1.1.2.2 Micrographically Controlled Surgery

To better ensure total removal of all tumor cells and, at the same time, minimize the size of the resulting scar, micrographically controlled surgery can be used. This procedure was initiated in the 1930s and first published in 1941 by Fredric Mohs who used zinc chloride paste for in vivo fixation of tissue. The method was later developed further by Mohs and Tromovich using freshly frozen tissues to examine the specimens ex vivo, which has now become the standard for most Mohs procedures [31]. In Mohs micrographic surgery, excised specimens are histologically examined in a fashion that allows visualization of the entire surgical margin, as opposed to only a fraction thereof, as in the traditional bread loaf sectioning method of histological specimens. This is traditionally achieved by excising the tumor in a saucer shape, placing the specimen flat on a slide, pressing the margins down and cutting the specimen from its under-surface. The specimen is then fixed with a cryostat, cut, and stained. The slides are read by the surgeon himself and examined for remaining tumor in the margins. If tumor cells are discovered in the margin, the corresponding area is marked on a map by the surgeon, reexcised, and the new specimen is processed in the same way. This process is repeated until clear margins can be confirmed. An alternative approach, more popular in Europe, is to embed the margins and the base of the specimen separately and fixate them using paraffin. These paraffin sections can then be read by a dermatopathologist 1–2 days later, and a reexcision is then performed, if necessary, or the wound is closed. This technique allows better visualization of tumor cells for some difficult tumors, i.e., neoplasms with spindle-cell histology or dedifferentiated tumors, and it can be performed in most existing infrastructures. However, it involves multiple patient visits for the different stages with the risk of complications such as wound infections between stages and problems with accuracy if the slides are not read by the surgeon herself [4, 45].

By using micrographically controlled surgery, 100% of the surgical margin can be examined, as opposed to only a small fraction thereof as in the classic bread loaf sectioning method [17]. Thus, this method achieves a markedly reduced recurrence rate and, at the same time, results in minimal scarring with optimal preservation of healthy tissue [44].

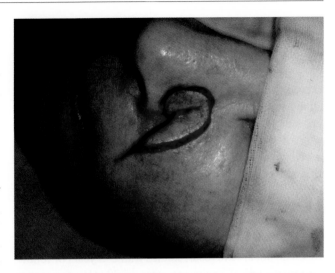

Fig. 4.1.2 Reconstruction of the defect with a modified island flap ("shark island pedicle flap" [9])

4.1.1.2.3 Reconstruction

The defects resulting from surgical excision of skin tumors can be reconstructed in many ways [29]. The easiest procedure is to allow the defect to granulate and heal by secondary intention. This requires no additional surgical intervention and leads to satisfying cosmetic results in many areas, especially in concave areas such as the nasal alar grove or the median canthus of the eye. However, large defects can require lengthy time periods to heal and, in many locations, the resulting scar will not be acceptable. Furthermore, the naturally occurring scar contraction can cause problems, especially in defects located near a free margin (i.e., eyelid, nasal ala).

Whenever possible, without causing too much tension in the tissue or distorting a free margin, the defect should be closed side-to-side, first bringing the defect into an elliptic or fusiform shape by excising dog ears and then adapting the edges. This can be done using dermal or intracutaneous sutures and a running suture or interrupted sutures. To support the tissue under tension, cause everted wound margins, and thus create a more pleasing scar, subcutaneous sutures with resorbable threads can be placed beforehand.

For larger defects, where direct closure would put too much tension on the tissue or distort a free margin, skin flaps must be used for wound closure. There is a vast array of possible sources of tissue movement to cover a defect with random pattern flaps such as burrows flaps, transposition flaps, rotation flaps, island flaps, or combinations thereof (Fig. 4.1.2). They provide the skilled dermatosurgeon with excellent options to close almost all defects with good cosmetic results. Another option, which can be used for a large number of defects, is a full thickness skin graft. Its long-term results provide satisfying cosmetic outcomes in many locations such as the tip of the nose or the temples.

4.1.1.2.4 Metastasizing Non-Melanoma Skin Cancer

The rare occurrences of metastasizing disease in NMSC must be treated in a multidisciplinary approach, involving head and neck surgeons or plastic surgeons, depending on the location of the metastases, for excision of metastases and radiotherapy [27].

4.1.1.2.5 Ablative Methods

Surgical treatment options for superficial epithelial tumors include ablative methods such as curettage/electrodessication [2, 10, 20, 32, 37, 47, 55], CO_2-laser [36], and cryosurgery [11–13, 15, 19, 22, 23, 28, 51, 56]. They are less invasive for the patient, can usually be performed very easily and quickly, and also allow for treatment in patients with contraindications for surgical interventions. Scarring is usually less pronounced than with surgical excision and often consists only of inconspicuous depressed whitish areas, but hypertrophic scarring is also possible. However, they have the major disadvantage of not allowing histological confirmation of the totality of the excision. They are therefore only feasible for superficial and low-risk skin tumors such as superficial BCC, M. Bowen and actinic keratoses.

4.1.1.3 Outcome

The most important outcome parameters in the treatment of non-melanoma skin cancer are the complete removal of the tumor as reflected in the recurrence rate, preserved function, and a cosmetically acceptable appearance. For surgical excision of BCCs, recurrence rates depend on the above mentioned risk factors, especially the margin of the excision, the type of margin control, and the histologic type of tumor. For primary low-risk BCCs, the rates for total clearance after excision with a 4-mm margin are approximately 95% [5, 54], although recurrence rates in two series were <2% [14, 50]. For sclerodermiform BCCs, clearance rates after excision with a 5-mm margin are only 82%, whereas for a 95% clearance rate margins of 13–15 mm are needed [5]. For relapsed BCCs, 5-year rates for further recurrence of 17% are reported for simple excision [40]. The lowest recurrence rates can be achieved with micrographically controlled surgery; cure rates of >99% are reported for primary BCCs [41, 46] and 93–96% for recurrent tumors [40, 46]. Incompletely excised BCCs do not always recur; studies with 2–5 years of follow-up report clinical recurrence rates of 30–41% for incompletely excised tumors [21, 26, 39, 53]. Reexcision is highly recommended for high-risk lesions, if skin flaps were used to repair the defect and if a deep margin was involved.

Successful outcomes for ablative treatments depend largely on careful selection of the lesions treated with these methods. If used for superficial low-risk tumors, 5-year cure rates of 92% have been reported for curettage and electrodessication [41], whereas residual tumor is found in a much higher percentage following treatment of lesions on the face or recurring lesions [20, 43]. On the other hand, cryosurgery for low-risk lesions yields cure rates of up to 99% and can, in some instances, even be used by experts for high-risk lesions [22, 23].

Cure rates for SCC after standard excision are slightly lower than for BCC and are around 92% for primary disease and 77% for recurrent lesions [42]. They are even lower for high-risk SCC such as tumors of the ear, SCC with perineural invasion, or poorly differentiated SCC. Recurrence rates can be reduced to 3% for primary lesions and 11% for recurrent lesions by using micrographically controlled surgery [35].

Fortunately, complications in skin cancer surgery are rare [18]. As in any surgical procedure, hematoma due to postoperative bleeding and wound infection can occur. Excessive tension can lead to flap or wound margin necrosis, which in turn favors wound infection. If complications arise, healing will be prolonged, and more pronounced scarring will result. Hypertrophic scarring can be the result of complications but also of a patient predisposition; it occurs more frequently in certain body areas such as the presternal area or the ears.

The cosmetic and functional outcome of skin cancer surgery, if performed properly by an experienced surgeon, is usually excellent. Appropriate selection of techniques, e.g., usage of a suitable flap for reconstruction and placing scar lines in existing facial lines or along relaxed skin tension lines, leads to inconspicuous scars. Standard excision can lead to sizeable defects due to the margins that must be used with certain tumor types. Esthetic results are usually best after Mohs micrographic surgery, as it allows tumor excision with a minimal margin.

4.1.2 Phototherapy, Laser and Radiation: Phototherapie

Günther F.L. Hofbauer

4.1.2.1 Indication

The first insights into photodestruction of tissue date back almost a century [1]. Nowadays, phototherapy has become an established treatment option for non-melanoma skin cancer (NMSC), applying visible light to photosensitized skin. The term photodynamic therapy (PDT) is used for intended tissue destruction, while the term fluorescence dynamic diagnosis (FDD) refers to visualizing areas of, e.g., NMSC without tissue destruction. Following the application of photosensitizers such as 5-aminolevulinic acid (5-ALA) or methyl aminolevulinate (MAL), protoporphyrin IX (PPIX) is formed within cells and renders these cells susceptible to destruction in the presence of oxygen by forming reactive oxygen species.

The depth of light wave penetration in the tissue determines the extent of PDT. In general, longer light waves more deeply penetrate the skin, and thus, red light-emitting lamps are frequently used. A second determining factor is the depth of photosensitizer penetration in the skin. Recent topical formulations using liposomal and nanoemulsions aim for deeper penetration of the photosensitizing agent, while systemic application can overcome this limitation at the expense of long-lasting photosensitization. Cancer cells take up more photosensitizer and accumulate more PPIX, the substrate for the photodynamic reaction, than the healthy surrounding tissues. The ensuing PDT will in turn damage cancer cells more than the surrounding normal tissue, resulting in a tumor-selective effect. PDT can be repeated at a later time point, yielding similar clinical success rates.

Taking these factors into account, PDT is a treatment method well suited for skin cancer. The topically applied MAL is registered for actinic keratosis (AK) and superficial BCC in the European Union and additionally for Bowen's disease (BD) in the UK and the US. Topical 20% ALA in a stick formulation has been approved for AK in the US. Beyond these registered indications, PDT has been employed for other skin cancers such as in situ and invasive squamous cell carcinoma, erythroplasia Queyrat, and cutaneous lymphoma. Beyond skin cancer and thus beyond the scope of this book, PDT has shown varying degrees of efficacy in skin diseases such as acne, warts, photodamaged skin, psoriasis, leishmaniasis, and sebaceous gland hyperplasia.

A tumor-selective effect for PDT has been reported repeatedly. PPIX accumulates more in tumor cells of the epidermis than in surrounding normal cells, possibly by facilitated penetration through rapidly proliferating, relatively iron-deficient tumor cells [2]. Following photosensitizer application, fluorescence of accumulated PPIX can be elicited in cells using light energy far below the levels needed to induce a photodynamic reaction. This process is referred to as FDD. Using Wood's light or, preferably, a digital contrast-enhancing camera system, FDD is used for clear delineation of tumor margins and follow-up of treatment success.

4.1.2.2 Technique

4.1.2.2.1 Preparation

Removal of hyperkeratosis and crusts covering the target is an important step to allow penetration of the photosensitizer. In the days leading up to PDT, a topical application of 10% urea can be administered repeatedly. Alternatively, curettage can be used to remove hyperkeratosis before application of the photosensitizer. Superficial curettage is usually performed to remove scales and crusts without bleeding. This procedure requires no anesthesia and carries a minimal risk of scarring. A deeper, bleeding curettage, however, improves the outcome of PDT but is not routinely recommended because of pain and scarring [3].

4.1.2.2.2 Application

The area of PDT application should be marked with a felt pen. The photosensitizer will then be evenly applied to cover the whole treatment field homogeneously. 5-ALA is typically used in a 20% oil-in-water emulsion to increase penetration. Penetration enhancers such as DMSO have been reported in small numbers [4, 5], and final 5-ALA preparations differ geographically. 5-ALA is left to incubate for 1–6 h, whereas incubation for 3 h is recommended for MAL, according to the manufacturer's instructions. This achieves a maximum of fluorescence with a maximum penetration of tumor [6]. The treatment field should then be covered with an occlusive dressing. The dressing should be impermeable to light to prevent photobleaching. At the end of the incubation, the remaining photosensitizer is removed with wet gauze.

4.1.2.2.3 Light Sources

Broadband and monochromatic light sources such as lasers, incandescent lamps, and light-emitting diodes can be employed in PDT. The maximum absorption for PPIX occurs at 400 nm, which suggests the use of blue light, frequently used in the US. Light penetration into the skin, however, is more profound in the red range of visible light. Light sources with an emission maximum around 630 nm have thus been used in most clinical studies. The dose of light recommended

for MAL PDT is 37 J/cm^2 from an LED lamp (peak 630 nm) or 75–100 J/cm^2 of a filtered incoherent lamp in the red waveband; the two show similar effects [7]. Light doses for 5-ALA vary with different study protocols.

4.1.2.2.4 Repetition, Precautions, and Adverse Events

Repeat application of PDT in the same treatment area 1 week following the first irradiation has been shown to increase treatment efficacy [8]. Patients should avoid sun exposure on the day of PDT on account of persistent photosensitivity. The most common adverse effects include acute pain during PDT as well as erythema and edema. Pain is a major concern and can be alleviated by premedication with, e.g., paracetamol, topical application of Emla or local anesthesia, and spray application of ice-cold water during PDT. The pain, however, seems comparable to other treatment modalities for AK [9]. Chronic adverse effects are rare as PDT generally achieves a very satisfying cosmetic outcome but comprise hypo- and hyperpigmentation, rarely hair loss within the treatment area and, very rarely, scarring.

4.1.2.3 Outcome

Numerous reports have studied the efficacy of PDT. Generally, studies using 5-ALA are more heterogeneous in quality and treatment protocols than those using MAL.

MAL PDT and cryosurgery were compared in a multicenter randomized prospective trial of AK. 193 patients with 699 lesions received MAL PDT or double-freeze cryosurgery. Complete response rates at 3 months were indistinct with 69% for MAL PDT and 75% for cryosurgery [10].

Two treatment sessions with MAL PDT led to 91% overall complete response at 3 months in 204 Australians and compared well to a single cryosurgery application with 68% and placebo with 30% [11]. A similar study of 80 US patients in a multicenter, double-blind, placebo-controlled design showed an 89% complete response of AK to MAL PDT and 38% to placebo at 3 months [12].

Thickness of AK lesions seems to matter: 211 patients with 413 thin to moderately thick AK underwent one or two MAL PDT weekly. Nineteen percent of AKs treated once showed an incomplete response and were retreated at 3 months. Thin lesions responded completely in 93% of single treatments and in 89% of repeated treatments. Thicker lesions, however, responded completely in 70% of single and 84% of repeated treatments. Eighty-eight percent of AK not cleared by a single treatment improved to a complete response after a second application of MAL PDT [13].

In a noteworthy study, there was a significant difference between treatment with blue light used in conjunction with

Levulan Kerastick and the placebo control. Of the patients showing significant AK clearance (≥75% of AKs clearing), significant clearance was observed in 77% at week 8 and 89% at week 12, compared to the placebo control arm, which revealed significant clearance in 18 and 13% at weeks 8 and 12, respectively. The week 12 response rates for the PDT group included 30% of the PDT-treated patients who received a second treatment [14].

Forty patients with BD were randomized to receive PDT or treatment with topical 5-fluorouracil (5-FU) and repeat treatment at 6 weeks for residual disease. Complete clearance was 88% for ALA PDT and 67% for 5-FU at 4 months and 82% for ALA PDT and 48% for 5-FU at 12 months [15].

Organ-transplant recipients (OTR) are a high-risk population for AK and SCC. AK or BD were treated with a single or repeated application of 20% 5-ALA PDT and showed comparable cure rates in OTR and immunocompetent patients at 4 weeks. At 12 and 48 weeks, however, OTR showed lower complete response rates [15]. Seventeen OTR with 129 mild-to-moderate AK were randomized to MAL PDT or placebo. Thirteen out of seventeen treatment areas were cleared of AK by MAL PDT, while no treatment area responded to placebo [8].

Superficial BCC was treated in 59 patients with 350 lesions and cleared in 89% at 3 months and 79% at 24-48 months [17]. Single MAL PDT for superficial BCC was compared to repeated cryosurgery in 180 patients. Incompletely responding lesions were retreated with repeat MAL PDT or cryosurgery at month 3. MAL PDT and cryosurgery reached complete response in 97 and 95%, respectively, at 3 months and 78 and

81% at 36-48 months [18]. Nodular BCC was treated with two MAL PDT or placebo after surgical debulking. Complete response was seen in 73% of MAL PDT and 21% of placebo-treated patients at 6 months [19]. Surgery was compared to two MAL PDT treatments for nodular BCC. At 3 months, complete response was 98% for surgery and 91% for MAL PDT. Recurrence rates were 10% for MAL PDT compared to 2% for surgery at 24 months with better cosmesis in MAL PDT [20]. Though not quite as effective as surgery, PDT may offer a good alternative for a large part of patients with difficult-to-treat superficial and/or nodular BCC. An open uncontrolled study followed 102 patients and reported complete response in 90% at 3 months and 78% at 24 months [21]. Another study reported similar success rates in 94 patients with 123 BCC [22].

In contrast to MAL PDT and Levulan Kerastick, 5-ALA has mainly been reported in smaller series, mostly uncontrolled, nonrandomized, with different light sources and doses, and thus, it is difficult to compare results side-to-side for the former two photosensitizers. However, it is generally recognized that PDT is not limited in the number of applications, does not lose efficacy on repeat application, and can successfully be used in previously photodamaged or therapeutically irradiated skin [23].

While pigmented or morpheic BCC does not respond well to PDT [24], basal cell nevus syndrome (Gorlin's syndrome) responds completely to ALA PDT in 85-98% [25].

In summary, PDT has established itself as a valid treatment option for superficial forms of NMSC and may be superior to other treatment modalities in select situations, while resulting in excellent cosmesis (Fig. 4.1.3).

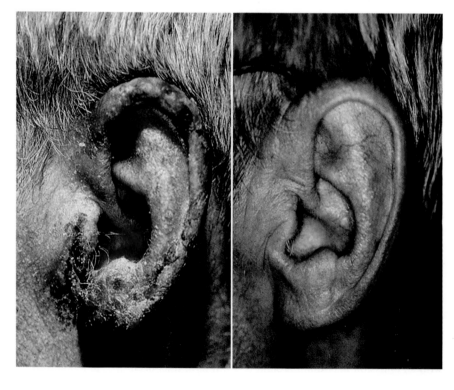

Fig. 4.1.3 Photodynamic therapy can provide very good clinical results in the treatment of intraepithelial squamous cell carcinoma of the skin with excellent cosmesis. In particular locations such as the ear, where radiation is difficult to apply due to varying distance from the source to the target field, or where self-administered treatments such as 5-fluorouracil or imiquimod may not be evenly used, photodynamic therapy can provide a superior solution to other alternative modalities. *Left panel* shows ear before, *right panel* shows ear after two sessions of 5-ALA PDT

4.1.3 Phototherapy, Laser and Radiation: Radiation

Antonio Cozzio

Non-melanoma skin cancer is the most frequent malignancy worldwide, and there are many treatment options available, such as curettage, cryosurgery, photodynamic therapy, application of immunmodulators such as Imiquimod, 5-fluorouracil, or surgery, including micrographic surgery. Radiotherapy for non-melanoma skin cancer in dermatology is often applied as surface-directed superficial radiotherapy, using voltages between 10 and 50 kV. In the last 30 years, superficial X-rays became less available, and electron beam therapy using high-energy electrons >4 MeV has been established. Both techniques are comparable with respect to local control and cosmesis. However, superficial X-ray therapy is safe, well-established, and may be performed in a dermatologist's private practice setting, or, as in our case, in a dermatology clinical setting.

Radiotherapy may be definitive in patients where the cosmetic and functional outcome is anticipated to be better with radiotherapy compared with surgery. It may be used in an adjuvant setting to reduce the risk of locoregional recurrences, and it may be palliative in advanced incurable disease stages. It has the advantage of being a rather painless intervention and can be performed in an outpatient-setting. The rather large safety margins that may be applied in radiotherapy, as compared to surgery, can be advantageous.

For non-melanoma skin cancers, using 40–50 Gy total dose, we generally apply superficial X-ray therapy only in patients older than 60 years due to comparatively less danger of late radiation sequelae compared to younger patients. There is a risk of permanent alopecia, using voltages equal or higher than 30 kV. X-ray therapy is not indicated for tumors secondary to osteomyelitis, chronic ulcers, or burn scars due to chronic wound healing issues.

4.1.3.1 Indication and Outcome

Radiotherapy may be used for basal cell carcinomas (BCC) and squamous cell carcinoma (SCC) as well as actinic keratosis (AK), Morbus Bowen and Bowen's carcinoma, and keratoacanthoma (KA). However, several factors have to be taken into account.

Basal cell carcinoma: BCC occurs mainly in the sun-exposed areas of the skin, such as head, neck, trunk [11]. It exhibits a low metastatic potential [5]. Based on clinical and histologic characteristics, three subtypes of BCC have been described: the superficial subtype, the nodular subtype, and the sclerosing (morphaeform) subtype [11]. In a study performed by Dummer and colleagues, the nodular BCC showed a lower recurrence rate than the superficial and sclerosing BCC (8.2 vs. 26.1 and 27.7%, respectively) [15]. However, other groups reported control rates up to 90–95% [4, 10]. It is thus generally accepted that the more aggressive sclerosing BCC type should not be primarily treated with radiotherapy, but rather by surgical intervention [8, 12].

Soft X-ray superficial radiotherapy is an excellent option in patients older than 60 years with BCC in mid-facial or nasal areas, or in the area of the inner canthus or lower eyelid. In these areas, management decisions often are based on several factors (cure rate, functional outcome, cosmetic outcome, number and duration of surgical interventions vs. radiotherapy sessions). With cosmesis judged >90% as excellent or good [10], radiotherapy remains an excellent therapy option in a definitive setting for BCC in mid-facial/nasal/ocular area.

In a study observing the course of incompletely excised BCC in the head/neck area, postoperative radiotherapy improved the 5-year local control rate from 61% (nonirradiated patients) to 91%. However, The 10-year actuarial probability of local control for the lesions immediately irradiated and observed was similar, 92 and 90%, respectively ($p = 0.5$) [3]. Thus, given certain circumstances such as advanced age, patient mobility issues, observation and an expectant treatment position may be taken. Recurrences are rarely associated with serious consequences, but more extensive salvage surgery may be required [13].

Squamous cell carcinoma: SCC has a higher propensity to spread to regional lymph nodes; thus, local control of the tumor is important. High-risk SCC are tumors with increased risk of local recurrence and/or metastatic disease. The British Association of Dermatologists defined the patients at greater risk based on six variables: site of tumor (lip, ear, non-sun-exposed sites), size (>2 cm,), depth (>4 mm), grade (poorly differentiated), host immunosuppression, and local recurrence [6]. There is good evidence that Mohs' micrographic surgery shows low incidence of local recurrence or metastatic disease in high-risk SCC, on the other hand, radiotherapy offers cure rates for SCC that are comparable with other treatments [2, 9, 10, 14]. Furthermore, the cosmetic and/or functional outcome after radiotherapy for lesions arising on the lip, nose, and ear, among others, is generally better than after surgery.

In situations with incomplete excision of SCC, expectant policy is not an option due to the metastatic potential of SCC. Radiotherapy and/or surgery may both be applied.

Generally, radiotherapy should not be applied for SCC with poor differentiation and only cautiously for SCC in patients with immunosuppression. Furthermore, SCC with perineural or lymphovascular infiltration should be treated with Mohs' micrographic surgery, as the extent of the local tumor spreading is not predictable and may well exceed the safety margins usually applied in radiotherapy (see below). As with surgical interventions, radiotherapy for SCC on the lower leg in older people shows higher incidence of prolonged wound healing [1]. Furthermore, tumors that do infiltrate subjacent cartilage/bone should not be treated with X-ray therapy.

M. Bowen, actinic keratosis: Both the in situ carcinoma of the Bowen type and the AK type are sensitive to ionizing radiation doses that are well tolerated by the surrounding tissue. Relatively low tube voltage effectively treats tumor spread and is an excellent choice for extensive or confluent areas of diseases such as AK on the scalp, where cryotherapy (painful treatment) or surgery may not be tolerated (patients with multiple health problems that cannot tolerate surgery or extended size of excision), or in patients in whom insufficient compliance may be a problem (imiquimod therapy). Local control rates up to 95–100% have been described for superficial X-ray therapy for M. Bowen or AK [1].

4.1.3.2 Technique

Lesion selection: NMSC for which surgery may lead to functionally or cosmetically insufficient results (lip, nose, ear, others). Exclusion of lesions in the lower leg. High histologic grading of tumor; exclusion of sclerosing BCC, exclusion of perineural invasion (or in this setting: adjuvant radiotherapy).

Lesion preparation: Hyperkeratotic areas may be removed chemically (20% salicylic acid in vaseline) or by curettage.

Lesion treatment: We use the settings described in Table 4.1.2 set forth by Panizzon [7]. We try to include a safety margin of 10 mm around the NMSC. Voltage of the tube is set according to the histologic depth of the NMSC (mm, Breslow), and the corresponding tissue half-value layer. Tissue half-value layer for 10, 30, 40, 50, and 100 kV is given below (Table 4.1.3), respectively.

During the radiation period, the lesions are treated with 1% Triclosan ointment. First check ups are scheduled 4 weeks after cessation of radiotherapy.

Table 4.1.2 Treatment guidelines for skin tumors

Diagnosis	Diameter (cm)	Voltage (kV)	Fractionation (Gy)	Total dose	Time interval
Actinic keratosis		10–12	5–7×6	30–42	2–7
M. Bowen		20	5–7×4	20–28	2–7
BCC	<2	20–50, according to histologic depth	5–6×8	40–48	7
SCC	2–5		10–12×4	40–48	2–7
Keratoacanthoma	>5		26–28×2	52–56	Daily

Table 4.1.3 Half-value-layer (cm) for Gulmay GM0205

Field diameter (cm)	10 kV	30 kV	40 kV	50 kV	100 kV
2	0.16	0.4	0.81	1.01	1.77
4	0.16	0.48	0.88	1.1	2.03
6	0.16	0.49	0.9	1.15	2.21
8	0.16	0.49	0.9	1.16	2.32
10	0.16	0.51	0.98	1.29	2.79
15	0.16	0.51	0.97	1.31	2.99

4.1.4 Phototherapy, Laser and Radiation: Lasers for Non-Melanoma Skin Cancer

Jürg Hafner

4.1.4.1 Indications

Cross-sectional studies amongst dermatologists' offices have confirmed that most actinic keratoses and a number of superficial epithelial skin cancers cannot be assessed with pathological records but instead are treated with ablative methods, such as cryotherapy, electrodessication with curettage, dermabrasion, or one of the more modern ablative lasers (CO_2-laser, ErYAG-laser) [1]. Ablative surgery is technically easy to perform. One of the main advantages of laser ablation of superficial epithelial skin tumors is the absence of significant bleeding, if the appropriate technique is used [7]. As a rule, solitary skin lesions, or in cases of very extensive or confluent epithelial skin lesions on UV-damaged skin ("field cancerization"), the most clinically worrisome sites, should be biopsied prior to destruction [7].

AK is a form of squamous cell carcinoma in situ that shows spontaneous remission in approximately 50% of cases, with rigorous UV protection as the only treatment. AK is one of the most accepted indications amongst non-melanoma skin cancers for treatment with non-excisional, "destructive" modalities. Ablative laser surgery achieves 12-month remission rates around 75–85% [12, 14].

BD is a form of more advanced squamous cell carcinoma in situ that shows close histological similarities with VIN, PIN, and AIN. Untreated, BD is slowly progressive and can eventually progress into invasive Bowen's carcinoma, a histological subtype of SCC. The Bowen cells typically extend into the infudibula of skin appendages, where reepithelization takes place after ablative laser surgery. Therefore,

ablative laser treatment of BD requires a more extensive procedure that usually will cause noticeable superficial scarring and hypopigmentation. Older clinical publications on electrodessication and curettage for basal cell carcinoma have stressed that secondary wound healing, by itself, may help clear residual epithelial skin cancer [11]. This may also apply to BD, since the reported complete remission rates of 75–85% at 12 months [5-6] are markedly higher than those in HPV-induced VIN (see below).

VIN, PIN (Erythroplasie of Queyrat), and AIN are typical indications for ablative laser surgery. For the same reasons as the treatment of BD, these procedures have to be performed to the mid-dermis or deep dermis to get a realistic chance of complete remission. At the typically diseased sites, depigmentation may play a minor role – except in skin of color. The treated patients must be motivated for regular surveillance, since recurrence rate at 12 months is around 40% for patients who had a technically correct laser treatment of VIN [3, 8], PIN, or AIN.

For anal condyloma acuminatum (CA), it has been shown in a small patient series that postinventional application of imiquimod anal tampons can reduce recurrence [9]. This concept (ablative laser surgery followed by imiquimod cream as soon as surgical wounds are healed) can also be transposed to VIN, PIN, and AIN.

CA is mainly caused by the noncarcinogenic HPV 11. The first line of treatment for multiple "pinhead-like" small, popular CA is topical podophyllotoxin or imiquimod cream. Larger or refractory CA can readily be debulked with the CO_2-laser [4], followed by topical imiquimod as a second step, to reduce the risk of recurrence. HPV 11 does not cause invasive skin cancer; however, CA can be a marker disease for infection with other, oncogenic HPV. The rare HPV 11-induced "giant" Buschke-Löwenstein tumors represent a subtype of low-grade squamous cell carcinoma. These tumors require excisional surgery and are – except in palliative situations – unsuitable for CO_2-laser surgery (Fig. 4.1.4).

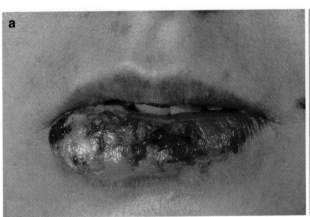
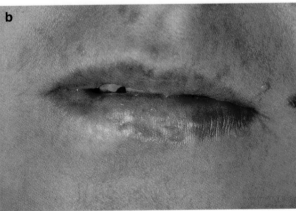

Fig. 4.1.4 (**a**) A 24-year-old female (war refugee) with untreated HPV-infection of the lip (histologically noninvasive). (**b**) Same patient after two sessions with the CO_2-laser under local anesthesia (technique as described above). Minimal scarring noticeable. By comparison, treatment with surgical excision and plastic repair would be rather complex to perform

Epidermodysplasia verruciformis (EV) of Lewandowski and Lutz is a rare, hereditary, autosomal-dominant skin disease (EVER 1 and EVER 2 mutation), in which patients become especially susceptible to infection with the oncogenic HPV 8. The typical, pityriasiform, circumscribed macules in the shoulder and scalp region typically increase in surface area without becoming invasive for several decades. Later in life, they can progress into invasive squamous cell carcinoma. Its histology is very specific, showing features of BD as well as so-called "blue cells" in the epidermis, which correspond to the virally infected keratinocytes. Cryotherapy as well as all ablative methods, including ablative lasers (CO_2 or ErYAG), can be used to control the multiple pityriasiform skin lesions. In our experience, EV also responds particularly well to imiquimod cream. Invasive squamous cell carcinoma in EV, however, requires micrographic surgery [2].

Extensive or refractory "common" warts in the immunosuppressed patient are mostly unresponsive to all first line treatment modalities, such as keratolysis and curettage and cryotherapy. Ablative CO_2-laser surgery has a rather exclusive position in the treatment of these conditions. It relieves the patients of the stigmatizing verrucous lesions in socially exposed skin areas and, more generally, reduces the HPV burden of their skin [10]. Organ-allotransplant recipients have a 70-fold elevated risk to develop SCC; however, the role of HPV as potential co-carcinogen in UV-light-exposed skin areas has remained controversial.

Laser treatment of organoid nevi can give satisfactory results from an esthetic perspective; however, the risk of transformation to invasive growth cannot be modified or eliminated. Therefore, epidermal nevi are particularly suitable for ablative laser treatment, whereas sebaceous nevi, that have an approximately 20–30% life-time risk of transformation to invasive epithelial skin cancer, particularly to trichoblastoma or syringocystadenoma papilliferum, should be excised.

4.1.4.2 Technique

For ablative laser surgery in non-melanoma skin cancer, the CO_2-laser is commonly used as standard treatment, and the more superficially acting ErYAG-laser can be employed as a second line treatment, e.g., in very thin skin areas. For the first pass, the CO_2-laser is applied in the defocused mode [7]. For this purpose, we recommend using a relatively high output power (e.g., 5 W superpulse mode instead 2 W) and holding the handpiece at a large distance from the skin lesion, i.e., 3–5 times the technically predefined focus (e.g., 6–10 cm distance instead of 2 cm according to the handpiece focus). This technique provokes a thermic blister limited to the epidermis, without significant thermal damage to the surrounding tissues. The ablated tissue layer can be cleansed off with moist cotton gauze, and one to two additional treatment layers will be sufficient to reach the superficial dermis and, therefore, completely remove in situ or superficially invasive epithelial processes. As in all ablative methods, postsurgical hypopigmentation cannot always be avoided, as melanocytes are very sensitive to temperature changes. This is certainly the main disadvantage of this otherwise very elegant method. In persons with a Fitzpatrick skin type 3–5 complexion, a test site can be treated for precaution before extending the procedure to a larger surface of diseased skin.

4.1.4.3 Outcome

Healing and recurrence rates of non-melanoma skin cancers after laser therapies have not been investigated with randomized, controlled studies until now. In published case series, ablative laser surgery results in a 12-month clearing rate of 75–85% for AK [12–14] and of 75–85% for BD [5-6]. The latter is markedly higher than the response rate of 60% in the HPV-induced "BD" of the anogenital area. For VIN [3, 8], PIN, and AIN, recurrence rates of 40% have to be expected after appropriate ablative laser surgery. Long-term results may be improved with postinterventional prophylactic application of topical imiquimod cream. This has been shown for AIN with an imiquimod suppository that was specifically designed to stop and dissolve at the height of the anal canal [9]. Pregnancy is not a contraindication for CO_2-laser surgery.

Surveillance: The relatively high recurrence rates after laser ablation for in situ and superficially invasive epithelial skin tumors underline the need to establish a reliable clinical surveillance system for patients who are treated with ablative laser surgery.

4.1.5 Drug Therapy for Non-Melanoma Skin Cancer

Mirjana Urosevic-Maiwald

4.1.5.1 Topical Therapy

4.1.5.1.1 5-Fluorouracil

5-Fluorouracil (5-FU) is a pyrimidine analog that inhibits the enzyme thymidylate synthase and thereby prevents DNA synthesis in tumor cells. This inhibits cellular proliferation and results in cell death, particularly in rapidly dividing neoplastic cells.

Indications and Dosages

Topical 5-FU has been successfully used in the treatment of actinic keratoses (AK). This medication is advantageous in treating large AK, numerous AK within a circumscribed area, and areas of severe actinic damage without clinically apparent lesions. In addition, 5-FU was also effectively employed in the treatment of Bowen's disease (BD) and erythroplasia of Queyrat. Occasionally, 5-FU was used in patients with xeroderma pigmentosum, arsenic, and radiation-induced keratoses, as well as in organ-transplant recipients. This medication is available in cream (0.5–5%) and solution (2–5%) form.

For AKs, 5-FU is applied once or twice daily for 2–6 weeks, depending on the formulation. Since the 1960s, numerous clinical studies have shown remission rates for AKs ranging from 75 to 86.6% [5, 11, 19]. Intermittent 5-fluorouracil treatment (2–4 times per week) was also shown to be effective, without causing significant irritation, but increases in healing time were observed with declining application frequency [12]. 0.5% 5-FU applied once daily seems to be as effective as 5% 5-FU applied twice daily in reducing the number of AKs as well as in reaching complete remission (both regimes approximately 43%), after 4 weeks of treatment [13]. Furthermore, if 5-FU is applied beyond the obvious clinical margin of the AKs, the chances of lateral residual disease decrease. On the dorsal hands, extension forearms, and shins, pretreatment with topical retinoids for reduction of hyperkeratoses several weeks prior to 5-FU application improves efficacy.

For BD, 5-FU is usually applied once or twice daily as a 5% cream for 1 week to 2 months to achieve disease control; if required, this protocol is repeated at intervals [2, 19]. After one cycle of once-daily application for 1 week followed by twice daily application for 3 weeks, a response rate of 67% was observed, with 48% remaining clear at 12 months [17]. Lower concentrations are considered less effective. Efficacy in BD can be improved with application under occlusion, use of

dinitrochlorobenzene (DNCB) as a vehicle, ionopheresis (improving follicular penetration), or laser pretreatment (ablating stratum corneum enhances the penetration of 5-FU) [2].

For erythroplasia of Queyrat, application of 5% 5-FU cream twice daily for 4–5 weeks has been recommended, but local irritation due to inflammation can often limit this treatment option [2, 19].

In organ-transplant recipients, 5-FU can be safely employed given its primarily chemotherapeutic and non-immunomodulatory action.

Side Effects and Limitations

During treatment, inflammation, necrosis, and even ulceration occur prior to re-epithelisation, which may take 2–4 weeks. This causes discomfort and cosmetic problems for most patients, reducing compliance. Thus, patients should be warned to discontinue treatment once significant erythema occurs. Whereas suppression of inflammation was initially thought to not affect efficacy, recent data suggest that inflammation is likely required to achieve a therapeutic effect [7]. The use of topical steroids may still be necessary in some cases in order to reduce local inflammation and irritation. Topical steroids are usually applied subsequent to 5-FU application once peak inflammation has been reached. In patients with background facial erythema or pigmentation, topical 5-FU does not cause hypopigmentation of the treated areas, as is often observed following cryotherapy.

The use of 5-FU is contraindicated in those with hypersensitivity to 5-FU or a dihydropyridine dehydrogenase deficiency as well as in pregnant and nursing women.

4.1.5.1.2 Diclofenac-Sodium

Diclofenac is a potent NSAID that selectively inhibits enzyme cyclooxygenaze (COX). COX is a key mediator in the proinflammatory cascade in which arachidonic acid is converted into prostaglandins [14]. Diclofenac primarily inhibits COX-2, which is physiologically induced in response to inflammatory and mitogenic stimuli as well as in UV-damaged skin. Increased levels of COX-2 have been found in actinic keratoses. The carcinogenic potential of COX-2 is attributed to its ability to induce angiogenesis, cell proliferation, and protect cells from apoptosis. Diclofenac is hypothesized to counteract these mechanisms independently or via COX-2 inhibition.

Indications and Dosage

Topical 3% diclofenac-sodium in 2.5% hyaluronic acid gel has been shown to effectively clear AKs [5, 11, 14, 19]. The hyaluronic acid vehicle represents an important component of this topical treatment, as it enhances epidermal diclofenac delivery and retention. Three percent diclofenac in 2.5% hyaluronic acid gel is applied twice daily for 60–90 days. Similar to 5-FU and Imiquimod, this formulation is advantageous in treating multiple lesions. Randomized studies report complete resolution of AK lesions following twice-daily application of 3% diclofenac in 2.5% hyaluronic acid gel in approximately 50% of patients.

Side Effects and Limitations

Treatment with 3% diclofenac in 2.5% hyaluronic acid gel shows good tolerability. The most frequent side effects are mild and include pruritus, dry skin, and inflammation at the application site.

The use of topical diclofenac is contraindicated in those with hypersensitivity to diclofenac or salicylic acid as well as during the last trimester of pregnancy.

4.1.5.1.3 Topical Retinoids

Photoaging as the consequence of UV-damage to the skin reduces expression of RXR-α and RAR-γ, two major receptors in keratinocytes, and also upregulates matrix metalloproteinases. Topical retinoids produce antiproliferative effects and promote cellular dedifferentiation and extracellular matrix synthesis, accompanied by an increase in hyaluronate acid. Histologically, this is reflected in compaction of the stratum corneum, epidermal hyperplasia (acanthosis), correction of atypia (e.g., in actinic keratoses), dispersion of melanin granules (evened tan), increases in dermal collagen synthesis, and angiogenesis [10].

Indications and Dosage

The most commonly used topical retinoid is tretinoin, available in various concentrations (0.01–0.1%) as a gel, cream, or solution. Tretinoin is usually applied once daily, preferentially in the evening. Studies show effective clearance of AK on the face using tretinoin 0.1% cream with an approximate response rate of 70% [19] Interestingly, lesions located in other regions such as the scalp and upper extremities do not seem to show such high responsiveness to this treatment. Other retinoid derivates such as 0.1% tazarotene gel and 0.1–0.3% adapalene gel have also been shown to significantly reduce the signs of photoaging, including the reduction in the number of AKs [18, 15]. Tazarotene 0.1% gel application once daily was also studied for treatment of superficial and nodular basal cell carcinoma (BCC) [1]. Complete regression of superficial BCCs was higher (64.8%)

than of nodular BCCs (28.3%). Nevertheless, total complete clearance rate for BCCs was 30.5%, making this option no bona fide treatment alternative for BCCs.

Side Effects and Limitations

By far the most common side effect of topical retinoids is skin irritation, characterized by pruritus, stinging, burning, dryness, scaling, and erythema. This so-called "retinoid dermatitis" occurs within the first month of treatment and tends to abate thereafter. The simplest way to relieve the irritation is to reduce the amount or frequency of retinoid application and to apply a moisturizer. As the perioral area of the face is the most sensitive to peeling, the use of topical retinoids should be limited or avoided in this area. The concomitant use of other abrasive topical products (e.g., soaps, cosmetics, scrubs, peeling lotions) is discouraged. In addition to irritation, many patients report an increase in photosensitivity shortly after sun exposure. Therefore, excessive sun exposure should be avoided during the treatment, even after applying sunscreens. Topical retinoids should not be used during pregnancy and nursing, primarily due to medicolegal issues associated with the teratogenic potential of oral isotretinoin.

4.1.5.2 Topical Immunotherapy

4.1.5.2.1 Imiquimod

Imiquimod belongs to the imidazoquinolone family, a group of low molecular weight synthetic compounds that are potent immunomodulators in vivo. Imiquimod directly activates innate immunity effectors, e.g., plasmacytoid dendritic cells, by triggering the Toll-like receptor 7/MyD88/NF-κB pathway and leading to induction, synthesis, and release of various cytokines, in particular IFN-α [22]. Combined with upregulation of the surface expression of costimulatory molecules on dendritic cells, imiquimod promotes migration and activation of skin Langerhans cells to the regional lymph nodes, enhancing antigen presentation and the development of naive T cells into T helper-1 cells, i.e., subsequent activation of adaptive cellular anti-tumor immunity. Moreover, imiquimod also promotes bcl-2 and caspase-dependent proapoptotic activity in different cell types [18].

Indications and Dosage

Imiquimod is commercially available as a 5% cream for the treatment of AKs and superficial BCC [23]. Randomized, double-blind trials have repeatedly demonstrated the superiority of imiquimod 5% cream, applied three times weekly for 12–16 weeks, over placebo in the treatment of immuno-competent patients with AKs. Complete clearance occurred in 45–57% of imiquimod recipients. Recurrence rates ranged between 8 and 43% in the follow-up period of up to 24 months. The current recommendations for the treatment of AKs with imiquimod depend on the area of registration (US or EU) and vary in frequency and length of treatment from two to three times per week over a course of up to 16 weeks.

Topical imiquimod 5% was also consistently superior to placebo in the treatment of immunocompetent patients with superficial BCC in randomized, double-blind trials. Complete clinical and histologically verified clearance of the tumors occurred in 79–87% of imiquimod-treated patients after application five-times-weekly or daily for 6–12 weeks. Sustained clearance rates taking recurrence into account were not assessed in these trials. Less robustly designed trials suggest sustained clearance rates of approximately 80% at 4 years and 65% at 5 years after imiquimod treatment. The current recommendation for the treatment of histologically proven superficial BCC is application five times per week for up to 6 weeks.

Similarly designed trials involving nodular BCCs were also performed, showing slightly lower histologically confirmed clearance rates, 70–76%, with application of imiquimod 5% cream five-times-weekly for 6–12 weeks. For BD, complete clearance was observed in 73% of patients applying topical 5% imiquimod daily for 16 weeks, compared to 0% of patients receiving placebo. No recurrence was seen in the following 6 months in the patients who achieved complete clearance. Other small noncomparative studies support this outcome. Treatment of non-melanoma skin cancer with topical imiquimod 5% has shown promising efficacy in immuno-compromised organ-transplant recipients. Furthermore, the use of imiquimod 5% cream has been reported in non-controlled case reports and series to be effective in arsenical keratoses, EV, porokeratosis of Mibelli, keratoacanthoma, xeroderma pigmentosum, nevoid BCC, different squamous cell carcinomas, extramammary Paget's disease, etc [21, 23]. The frequency of application for other "off-label" indications is variable and depends on the indication itself.

Side Effects and Limitations

The most common side effects of the topical imiquimod treatment are restricted to the site of application and include development of local inflammation with erythema, edema, ulceration, and scaling. These are often managed with a drug holiday. In cases of "field cancerization," most commonly involving the face and scalp, application of imiquimod was reported to unmask clinically unapparent AKs, leading to initial worsening and extension of the inflammation to clinically uninvolved areas. The patient should be informed in detail

about the local side effects to ensure full compliance. The inflammatory reaction seems to be necessary for the clearance of the treated lesion [22]. Systemic side effects, caused by the production of inflammatory cytokines, are reflected in flu-like symptoms (i.e., fatigue, headache, fever, myaligas, and diarrhea) described in approximately 1–2% of patients and tend to occur while treating larger skin areas. Patients using topical imiquimod may develop a flare of psoriasis.

No contraindications are currently known for the use of topical imiquimod. Imiquimod 5% cream should not be used in pregnancy, unless absolutely necessary. It is not known whether topically applied imiquimod is excreted in breast milk.

4.1.5.3 Systemic Therapy

4.1.5.3.1 Interferons

Interferons (IFNs) are a group of naturally occurring glyco-proteins exerting antiviral, antiproliferative (control of cell growth/differentiation, induction of apoptosis), and immuno-regulatory (modulation of humoral and cellular immunity) effects [3, 16]. There are three antigenically distinct IFNs, originally described as leukocyte (α), fibroblast (β), and immune (γ). The development of recombinant DNA technology has enabled production of large quantities of highly purified human IFN by *E. coli*. There are over 30 different species of IFN-α that share similar amino acid sequences. IFN-α_{2a} and IFN-α_{2b} differ in just a single amino acid, whereas IFN-β shares 29% structural homology with IFN-α. IFN-γ has no statistically significant structural homology to either IFN-α or IFN-β. In addition to standard parenteral application, IFNs can also be injected intralesionally.

Indications and Dosage

Intralesional IFN-α can be regarded as an alternative to surgery for BCC and squamous cell carcinoma (SCC) of the skin in highly selected patients. In some countries (e.g., in Switzerland), intralesional IFN-α2b is even registered for therapeutically difficult BCC with a minimal recommended dose of 1.5 million IU to be administered three times per week (average dose three million IU per injection). Results from non-randomized, occasionally controlled clinical studies, small series, and case reports indicated that IFN-α, β and γ are effective in the treatment of BCC and SCC (most important studies summarized in [20]). In BCC patients, overall remission rates for multiple intralesional IFN-α injections were reported between 70 and 100%. Five- and ten-year follow-up showed no recurrences in BCC patients with complete response to intralesional IFN-α treatment. For IFN-β, remission rates between 50 and 100% were reported, with the advantages of lower total doses inducing complete BCC remission and less frequent side effects, when compared to IFN-α. Available data on the use of IFN-γ in BCC treatment are somewhat contradictory, with no cure rate above 50% and frequent side effects. Of note is that the tumor type and size must be considered before the therapy, due to the lower efficacy (40%) of interferons in morpheaform BCC.

SCCs have also been treated successfully with intralesional IFN-α, showing response rates up to 98%. Ikic et al. treated 52 patients with SCC, of whom 32 were in their early eighties, using intratumoral application of IFN. After one decade of observation, only two recurrences occurred at the site of original lesion, suggesting that IFN may offer a persistent cure for patients with SCC [6]. IFN-α treatment may not only be used in patients with actinically induced SCC but also in patients with human papillomavirus (HPV)-associated SCC who are not candidates for surgical excision or are not amenable to surgery [4]. The dosing schedule for IFN-α in these cases is similar to that of BCC.

Side Effects and Limitations

The main advantage of locally injected IFNs is probably the superior cosmetic result, but the treatment is inconvenient since injections are commonly given three times per week for several weeks (average 3 weeks). Side effects of IFN treatment are dose-dependent and generally improve or remit during the course of treatment or following dose reduction. The most common side effects include flu-like symptoms (i.e., fever, chills, fatigue, myalgias, arthralgias, and headache). Prophylactic (1–2 h prior to injection) administration of paracetamol/acetaminophen, aspirin, or nonsteroidal anti-inflammatory drugs (e.g., ibuprofen) helps to prevent these effects. Plaque of psoriasis may develop at the sites of injection of IFN, as can flares of psoriasis. Gastrointestinal disturbances such as nausea, vomiting, and diarrhea can occur, as can anorexia and hepatitis. Bone marrow suppression can also be a problem, particularly in patients who have other reasons for bone marrow suppression (e.g., concomitant use of myelosuppressive drugs or zidovudine). Autoimmune thyroiditis with hypo- or hyperthyroidism was also described in patients receiving IFN. Serial evaluation of liver and thyroid function tests as well as complete blood counts is recommended.

Hypersensitivity to an IFN formulation represents an absolute contraindication. Relative contraindications are cardiac arrhythmias, depression and other psychiatric disorders, leucopenia, coagulopathies, and previous organ transplantation. IFN should not be used during pregnancy, unless absolutely necessary. It is not unknown whether IFN is excreted into human milk; it is however excreted into mouse milk.

References

Surgery

1. Alcalay, J., Alkalay, R.: Controversies in perioperative management of blood thinners in dermatologic surgery: continue or discontinue? Dermatol. Surg. **30**(8), 1091–1094 (2004), discussion 4
2. Barlow, J.O., Zalla, M.J., Kyle, A., DiCaudo, D.J., Lim, K.K., Yiannias, J.A.: Treatment of basal cell carcinoma with curettage alone. J. Am. Acad. Dermatol. **54**(6), 1039–1045 (2006)
3. Bath-Hextall, F.J., Perkins, W., Bong, J., Williams, H.C.: Interventions for basal cell carcinoma of the skin. Cochrane Database Syst. Rev. (1):CD003412 (2007)
4. Breuninger, H.: Micrographic surgery of malignant skin tumors: a comparison of the frozen technique with paraffin sectioning. Facial Plast. Surg. **13**(2), 79–82 (1997)
5. Breuninger, H., Dietz, K.: Prediction of subclinical tumor infiltration in basal cell carcinoma. J. Dermatol. Surg. Oncol. **17**(7), 574–578 (1991)
6. Breuninger, H., Sebastian, G., Kortmann, R.D., Wolff, K., Bootz, F., Garbe, C.: Brief guidelines: squamous cell carcinoma of the skin, lip and eyelids. J. Dtsch. Dermatol. Ges. **4**(3), 260–262 (2006)
7. Burg, G., Hirsch, R.D., Konz, B., Braun-Falco, O.: Histographic surgery: accuracy of visual assessment of the margins of basal-cell epithelioma. J. Dermatol. Surg. **1**(3), 21–24 (1975)
8. Chiller, K., Passaro, D., McCalmont, T., Vin-Christian, K.: Efficacy of curettage before excision in clearing surgical margins of nonmelanoma skin cancer. Arch. Dermatol. **136**(11), 1327–1332 (2000)
9. Cvancara, J.L., Wentzell, J.M.: Shark island pedicle flap for repair of combined nasal ala-perialar defects. Dermatol. Surg. **32**(5), 726–729 (2006)
10. Edens, B.L., Bartlow, G.A., Haghighi, P., Astarita, R.W., Davidson, T.M.: Effectiveness of curettage and electrodesiccation in the removal of basal cell carcinoma. J. Am. Acad. Dermatol. **9**(3), 383–388 (1983)
11. Giuffrida, T.J., Jimenez, G., Nouri, K.: Histologic cure of basal cell carcinoma treated with cryosurgery. J. Am. Acad. Dermatol. **49**(3), 483–486 (2003)
12. Goncalves, J.C.: Fractional cryosurgery. A new technique for basal cell carcinoma of the eyelids and periorbital area. Dermatol. Surg. **23**(6), 475–481 (1997)
13. Graham, G.F.: Statistical data on malignant tumors in cryosurgery: 1982. J. Dermatol. Surg. Oncol. **9**(3), 238–239 (1983)
14. Griffiths, R.W., Suvarna, S.K., Stone, J.: Do basal cell carcinomas recur after complete conventional surgical excision? Br. J. Plast. Surg. **58**(6), 795–805 (2005)
15. Holt, P.J.: Cryotherapy for skin cancer: results over a 5-year period using liquid nitrogen spray cryosurgery. Br. J. Dermatol. **119**(2), 231–240 (1988)
16. Johnson, T.M., Tromovitch, T.A., Swanson, N.A.: Combined curettage and excision: a treatment method for primary basal cell carcinoma. J. Am. Acad. Dermatol. **24**(4), 613–617 (1991)
17. Kimyai-Asadi, A., Goldberg, L.H., Jih, M.H.: Accuracy of serial transverse cross-sections in detecting residual basal cell carcinoma at the surgical margins of an elliptical excision specimen. J. Am. Acad. Dermatol. **53**(3), 469–474 (2005)
18. Kimyai-Asadi, A., Goldberg, L.H., Peterson, S.R., Silapint, S., Jih, M.H.: The incidence of major complications from Mohs micrographic surgery performed in office-based and hospital-based settings. J. Am. Acad. Dermatol. **53**(4), 628–634 (2005)
19. Kokoszka, A., Scheinfeld, N.: Evidence-based review of the use of cryosurgery in treatment of basal cell carcinoma. Dermatol. Surg. **29**(6), 566–571 (2003)

20. Kopf, A.W., Bart, R.S., Schrager, D., Lazar, M., Popkin, G.L.: Curettage-electrodesiccation treatment of basal cell carcinomas. Arch. Dermatol. **113**(4), 439–443 (1977)
21. Koplin, L., Zarem, H.A.: Recurrent basal cell carcinoma. A review concerning the incidence, behavior, and management of recurrent basal cell carcinoma, with emphasis on the incompletely excised lesion. Plast. Reconstr. Surg. **65**(5), 656–664 (1980)
22. Kuflik, E.G.: Cryosurgery for skin cancer: 30-year experience and cure rates. Dermatol. Surg. **30**(2 pt 2), 297–300 (2004)
23. Kuflik, E.G., Gage, A.A.: The five-year cure rate achieved by cryosurgery for skin cancer. J. Am. Acad. Dermatol. **24**(6 pt 1), 1002–1004 (1991)
24. Lewis, K.G., Dufresne Jr., R.G.: A meta-analysis of complications attributed to anticoagulation among patients following cutaneous surgery. Dermatol. Surg. **34**(2), 160–164 (2008), discussion 4–5
25. Licitra, L., Bossi, P., Locati, L.D.: A multidisciplinary approach to squamous cell carcinomas of the head and neck: what is new? Curr. Opin. Oncol. **18**(3), 253–257 (2006)
26. Liu, F.F., Maki, E., Warde, P., Payne, D., Fitzpatrick, P.: A management approach to incompletely excised basal cell carcinomas of skin. Int. J. Radiat. Oncol. Biol. Phys. **20**(3), 423–428 (1991)
27. Lo, J.S., Snow, S.N.: Metastatic basal cell carcinoma. J. Am. Acad. Dermatol. **27**(5 pt 1), 788–789 (1992)
28. Mallon, E., Dawber, R.: Cryosurgery in the treatment of basal cell carcinoma. Assessment of one and two freeze-thaw cycle schedules. Dermatol. Surg. **22**(10), 854–858 (1996)
29. Marchac, D., Papadopoulos, O., Duport, G.: Curative and aesthetic results of surgical treatment of 138 basal-cell carcinomas. J. Dermatol. Surg. Oncol. **8**(5), 379–387 (1982)
30. Miller, S.J.: The National Comprehensive Cancer Network (NCCN) guidelines of care for nonmelanoma skin cancers. Dermatol. Surg. **26**(3), 289–292 (2000)
31. Mohs, F.E.: Chemosurgery for skin cancer: fixed tissue and fresh tissue techniques. Arch. Dermatol. **112**(2), 211–215 (1976)
32. Motley, R.J., Gould, D.J., Douglas, W.S., Simpson, N.B.: Treatment of basal cell carcinoma by dermatologists in the United Kingdom. British Association of Dermatologists Audit Subcommittee and the British Society for Dermatological Surgery. Br. J. Dermatol. **132**(3), 437–440 (1995)
33. Nelson, B.R., Railan, D., Cohen, S.: Mohs' micrographic surgery for nonmelanoma skin cancers. Clin. Plast. Surg. **24**(4), 705–718 (1997)
34. Neville, J.A., Welch, E., Leffell, D.J.: Management of nonmelanoma skin cancer in 2007. Nat. Clin. Pract. Oncol. **4**(8), 462–469 (2007)
35. Nguyen, T.H., Ho, D.Q.: Nonmelanoma skin cancer. Curr. Treat. Options Oncol. **3**(3), 193–203 (2002)
36. Nouri, K., Chang, A., Trent, J.T., Jimenez, G.P.: Ultrapulse CO_2 used for the successful treatment of basal cell carcinomas found in patients with basal cell nevus syndrome. Dermatol. Surg. **28**(3), 287–290 (2002)
37. Nouri, K., Spencer, J.M., Taylor, J.R., Hayag, M., DeVoursney, J., Shah, N.: Does wound healing contribute to the eradication of basal cell carcinoma following curettage and electrodessication? Dermatol. Surg. **25**(3), 183–187 (1999), discussion 7–8
38. Otley, C.C.: Perioperative evaluation and management in dermatologic surgery. J. Am. Acad. Dermatol. **54**(1), 119–127 (2006)
39. Richmond, J.D., Davie, R.M.: The significance of incomplete excision in patients with basal cell carcinoma. Br. J. Plast. Surg. **40**(1), 63–67 (1987)
40. Rowe, D.E., Carroll, R.J., Day Jr., C.L.: Mohs surgery is the treatment of choice for recurrent (previously treated) basal cell carcinoma. J. Dermatol. Surg. Oncol. **15**(4), 424–431 (1989)
41. Rowe, D.E., Carroll, R.J., Day Jr., C.L.: Long-term recurrence rates in previously untreated (primary) basal cell carcinoma: implications for patient follow-up. J. Dermatol. Surg. Oncol. **15**(3), 315–328 (1989)
42. Rowe, D.E., Carroll, R.J., Day Jr., C.L.: Prognostic factors for local recurrence, metastasis, and survival rates in squamous cell carcinoma of the skin, ear, and lip. Implications for treatment modality selection. J. Am. Acad. Dermatol. **26**(6), 976–990 (1992)
43. Salasche, S.J.: Curettage and electrodesiccation in the treatment of midfacial basal cell epithelioma. J. Am. Acad. Dermatol. **8**(4), 496–503 (1983)
44. Shriner, D.L., McCoy, D.K., Goldberg, D.J., Wagner Jr., R.F.: Mohs micrographic surgery. J. Am. Acad. Dermatol. **39**(1), 79–97 (1998)
45. Skaria, A.M., Salomon, D.: Mohs' surgery of periocular basal cell carcinoma using formalin-fixed sections and delayed closure. Br. J. Dermatol. **140**(4), 775 (1999)
46. Smeets, N.W., Kuijpers, D.I., Nelemans, P., Ostertag, J.U., Verhaegh, M.E., Krekels, G.A., et al.: Mohs' micrographic surgery for treatment of basal cell carcinoma of the face–results of a retrospective study and review of the literature. Br. J. Dermatol. **151**(1), 141–147 (2004)
47. Spencer, J.M., Tannenbaum, A., Sloan, L., Amonette, R.A.: Does inflammation contribute to the eradication of basal cell carcinoma following curettage and electrodesiccation? Dermatol. Surg. **23**(8), 625–630 (1997), discussion 30–31
48. Stasko, T., Brown, M.D., Carucci, J.A., Euvrard, S., Johnson, T.M., Sengelmann, R.D., et al.: Guidelines for the management of squamous cell carcinoma in organ transplant recipients. Dermatol. Surg. **30**(4 pt 2), 642–650 (2004)
49. Telfer, N.R., Colver, G.B., Morton, C.A.: Guidelines for the management of basal cell carcinoma. Br. J. Dermatol. **159**(1), 35–48 (2008)
50. Walker, P., Hill, D.: Surgical treatment of basal cell carcinomas using standard postoperative histological assessment. Australas. J. Dermatol. **47**(1), 1–12 (2006)
51. Wang, I., Bendsoe, N., Klinteberg, C.A., Enejder, A.M., Andersson-Engels, S., Svanberg, S., et al.: Photodynamic therapy vs. cryosurgery of basal cell carcinomas: results of a phase III clinical trial. Br. J. Dermatol. **144**(4), 832–840 (2001)
52. Williford, P.M., Feldman, S.R.: Surgery for basal-cell carcinoma of the face. Lancet **364**(9447), 1732–1733 (2004)
53. Wilson, A.W., Howsam, G., Santhanam, V., Macpherson, D., Grant, J., Pratt, C.A., et al.: Surgical management of incompletely excised basal cell carcinomas of the head and neck. Br. J. Oral Maxillofac. Surg. **42**(4), 311–314 (2004)
54. Wolf, D.J., Zitelli, J.A.: Surgical margins for basal cell carcinoma. Arch. Dermatol. **123**(3), 340–344 (1987)
55. Wu, J.K., Oh, C., Strutton, G., Siller, G.: An open-label, pilot study examining the efficacy of curettage followed by imiquimod 5% cream for the treatment of primary nodular basal cell carcinoma. Australas. J. Dermatol. **47**(1), 46–48 (2006)
56. Zacarian, S.A.: Cryosurgery of cutaneous carcinomas. An 18-year study of 3,022 patients with 4,228 carcinomas. J. Am. Acad. Dermatol. **9**(6), 947–956 (1983)

Phototherapy, Laser and Radiation: Phototherapie

1. Meyer-Betz, F.: Untersuchungen über die biologische (photodynamische) Wirkung des Haematoporphyrins und anderer Derivative des Blut- und Gallenfarbstoffs. Dtsch Arch. Klin. Med. **112**, 476–503 (1913)
2. Svanberg, K., Andersson, T., Killander, D., et al.: Photodynamic therapy of non-melanoma malignant tumors of the skin using topical delta-amino levulinic acid sensitization and laser irradiation. Br. J. Dermatol. **130**, 743–751 (1994)
3. Thissen, M.R., Schroeter, C.A., Neumann, H.A.: Photodynamic therapy with delta-aminolaevulinic acid for nodular basal cell carcinomas using a prior debulking technique. Br. J. Dermatol. **142**, 338–339 (2000)

4. Fijan, S., Honigsmann, H., Ortel, B.: Photodynamic therapy of epithelial skin tumors using delta-aminolaevulinic acid and desferrioxamine. Br. J. Dermatol. **133**, 282–288 (1995)

5. Peng, Q., Warloe, T., Moan, J., et al.: Distribution of 5-aminolevulinic acid-induced porphyrins in noduloulcerative basal cell carcinoma. Photochem. Photobiol. **62**, 906–913 (1995)

6. Peng, Q., Soler, A.M., Warloe, T., Nesland, J.M., Giercksky, K.E.: Selective distribution of porphyrins in skin thick basal cell carcinoma after topical application of methyl 5-aminolevulinate. J. Photochem. Photobiol. B **62**, 140–145 (2001)

7. Clark, C., Bryden, A., Dawe, R., Moseley, H., Ferguson, J., Ibbotson, S.H.: Topical 5-aminolaevulinic acid photodynamic therapy for cutaneous lesions: outcome and comparison of light sources. Photodermatol. Photoimmunol. Photomed. **19**, 134–141 (2003)

8. Dragieva, G., Prinz, B.M., Hafner, J., et al.: A randomized controlled clinical trial of topical photodynamic therapy with methyl aminolaevulinate in the treatment of actinic keratoses in transplant recipients. Br. J. Dermatol. **151**, 196–200 (2004)

9. Kurwa, H.A., Yong-Gee, S.A., Seed, P.T., Markey, A.C., Barlow, R.J.: A randomized paired comparison of photodynamic therapy and topical 5-fluorouracil in the treatment of actinic keratoses. J. Am. Acad. Dermatol. **41**, 414–418 (1999)

10. Szeimies, R.M., Karrer, S., Radakovic-Fijan, S., et al.: Photodynamic therapy using topical methyl 5-aminolevulinate compared with cryotherapy for actinic keratosis: A prospective, randomized study. J. Am. Acad. Dermatol. **47**, 258–262 (2002)

11. Freeman, M., Vinciullo, C., Francis, D., et al.: A comparison of photodynamic therapy using topical methyl aminolevulinate (Metvix) with single cycle cryotherapy in patients with actinic keratosis: a prospective, randomized study. J. Dermatolog. Treat. **14**, 99–106 (2003)

12. Pariser, D.M., Lowe, N.J., Stewart, D.M., et al.: Photodynamic therapy with topical methyl aminolevulinate for actinic keratosis: results of a prospective randomized multicenter trial. J. Am. Acad. Dermatol. **48**, 227–232 (2003)

13. Tarstedt, M., Rosdahl, I., Berne, B., Svanberg, K., Wennberg, A.M.: A randomized multicenter study to compare two treatment regimens of topical methyl aminolevulinate (Metvix)-PDT in actinic keratosis of the face and scalp. Acta Derm. Venereol. **85**, 424–428 (2005)

14. Piacquadio, D.J., Chen, D.M., Farber, H.F., et al.: Photodynamic therapy with aminolevulinic acid topical solution and visible blue light in the treatment of multiple actinic keratoses of the face and scalp: investigator-blinded, phase 3, multicenter trials. Arch. Dermatol. **140**, 41–46 (2004)

15. Salim, A., Leman, J.A., McColl, J.H., Chapman, R., Morton, C.A.: Randomized comparison of photodynamic therapy with topical 5-fluorouracil in Bowen's disease. Br. J. Dermatol. **148**, 539–543 (2003)

16. Dragieva, G., Hafner, J., Dummer, R., et al.: Topical photodynamic therapy in the treatment of actinic keratoses and Bowen's disease in transplant recipients. Transplantation **77**, 115–121 (2004)

17. Soler, A.M., Warloe, T., Berner, A., Giercksky, K.E.: A follow-up study of recurrence and cosmesis in completely responding superficial and nodular basal cell carcinomas treated with methyl 5-aminolaevulinate-based photodynamic therapy alone and with prior curettage. Br. J. Dermatol. **145**, 467–471 (2001)

18. Basset-Seguin, N., Ibbotson, S.H., Emtestam, L., et al.: Topical methyl aminolaevulinate photodynamic therapy versus cryotherapy for superficial basal cell carcinoma: a 5 year randomized trial. Eur. J. Dermatol. **18**, 547–553 (2008)

19. Foley, P.: Clinical efficacy of methyl aminolevulinate (Metvix) photodynamic therapy. J. Dermatolog. Treat. **14**(suppl 3), 15–22 (2003)

20. Rhodes, L.E., de Rie, M., Enstrom, Y., et al.: Photodynamic therapy using topical methyl aminolevulinate vs surgery for nodular basal cell carcinoma: results of a multicenter randomized prospective trial. Arch. Dermatol. **140**, 17–23 (2004)

21. Vinciullo, C., Elliott, T., Francis, D., et al.: Photodynamic therapy with topical methyl aminolevulinate for 'difficult-to-treat' basal cell carcinoma. Br. J. Dermatol. **152**, 765–772 (2005)

22. Horn, M., Wolf, P., Wulf, H.C., et al.: Topical methyl aminolaevulinate photodynamic therapy in patients with basal cell carcinoma prone to complications and poor cosmetic outcome with conventional treatment. Br. J. Dermatol. **149**, 1242–1249 (2003)

23. Guillen, C., Sanmartin, O., Escudero, A., Botella-Estrada, R., Sevila, A., Castejon, P.: Photodynamic therapy for in situ squamous cell carcinoma on chronic radiation dermatitis after photosensitization with 5-aminolaevulinic acid. J. Eur. Acad. Dermatol. Venereol. **14**, 298–300 (2000)

24. Calzavara-Pinton, P.G.: Repetitive photodynamic therapy with topical delta-aminolaevulinic acid as an appropriate approach to the routine treatment of superficial non-melanoma skin tumors. J. Photochem. Photobiol. B **29**, 53–57 (1995)

25. Oseroff, A.R., Shieh, S., Frawley, N.P., et al.: Treatment of diffuse basal cell carcinomas and basaloid follicular hamartomas in nevoid basal cell carcinoma syndrome by wide-area 5-aminolevulinic acid photodynamic therapy. Arch. Dermatol. **141**, 60–67 (2005)

Phototherapy, Laser and Radiation: Radiation

1. Dupree, M.T., Kiteley, R.A., et al.: Radiation therapy for Bowen's disease: lessons for lesions of the lower extremity. J. Am. Acad. Dermatol. **45**(3), 401–404 (2001)

2. Freeman, R.G., Knox, J.M., et al.: The treatment of skin cancer. A statistical study of 1, 341 skin tumors comparing results obtained with irradiation, surgery, and curettage followed by electrodesiccation. Cancer **17**, 535–538 (1964)

3. Liu, F.F., Maki, E., et al.: A management approach to incompletely excised basal cell carcinomas of skin. Int. J. Radiat. Oncol. Biol. Phys. **20**(3), 423–428 (1991)

4. Locke, J., Karimpour, S., et al.: Radiotherapy for epithelial skin cancer. Int. J. Radiat. Oncol. Biol. Phys. **51**(3), 748–755 (2001)

5. Malone, J.P., Fedok, F.G., et al.: Basal cell carcinoma metastatic to the parotid: report of a new case and review of the literature. Ear Nose Throat J. **79**(7), 511–515 (2000). 518–519

6. Motley, R., Kersey, P., et al.: Multiprofessional guidelines for the management of the patient with primary cutaneous squamous cell carcinoma. Br. J. Dermatol. **146**(1), 18–25 (2002)

7. Panizzon, R.G.: Dermatologic radiotherapy. Hautarzt **58**(8), 701–710 (2007). quiz 711

8. Rippey, J.J., Rippey, E.: Characteristics of incompletely excised basal cell carcinomas of the skin. Med. J. Aust. **166**(11), 581–583 (1997)

9. Rowe, D.E., Carroll, R.J., et al.: Prognostic factors for local recurrence, metastasis, and survival rates in squamous cell carcinoma of the skin, ear, and lip. Implications for treatment modality selection. J. Am. Acad. Dermatol. **26**(6), 976–990 (1992)

10. Schulte, K.W., Lippold, A., et al.: Soft x-ray therapy for cutaneous basal cell and squamous cell carcinomas. J. Am. Acad. Dermatol. **53**(6), 993–1001 (2005)

11. Scrivener, Y., Grosshans, E., et al.: Variations of basal cell carcinomas according to gender, age, location and histopathological subtype. Br. J. Dermatol. **147**(1), 41–47 (2002)

12. Telfer, N.R., Colver, G.B., et al.: Guidelines for the management of basal cell carcinoma. British Association of Dermatologists. Br. J. Dermatol. **141**(3), 415–423 (1999)

13. Veness, M.J.: The important role of radiotherapy in patients with non-melanoma skin cancer and other cutaneous entities. J. Med. Imaging Radiat. Oncol. **52**(3), 278–286 (2008)
14. Veness, M.J., Ong, C., et al.: Squamous cell carcinoma of the lip. Patterns of relapse and outcome: Reporting the Westmead Hospital experience, 1980–1997. Australas. Radiol. **45**(2), 195–199 (2001)
15. Zagrodnik, B., Kempf, W., et al.: Superficial radiotherapy for patients with basal cell carcinoma: recurrence rates, histologic subtypes, and expression of p53 and Bcl-2. Cancer **98**(12), 2708–2714 (2003)

Phototherapy, Laser and Radiation: Lasers for Non-Melanoma Skin Cancer

1. Bernard, P., Dupuy, A., Sasco, A., Brun, P., Duru, G., Nicoloyannis, N., Grob, J.J.: Basal cell carcinomas and actinic keratoses seen in dermatological practice in France: a cross-sectional study. Dermatology **216**, 194–199 (2008)
2. Bogdan, I., Schärer, L., Rüdlinger, R., Hafner, J.: Epidermodysplasia verruciformis in two brothers developing aggressive squamous cell carcinoma. Dermatol. Surg. **33**, 1525–1528 (2007)
3. Bruchim, I., Gotlieb, W.H., Mahmud, S., Tunitsky, E., Grzywacz, K., Ferenzy, A.: PPV-related vulvar intraepithelial neoplasia: outcome of different management modalities. Int. J. Gynaecol. Obstet. **99**, 23–27 (2007)
4. Carrozza, P.M., Merlani, G.M., Burg, G., Hafner, J.: CO2 laser surgery for extensive, cauliflower-like anogenital condylomata acuminata: retrospective long-term study on 19 HIV-positive and 45 HIV-negative men. Dermatology **205**, 255–259 (2002)
5. Covadonga Martinez-Gonzalez, M., del Pozo, J., Paradela, S., Fernandez-Jorge, B., Fernandez-Torres, R., Fonseca, E.: Bowen's disease treated by carbon dioxide laser. A series of 44 patients. J. Dermatol. Treat. **19**, 293–299 (2008)
6. Gordon, K.B., Garden, J.M., Robinson, J.K.: Bowen's disease of the distal digit. Outcome of treatment with carbon dioxide laser vaporization. Dermatol. Surg. **22**, 723–728 (1996)
7. Hafner, J.: CO_2-laser und Er-YAG-laser. In: Dummer, R. (ed.) Physikalische Therapiemassnamen in der Dermatologie. Steinkopff, Darmstadt (2006)
8. Hillemanns, P., Wang, X., Staehle, S., Michels, W., Dannecker, C.: Evaluation of different treatment modalities for vulvar intraepithelial neoplasia (VIN): CO_2 laser vaporization, photodynamic therapy, excision and vulvectomy. Gynecol. Oncol. **100**, 271–275 (2006)
9. Kaspari, M., Gutzmer, R., Kaspari, T., Kapp, A., Brodersen, J.P.: Application of imiquimod by suppositories (anal tampons) efficiently prevents recurrences after ablation of anal canal condyloma. Br. J. Dermatol. **147**, 757–759 (2002)
10. Läuchli, S., Dragieva, G., Kempf, W., Hafner, J.: CO2-laser treatment of warts in immunosuppressed patients. Dermatology **206**, 148–152 (2003)
11. Nouri, K., Spencer, J.M., Taylor, J.R., Hayag, M., de Voursney, J., Shah, N.: Does wound healing contribute to the eradication of basal cell carcinoma following curettage and electrodessication? Dermatol. Surg. **25**, 183–188 (1999)
12. Trimas, S.J., Ellis, D.A., Metz, R.D.: The carbon dioxide laser: an alternative for the treatment of actinically damaged skin. Dermatol. Surg. **23**, 885–889 (1997)
13. Weyandt, G.H., Benoit, S., Becker, J.C., Bröcker, E.B., Hamm, H.: Controlled layered removal of anogenital warts by argon-plasma coagulation. JDDG **3**, 271–275 (2005)
14. Wollina, U., Konrad, H., Karamfilov, T.: Treatment of common warts and actinic keratoses by Er:YAG laser. J. Cutan. Laser Ther. **3**, 63–66 (2001)

Drug Therapy for Non-Melanoma Skin Cancer

1. Bianchi, L., Orlandi, A., Campione, E., et al.: Topical treatment of basal cell carcinoma with tazarotene: a clinicopathological study on a large series of cases. Br. J. Dermatol. **151**, 148–156 (2004)
2. Cox, N.H., Eedy, D.J., Morton, C.A.: Guidelines for management of Bowen's disease: 2006 update. Br. J. Dermatol. **156**, 11–21 (2007)
3. Dunn, G.P., Koebel, C.M., Schreiber, R.D.: Interferons, immunity and cancer immunoediting. Nat. Rev. Immunol. **6**, 836–848 (2006)
4. Edwards, L., Berman, B., Rapini, R.P., et al.: Treatment of cutaneous squamous cell carcinomas by intralesional interferon alfa-2b therapy. Arch. Dermatol. **128**, 1486–1489 (1992)
5. Hengge, U.R.: Topical therapy of squamous cell carcinoma. Hautarzt **58**, 412–418 (2007)
6. Ikić, D., Padovan, I., Pipić, N., et al.: Interferon reduces recurrences of basal cell and squamous cell cancers. Int. J. Dermatol. **34**, 58–60 (1995)
7. Jury, C.S., Ramraka-Jones, V.S., Gudi, V., et al.: A randomized trial of topical 5% 5-fluorouracil (Efudix cream) in the treatment of actinic keratoses comparing daily with weekly treatment. Br. J. Dermatol. **153**, 808–810 (2005)
8. Kang, S., Goldfarb, M.T., Weiss, J.S., et al.: Assessment of adapalene gel for the treatment of actinic keratoses and lentigines: a randomized trial. J. Am. Acad. Dermatol. **49**, 83–90 (2003)
9. Kligman, A., Thorne, E.: Topical therapy of actinic keratoses with tretinoin. In: Marks, R. (ed.) Retinods in Cutaneous Malignancy. Blackwell Scientific, Oxford (1991)
10. Kuenzli, S., Saurat, J.: Retinoids. In: Bolognia, J.L., Jorizzo, J.L., Rapini, R.P. (eds.) Dermatology. Mosby Elsevier, Philadelphia (2008)
11. Kunte, C., Konz, B.: Current recommendations in the treatment of basal cell carcinoma and squamous cell carcinoma of the skin. Hautarzt **58**, 419–426 (2007)
12. Labandeira, J., Pereiro, M.J., Valdés, F., et al.: Intermittent topical 5-fluorouracil is effective without significant irritation in the treatment of actinic keratoses but prolongs treatment duration. Dermatol. Surg. **30**, 517–520 (2004)
13. Loven, K., Stein, L., Furst, K., et al.: Evaluation of the efficacy and tolerability of 0.5% fluorouracil cream and 5% fluorouracil cream applied to each side of the face in patients with actinic keratosis. Clin. Ther. **24**, 990–1000 (2002)
14. Merk, H.F.: Topical diclofenac in the treatment of actinic keratoses. Int. J. Dermatol. **46**, 12–18 (2007)
15. Phillips, T.J., Gottlieb, A.B., Leyden, J.J., et al.: Efficacy of 0.1% tazarotene cream for the treatment of photodamage: a 12-month multicenter, randomized trial. Arch. Dermatol. **138**, 1486–1493 (2002)
16. Platanias, L.C.: Mechanisms of type-I- and type-II-interferon-mediated signalling. Nat. Rev. Immunol. **5**, 375–386 (2005)
17. Salim, A., Leman, J.A., McColl, J.H., et al.: Randomized comparison of photodynamic therapy with topical 5-fluorouracil in Bowen's disease. Br. J. Dermatol. **148**, 539–543 (2003)
18. Schön, M.P., Schön, M.: TLR7 and TLR8 as targets in cancer therapy. Oncogene **27**, 190–199 (2008)
19. Szeimies, R., Karrer, S., Bäcker, H.: Therapeutic options for epithelial skin tumors. Actinic keratoses, Bowen disease, squamous cell carcinoma, and basal cell carcinoma. Hautarzt **56**, 430–440 (2005)
20. Urosevic, M., Dummer, R.: Immunotherapy for nonmelanoma skin cancer: does it have a future? Cancer **94**, 477–485 (2002)
21. Urosevic, M., Dummer, R.: Role of imiquimod in skin cancer treatment. Am. J. Clin. Dermatol. **5**, 453–458 (2004)
22. Urosevic, M., Dummer, R., Conrad, C., et al.: Disease-independent skin recruitment and activation of plasmacytoid predendritic cells following imiquimod treatment. J. Natl. Cancer Inst. **97**, 1143–1153 (2005)
23. Wagstaff, A.J., Perry, C.M.: Topical imiquimod: a review of its use in the management of anogenital warts, actinic keratoses, basal cell carcinoma and other skin lesions. Drugs **67**, 2187–2210 (2007)

Melanoma

4.2

Merlin Guggenheim, Pietro Giovanoli, Brigitta G. Baumert,
Thomas Kurt Eigentler, Claus Garbe, Joanna Mangana,
and Reinhard Dummer

4.2.1 Surgery

Merlin Guggenheim and Pietro Giovanoli

4.2.1.1 Indications

4.2.1.1.1 Primary Excision

Diagnosis should be based on a full-thickness excisional biopsy, with a small side margin. Suspicious melanocytic lesions should be excised completely, with a narrow clinical margin [7].

4.2.1.1.2 Wide Excision

Wide local excision of a cuff of normal tissue after an excision biopsy reduces local recurrence rates. Up until the 1980s, radical disfiguring wide local excision margins of 4–5 cm were used on the basis of anecdotal evidence from 1907 [8]. Meanwhile, surgical management of early-stage melanomas is guided mainly by the Breslow thickness of the lesion

M. Guggenheim (✉) and P. Giovanoli
Department of Surgery, Division of Plastic and Reconstructive Surgery, University Hospital Zurich, 8091 Zurich, Switzerland
e-mail: merlin.guggenheim@usz.ch

B.G. Baumert
Department of Radiation-Oncology (MAASTRO), GROW (School for Biology and Developmental Biology), Maastricht University Medical Centre (MUMC), 6229 ET Maastricht, The Netherlands
e-mail: brigitta.baumert@maastro.nl

T.K. Eigentler and C. Garbe
Division of Dermatooncology, Department of Dermatology, University Medical Center, Liebermeisterstrasse 25, 72076 Tübingen, Germany
e-mail: thomas.eigentler@med.uni-tuebingen.de

J. Mangana and R. Dummer
Deparment of Dermatooncology, Department of Dermatology, University Hospital of Zürich, Gloriastrasse 31, 8091 Zürich, Switzerland
e-mail: joannamangana@gmail.com; reinhard.dummer@usz.ch

(Table 4.2.1). The current guidelines have been developed based on five randomized trials in both Europe and the United States. The first of these trials, conducted by the World Health Organization (WHO) [9], showed that 1 and 3-cm margins were equivalent in terms of recurrence and survival. Moreover, a 1-cm margin for melanomas less than 2.0-mm thick was found to be safe. In contrast, the other two trials looked at 2- vs. 5-cm margins in melanoma with a Breslow thickness of less than 2.0-mm and concluded that 2 cm was just as safe as 5 cm [10, 11]. Two further studies focused on thicker melanoma, with Breslow thickness ranging from 1- to 4-mm and more than 2.0 mm, respectively. The Intergroup Melanoma Trial showed that a 2-cm margin was equivalent to 4 cm in terms of locoregional recurrvence and overall survival [12]. In the fifth trial, from the United Kingdom [13], a significantly worse local recurrence and disease-free survival (DFS) rate were observed in the 1-cm arm when compared to the 3-cm arm, for melanoma more than 2.0-mm thick. However, no overall survival difference was seen; thus, the conclusion was that a 1-cm margin was not safe for melanoma with a Breslow thickness >2.0 mm because of the increased risk of locoregional recurrence and a possible increase in mortality. Decisions on the size of the margins in facial and acral melanoma should be made by members of the multidisciplinary team, who balance the morbidity of the procedure with the potential benefit to the patient.

4.2.1.1.3 Sentinel Lymph Node Biopsy

In the past decade, sentinel lymph node biopsy (SLNB) has become the standard for staging patients diagnosed with cutaneous malignant melanoma. The method's accuracy and reliability and the status of the SLN as the single most important prognostic factor for recurrence and survival in melanoma patients have been proven beyond any reasonable doubt [5, 14]. Nevertheless, the impact of SLNB on survival remains unclear. Recently, Morton et al. [15] reported an increased DFS with SLNB but no significant impact on overall survival, raising the question whether lymph node dissection is necessary in cases of positive SLN. Nevertheless,

R. Dummer et al. (eds.), *Skin Cancer – A World-Wide Perspective*,
DOI: 10.1007/978-3-642-05072-5_4.2, © Springer-Verlag Berlin Heidelberg 2011

Table 4.2.1 Excision safety margins for surgical treatment of primary melanoma (pT1–4N0M0) [7]

Tumor thickness (Breslow)	Excision safety margin (cm)
Melanoma in situ (tumor thickness is not indicated) (plisN0M0)	0.5
<2 mm (pT1–2N0M0)	1
>2 mm (pT3–4N0M0)	2

there is a general agreement that SLNB helps to identify patients who might benefit from further therapy, such as CLND and/or adjuvant interferon therapy [5, 6], even if clinical trials aiming to determine the impact of these adjuvant measures are still ongoing. The recently published proceedings of an expert panel clarify the indication of SLNB as a staging tool [16]: SLNB should be discussed with and offered to all patients with primary melanoma with Breslow thickness equal to or greater than 1.0 mm and clinically normal regional lymph nodes (determined by physical examination when the criteria described above are met). Many experts recommend discussing and offering SLNB to patients whose melanomas are not thicker than 1.0 mm but have characteristics that increase the likelihood of regional node micrometastasis (Clark level of invasion, mitotic index, vertical growth phase, male gender, ulceration of the primary tumor, young age, regression, and discordancy between clinical findings and biopsy findings). Although unanimous consensus was not reached for all criteria, many experts recommend the procedure for patients with T1 melanoma with primary tumor ulceration, a mitotic rate greater than or equal to 1 per millimeter [17], and/or Clark level IV/V invasion, especially if tumor thickness exceeds 0.75 mm. Whereas tumor thickness is regarded by some as the sole criterion for SNB, ulceration, mitotic rate, and Clark level are especially relevant in patients who have no significant comorbidity, who are younger than 40–45 years [18], or whose primary tumor depth is uncertain because of tumor-positive deep margins in the biopsy specimen. As the incidence of sentinel positivity for primary melanoma with Breslow thickness of 0.75–1.00 is reduced, in addition to the fact that further positive nonsentinel lymph nodes in this group are found only occasionally [19], many national guidelines recommend SLNB only for melanomas with a Breslow thickness of ≥1 mm. Nonetheless, sentinel lymphadenectomy in thin melanomas remains controversial, and there are currently no phase III randomized studies supporting any treatment recommendation for this group of patients. Several single-center retrospective studies have examined histopathologic factors that would predict sentinel node positivity in thin melanomas, and one study found that the sentinel node status was significant for disease and overall survival in a group of 631 patients with thin melanomas; the incidence of sentinel node positivity in these studies ranged from 3.6 to 6.5%, possibly indicating at least some need for sentinel lymphadenectomy thin melanoma [20].

4.2.1.1.4 Completion Lymph Node Dissection

In the presentinel era, melanoma patients were subject to ELND, which, however, did not produce a statistically significant survival benefit [21]. Today, CLND is only recommended, according to the Augsburg Consensus guidelines [19], to patients with a positive SLN. Thus, roughly 80% of all patients, who are sentinel-negative, are spared elective lymph node dissection. Whereas SLNB is a minimally invasive procedure with limited morbidity, CLND, much like ELND, is associated with considerable complications and socioeconomic costs [22]. Whereas dissection of the regional lymph node basins has been shown to delay nodal recurrence [23], thereby potentially prolonging DFS, no sound scientific evidence exists demonstrating a benefit in melanoma-specific survival for patients undergoing any form of lymph node surgery. Sixty-seven to ninety percent of SLN-positive patients have no further non-SLNs that contain tumor deposits in the CLND specimens [24, 25]. As a consequence, the majority (80%) of SLN-positive patients undergo unnecessary surgery associated with considerable morbidity [25]. Therefore, several authors have tried to identify patient, tumor, and SLN characteristics predicting further non-SLN positivity to safely avoid CLND [25]. Although CLND has not yet been proven to positively influence overall melanoma-specific survival, Cascinelli et al. [26] have recently shown that CLND is necessary to achieve the best assessment of prognosis in stage IB and II melanoma and to identify those patients who, having only positive sentinel nodes and negative nonsentinel nodes, have a good prognosis. Although previous studies have failed to consistently identify the same clinicopathological features as indicators for additional non-SLN positivity upon CLND or for DFS [27], SLN tumor load was uniformly confirmed by all of these studies as prognosticator for non-SLN positivity and recurrence. There is considerable debate as to how to stratify SLN tumor burden; Satzger et al. [28] found that isolated immunohistochemically positive tumor cells are without prognostic significance, and DFS of these patients did not differ from that of SLN-negative patients, an observation that is supported in a broader sense by Van Akkooi et al. [24]. In their study, no patient with an SLN tumor load of <0.1 mm had additional non-SLN positivity upon CLND, and 5-year overall survival was 100%. On the basis of these data, they suggested that such patients be considered SLN-negative and should be spared CLND.

4.2.1.1.5 Systemic Metastases

Metastases can occur virtually anywhere and at any time after a diagnosis of melanoma. Common sites for systemic melanoma metastases are nodal basins, liver, lung, bone, and brain. All new diagnoses of metastatic disease should be discussed by the specialist multidisciplinary team [20]. In advanced disease, no intervention has been shown to have a significant effect on overall survival. Metastasectomy in oligometastatic relapse may be considered in highly selected patients who have been disease-free for a long time [29]. Surgery of visceral metastases may be appropriate for select cases of good patient performance status and isolated tumor manifestation. In all surgically treated patients, in principle, R0-resections should be attempted [30]. Cutaneous metastases, in-transit metastases (deposits from a focus of cells moving along regional lymphatics), and nodal metastases in oligo- and poymetastatic patients are generally treated surgically with palliative intent. Multiple cutaneous deposits in a single limb (with no distant metastases) can be treated with isolated limb perfusion or infusion using melphalan as a single agent or combined with other cytotoxic and biological agents [31]. This can have excellent results in appropriately selected patients but can cause considerable morbidity. Metastases to the central nervous system carry a poor prognosis. Surgery may be indicated for isolated lesions if amenable [32]. Stereotactic radiotherapy, including newer techniques such as gamma-knife treatment, can also be employed [33].

4.2.1.2   Technique

4.2.1.2.1   Primary Excision

Suspicious lesions are characterized by asymmetry, border irregularities, color heterogeneity, and dynamics (evolution of color, elevation, or size) ("ABCDE rule"). Diagnosis should be based on a full-thickness excisional biopsy with a small side margin. Processing by an experienced pathology institute is mandatory. The histology report should follow the WHO classification and include maximum thickness in millimeters (Breslow), level of invasion (Clark level I–V), presence of ulceration, presence and extent of regression, and clearance of the surgical margins [30]. This allows for confirmation of the diagnosis by an examination of the entire lesion, so that definitive treatment can be based upon histological features. Shave biopsies are discouraged because they may lead to sampling errors, incorrect diagnosis, and inaccurate pathological staging. Incisional or punch biopsies are sometimes acceptable – for example, in the differential diagnosis of lentigo maligna of the face or of acral melanoma – but incisional biopsy of a suspicious pigmented lesion has no place outside the multidisciplinary skin cancer team.

4.2.1.2.2   Wide Excision

Wide excisions should be performed with an elliptic incision carrying the primary excision scar with a length-to-width ratio of approximately 3:1. As outlined above, an appropriate surgical margin must be selected according to the Breslow thickness of the primary tumor. The excision is carried down to the muscle fascia and closure, usually accomplished with direct closure. For those lesions not amenable to an elliptic incision or direct closure, a rotational flap or split thickness graft can be used. The skin graft donor site should be placed outside any potential areas of locoregional recurrence [20]. It is very important to mark the excisied specimen unequivocally for the pathologic workup, so excision margins containing residual tumor cells can be identified and reexcised safely. For reasons of oncosurgical safety, wide excision should only be carried out after harvesting of the SLNs is complete. Lymphatic drainage of blue dye injected into the primary excision scar should not be disturbed prematurely, and contamination of the regional nodal basin with tumor cells potentially remaining in the primary excision site should be avoided.

4.2.1.2.3   Sentinel Lymph Node Biopsy

SLNs are identified through a combination of preoperative cutaneous lymphoscintigraphy and intraoperative intradermal injection of vital blue dye. Preoperative cutaneous lymphoscintigraphy is performed with either technetium-99m (99mTc)-labeled albumin colloid, 99mTc sulfur colloid, or 99mTc human serum albumin; colloidal antimony sulfide is often used in Australia, and human albumin nanocolloid is commonly used in European centers. Approximately 18.5–30 MBq (0.5–0.8 mCi) of radiopharmaceutical is injected at the site of the primary excision or primary tumor, if not previously excised. A scintillation camera documents the drainage pattern from this site through the dermal lymphatics to the regional lymph node basin or basins. Due to ectopic drainage patterns, particulary of truncal melanoma, all potentially draining nodal basins must be examined with the scintillation camera. The skin overlying the SLN is marked cutaneously in two perpendicular views, outlining the plane in which the SLNs are situated. Due to varying transition speed of various radiopharmaceutical agents and the distance from the injection site to the regional basin, dynamic imaging is essential to differentiate SLNs from secondary echelon non-SLNs. In general, SLNs are identified within the first 30 min following injection; often after 4 h, SLNs and non-SLNs can no longer be differentiated because of migration of the radiocolloid to secondary echelon nodes beyond the SLN. Recently, hybrid imaging combining single photon emission computed tomography (SPECT) and computed tomography (SPECT/CT) has been recommended not as replacement but as an adjunct to dynamic lymphoscintigraphy [34]. SPECT/CT provides advantages over planar lymphoscintigraphic imaging. These include higher sensitivity for SLN detection, facilitated detection of SLNs in cases of ectopic drainage, improved detection of SLNs situated near the injection site, detection of deep pelvic SLNs in patients with leg melanomas, and improved surgical location of SLNs by providing exact anatomical location.

The surgical procedure can be performed under general or regional anesthesia, immediately preceded by a single intradermal injection of 1–2 mL of vital blue dye (patent blue or isosulfan blue) into and around the primary excision scar (or primary tumor if not previously excised). Some authors advocate gently massaging the injection site for several minutes before incising the regional lymph basin [35]. Placement and orientation of this incision are based on the anatomy of the regional basin, allowing for inclusion by excision in a subsequent CLND, if mandated by a positive SLNB. Ideally, visual identification of the blue-stained lymphatics from the edge of the wound to the SLN(s) is possible, while determining the exact location of the SLNs by means of a handheld γ-probe. If an SN is not identified within 20 min, a second injection of blue dye can be administered. All blue-stained and/or radioactive SLNs are excised. All lymph nodes issuing counts of 10% or more of the most active ("hottest") node must be excised; thus, the procedure can only be terminated once the residual activity in the RNB stage has dropped below 10% of the most active SLN. If the sentinel workup, according to institutional protocol [36], reveals metastases to one or more SLNs, CLND is recommended. Recently, Van Akkooi et al. (2006) reported that micrometastases of <0.1 mm are not associated with additional non-SLN positivity upon CLND, and 5-year overall survival was 100%. On the basis of these data, they suggested that such patients be considered SLN-negative and should be spared CLND.

4.2.1.2.4 Completion Lymph Node Dissection

Many controversies exist concerning the extent and radicality of CLND. In neck dissection, there is no current consensus on the appropriate extent of surgery. Several series, in part with contradictory results, have been published with wildly varying results for selective, modified radical, and radical neck dissections. Mack and McKinnon summarized, in a review on the subject, that evidence suggests that for microscopic disease, a category into which arguably most of all SLNs fall, modified radical neck dissection may be adequate, but controversies about the extent of parotidectomy remain [37]. Similar debates are found in the literature on axillary dissection. Though many authors concur that in melanoma patients, axillary dissection should include levels I–III, others include level III only when suspicious nodes are evident upon intraoperative palpation [38]; these protocols show similar rates of axillary nodal recurrences, indicating

that a less radical approach in axillary dissection suffices to obtain local tumor control. It is surmised that a minimum of ten nodes are required to safely assess the axillary nodal status [39]. The appropriate management of patients with metastatic melanoma involving the groin remains fraught with considerable uncertainty. Although there is no definitive statistical difference between deep and superficial groin dissections in overall survival and possibly a still unproven difference in overall morbidity, a combined deep and superficial lymphadenectomy is considered prudent in cases of clinically palpable disease, given the observation that 30–40% of these patients will have positive deep pelvic nodes, which may be associated with a higher overall recurrence rate [38]. In contrast, patients with nonpalpable disease are a separate group. Despite the fact that several studies have shown that patients with positive superficial lymph nodes in ELND have a 9–67% risk of harboring deep nodal metastases, the proportion of patients with positive deep pelvic nodes after only one positive SLN is small [37]. The practice of performing combined ilioinguinal lymphadenectomies after positive groin SLNs is still widespread, but several authors have recently stated that they consider superficial dissection sufficient in cases where metastatic disease in the SLNs is discovered only through immunohistochemical means [38].

4.2.1.2.5 Therapeutic Lymph Node Dissection

Patients in whom the nodal basins were not previously staged or in whom SLN biopsies were negative qualify for therapeutic lymph node dissection (TLND), if no further evidence of metastatic tumor spread is found in staging examinations. Essentially, these procedures are similar to CLND, but generally, more extensive procedures are recommended. Frequently, TLND specimens reveal more positive non-SLN positivity than CLND specimens and are associated with more morbidity. The number of lymph nodes removed is of prognostic significance in TLND; overall 5-year survival is increased for patients undergoing TLND when patients from the highest quartile of number of nodes excised at surgery are compared to patients from the lowest quartile [40].

4.2.1.3 Outcome

As 80% of melanoma patients present themselves at an early stage, they can effectively be treated with surgery alone, with 5- and 10-year survival rates of 91 and 89%, respectively; overall, localized melanomas have a 99% 5-year survival rate [7]. On the other hand, the 5-year survival rates of regional and distant disease are 65 and 15%, respectively [7].

As with many cancers, surgery represents only one of several therapeutic modalities for melanoma and should, therefore, be firmly embedded in a multidisciplinary context.

4.2.2 Radiation

Brigitta G. Baumert

4.2.2.1 Radiation Therapy

The role of radiation therapy (RT) in the treatment for melanoma, both as primary and adjuvant therapy, is discussed controversially. Clinical studies, however, suggest that RT is effective and has a place in the management of malignant melanoma. Numerous studies indicate that melanoma is generally responsive to radiation, in contrast to earlier publications stating that melanoma was radioresistant. Defining indications for RT should be part of a multidisciplinary treatment approach, and patients should be treated by a specialized multidisciplinary oncology team. Despite the fact that the impact of adjuvant RT on survival is reported as being minimal, greater incorporation of radiotherapy into the multidisciplinary management of melanoma is important because of the typical oncological history of the disease (locoregional recurrence and distant metastases) and its poor response to systemic treatment [51].

4.2.2.2 Indication

4.2.2.2.1 Adjuvant Radiotherapy of the Primary Tumor

The impact of RT on the development of distant disease and overall survival has not been established, but despite the high incidence of distant metastasis, locoregional control remains an important goal in the management of melanoma. The role of adjuvant radiotherapy is not clear but may be advisable in cases of resection margins <1 cm.

4.2.2.2.2 Primary Radiotherapy in Lentigo Maligna/ Melanoma

Even though excision is the treatment of choice for lentigo maligna, primary radiation therapy can achieve adequate tumor control with good cosmetic and functional results.

4.2.2.2.3 Adjuvant Radiation Therapy Following Lymph Node Dissection

Adjuvant radiation therapy is not considered a standard treatment following lymph node dissection, as it improves

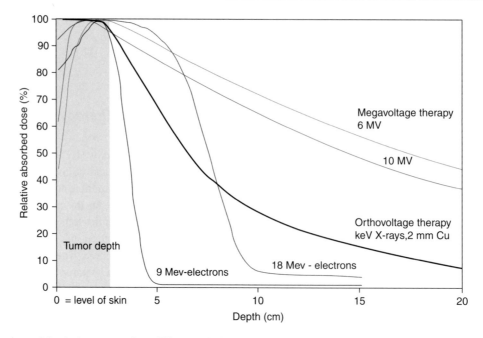

Fig. 4.2.1 Comparison of depth–dose curves from different radiation treatment modalities. Examples of megavoltage radiotherapy, orthovoltage, and treatment with corpuscular radiation with electrons are shown. Depending on the depth of tumor infiltration, the appropriate treatment modality can be chosen. An example of a tumor with approximately 2.5-cm depth is shown; in order to cover the full tumor, elec- trons with an energy of 9 MeV or orthovoltage with 2 mm Cu would be a good choice. Megavoltage treatment can also be applied but needs additional application of bolus material on the skin in order to modify the depth–dose (the maximum dose of megavoltage therapy lies ca. one to three centimeter below the surface, 0 cm representing the skin surface)

regional control, but has no impact on survival. However, a regional recurrence can cause significant morbidity. The risk of recurrent disease after lymph node dissection is increased if the following risk factors are present: extracapsular exten- sion, multiple (>2–4) involved lymph nodes, large lymph nodes (≥3 cm), irradical resection, and in cases of recurrent disease after complete lymph node dissection. Adjuvant RT should then be considered.

4.2.2.2.4 Radiation Therapy in Metastases

Palliative radiation therapy may provide relief of symptoms. Retrospective studies have shown that patients with brain metastases, bone metastases, and spinal cord compression may achieve symptom relief and tumor response with radia- tion therapy.

4.2.2.3 Technique

For the treatment of melanoma, different radiotherapy treat- ment modalities are available. The technique is selected based on size, extent, depth, and anatomical location of the tumor. It is essential to choose the right radiation technique in order to reach the best dose distribution in relation to the target volume. The treatment goal is to apply the desired dose in the tumor, while simultaneously sparing as much healthy tissue as possible.

The energy of the radiation determines the penetration depth (Fig. 4.2.1). Radiation with an energy of <20 kilovolt (KV) is defined as Grenz ray therapy, with 30–100 KV as superficial therapy. Radiotherapy with energies of 100– 300 KV is called Orthovoltage therapy, and radiation with high energies over 1 Megavolt (MeV) is defined as megavolt- age therapy (applied with a linear accelerator or 60-Cobalt).

Most modern linear accelerators allow for radiation with electrons (corpuscular radiation), with which superficially located tumors can also be irradiated. Usually, electrons with energies of 6 or 9 MeV are applied, with circa one third of the energy of the effective penetration depth in cm (i.e., at 6 MeV:2 cm). Radiotherapy with electrons represents an alternative to orthovoltage therapy, where the beam energy can be adapted to the depth of the tumor growth: lower ener- gies for more superficial tumors and higher energies for infil- trating tumors, to ensure a sufficient dose at the depth of the tumor (Fig. 4.2.1). Another treatment option for superficial skin tumors, e.g., melanoma, is brachytherapy or interstitial radiotherapy with a mould application (with or without hyperthermia). For brachytherapy, sealed radioactive sources are precisely placed in the treated area; the most commonly used source of radiation is Iridium-192, with only superfi- cially penetrating radiation.

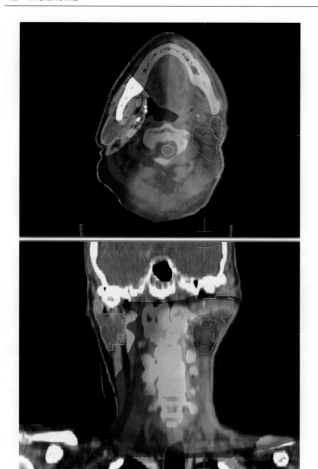

Fig. 4.2.2 Radiation treatment plan (intensity-modulated radiotherapy) of adjuvant RT after resection of cervial lymph nodes of a melanoma. The area colored in *yellowish-green* on the axial and coronal images shows the dose to the unilateral loco-regional lymph nodes (adjuvant radiotherapy to a total dose of 50 Gy). The area at high risk of recurrence (*red area*=area of resected lymph node) receives a higher RT dose (total dose of 66 Gy). The higher dose level is given simultaneously with the low dose (integrated boost). *Blue areas* represent a low RT dose

For tumors deeply infiltrating neighboring structures (e.g., bone, nerve), those in the vicinity of critical organs (e.g., brain), and in cases of lymph node metastases, high energy photons are used. The method of radiation delivery is determined with CT-based radiotherapy treatment planning and/or treatment simulation. RT planning defines radiation fields and calculates the dose distribution. Figure 4.2.2 demonstrates an example of an irradiation plan for the cervical region (unilateral radiation) after resection of lymph node metastases in a case of melanoma. In this case, intensity-modulated radiotherapy (IMRT) was applied. IMRT is an advanced type of three-dimensional radiotherapy. IMRT allows the RT dose to better conform to concave tumor shapes, e.g., in cases where the tumor is wrapped around a vulnerable structure such as the spinal cord. The radiation dose is modulated in three dimensions

consistent with the shape of the tumor. This is achieved by controlling, or modulating, the radiation beam's intensity. The intensity of radiation is high in the gross tumor volume, while radiation in the neighboring healthy tissue is low or completely avoided. Another highly precise radiation technique is stereotactic radiosurgery (SRS), which is used to target lesions in the brain. SRS is usually applied in a single session with a single high dose. Its precision is based on highly precise neuronavigation or stereotactic-radiotherapy-planning devices. Multiple beams are centered on the intracranial lesion to be treated. In this way, radiation of healthy tissues around the target is avoided. Figure 4.2.3 shows an example of a radiosurgery plan for treatment of a brain metastasis.

Not only the type of radiation but also an appropriate fractionation schedule should also be chosen, taking into account the tolerance of the surrounding healthy tissue and the cosmetic result. The relationship between the radiation energy, volume, dose, time, tumor size, and the radiation tolerance of adjacent tissues has been investigated [35, 54] (Table 4.2.2). Other hypofractionated schedules were also explored, e.g., 30–36 Gy in 5–7 fractions (see below for more details). For larger RT volumes, conventionally fractionated schedules are preferable with a total dose of approximately 50–65 Gy in fractions of 1.8–2.0 Gy over 5–6 weeks.

4.2.2.4 Outcome

4.2.2.4.1 Adjuvant Radiotherapy of the Primary Tumor

The impact of RT on the development of distant disease and overall survival has not been established, but despite the high incidence of distant metastasis, locoregional control remains an important goal of melanoma management. The role of adjuvant radiotherapy is not clear but can be recommended in cases of resection margins <1 cm for melanoma with neurotropism. Adjuvant RT may have been effective in reducing the rate of local recurrence (3-year recurrence-free rate 93%) in a study of 24 patients with desmoplastic melanoma of the head and neck region who received RT as part of the primary treatment [24].

A larger study of 174 patients with locally advanced melanoma where postoperative RT was given reported improved local control when compared to published surgical data (median survival 13 and 35 months for those with and without infield recurrence, $p < 0.0001$) [51]. Adjuvant RT given with a hypofractionated schedule (30–36 Gy in 5–7 fractions) was effective in reducing local recurrence in patients at high risk of locoregional failure. High risk of locoregional failure was defined by the presence of microscopically positive surgical margins, desmoplasia with neurotropism,

Fig. 4.2.3 Stereotactic radiosurgery treatment plan of a brain metastasis. A solitary metastasis with isodoses of several dose levels is shown. Note the steep dose fall-off between the 80 and 90% isodose. The *pink line* is the prescription dose to the tumor margin, which is lower than the central dose (margin dose 18 Gy, central dose >24 Gy, *green* and *pink*). The image in the *upper left* shows a fused MRI and CT scan and the relation of the metastasis to potential organs-at-risk, which should not be irradiated, as well as three other metastases irradiated earlier and a good local control

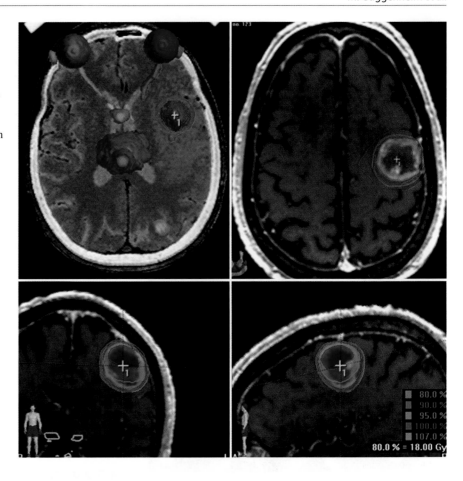

Table 4.2.2 Recommended dose of radiotherapy for skin tumors modified after Miescher [35]

Diagnosis	Radiation field size (cm)	Fractionation (Gy)	Total dose (Gy)	Time interval (days)	Technique
Lentigo maligna	<2	5–6×20	100–120	4–7	Grenz rays
	>2	10–12×10	100–120	3–4	
Basalioma/spinalioma	<2	5–6×8	40–48	4–7	Grenz rays.,
	2–5	10–12×4	40–48	3–4	Orthovoltage, or megavoltage RT (with electrons)
	>5	26–28×2	52–56	Daily	
Mycosis fungoides/cutaneous T-cell-lymphoma		3–7×2	6–14	3–4	All (depending on infiltrating tumor depths)
		4–10×1	4–10	3–7	
Lentigo maligna – melanoma, melanoma metastases		7–9×6	42–54	4–7	All (depending on infiltrating tumor depths)
Kaposi sarcoma	<2	3–5×8	24–40	4–7	Grenz rays, orthovoltage, electrons
	>2	5–10×4	20–40	3–4	

multiple lymph node involvement, and large lymph nodes with extracapsular growth [50]. The use of higher RT doses per fraction has already been shown to improve local control (<4 Gy 25% local control vs. >4 Gy 71% local control) [31].

The lentigo maligna and lentigo maligna melanoma literature reports best results for the use of primary RT. Even though excision is the treatment of choice for lentigo maligna, radiation therapy can achieve adequate tumor control with

good cosmetic and functional results in difficult areas of the face, especially in elderly individuals. For example, in elderly patients with significant comorbidities and large lesions on the face, radiotherapy may be warranted. Grenz or soft X-ray therapy with 20 KV is often used with a local control rate of >90% [15, 19, 21, 28–30, 47, 52]. The cosmetic results are almost always very good [15, 19, 21, 47], especially in acral melanoma [29]. Either electron beams or soft radiographs can be used in conventional fractions with a total dose of

50–60 Gy and individual doses of 2–6 Gy. Lesions may take up to 2 years to completely regress, and careful clinical follow-up is required.

4.2.2.4.2 Adjuvant Radiation Therapy Following Lymph Node Dissection

Adjuvant radiation therapy is not considered a standard treatment following lymph node dissection. RT improves regional control but does not prolong survival. Whether radiation therapy is applied and how it is applied depends on the prognosis and the risk of recurrent disease in the area of the removed lymph nodes. A small retrospective study concluded that RT may provide relatively long-term local control in patients with clinical perineural invasion [38]. Another study of 44 patients diagnosed with a desmoplastic malignant melanoma showed that adjuvant RT was effective in recurrent disease and proposed consideration of RT as part of initial treatment, especially in cases where surgical margins are not clear of the residual tumor [55]. None of 15 patients who received adjuvant irradiation had recurrences during a mean follow-up of 64.7 months [55]. The majority of lesions were diagnosed in the head and neck area.

One randomized trial using substandard technique in the mid-1970s showed no benefit [18]. Several studies recommend postoperative RT for patients at high risk of regional recurrence, defined as the presence of multiple nodes, extracapsular extension, large lymph nodes (3 cm), recurrent nodal disease, and in cases of irradical resection [3, 4, 8, 11, 14, 16, 17, 34, 39]. This is supported by prospective studies [2, 3, 13]. Others found no evidence to support the use of adjuvant RT in the lymph nodes [25, 36]. Retrospective studies looking at different anatomic lymph node areas generally recommend adjuvant RT after resection of cervical and axillar nodes, especially if the above listed risk factors are present [4, 5, 7, 9, 10]. Some of them even propose elective regional RT as alternative to lymph node dissection [7, 10]. In axillary lymph nodes, there is an expected control rate of 87% for RT, compared to a control rate of 50–70% with surgery alone [4]. RT in inguinal lymph node metastases improved local control [6].

The total RT dose prescribed and fractionation schedules vary throughout the literature. Ideally, the fractionation scheme should be based on the tolerance of adjacent normal tissues, e.g., the peripheral nerves. A total dose of 50–65 Gy with individual doses of 1.8–2.0 Gy is recommended. Different hypofractionation schemes have been used and were reported to be safe and result in the same local control rates as conventional RT schedules [2, 3, 9, 14, 37, 50]. The most commonly used schemes were 30 Gy in 5 fractions and 36 Gy in 6 fractions [2, 3, 9, 14]. Only one study reported higher single doses as offering no advantages over conventionally fractionated schedules [22].

4.2.2.4.3 Hyperthermia

For hyperthermia therapy, tissue is locally exposed to high temperatures to sensitize cancer cells to the effects of ionizing radiation. Hyperthermia is useful in the treatment of malignant melanoma. According to retrospective reports, it increases the effectiveness of radiation therapy with a factor of 1.4, resulting in control rates ranging from 50 to 70% [20, 40, 44, 49]. A prospective, randomized trial investigating the value of hyperthermia as an adjuvant to radiotherapy in the treatment of malignant melanoma reported control rates of 46% [42]. Treatment was randomized for 134 metastatic and recurrent malignant melanoma lesions between radiotherapy alone (3 fractions in 8 days) and RT followed by hyperthermia (aimed for 43°C for 60 min). The most important prognostic parameters were hyperthermia, tumor size, and radiation dose [42]. The use of hyperthermia is limited by availability and technical factors. It is indicated mainly in the treatment of superficial tumors.

4.2.2.4.4 Radiation Therapy in Metastases

Palliative radiation therapy may provide relief of symptoms. Retrospective studies have shown that RT achieves symptom relief in patients with multiple brain metastases, bone metastases, and spinal cord compression in up to 85% of cases and can also provide local control [32, 43, 48]. The response of metastatic deposits to radiation varies with tumor volume, total dose, and dose per fraction. Optimal fractionation depends on tumor site and the patient's survival expectation. A general review recommends 36 Gy in 6 fractions, twice weekly for unresectable local disease; for large axillary or inguinal metastases, 50 Gy in 20 fractions is recommended to reduce the risk of limb oedema and neuropathy, for brain metastases 30 Gy in 10 fractions (consider radiosurgery, see below), and for other sites 20 Gy in 5 fractions or 30 Gy in 10 fractions [26].

The most effective dose-fractionation schedule for palliation of melanoma metastatic to the bone or spinal cord is unclear, but retrospective studies report that high-dose-per-fraction schedules are sometimes used to overcome tumor resistance. Two randomized trials showed no difference in response between the two fractionation schedules. One trial randomized patients with metastatic or recurrent malignant melanoma between 9 Gy × 3 fractions or 5 Gy × 8 fractions, twice weekly [41]. The other trial, conducted by the Radiation Therapy Oncology Group in patients with a primary melanoma (RTOG 83–05) [46], randomized between 32 Gy in 4 fractions of 8 Gy and 50 Gy in 20 fractions of 2.5 Gy. The use of larger doses per fraction does not result in improved local control rates, despite the many retrospective reports implicating improved local control with higher doses per fraction [46].

Brain Metastases

Brain metastases are common in melanoma, with melanoma being the third most common cause of brain metastases (after lung and breast). In general, patients presenting with multiple brain metastases should be treated with whole brain radiotherapy (30 Gy in 10 fractions or 20 Gy in 4 fractions). Differences in outcome are based mainly on additional prognostic factors, e.g., the presence or absence of other visceral metastasis and performance status [33, 45]. In a retrospective evaluation of 686 patients with melanoma brain metastases, a median survival of 8.9 months after surgery and RT, 8.7 months after surgery alone, 3.4 months after RT alone, and 2.1 months after supportive care was reported [23]. Multivariate analysis revealed that the type of treatment and the presence of other metastases were the most important predictors of survival. Median survival was dependent upon patient selection, based on clinical prognostic factors [23]. A set of 479 patients with brain metastases from different primary sites was analyzed to determine the influence of the primary site on prognostic factors and grading systems on overall survival, in patients treated with SRS (precise single high-dose radiation therapy) for brain metastases [27]. In subgroup multivariate analysis, favorable prognostic factors were Karnofsky performance status ≥70, primary tumor control, and ≤3 melanoma brain metastases. It was further shown that prognostic grading systems varied depending on primary tumor site. Therefore, for defined prognostic patient groups with a longer estimated median survival (≤3 cerebral metastases, good clinical condition, and a stable or controlled primary), a more aggressive approach can be chosen, consisting of a combination of either resection followed by whole brain radiotherapy or SRS. This approach was also shown to be valid in randomized studies of patients with solitary brain metastases; however, in these studies, the primary tumor was not demonstrated to be of prognostic value [1, 53].

4.2.3 Drug Therapy

Thomas Kurt Eigentler and Claus Garbe

4.2.3.1 Topical Treatment

4.2.3.1.1 Indication

The management of skin and soft-tissue metastases of melanoma can be a major challenge, particularly in cases of rapidly progressive disease and multiple consecutive recurrences. To date, there is no recommended standard therapy for advanced melanoma with skin and soft-tissue metastases, though a number of therapies are currently used under these circumstances.

4.2.3.1.2 Technique and Outcome

Definitive surgical resection of skin and soft-tissue metastases is usually considered the treatment of choice but is restricted to cases of limited disease burden [40]. Other ablative options with comparable indications include cryosurgery and carbon dioxide laser surgery [48].

The studies evaluating the palliative effects of radiation treatment revealed overall response rates ranging up to 75% in stage III disease [99]. However, while appropriate protocols for radiation are variable in dose per fraction, number of fractions, and time course of fractionated therapy, symptomatic control is obtained for the majority of patients. Moreover, the application of adjuvant hyperthermia seems to confer a significant local control benefit in patients receiving radiation therapy [52]. Recent reports also indicate local disease control for patients treated with electrochemotherapy [88]. This therapeutic procedure uses short, high-intensity electrical pulses to create cell membrane defects or porations enabling the increase in uptake of cytotoxic drugs (Bleomycin, Cisplatin) that are administered prior to the electrical pulsations. Overall response rates were reported to be up to 93% [88], whereas small lesions <1 cm seem to respond much better than larger metastases.

Hyperthermic-isolated limb perfusion is a regional treatment for skin and soft-tissue metastases, which uses high-dose chemotherapy or biochemotherapy and bypasses systemic complications. The surgical procedure compromises dissecting and isolating the external iliac vessels for the lower extremity or the axillary vessels for the upper extremity. The vessels are tapped directly, and the limb is isolated via a tourniquet. The chemotherapeutic agent (mainly melphalan ± TNF-α) is infused and recirculated through the limb via a cardiopulmonary bypass machine, which reheats and re-oxygenates the removed blood. In contrast to other therapeutic modalities, hypothermic-isolated limb perfusion allows for treatment of the whole extremity in one step. Overall response rates are reported to be around 65%, whereas the beneficial effect of additional TNF-α is still controversially discussed [19]. Isolated limb perfusion without hyperthermia is less demanding and might have a similar efficiency [108].

4.2.3.2 Topical Immunotherapy

4.2.3.2.1 Indication

In addition to the surgical, radio-, and chemotherapeutic options, a number of topical immunotherapeutic agents have been investigated in skin and soft-tissue metastases. Most of them are also available for patients with limited disease burden.

4.2.3.2.2 Technique and Outcome

Intratumoral Treatment with Interleukin-2

Intratumoral treatment with Interleukin-2 was reported to be an effective treatment option in case of small (<1 cm) in-transit metastases [89]. Depending on the number of lesions (up to 100), a cumulative dosage of 16 MIU IL-2 was applied three times a week for 4–6 weeks. Eighty percent of the patients seemed to respond to this treatment, whereas 60% demonstrated a complete response in the treated lesions [89]. Only injected lesions respond to this treatment; however, simultaneous or subsequent treatment of up to 100 metastases revealed to be feasible and safe. We see this as a preferred treatment modality for satellite and in-transit metastases, particularly if the lesions are still small and early treatment is possible. The proposed treatment regimen is given in Table 4.2.3; the dosages refer to a single metastasis and may multiply when injected into multiple metastases. The dosage for one treatment session should not exceed 12–16 MIU. Treatment is applied three times a week.

Table 4.2.3 Treatment regimen for intratumoral application of interleukin-2 in respect to single lesions, for the preparation of stock solution, see Radny et al. [89]

Lesion size: maximal diameter (mm)	Single dose (MIU)	Milliliter of stock solution	Duration of treatment (weeks)
<5	0.6	0.2	2
>5	1.2	0.4	3
>10	3.0	1.0	4
>15	6.0	2.0	4

Topical Treatment with Imiquimod

Imiquimod is a toll-like receptor-7-agonist, which enhances the innate immune response, enhances dendritic cells survival, and promotes tumor antigen specific T-cell priming [87]. A number of case series and reports observed complete remissions of lentigo maligna under imiquimod treatment [54, 78, 86]. Treatment with topical imiquimod was also investigated in cutaneous in-transit metastases, and complete responses were achieved in about 2/3 of patients under occlusive application for up to 28 weeks [11, 114, 115]. A combined treatment with imiquimod and intralesional interleukin-2 did not exceed treatment results of either substance alone when compared to the reports on intratumoral interleukin-2 or imiquimod in the literature [43].

2-4 Dinitrochlorobenzene

2-4 Dinitrochlorobenzene (DNCB) is a potent and obligatory contact sensitizer eliciting a delayed hypersensitivity response. In the case of skin metastases, it can be applied to induce a contact dermatitis and an allergic, immunologic reaction at the treatment site eliciting a simultaneous immunologic response against the cutaneous melanoma metastases [70, 110]. Some studies used topical treatment with DNCB in combination with systemic dacarbazine for the therapy of visceral metastases [107]. The largest trial reported is a retrospective survey of 72 patients from nine centers treated with a course of combined DNCB and dacarbazine [107]. In stage III melanoma patients with in-transit and satellite metastases ($n=39$), the objective response rate was 62% (complete responses 39%). In stage IV melanoma ($n=33$), the objective response rate was only 9% (CR 3%). Thus, the analysis of the trial patients showed that responses were rare in distant metastases but more frequent and long-lasting in locoregional disease.

Emerging Therapies

Recently, some new immunological treatment modalities for skin and soft-tissue metastases have been evaluated in phase I/II trials. Allovectin™ (Vical Incorporated, San Diego, California, USA) is a plasmid DNA encoding the MHC heavy chain class I antigen HLA-B7 and β2 microglobulin proteins. Intralesional injection is believed to result in synthesis and expression of the complete MHC complex on the surface of the cell. The plasmid is a complex with a cationic lipid mixture, which, when combined with DNA, facilitates transfection of plasmid DNA and may induce a potent proinflammatory response. Results from a phase II trial indicated an overall response rate of 9.1%, including some patients with durable response [42].

Another experimental treatment option is the intralesional injection of OncoVEX^GM-CSF (BioVex Ltd, Oxon, United Kingdom), a second generation, GM-CSF-encoding, oncolytic herpesvirus. Recently, presented data showed an overall response of 28% including patients with a durable response up to 27 months [101].

Both agents are currently being investigated in further phase II and III studies.

4.2.3.3 Systemic Therapy

4.2.3.3.1 Indication

Adjuvant Therapy

Patients with thick primary melanoma and regional lymph node metastases have a high risk of recurrence and death following surgery [49]. Current recommendations for patients with stage IIb (>4 mm, but negative nodes) melanoma are adjuvant therapy or enrollment in a clinical trial. The primary treatment recommendations for patients with stage III melanoma vary, but the secondary treatment recommendation is adjuvant therapy or enrollment in a clinical trial.

Adjuvant therapies for high-risk (stage IIb, III) patients have shifted over the past 10–15 years from adjuvant radiotherapy or unspecific immune-stimulants like Bacillus Calmette Guerin (BCG) and levamisole to treatment with the cytokine interferon-α [56].

Treatment of Metastatic Melanoma

Among patients with AJCC stage IV metastatic melanoma, median survival time is estimated to be approximately 8 months, and only about 5–10% of patients survive more than 5 years after diagnosis [39]. Current guidelines state that there is no single standard therapy for metastatic melanoma [39], and there are few effective therapies. No systemic therapies have yet been shown to significantly prolong survival of

patients with advanced-stage IV melanoma [31]. The poor prognosis for these patients creates an urgent need for new treatment approaches. An increased understanding of tumor biology and immune regulation has led to the development of novel agents.

4.2.3.3.2 Outcome

Adjuvant Therapy

Interferon-α

Interferon-α2a and interferon-α2b are currently the only two approved drugs for the adjuvant treatment of high-risk melanoma; both substances are very similar in their efficacy and toxicity. Additionally, pegylated compounds of both cytokines, with much longer half lives, are meanwhile on the market; they are only administered once a week. There are currently no generally accepted recommendations for the adjuvant treatment and medical management of high-risk melanoma; it varies in different countries. Different dosage regimens for interferon-α treatment are summarized in Table 4.2.4.

Interferon alfa-2b (IFN-α2b, Intron A, Schering-Plough Corporation, Kenilworth, New Jersey) was the first agent to show a significant survival benefit in patients with high-risk melanoma in a randomized, controlled trial [63]. Patients ($N=287$) with high-risk resected cutaneous melanoma were randomized to receive IFN-α2b (20 MU/m²/day) intravenously for 1 month and 10 MU/m² subcutaneously three times a week for 48 weeks or observation. Overall survival (OS) was significantly prolonged with IFN-α2b, after a median follow-up time of 6.9 years (median survival, 3.82 years with IFN-α2b vs. 2.78 years with observation only; 1-sided log-rank p value=0.0237) [63].

Subsequent to this first trial, a number of studies have attempted to optimize the dose level and schedule for IFN for adjuvant therapy. In a subsequent trial comparing patients ($N=642$) receiving high-dose IFN-α2b for 1 year (HDI), low-dose IFN-α2b for 2 years (LDI), or observation, relapse-free survival (RFS) was significantly enhanced with HDI vs.

Table 4.2.4 Dosage schedules for adjuvant therapy of melanoma with interferon-α

Schedule	Dose	Frequency	Duration	Indication
Low dose	3 Million IU s.c.	Days 1, 3 and 5 every week	18 Months	Stage II–III
High dose				
Initiation	20 Million IU/m² i.v. rapid infusion	Day 1–5 every week	4 Weeks	Stage III
Maintenance	10 Million IU/m² s.c.	Days 1, 3 and 5 every week	11 Months	Stage III
Pegylated				
Initiation	6 µg/kg body weight s.c.	Day 1 every week	8 Weeks	Stage III
Maintenance	3 µg/kg body weight s.c.	Day 1 every week	Total 5 years	Stage III

observation ($p=0.03$), but OS was not improved [61]. LDI was associated with a greatly reduced incidence of grade 3/4 adverse events compared with high-dose IFN-α2b (1 vs. 17 grade 4 AEs, respectively), and the RFS was equivalent to HDI after 3 and 4 years, and there was no statistical difference in RFS between the LDI and HDI arm. However, the authors interpreted LDI to be ineffective, because RFS failed to achieve statistical significance for RFS, though hazard ratios for RFS were very similar for HDI and LDI (608 eligible cases: HDI vs. obs. HR = 1.27, $p=0.068$; LDI vs. obs. HR = 1.23, $p=0.115$).

In a randomized controlled trial in patients ($N=1,388$) treated with intermediate-dose IFN-α2b (5 weekly doses with 10 MU for 4 weeks, followed by 3 weekly doses of 10 MU for 1 year or 5 MU for 2 years) for 13 or 25 months or observation, intermediate-dose IFN-α2b did not significantly improve distant metastasis-free interval or OS outcomes [30]. Low-dose IFN-α also failed to improve survival outcomes compared to observation alone when patients were treated two times weekly with 3 MU for 6 months ($N=95$) or three times weekly with 3 MU for 2 years ($N=674$) or 3 years ($N=427$) [12, 15, 47]. However, low-dose IFN-α did improve prolonged disease-free survival over observation alone when patients ($N=311$) received 3 MU daily for 3 weeks and were treated three times weekly for 1 year ($p=0.02$) and when patients ($N=499$) were treated with 3 MU three times weekly for 18 months ($p=0.038$) [44, 84].

The large number of clinical trials with variations in dose level, schedule of IFN administration, as well as patient populations has led to several attempts to consolidate and review available data [39, 67, 113]. A large meta-analysis of the available randomized clinical trial data was reported in 2007, summarizing event-free survival and OS in patients with high-risk melanoma treated with IFN-α adjuvant therapy [112]. Clinical data were sorted by IFN dose: high ($20\ MU/m^2$), intermediate ($5-10\ MU/m^2$), low ($3\ MU/m^2$), and very low ($1\ MU/m^2$) doses. Groups were also stratified by duration of treatment (<6, 12–18, or >24 months). Although there was a statistically significant OS benefit in patients administered IFN-α ($p=0.008$), there was no evidence of a clear difference in OS between different dose levels ($p=0.8$) or durations of treatment ($p=0.9$). In subgroup analyses, age, sex, tumor size, Breslow thickness, number of nodes, or disease stage did not affect response to IFN, although patients with ulcerated tumors did appear to have a greater benefit than those without ulcerations [112]. Another meta-analysis is shown in Table 4.2.5 for progression-free survival (PFS) and OS including high-dose, intermediate-dose, and low-dose schedules as well as a trial with pegylated interferon-α. In summary, adjuvant IFN improves OS in patients with high-risk melanoma, though the absolute survival benefit of IFN is small (~3%, with a confidence interval [CI] of 1–5%).

Combination therapies with low-dose IFN-α have also been investigated. In a recent prospective, randomized trial in patients ($N=252$) with totally resected cutaneous melanoma (248 patients with stage II/III and 4 patients with stage IV) receiving DTIC with or without subsequent IFN-α (3 MU) administered three times weekly for 6 months, adjuvant therapy improved OS (hazard ratio [HR] = 0.71; $p=0.052$) [105].

Clinical trials based in the United States have primarily applied high-dose schedules of IFN treatment, because this is the only dose level approved by the US Food and Drug Administration. High-dose IFN-α2b is associated with acute constitutional symptoms, chronic fatigue, myelosuppression, elevated liver enzyme levels, and neurologic symptoms (e.g., depression) [64]. Both high- and low-dose IFN-α have been approved in Europe, but low-dose IFN-α is preferentially used [39]. Currently, common practice in Europe for adjuvant therapy in patients with high-risk, resected stage II/III melanoma is low-dose IFN-α for 18–24 months. Particularly in light of the recent data showing dose level and regimen do not significantly affect the survival benefit of adjuvant IFN therapy [112], there is stronger rationale for use of low-dose IFN to provide survival benefit without the added toxicities of high-dose IFN. European studies continue to determine how best to apply IFN-α in the adjuvant setting for patients with stage II/III disease. Current trials are assessing the tolerability and efficacy of a shorter but more intense dosing regimen of IFN-α2b[18] and pegylated interferon (peginterferon-α2a and pegylated IFN-α2b) [29].

Vaccines

The goal of cancer vaccines is to enhance presentation of tumor antigens and elicit a durable memory T-cell response [59]. Increased knowledge of antigenic epitopes and antitumor immunity has prompted a variety of vaccine approaches. Although vaccines are well-tolerated, they have rarely demonstrated robust antitumor activity [118].

A randomized, phase III study (ECOG 1694) compared high-dose IFN with the ganglioside vaccine GMK (ganglioside conjugate [GM2] coupled to keyhole limpet hemocyanin [KLH] and formulated with adjuvant QS-21; (Progenics Pharmaceuticals, Tarrytown, New York)) as adjuvant therapies for patients with high-risk melanoma [62]. The GMK vaccination induces antibodies against GM2 capable of specifically killing melanoma cells, and patients with these antibodies were known to have improved survival [65]. However, the study was terminated early when interim analyses detected a markedly inferior survival in the GMK arm compared to the IFN arm [104]. Subsequent analyses comparing pre- and posttreatment patient sera found that GMK had induced persistent (for at least 1 year) antibodies in approximately 80% of vaccinated patients, so these results were not explained by a lack of antibody titer generation. While these results were interpreted by the authors as improvement in survival with

Table 4.2.5 Meta-analysis of randomized trials of adjuvant treatment with interferon-α in stage II and III melanoma patients (A) progression-free survival (B) Overall survival

Study	Treatment (n/N)	Control (n/N)	OR fixed (95%)	Weight (%)	OR fixed (95%)
High-dose interferon-α					A
Creagan et al. [22]	77/131	85/131		4.54	0.77 [0.47, 1.27]
Kirkwood et al. [63]	90/143	103/137		5.06	0.56 [0.33, 0.94]
Kirkwood et al. [61]	114/215	127/212		7.79	0.76 [0.51, 1.11]
Subtotal (95% CI)	281/489	315/480		17.40	0.70 [0.54, 0.91]
Test for heterogeneity: $Chi^2=1.01$, df=2 ($p=0.60$), $I^2=0\%$					
Test for overall effect: $Z=2.64$ ($p=0.008$)					
Intermediate-dose interferon-α					
Eggermont et al. [30]	679/1,109	183/279		14.71	0.83 [0.63, 1.09]
Subtotal (95% CI)	679/1,109	183/279		14.71	0.83 [0.63, 1.09]
Test for heterogeneity: not applicable					
Test for overall effect: $Z=1.51$ ($p=0.18$)					
Low-dose interferon-α					
Cameron et al. [12]	32/46	35/49		1.34	0.91 [0.38, 2.21]
Cascinelli et al. [15]	162/225	158/219		5.82	0.99 [0.66, 1.50]
Garbe et al. [38]	86/146	104/147		5.52	0.59 [0.36, 0.96]
Grob et al. [44]	100/244	119/245		9.09	0.74 [0.51, 1.05]
Hancock et al. [47]	211/338	215/336		10.51	0.94 [0.68, 1.28]
Kirkwood et al. [61]	122/215	127/212		7.18	0.88 [0.60, 1.29]
Pehamberger et al. [84]	37/154	57/157		5.56	0.55 [0.34, 0.91]
Subtotal (95% CI)	750/1,368	815/1,365		45.02	0.80 [0.69, 0.94]
Test for heterogeneity: $Chi^2=6.11$, df=6 ($p=0.41$), $I^2=1.8\%$					
Test for overall effect: $Z=2.73$ ($p=0.006$)					
Pegylated interferon-α					
Eggermont et al. [29]	326/627	368/629		22.88	0.77 [0.61, 0.96]
Subtotal (95% CI)	326/627	368/629		22.88	0.77 [0.61, 0.96]
Test for heterogeneity: not applicable					
Test for overall effect: $Z=2.32$ ($p=0.02$)					
Total (95% CI)	2,036/3,593	1,554/2,541		100.00	0.83 [0.75, 0.92]
Test for heterogeneity: $Chi^2=8.06$, df=11 ($p=0.71$), $I^2=0\%$ Test for overall effect: $Z=4.54$ ($p<0.0001$)			0.2 0.5 1 2 5		
High-dose interferon-α					B
Creagan et al. [22]	68/131	72/131		4.79	0.88 [0.54, 1.44]
Kirkwood et al. [63]	81/143	90/137		5.51	0.68 [0.42, 1.11]
Kirkwood et al. [61]	98/215	93/212		7.05	1.07 [0.73, 1.57]
Subtotal (95% CI)	247/489	255/480		17.35	0.90 [0.70, 1.16]
Test for heterogeneity: $Chi^2=2.07$, df=2 ($p=0.36$), $I^2=3.4\%$					
Test for overall effect: $Z=0.84$ ($p=0.40$)					
Intermediate-dose interferon-α					
Eggermont et al. [30]	535/1,109	146/279		16.70	0.85 [0.65, 1.10]
Subtotal (95% CI)	535/1,109	146/279		16.70	0.85 [0.65, 1.10]
Test for heterogeneity: not applicable					
Test for overall effect: $Z=1.51$ ($p=0.18$)					

Table 4.2.5 (continued)

Study	Treatment (n/N)	Control (n/N)	OR fixed (95%)	Weight (%)	OR fixed (95%)
Low-dose interferon-α					
Cameron et al. [12]	31/46	36/49		1.57	0.75 [0.31, 1.81]
Cascinelli et al. [15]	146/225	138/219		6.79	1.08 [0.74, 1.60]
Garbe et al. [38]	62/146	85/147		6.74	0.54 [0.34, 0.86]
Grob et al. [44]	59/244	76/243		7.99	0.70 [0.47, 1.04]
Hancock et al. [47]	151/338	156/336		11.97	0.93 [0.69, 1.26]
Kirkwood et al. [61]	96/215	93/212		7.17	1.03 [0.70, 1.51]
Pehamberger et al. [84]	17/154	21/157		2.56	0.80 [0.41, 1.59]
Subtotal (95% CI)	562/1,368	605/1,363		44.80	0.86 [0.73, 1.01]
Test for heterogeneity: $Chi^2 = 7.59$, df=6 ($p=0.27$), $I^2=21.0\%$					
Test for overall effect: $Z=1.89$ ($P=0.06$)					
Pegylated interferon-α					
Eggermont et al. [29]	262/627	263/629		21.14	1.00 [0.80, 1.25]
Subtotal (95% CI)	262/627	263/629		21.14	1.00 [0.80, 1.25]
Test for heterogeneity: not applicable					
Test for overall effect: $Z=0.01$ ($p=0.99$)					
Total (95% CI)	1,606/3,593	1,176/2,539		100.0	0.88 [0.79, 0.99]
Test for heterogeneity: $Chi^2 = 10.49$, df=10 ($p=0.40$), $I^2=4.7\%$ Test for overall effect: $Z=2.21$ ($p=0.03$)			0.2 0.5 1 2 5		

HDI treatment, in the light of new results from vaccination trials (see below), it was more likely that the vaccination treatment led to deterioration of the patients' outcome.

In another randomized, phase III trial, postoperative adjuvant therapy with BCG alone or in combination with an allogenic melanoma vaccine (Canvaxin™; Micromet, Munich, Germany) for treatment of patients with stage III ($n=1,160$) or IV ($n=496$) melanoma was terminated due to the low probability of demonstrating significant improvement in survival [77]. Furthermore, survival was actually significantly worse, both in terms of RFS and OS in the BCG + vaccine arm vs. the BCG-alone cohort, suggesting that the cancer vaccine may have increased tumor tolerance instead of tumor immunity. This interpretation is supported by preliminary results from another large adjuvant trial of tumor vaccination in high-risk melanoma patients. The EORTC18961 trial of 1,312 patients in stage II was testing a ganglioside M2 vaccination against observation (similar to the above described ECOG 1694 trial) and was prematurely stopped after the second interim analysis (with a median follow-up of 1.8 years), because survival in the vaccination arm was significantly worse both in terms of distant metastasis-free survival and OS ($p<0.02$) [27].

Thus, despite many years of research, no vaccine is currently approved for the treatment of melanoma [34]. Furthermore, with these vaccination trials, it has been observed, for the first time, that the prognosis of melanoma patients can be deteriorated by application of an adjuvant treatment. Interestingly, this phenomenon was not observed in a vaccination trial using dendritic cells and antigeneic melanoma peptides; however, this trial did not show any benefit in comparison to DTIC treatment [98].

Treatment of Metastatic Melanoma

Chemotherapy

Chemotherapy is presently the only established therapy for stage IV metastatic disease, while cytokine treatments in disseminated melanoma are uncommon in Europe. Monochemotherapy is, in general, currently recommended as the first line treatment for disseminated melanoma outside of clinical trials. Single agent regimens are given in Table 4.2.6.

DTIC is the most widely used chemotherapy for the treatment of metastatic melanoma [68]. DTIC yields objective responses in approximately 20–25% of patients according to older phase II trials and 5–12% in newer phase III trials. However, most responses are transient; only 1–2% of patients achieve a long-term durable response to chemotherapy [9, 28]. There is little evidence that DTIC treatment offers a significant survival advantage over supportive care. Other chemotherapies used for patients with metastatic melanoma include temozolomide and fotemustine. Temozolomide has been demonstrated to be at least as effective as DTIC in a phase III study and is an oral alternative to DTIC [73], while fotemustine significantly improved response rate and tended to prolong median OS when compared to DTIC (7.3 vs. 5.6 months; $p=0.067$) in a phase III trial [7].

The antitumor activity of some combinations of chemotherapeutic agents has also been evaluated. In general, polychemotherapy regimens achieve higher objective response rates, mainly in the range of 20–30%. Their possible

Table 4.2.6 Single agent therapies for advanced cutaneous melanoma described in prospective randomized trials or phase II studies

Drug	Dose	Response rate (%)
Dacarbazine		
Ringborg et al. [95], Middleton et al. [73]	250 mg/m² i.v. daily for 5 days every 3–4 weeks	12.1–17.6
Chiarion Sileni et al. [17], Young et al. [117]	800–1,200 mg/m² i.v. daily on 1 day every 3–4 weeks	5.3–23
Temozolomide		
Bleehen et al. [10], Middleton et al. [73]	150–200 mg/m² p.o. daily for 5 days every 4 weeks	13.5–21
Fotemustine		
Jacquillat et al. [51], Mornex et al. [76]	100 mg/m² i.v. on days 1, 8 and 15; then 5 week pause, then repeat single dose every 3 weeks	7.4–24.2
Vindesine		
Nelimark et al. [80], Carmichael et al. [13]	3 mg/m² i.v. every 14 day	12–26
Interferon-α[a]		
Robinson et al. [96], Miller et al. [74]	9–18 million IU/m² s.c. 3 × weekly	13–25
Interleukin-2[a]		
Dorval et al. [25], Legha et al. [66], Atkins et al. [4]	600,000 IU/kg as 15 min infusion i.v. every 8 h for 5 days (total of 14 doses).	16–21.6
	Repeat every 2 weeks	

[a]If phase III trials were not available

indication is second line treatment after progressive disease under a first line regimen or first line treatment of very rapidly and aggressively growing metastases. However, polychemotherapies tested in phase III trials (e.g., Dartmouth regimen: cisplatin/vinblastine/DTIC) have also failed to demonstrate a survival benefit when compared to DTIC alone [31, 68]. Thus, their indication as first line treatments has to be considered carefully. The best established regimens of polychemotherapy or combinations with interferon-α are listed in Table 4.2.7.

Special Case: Metastatic Uveal Melanoma

Melanomas of the eye involving the uvea, ciliary body, or the retina have a different pattern of metastasis than cutaneous melanomas. Since the eye does not have a lymphatic system, almost all metastases are found in the liver due to direct hematologic spread. For this reason, the prognosis of metastatic ocular melanoma is generally much worse than that of cutaneous lesions. However, when patients with liver metastases from ocular and skin melanomas are compared, there are no prognostic differences.

Because of preferential metastasis to the liver, patients with ocular melanoma and liver metastases may be candidates for local-regional (ablative) therapeutic measures. Few systemic schedules have been reported with objective responses shown in Table 4.2.8.

Cytokine Therapy

Two cytokines are predominantly used to treat patients with metastatic melanoma: IL-2 and IFN-α. These immunotherapies have no direct cytotoxic effects on melanoma and require immune system cells to promote an antitumor effect [92].

Cytokine therapy with high-dose IL-2 (aldesleukin, Proleukin; Chiron, Emeryville, California) was approved for the treatment of patients with metastatic melanoma in the United States in 1998. An objective response rate of approximately 20% was observed in a phase II trial in patients ($N = 47$) with metastatic melanoma receiving single-agent therapy with 600,000 U/kg IL-2. Although a small percentage of patients (~5%) experience long-term, durable, complete responses with IL-2, it is not associated with improved survival in the overall patient population [5, 57]. In addition, IL-2 is poorly tolerated; treatment-related toxicity is severe and routinely requires inpatient intensive care [4]. Common dose-limiting toxicities include hemodynamic toxicity (e.g., hypotension, edema, weight gain, decreased renal function), respiratory insufficiency, and neurotoxicity [4]. Because of the severe toxicity associated with administration of IL-2 and the lack of improvement in survival, EU guidelines do not recommended IL-2 for the routine treatment of metastatic melanoma, and in the US, IL-2 treatment is limited to younger patients (<50 years) and is performed by only a few centers.

High-dose IFN-α2a (Roferon; Roche Pharmaceuticals, Nutley, NJ) is no more effective than single-agent DTIC in patients with malignant melanoma [79]. In phase II trials, the overall response rates of patients with advanced melanoma to IFN-α2a were 8–22%, but responses were rarely durable [21, 79]. Simultaneous administration of low-dose IFN-α and temozolomide was shown to significantly enhance objective response rates when compared to temozolomide alone ($p = 0.036$). However, median survival was not significantly improved by the simultaneous addition of low-dose IFN-α to chemotherapy ($p = 0.16$) [55].

Biochemotherapy

Biochemotherapy (e.g., cisplatin, vinblastine, and DTIC combined with IFN-α ± IL-2) dramatically increases response rates but has not been shown to significantly improve survival

Table 4.2.7 Polychemotherapy and chemoimmunotherapy of advanced cutaneous melanoma from prospective randomized trials or phase II trials[a]

Regimen	Dose	Response rate (%)
DTIC (Temozolomide) + interferon-α Bajetta et al. [8], Falkson et al. [33], Kaufmann et al. [55]	DTIC 850 mg/m² i.v. day 1 (or temozolomide 150 mg/m² p.o. day 1–5) Interferon-α2a/b 3 million IU/m² s.c. days 1–5; then Interferon-α2a/b 5 million IU/m² s.c. 3× weekly in weeks 2–4; repeat every 4 weeks	14–27.7
Vindesine + interferon-α Smith et al. [103]	Vindesine 3 mg/m² i.v. day 1 Interferon-α2a/b 5 million IU/m² s.c. 3× weekly; repeat every 2 weeks	24
BHD Carter et al. [14], Costanzi et al. [20]	BCNU 150 mg/m² i.v. day 1 in every other cycle; Hydroxyurea 1,500 mg/m² p.o. days 1–5 DTIC 150 mg/m² i.v. days 1–5 every 4 weeks	12.7–30.4
BOLD Seigler et al. [100], York et al. [116]	Bleomycin 15 mg i.v. days 1+4 Vincristine 1 mg/m² i.v. days 1+5 CCNU 80 mg/m² p.o. day 1 DTIC 200 mg/m² i.v. days 1–5 every 4–6 weeks	22–40
DVP Gunderson et al. [45], Pectasides et al. [83], Jungnelius et al. [53]	DTIC 250 mg/m² i.v. days 1–5 Vindesine 3 mg/m² i.v. day 1 Cisplatin 100 mg/m² i.v. day 1 every 3–4 weeks	31.4–45
DVP Verschraegen et al. [109]	DTIC 450 mg/m² i.v. days 1+8 Vindesine 3 mg/m² i.v. days 1+8 Cisplatin 50 mg/m² i.v. days 1+8 every 3–4 weeks	24
DBCT McClay et al. [71], Chapman et al. [16], Creagan et al. [23]	DTIC 220 mg/m² i.v. days 1–3 BCNU 150 mg/m² i.v. day 1 of every other cycle. Cisplatin 25 mg/m² i.v. days 1–3 Tamoxifen 2×10 mg p.o. daily every 3–4 weeks	18.5–31.9
CarboTax Rao et al. [90]	Carboplatin AUC6 i.v. day 1, after four cycles reduce to AUC4 Paclitaxel 225 mg/m² i.v. day 1 every 3 weeks, after four cycles reduce to 175 mg/m²	12.1 (second line)

[a]If no phase III trials are available

Table 4.2.8 Chemotherapy for advanced ocular melanoma

Drug/regime	Dose	Response rate (%)
Fotemustine Leyvraz et al. [69], Egerer et al. [26], Siegel et al. [102]	Induction cycle 100 mg/m² intraarterial (hepatic artery) over 4 h weekly for 4 weeks; then 5 week pause; then repeat every 3 weeks	30–40
Treosulfan/gemcitabine Pföhler et al. [85]	Treosulfan 5 g/m² i.v. day 1 Gemcitabin 1 g/m² i.v. day 1 Repeat every 3 weeks	28.6

when compared with DTIC alone or polychemotherapy in randomized phase III trials [3]. In a systematic review of 41 randomized clinical trials of patients with melanoma receiving various biochemotherapy regimens, none of the treatment schedules improved OS [31]. Furthermore, the addition of IL-2 does not significantly enhance the efficacy of biochemotherapy with DTIC/IFN [52] or DTIC/cisplatin/IFN-α2b [58]. To date, biochemotherapy has demonstrated significant clinical benefit neither in adjuvant trials [60] nor in the metastatic setting [3], and biochemotherapy is associated with additive toxicity. For these reasons, biochemotherapy regimens have not entered into standard clinical practice.

Although in a recent meta-analysis of 18 trials and nearly 2,500 patients with metastatic melanoma, there was a clear benefit of biochemotherapy in terms of objective response and there was no benefit for addition of IFN or IL-2 to chemotherapy in terms of OS ($p=0.9$) [54]. Therefore, the results from this meta-analysis revealed no reasons (with the exception of enrollment in clinical trials) to change the present concept of first line monochemotherapy for patients with metastatic melanoma [50].

Emerging Therapies

Several approaches to overcoming tolerance that appear promising in clinical trials include downregulation of anti-apoptotic proteins, inhibition of oncogenic kinase pathways, and downregulation of inhibitory receptors/cytokines. These and other emerging therapies are still in the early stages of development and may yield incremental improvements in the treatment of metastatic melanoma.

Oblimersen

Oblimersen (G3139, Genasense; Genta, Inc, Berkeley Heights, NJ) is an antisense oligonucleotide that selectively targets Bcl-2 RNA for degradation, decreasing Bcl-2 protein production. The normal role of Bcl-2 is prevention of apoptosis, and its activity plays a role in resistance to chemotherapy. Bcl-2 is overexpressed in many cancers, and the reduction of Bcl-2 protein in cancer cells through the use of oblimersen may synergistically enhance the antitumor activities of standard therapies [1, 106]. An initial phase III study of oblimersen and DTIC tended to show improved survival over DTIC alone (9.1 months with combination therapy vs. 7.9 months with DTIC alone, $p=0.18$) [75]. A subsequent phase III study of patients with melanoma randomized to receive DTIC alone or in combination with oblimersen pretreatment found a significant increase in objective responses and significant prolongation of PFS but failed to show a significant OS advantage with the addition of oblimersen to DTIC therapy (median survival at minimum follow-up 24 months, 9.0 vs. 7.8 months; $p=0.077$) [9]. Interestingly, all three endpoints became significant in the subgroup of patients with normal levels of lactate dehydrogenase (LDH). Presently, another study is being conducted with the intent to confirm the survival advantage in patients with low LDH.

Elesclomol

Elesclomol (STA-4783, Synta Pharmaceuticals, Lexington, MA) is a *bis*-thiobenzoylhydrazide small molecule that induces heat shock protein 70 (hsp70). STA-4783 is thought to cause cell death by increasing the level of oxidative stress beyond a sustainable threshold. This may occur through activation of natural killer (NK) cells or through intracellular stress-activated pathways. A randomized, double-blinded, controlled, phase II study ($N=81$) has shown that combination therapy with STA-4783 and paclitaxel increases the duration of PFS in patients with metastatic cutaneous melanoma when compared to paclitaxel treatment alone (median PFS of 3.7 months for patients treated with combination therapy vs. 1.8 months for patients treated with paclitaxel alone; $p=0.035$) [82]. Subgroup analysis showed that chemotherapy-naive patients ($N=23$) treated with combination therapy had a median PFS of 8.3 vs. 2.4 months in the paclitaxel-only arm ($n=9$) [82].

Sorafenib

Sorafenib (Nexavar, BAY 43-9006; Bayer Pharmaceuticals Corporation, West Haven, Connecticut) is an oral multikinase inhibitor that is being investigated in patients with metastatic melanoma. The most frequently (60–70%) mutated oncogene identified to date in melanoma is BRAF, an upstream mediator of the mitogen-activated protein kinase (MAPK) pathway [35]. Increased activation of the MAPK pathway is implicated in melanoma tumorgenesis and is enhanced in advanced-stage melanoma [97]. Sorafenib is the only agent with BRAF inhibitory activity that has reached clinical testing, so far [35]. Results from clinical studies of sorafenib vary. Although well-tolerated when combined with IFN or dacarbazine in phase I trials, a phase II randomized discontinuation trial of patients ($N=37$) with advanced melanoma treated twice daily with single-agent, oral sorafenib therapy found that while the drug was well-tolerated, there was little or no antitumor activity [32]. Another phase II study ($N=90$) of sorafenib in combination with temozolomide vs. temozolomide alone found no advantage with the addition of sorafenib [2]. However, a single-arm, phase II trial of sorafenib in combination with carboplatin and paclitaxel found an objective response rate (31%) that was surprisingly high for this disease population ($N=35$) [36]. In another phase II trial of treatment-naive patients ($N=101$) with advanced melanoma, either DTIC alone or in combination with sorafenib was administered, and improved PFS (11.7 vs. 21.1 weeks) and greater response rates (12 vs. 24%) were observed with the addition of sorafenib [72]. This treatment regimen is being evaluated further in larger clinical trial settings.

Cytotoxic T-Lymphocyte-Associated Antigen 4 Blockade

Full T-cell activation requires stimulation of the T-cell receptor as well as a costimulatory signal provided by the binding of B7 on the antigen-presenting cell (e.g., dendritic cell) to CD28 on the T cell. Cytotoxic T-lymphocyte-associated antigen 4 (CTLA4) is a homologue of CD28 and is an inhibitory receptor on the T cell that is upregulated following T-cell activation. The normal function of CTLA4 is to compete with CD28 to bind B7 and turn off T-cell activation, thus, acting as a natural "brake" by removing the costimulatory signal. The CTLA4-B7 interaction can be blocked with an anti-CTLA4 monoclonal antibody (mAb), which has a higher affinity for CTLA4 than B7. Thus, the inhibitory signal is prevented and the "brake" on T-cell activation released. Two fully human anti-CTLA4 mAbs that block CTLA4 and potentially prolong T-cell activation are currently in clinical development: tremelimumab (CP-675,206; Pfizer Inc., New York, NY) and ipilimumab (MDX-010; Medarex, Inc./ Bristol-Myers Squibb). Objective response rates of patients with metastatic melanoma treated with either of the two anti-CLTA4 mAbs as single agents are similar (~10%) [6, 46, 94, 111] and resemble the response rates found in patients treated with high-dose IL-2. Responses to anti-CTLA4 mAbs are durable (as much as 70%) [93, 111] but may take as long as 12 weeks or more to develop [81], and late-onset ORs are sometimes preceded by months of stable disease. Early trials also indicate that CTLA4 blockade may increase OS compared to historical controls [41]. Side effects of CTLA4 blockade are less severe than exogenous cytokine therapy and are manageable. Commonly reported AEs include diarrhea/colitis and rash/pruritus. Several randomized studies are ongoing to assess whether these early observations of durable responses will translate into an OS benefit.

Other Treatments in the Early Stages of Development

Thymalfasin (Zadaxin™; SciClone Pharmaceuticals, Intl., Hong Kong) is a synthetic version of thymosin α1, an endogenous substance secreted by the thymus. Endogenous thymosin-α1 increases the number of T cells and NK cells by stimulating their differentiation, slowing their apoptosis, and enhancing specific cytokine production to protect the body against infectious diseases. Thymalfasin thus acts as an immunomodulator that may be therapeutic for multiple clinical conditions, including metastatic melanoma. Addition of thymalfasin and IFN to DTIC in a phase II trial more than doubled the objective response rates seen in patients with metastatic melanoma treated with DTIC alone (50% had objective responses, 25% CRs; median survival was 11.5 months) [37, 91].

AZD6244 (ARRY-142886; AstraZeneca, Wilmington, Delaware) is a potent, selective inhibitor of MAPK/ERK 1/2 kinase [24]. This is downstream but in the same signaling pathway as the kinase targeted by sorafenib. AZD6244 is currently being tested in a phase II, multicenter, open-label, randomized study comparing its antitumor activity with that of temozolomide for patients with stage III or IV malignant melanoma.

4.2.3.4 Conclusion

Despite decades of clinical research, patients with advanced melanoma continue to have a poor prognosis, and few agents consistently demonstrate increased OS. For high-risk, resected disease, adjuvant therapy with IFN-α has been shown to increase RFS and in some studies OS as well, but the probability of an absolute survival benefit at 5 years is small. The standard treatment for patients with metastatic melanoma is still chemotherapy, which offers only transient efficacy. Due to the potential benefits of new targeted drugs and immunotherapies, treatment guidelines for melanoma recommend the inclusion of patients with metastatic melanoma in clinical trials.

Several agents have demonstrated promising antitumor activity with manageable side effects in patients with melanoma. These include oblimersen, elesclomol, sorafenib, the anti-CTLA4 mAbs tremelimumab and ipilimumab, thymalfasin, and AZD6244. Early clinical trials have indicated that while none of these products seems to offer a "breakthrough" in terms of antitumor activity, each could offer incremental improvements in the standard of care. Ongoing clinical trials will elucidate whether these therapeutics, as single agents or in combination with other therapies, will provide substantial survival benefit to patients with melanoma.

4.2.4 Adjuvant Immunotherapy in Melanoma: Pegylated Interferons: A New Perspective

Joanna Mangana and Reinhard Dummer

4.2.4.1 Interferons Type I and II and Their Receptors: Overview

Since the discovery of IFNs by Isaacs and Lindemann [1], when they were originally described as agents that interfere with influenza virus replication, a tremendous amount of studies using predominantly type I IFNs have been conducted. It was only in 1978 when IFN was purified in amounts that allowed physical and chemical characterization.

Interferons are pleiotropic cytokines. They inhibit viral replication within host-cells through the induction of proteins and activation of specific signaling pathways [2–6].

Moreover, they interfere with immune functions by activating natural killer (NK) cells and macrophages – though they protect the unaffected cells from NK cell-mediated lysis – [7] and they augment antigen presentation to lymphocytes. These activities explain their implications in autoimmunity.

The central role of plasmacytoid dendritic cells (pDCs) to innate antiviral response system by producing type I IFNs has been documented [8, 9]. They regulate and link the adaptive and innate immune response [10, 11]. Human pDCs induce also the production of IFN-γ in NK cells through interleukin-2 (IL-2) secretion. They express a subset of toll-like receptors (TLRs), including TLR-7 and TLR-9, which allow them to detect presence of DNA and RNA viruses [12]. Furthermore, it has been demonstrated that pDCs infiltrate solid tumors [13, 14]. This observation opened intriguing questions about their potency in antitumor response. Recently, it has been shown that pDCs are themselves capable of inducing antitumor immunity by activating NK and Tcells [15]. In addition to their antiviral and immunomodulatory effects, IFNs are considered to be antiangiogenic [4, 16].

Recently, the involvement of both IFN type I and II in the elimination phase of cancer immunoediting has been identified [17, 18]. IFN-unresponsive hosts show an increased tumor incidence ,and the tumors that arise in IFN-unresponsive environments are highly antigenic.

Although first approval was for hairy cell leukemia and for Kaposi sarcoma, [19] they are widely used as a first line therapy in the treatment of many diseases such as chronic hepatitis-C and -B, multiple sclerosis (IFN-β), and melanoma (IFN-α). Despite the fact that their efficacy has been also demonstrated in other diseases such as follicular non-Hodgkins Lymphoma, condylomata acuminata, basal cell carcinoma, chronic phase Philadelphia (PH) chromosome-

positive chronic myelogenous leukemia (CML), and renal cell carcinoma [20–24], they are not regularly used as a first line treatment in these malignancies.

4.2.4.1.1 Types of Interferons

Interferons belong to the large class of glycoproteins known as cytokines. In 1980s, IFNs were simply classified in three groups: IFN-α, IFN-β, and IFN-γ [25]. This categorization was based on antigenic specificity. Today, they are classified according to their structural and functional properties in interferon type I, interferon type II, and interferon-like cytokines.

Type I interferons. There are 13 IFN-α [26] members and a single member of each IFN-β, IFN-ε, IFN-κ, IFN-ω, IFN-δ, and IFN-τ [27–29]. The genes encoding all members of IFN type I family are situated on chromosome 9 [30].

The molecular structure of the two recombinant IFNs-2α (IFNα-2α and IFNα-2b) differs from one another only by one single amino-acid at position 23 [31]. IFNα-2α and IFNα-2b show the same efficacy in the treatment of chronic hepatitis-C, hairy cell leukemia, and Kaposi's sarcoma.

All type I IFNs exert their biologic activities by binding to a specific cell surface receptor complex, known as the IFN-α receptor (IFNα-R). IFN-α receptor is the same for all members of type I IFN family. It consists of a subunit of a 135 kilo Daltons (kDa) IFNα-R1 and of a subunit of 115 kDa INFα-R2 chains. Both receptors are located in chromosome 9 [32, 33]. The primary signaling pathway activated by IFNs is the Jak-Stat pathway [34–36]. The IFNα-R1 and IFNα-R2 receptors bind to Janus-activated kinase (Jak) molecules, Tyk2 and Jak1, respectively [37–39]. This leads to activation of signal transducers and activators of transcription (Stats), Stats 1 and Stats 2, which are phosphorylated by the Jaks. The phosphorylated Stats translocate to the nucleus and activate the transcription of IFN-stimulated genes (ISGs). Interferon-Stimulated Gene Factor 3 (ISGF3) is an important transcription factor, which is induced by type I IFNs [40].

Although IFN-α predominantly signals through Stat-1 and -2 [41], its pathway can involve Stat-3, Stat-5, Stat-4, and Stat-6 [38, 42–48]. Stat-1 plays a prominent role in immune response, while Stat-3 is implicated in tumor progression. Stat-4 and Stat-6 are activated in certain cells, such as endothelial cells and lymphoid cells [46, 48].

Except Jak-Stat, other pathways activated by interferons have been recognized. Of the various Mitogen-activated protein kinase (MAPK) pathways, the p38 signaling has the most important role in the generation of IFN-mediated signals [49–51]. Other pathways include the phosphatidyl-inositol 3-kinase (PI3K) signaling pathway [52] and the CRK family of adaptor proteins [53]. Nevertheless, it is now understood that no signaling activation cascade alone is sufficient for the generation of IFN's biological properties.

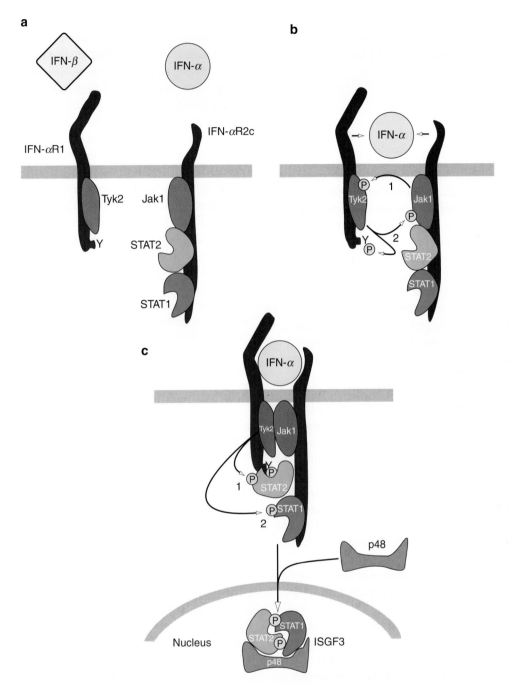

Fig. 4.2.4 Signaling pathways activated during engagement of the type I IFN receptor. IFN-a R1 and IFN-aR2 bind to Tyk2 and Jak1 respectively. After the phosphorylation of the receptor molecule signal transducers and activators of transcription (Stats) are activated

Cooperative function of this network of cytokines is needed for IFN-mediated immune response (Fig. 4.2.4).

Type II interferons. Only one member belongs in these class II interferons, IFN-γ [24, 54]. It is pharmacologically and chemically distinct from type I IFN. IFN-γ is a dimerized cytokine produced by NK and T cells located on human chromosome 12.

IFN-γ is structurally different from type I IFN, binds to a different receptor, and is encoded in a different chromosome.

IFN-γ is approved by the United States Food and Drug Administration (FDA) for use in chronic granulomatous disease. In Japan, IFN-γ was registered for cutaneous T-cell lymphoma in 1997 [55].

IFN-lambda. Another group of cytokines – consisting of IL-28 and IL-29 – was recognized as a third class of interferons, which are produced by lymphocytes. The genes encoding this family of cytokines are clustered on human chromosome 19. The group consists of three members

IFNλ1, IFNλ2 and IFNλ3. It expresses its activity by signaling through a receptor complex consisting of IL10R2 (also designated as CRF2-4) and of IFNλ-R1 (also designated as CRF2-12) [30].

4.2.4.2 Interferon Biomarkers and Resistance

A number of surrogate markers have been investigated in order to define the dose–response relationship of IFN-α. (2-5 oligoadenylate Synthetase), an enzyme induced by both IFN-α and IFN-γ, seem to play a role in IFN response. Increased levels of this enzyme were shown to correlate with decreased cell cycling in melanoma cell cultures treated with IFN [56]. Other markers such as neopterin and β2 microglobulin were used to evaluate this hypothesis. Studies in melanoma [57–59] provide conflicting data on the utility of neopterin levels in predicting response to immunotherapy. In aggregate, these markers may show laboratory confirmation of stimulation of IFN but do not provide consistent predictive information on the outcome of IFN therapy.

Another protein called Mx protein, associated with antiviral properties of IFN therapy, specifically type I and II IFN in vivo and in vitro, has been identified [60]. The Mx family, a subclass of high molecular weight GTPase, comprises MxA and MxB in humans and Mx1 and Mx2 in mice [61]. MX family is encoded in human chromosome 21, which is synergic to mouse chromosome 16 [62, 63]. MxA is induced selectively by type I IFNs, and its expression requires STAT 1 signaling [64]. As a result, MxA protein is used as a surrogate marker for type I IFN activity in various experimental and clinical settings [65].

The role of Mx as a predictive marker of anti-proliferative effect of IFN-α in melanoma has been studied [66, 67], with also conflicting results.

Yurkovetsky et al. tried to evaluate specific predictive markers of clinical outcome and of IFNα-2b response in patients with high-risk melanoma [68]. Differences in serum concentrations in 29 cytokines, angiogenic and growth factors in melanoma patients before and after high-dose IFNα-2b therapy and in healthy control groups were analyzed [68]. A statistically significant increase in 15 proteins was observed in melanoma patients compared to healthy individuals. IFN-α therapy decreased levels of angiogenic and growth factors (vascular endothelial growth factor VEGF, epidermal growth factor EGF, hepatocyte growth factor HGF), as it was noticed 3 months after the induction of therapy. However, this did not seem to correlate with changes in recurrence-free survival (RFS) among this population. It has also been shown that pretreatment levels of proinflammatory cytokines (IL-1α, IL-1β, IL-6, tumor necrosis factor TNF-α and macrophage inflammatory protein MIP-1α, MIP-1β) were higher in patients treated with IFN who had a RFS longer than 5 years compared to those with shorter RFS.

Furthermore, Lee et al. [69] studied defects in T-cell signaling (IFN signaling) in advanced melanoma patients, likely arising from their impaired response to IFN therapy. The reduced responses to IFNs could be involved in the susceptibility of lymphocytes to spontaneous apoptosis in the cancer state, which is critical of tumor immune dysfunction. These effects were normalized in vitro by exposure to high-dose IFN-α.

Finally, it has recently been demonstrated that silencing the suppressor of cytokine signaling (SOCS) proteins on tumor cells results in enhancement of the anti-proliferative effect of IFN-α and IFN-γ [70]. SOCS proteins are negative regulators of IFN signaling [71]. It has been shown that increased levels of them render cells resistant to IFN-α therapy [72].

Further investigations are required to identify the mechanisms of responsiveness to IFN therapy and to understand the possible mechanisms of resistance. Establishment of response markers would be helpful for the identification of patients who would be more likely benefited from IFN-α therapy.

4.2.4.2.1 Interferon-Induced Autoimmunity

The presence of autoantibodies or other clinical manifestations of autoimmunity after interferon treatment was shown to be associated with a prolongation in relapse-free survival [73].

Gogas et al. [73] investigated the appearance of autoantibodies or other clinical manifestation of autoimmunity in a group of 200 patients in a sub-study of a larger randomized trial [73]. Patients were enrolled in two groups: in the first group, they received IFNα-2b 15 MIU per square meter (m²) i.v. daily 5 days/week for 4 weeks while in the other, they received the same induction dose followed by s.c. injections of 10 MIU IFNα-2b thrice weekly for additional 48 weeks.

Detection of autoantibodies was associated with statistically significant improvement in relapse free survival (RFS) survival and overall survival (OS). Median relapse free survival (MRFS) was 16 months among patients without autoimmunity (108 out of 148) and was not reached among patients with autoimmunity (7 out of 52 had a relapse). MRFS Median relapse-free survival in patients without autoimmunity was 16 months (range between 0.3 and 74.3, whereas it was not reached during follow-up in patients with autoimmunity (range between 3.5 and 84.7 months) [73]. An evaluation of the presence of autoantibodies in patients who participated in the European Organisation for Research and Treatment of Cancer (EORTC) 18952 did not confirm the previous observations [74].

Nevertheless, the role of autoimmunity including vitiligo-like depigmentation in patients with melanoma is not a today observation as it occurs spontaneously or during chemotherapy. Spontaneous vitiligo was considered a favorable prognostic factor even before the advent of treatment with IL-2 [75].

4.2.4.3 Pegylation

The need for a substance with broader therapeutic effect and more convenient pharmacokinetic profile with less toxicity than conventional interferon led to pegylation of IFN-α.

The term pegylation describes the conjugation of a molecule with polyerthylene-glycol (PEG), which is used to alter the physical and chemical profile of molecule.

Pegylation increases the stability and solubility of the drug. Pegylation prolongs the drug's activity, delays its clearance, and reduces protein's immunogenicity. As a result, the administration frequency can be reduced; the pegylated form is injected once weekly, rather than three times per week for conventional interferon-α.

FDA recently approved two pegylated interferon-α preparations for the treatment of chronic hepatitis (PegIFNα-2b was approved in January 2001 while PegIFNα-2a was approved in October 2002). Unfortunately, PegIFNs are not yet officially approved for the treatment of melanoma.

4.2.4.3.1 Pegylated IFNα-2b (Pegintron)

PegIFNα-2b presents as a derivate of recombinant IFNα-2b conjugated with polyethylene-glycol [76]. The molecular weight of the PEG moiety is 12 kDa, and it is attached to a linkage to histidine-34 on IFNα-2b [77]. The average molecular weight of PegIFNα-2b is 31 kDa [78].

4.2.4.3.2 Pegylated IFNα-2α (Pegasus)

PegIFNα-2α is recombinant IFNα-2a conjugated with a 40 kDa-branched PEG moiety, and it consists of major isomers [76]. It is linked to the recombinant interferon via a stable amine to lysine bond [79]. PegIFNα-2α has an approximate molecular weight of 60 kDa [79].

Drugs with a large volume of distribution require adjustment of a dose according to the prevailing body weight. As a result, the 12 kDa PegIFNα-2b is dosed on a weight-basis, whereas the 40 kDa PegIFNα-2α is given as a flat dose.

Half time, mean peak concentration time, and clearing of conventional IFN and of PegIFNα-2b and PegIFNα-2α are compared in a table above (Table 4.2.9).

Table 4.2.9 Comparing pharmacology between conventional IFN and two pegylated IFN preparations

	Conventional IFN	12 kDa PEG IFN	40 kDa PEG IFN
Volume of distribution	25–30	20–40	8
Half time (h)	3–8	54	65
Time to serum peak	7–12	20	80
Clearing	Renal	Renal	Hepatic and renal

4.2.4.3.3 Pegylated Interferon in the Adjuvant Setting

The most important factor to determine survival in melanoma patients is disease stage. Measurement of tumor thickness with Breslow index and ulceration are used to determine the prognosis of the primary tumor in stage I and II melanoma patients [80].

For stage III melanoma patients, there are four major criteria of outcome determination: number of metastatic lymph nodes, tumor burden (microscopic or macroscopic), the presence or absence of ulceration of the primary tumor, and the presence or absence of in-transit or satellite metastases [80].

Five-year survival (5-year) for tumors with a thick Breslow index without involvement of lymph nodes ranges between 27 and 70% while it is decreased to 10–19% in patients with positive lymph nodes [70]. One-year survival in patients with distant metastases is 41–59% [80] while 10-year survival rate of 30% in patients with locoregional metastases in lymph nodes and of less than 5% in those with distant metastases [81].

With these features in mind, effective, adjuvant, postsurgical treatment following surgical interventions is urgently needed. Adjuvant chemotherapy and irradiation therapy failed to improve survival. Immunotherapy offers at least some promises.

A number of prospective randomized trials have been performed using adjuvant treatment with IFN in patients with cutaneous melanoma (see Chap. 4.2). Treatment with low, intermediate, and high doses of IFN-α after resection of primary tumor has improved RFS recurrence-free survival (RFS), but without confirmed significant effects on OS [82–84]. Based on ECOG 1684[85] , the first trial that showed a positive effect in OS, high-dose adjuvant IFN-α won US FDA approval. It was then proposed that IFN might exert its best effect in long-term therapy [84]. Definite clarification of the role of high-dose IFN would need a large prospective trial comparing it to long low-dose IFN therapy.

Since PegIFN-α is suitable for long-term therapy, the EORTC has designed a large prospective randomized trial to investigate the potent positive effect of PegIFNα-2b in adjuvant setting in patients with stage III melanoma. The largest trial ever conducted with pegylated interferon (EORTC 18991 study) was recently published in *Lancet* [86]. One thousand two hundred and fifty-six patients from 99 centers in 17 countries with resected stage III melanoma were randomized to receive observation or pegylated interferon-α therapy [86]. Randomization was stratified for microscopic (N1) vs. macroscopic (N2) nodal involvement, number of positive nodes, ulceration, and tumor thickness. RFS (primary endpoint), distant-metastases-free survival (DMFS), and OS were analyzed for the intent-to-treat population.

The interferon group received an induction interferon dose of weekly dose of 6 μg/kg for the first 8 weeks, and then the dose was reduced to 3 μg/kg/week for 5 years [86].

At 3.8 years of median follow-up, RFS was significantly reduced by 18% in the PegIFNα-2b arm compared with observation; the 4-year RFS rate was 45.6 vs. 38.9%. DMFS was improved but nonsignificantly ($p=0.11$). OS was unchanged in the two groups. In stage III-N1a (micrometastases detected in the sentinel node), both RFS (HR 0.72, 57.7 vs. 45.4%, $p=0.01$) and DMFS (HR 0.73, 60.5 vs. 52.6%, $p=0.01$) were prolonged in the PegIFNα-2b arm, whereas in stage III-N1b (macroscopic metastases), there was no benefit [86].

This trial showed that a prolonged adjuvant treatment with IFN-α improved the RFS period and DMFS in a subgroup of patients with low tumor burden. According to this, further search for predictive clinical or biological markers that can identify patients who are more likely to benefit from IFN treatment is encouraged [86].

Safety and efficacy of adjuvant treatment with PegIFNα-2α 100 μg s.c. weekly for 36 months vs. conventional 3 MIU IFNα-2α thrice weekly for 18 months are investigated in another European, multicenter, prospective trial performed by the Dermatologic Cooperative Oncology Group (EADO). Eight hundred and eighty patients with melanoma stage IIA–IIIB are randomized to receive adjuvant treatment after surgical excision. Inclusion criteria were tumor thickness >1.5 mm and absence of regional nodal macrometastases as assessed either by clinical examination or if, sentinel lymph node dissection (SLND) or elective node dissection (ELND) are performed by the absence of macroscopic evidence of disease. Patients with evidence of nodal macrometastasis by SLND or ELND are eligible. The primary endpoint of the study is 5-year-disease-free survival. The results of it are pending.

In addition, there is another randomized European trial initiated by the German Dermatologic Cooperativ Group (DeCoG) that investigates PegIFNα-2a in a dose of 180 μg/week for 24 weeks vs. IFNα-2α 3MI thrice per week also for 24 months. At this time point, no results of this study are available.

4.2.4.3.4 Pegylated Interferon in Palliative Disease (Stage IV Melanoma)

As referred above, stage IV malignant melanoma remains a rapidly fatal disease despite treatment [81]. Surgical excision, systemic chemotherapy, irradiation, immunotherapy, or combinations are offered to the patients without any proven evidence for an impact on survival. Therefore, participation in clinical trials is recommended.

Pegylated Interferon as Monotherapy in Stage IV

The use of PegIFN as monotherapy was evaluated in the study reporting a multicenter randomized dose comparing phase II trial [87]. This multicenter trial evaluated the efficacy of pegylated interferon monotherapy in patients with stage IV metastatic melanoma. One hundred and fifty patients were randomized to receive PegIFN in three different dose schedules. One group received 180 μg once a week; other groups received 360 or 450 μg weekly. The treatment phase was 24 weeks, followed by an 8-week follow-up time. Patients with previous chemotherapy or immunotherapy with IL-2 for stage IV melanoma were excluded. Approximately 20% of the patients had received IFN as adjuvant therapy in the past [87]. Tumor responses were confirmed by an independent radiology review board. The overall response rate (complete or partial response) was 6, 8, and 12% for each of the three groups, respectively. The difference between the dose groups was not statistically significant. In addition, there was a tendency that low-dose-treated patients presented a higher tumor burden. There was also no significant difference between stable and progressive disease among three groups [300].

Unfortunately, this trial does not clarify whether there is a true dose–response relationship with PegIFN in patients with metastatic melanoma due to the small number of the patients recruited in this study. The overall response rate in this trial is very similar to the response rate in a comparable patient population treated with DTIC monochemotherapy [88, 89]. It is challenging to argue that the targeted population includes a minority of patients who are able to respond to a therapeutic intervention, independent of its nature.

Pegylated Interferon in Combination with Chemotherapy

The combination of PegIFN and chemotherapy has been evaluated in different types of cancers [90, 91]. Several studies have been performed to evaluate the efficacy of combined chemotherapy and immunotherapy in patients with melanoma.

Hwu et al. enrolled thirty-five patients with stage IV melanoma to receive 0.5 µg/kg/weekly PegIFNα-2b plus TMZ 75 mg/m^2 daily for 6 days/week with a 2-week break between the cycles [92]. Patients with brain metastases, pregnant, or lactating patients or patients with evidence of other tumor except nonmelanoma skin or in situ cervical cancer were excluded. Median number of metastatic sites was 3, and the most common sites of metastasis were soft tissue, lymph nodes, and lungs, indicating a selection of patients with a relatively favorable prognosis. No patient had received chemotherapy in the past. Thirty-one percent of the patients experienced objective response (complete and partial) while 6% had stable disease (SD), which is surprising ratio. Sixty-three percent of the patients had progressive disease. At the time of the last follow-up, 27 out of 35 patients had died of their disease. The median survival for the responders (both CR and PR) was 20.2 months, and the median survival time for nonresponders was 6.9 months [92]. This study reported a very high response rate, which was not confirmed by independent radiology assessment. The survival reported is longer than with dacarbazine or temozolomide alone [93] but again needs confirmation in a randomized trial.

No grade IV hematological adverse effects (AEs) were experienced in the study. Other grade IV adverse effects were CNS hemorrhage and thrombosis/pulmonary embolism reported in one case (3%). This seemed to be neither PegIFN dose-related nor disease-dependent (hemorrhagic stroke in the absence of thrombocytopenia or clinical evidence of brain metastasis).

The efficacy of PegIFNα-2b combined with monochemotherapy was investigated in another study performed by Spieth et al. [94]. The study was designed based on previously published results from DECOG using combination of immunotherapy and chemotherapy [95]. One hundred and twenty-four patients with metastatic melanoma were included in the study. The patients received oral TMZ 200 mg/m^2 for 5 days every 28 days. In addition, subcutaneous injections of 100 µg PegIFNα-2b were performed once a week [94]. Patients with brain metastases as well patients with severe cardiac, pulmonary, psychiatric, or metabolic diseases were excluded. No patient had received prior systemic chemotherapy. In all patients, 18.1% showed complete or partial response, 25% achieved SD, while in 56.9% of the patients, the disease was progressive [94]. Median overall survival (MOS) in responders was 15.2 and in nonresponders was 8.6 months. Fifty out of one hundred and sixteen patients had an adjustment in the treatment due to adverse effects [307]. Grade 3 and grade 4 toxicities included leukopenia (23.3%) and thrombocytopenia (41.4%), which is more than observed with TMZ alone. One patient was diagnosed with sarcoidosis shortly after initiation of treatment.

Twenty-eight patients with stage IV malignant melanoma without brain metastases were enrolled in a multicenter phase II study [96]. Patients were treated with 850 mg/m^2 DTIC every 3 weeks combined with 180 µg PegIFNα-2α weekly. Only 50% of the patients participating in the study had received adjuvant therapy with IFN-α in the past. This study was initiated to evaluate the efficacy and tolerability of the combination. Primary endpoint was objective response (OR).

Two patients (8%) achieved CR, which lasted for more than 480 days and for 746 days, respectively. Four patients (16%) had a PR and another patient developed SD, which means that 24% of the patients achieved PR or CR. Median progression-free survival was 56 days, median duration of response was 236 days, and the OS time was 403 days [96]. Interesting is that 6 out of 7 patients that showed CR or PR or developed SD had neither received IFN adjuvant treatment in the past nor progressed to stage IV melanoma during interferon treatment.

One patient had to discontinue the treatment due to serious adverse effect (dizziness). The patient discontinued the treatment after shown complete response of her lung metastases.

This combination was well-tolerated. Based on the design, the impact on survival cannot be assessed. The long-term remission observed in IFN naïve patients suggests that combination of chemotherapy with IFN might be especially promising in this population.

Vaishampayan et al. aimed to evaluate the efficacy of PegIFNα-2b combined with thalidomide in patients with stage IV metastatic melanoma. Eighteen patients were enrolled to receive 0.5 µg/Kg s.c. daily plus 250 mg thalidomide orally [97]. Nine out of eighteen patients had received adjuvant treatment in the past, while 16 out of 18 patients had also received chemotherapy in the past [97]. No objective responses were noted; three patients demonstrated disease stabilization for a rate of 3/18=17% (90% confidence intervals CI, 0.06–0.35) [97]. The SD durations were 4, 5, and 15 months. The median survival was 7.2 months, with 90% CI, 4.1–13.6 months [97]. The 6-month and 1-year OS rates were 58 and 35%, respectively. Grade IV toxicity was hematologic toxicity (anemia and thrombocytopenia), which was experienced in 3 of 18 (16.6%) patients. The combination was well-tolerated, though without clinical efficacy.

Side Effects of PegIFNs

IFN-α therapy is associated with a wide spectrum of side effects that present in various severities depending on dose and individual susceptibility. Unfortunately, there are no clinical or laboratory constellations predicting the individual tolerability. FDA defines a serious adverse event to be life-threatening or to cause death, or initial or prolonged hospitalization or when one AE causes significant, persistent, or permanent disability, impairment, or disruption in the patient's body structure, physical activities, or quality of life [98]. An AE is also considered as serious when it requires intervention to prevent permanent damage [98].

Initially, the patients who are candidates for IFN therapy need detailed information about the nature of the drug. Understanding IFN as a biologic medication and not another cytostatic drug contributes to a better acceptance of the most prominent flue-like side symptoms. It is also helpful to encourage variations in the treatment schedule that interfere as little as possible with the daily activity of the individual.

Several interventions to alleviate the constitutional side effects such as dose decrement or cessation of treatment interruptions are necessary. Premedication with acetaminophen, ibuprofen, or other nonsteroidal anti-inflammatory drugs (NSADs) and/or anti-emetics is believed to reduce the severity of flue-like symptoms [99]. IFN administration at bedtime can also help [100]. Patients are also advised to avoid hepatotoxic agents and large quantities of alcohol while are on treatment with IFN. Regular hematological and biochemical tests (including thyroid antibodies) need to be drawn at baseline, monthly for the first 3 months and afterwards every 3 months when patients are treated with PegIFN-α [78, 79].

4.2.4.4 Summary and Conclusions

PegIFNs have been successfully introduced into melanoma therapy. Their pharmacologic profile allows a comfortable once weekly injection schedules. In the adjuvant setting, PegIFNα-2b is the preferred medication for long-term therapy that increases DMFS in patients with microscopic node involvement. Especially, young patients with no significant comorbidities are candidates for this approach. Side effects of PegIFNs are substantial. Therefore, there is a strong need for a detailed discussion of the pros and cons with the patient before therapy. The most common adverse effects include constitutional, neuropsychiatric, hematologic, and hepatic toxicity. Side effects are dose-dependent, and they impact on patient's quality of life. An ongoing dialog must occur between the patient and the physicians to ensure that all aspects of toxicity-related PegIFN are anticipated and treated. Autoimmunity phenomena induced by interferon treatment may be important surrogate markers for successful antitumor effect. However, additional predictive markers are necessary to identify the melanoma population who will benefit most from this immunotherapy.

Large multicenter trials in specialized centers are encouraged to address this issue by the collection of biological samples in large bio-banks.

References

Surgery

1. Mackie, R.M., Bray, C., Vestey, J., et al.: Melanoma incidence and mortality in Scotland 1979–2003. Br J Cancer **96**, 1772 (2007)
2. Cancer Facts and Figures. Available at: http://www.cancer.org (2007)
3. McMasters, K.M., Swetter, S.M.: Current management of melanoma: benefits of surgical staging and adjuvant therapy. J Surg Oncol **82**, 209 (2003)
4. Morton, D.L., Wen, D.R., Wong, J.H., et al.: Technical details of intraoperative lymphatic mapping for early stage melanoma. Arch Surg **127**, 392 (1992)
5. Balch, C.M., Soong, S.J., Gershenwald, J.E., et al.: Prognostic factors analysis of 17,600 melanoma patients: validation of the American Joint Committee on Cancer melanoma staging system. J Clin Oncol **19**, 3622 (2001)
6. Eggermont, A.M., Santinami, M., Kruit, W., et al.: Therapy with pegylated interferon α-2b versus observation in resected stage III melanoma: final results of EORTC 18991, a randomised phase 3 trial. Lancet (2008)
7. Dummer, R., Panizzon, R., Bloch, P.H., Burg, G.: Updated Swiss guidelines or the treatment and follow-up of cutaneous melanoma. Dermatology **210**, 39 (2005)
8. Handley, W.: The pathology of melanotic growths in relation to their operative treatment. Lancet **1**, 927–933 (1907)
9. Veronesi, U., Cascinelli, N., Adamus, J., et al.: Thin stage I primary cutaneous malignant melanoma. Comparison of excision with margins of 1 or 3 cm. N Engl J Med **318**, 1159–1162 (1988)
10. Cohn-Cedermark, G., Lars, E.R., Andersson, R., et al.: Long term results of a randomized study by the Swedish melanoma study group on 2-cm versus 5-cm resection margins for patients with cutaneous melanoma with a tumor thickness of 0.8–2.0mm. Cancer **89**(7), 1495–1501 (2000)
11. Khayat, D., Rixe, O., Martin, G.: Surgical margins in cutaneous melanoma (2 cm versus 5 cm for lesions measuring less then 2.1-mm thick). Long-term results of a large European multicentric phase III study. Cancer **97**, 941–1946 (2003)
12. Balch, C.M., Urist, M.M., Karakousis, C.P., et al.: Efficacy of 2-cm surgical margins for intermediate-thickness melanomas (1 to 4 MM). Results of a multi-institutional randomized surgical trial. Ann Surg **218**, 262–269 (1993)
13. Thomas, J.M., Newton-Bishop, J., A'Hern, R., et al.: Excision margins in high-risk malignant melanoma. N Engl J Med **350**, 757–766 (2004)
14. Morton, D.L., Thompson, J.F., Essner, R., et al.: Validation of the accuracy of intraoperative lymphatic mapping and sentinel lymphadenectomy for early-stage melanoma: a multicenter trial. Multicenter Selective Lymphadenectomy Trial Group. Ann Surg **230**, 453–463 (1999)
15. Morton, D.L., Thompson, J.F., Cochran, A.J., Mozzillo, N., Elashoff, R., Essner, R., Nieweg, O.E., Roses, D.F., Hoekstra, H.J., Karakousis, C.P., Reintgen, D.S., Coventry, B.J., Glass, E.C., Wang, H.J.: Sentinel-node biopsy or nodal observation in melanoma. N Engl J Med **355**, 1307 (2006)
16. Balch, C.M., Morton, D.L., Gershenwald, J.E., et al.: Sentinel node biopsy and standard of care for melanoma. J Am Acad Dermatol **60**, 872–875 (2009)
17. McMasters, K.M.: What good is sentinel lymph node biopsy for melanoma if it does not improve survival? Ann Surg Oncol **11**, 810–812 (2004)
18. Bleicher, R.J., Essner, R., Foshag, L.J., et al.: Role of sentinel lymphadenectomy in thin invasive cutaneous melanomas. J Clin Oncol **21**, 1326–1331 (2003)

19. Cochran, A.J., Balda, B.R., Starz, H., et al.: The Augsburg Consensus. Techniques of lymphatic mapping, sentinel lymphadenectomy, and completion lymphadenectomy in cutaneous malignancies. Cancer **89**, 236–241 (2000)

20. Yao, K., Balch, G., Winchester, D.J.: Multidisciplinary treatment of primary melanoma. Surg Clin North Am **89**, 267–281 (2009)

21. Pharis, D.B.: Cutaneous melanoma: therapeutic lymph node and elective lymph node dissections, lymphatic mapping and sentinel lymph node biopsy. Dermatol Ther **18**, 397–406 (2005)

22. Wrightson, W.R., Wong, S.L., Edwards, M.J., et al.: Complications associated with sentinel lymph node biopsy for melanoma. Ann Surg Oncol **10**, 676–680 (2003)

23. Gutzmer, R., Al Ghazal, M., Geerlings, H., et al.: Sentinel node biopsy in melanoma delays recurrence but does not change melanoma-related survival: a retrospective analysis of 673 patients. Br J Dermatol **153**, 1137–1141 (2005)

24. Van Akkooi, A.C., De Wilt, J.H., Verhoef, C., et al.: Clinical relevance of melanoma micrometastases (<0.1mm) in sentinel nodes: are these nodes to be considered negative? Ann Oncol **17**, 1578 (2006)

25. Guggenheim, M., Dummer, R., Jung, F.J., et al.: The influence of sentinel lymph node tumor burden on additional lymph node involvement and disease-free survival in cutaneous melanoma–a retrospective analysis of 392 cases. Br J Cancer **98**, 1922–1928 (2009)

26. Cascinelli, N., Bombardieri, E., Bufalino, R., Camerini, T., Carbone, A., Clemente, C., Lenisa, L., Mascheroni, L., Maurichi, A., Pennacchioli, E., Patuzzo, R., Santinami, M., Tragni, G.: Sentinel and nonsentinel node status in stage IB and II melanoma patients: two-step prognostic indicators of survival. J Clin Oncol **24**, 4464 (2006)

27. Scolyer, R.A., Murali, R., Gershenwald, J.E., et al.: Clinical relevance of melanoma micrometastases in sentinel nodes: too early to tell. Ann Oncol **18**, 806 (2007)

28. Satzger, I., Volker, B., Meier, A., et al.: Prognostic significance of isolated HMB45 or Melan A positive cells in Melanoma sentinel lymph nodes. Am J Surg Pathol **31**, 1175 (2007)

29. Meyer, T., Merkel, S., Goehl, J., Hohenberger, W.: Surgical therapy for distant metastases of malignant melanoma. Cancer **89**, 1983–1991 (2000)

30. Dummer, R., Hauschild, A., Jost, L.: ESMO Guidelines Working Group. Cutaneous malignant melanoma: ESMO clinical recommendations for diagnosis, treatment and follow-up. Ann Oncol **19**(suppl 2), ii86–ii88 (2008)

31. Kroon, H.M., Thompson, J.F.: Isolated limb infusion: a review. J Surg Oncol **100**, 169–177 (2009)

32. Zacest, A.C., Besser, M., Stevens, G., et al.: Surgical management of cerebral metastases from melanoma: outcome in 147 patients treated at a single institution over two decades. J Neurosurg **96**, 552–558 (2002)

33. Selek, U., Chang, E.L., Hassenbusch III, S.J., et al.: Stereotactic radiosurgical treatment in 103 patients for 153 cerebral melanoma metastases. Int J Radiat Oncol Biol Phys **59**, 1097–1106 (2004)

34. Uren, R.F.: SPECT/CT lymphoscintigraphy to locate the sentinel lymph node in patients with melanoma. Ann Surg Oncol **16**, 1459–1460 (2009)

35. Morton, D.L., Thompson, J.F., Essner, R., et al.: Validation of the accuracy of intraoperative lymphatic mapping and sentinel lymphadenectomy for early-stage melanoma. A multicenter trial. Ann Surg **230**, 453 (1999)

36. Cook, M.G., Green, M.A., Anderson, B., et al.: The development of optimal pathological assessment of sentinel lymph nodes for melanoma. J Pathol **200**, 314 (2003)

37. Mack, L.A., McKinnon, J.G.: Controversies in the management of metastatic melanoma to regional lymphatic basins. J Surg Oncol **86**, 189–199 (2004)

38. Guggenheim, M.M., Hug, U., Jung, F.J., et al.: Morbidity and recurrence after completion lymph node dissection following sentinel lymph node biopsy in cutaneous malignant melanoma. Ann Surg **247**, 687 (2008)

39. Karakousis, C.P., Hena, M.A., Emrich, L.J., et al.: Axillary node dissection in malignant melanoma: results and complications. Surgery **108**, 10–17 (1990)

40. Chan, A.R., Essner, R., Wanek, L.A., et al.: Judging the therapeutic value of lymph node dissections in melanoma. J Am Coll Surg **191**, 16–23 (2000)

Radiation

1. Andrews, D.W., Scott, C.W., Sperduto, P.W., et al.: Whole brain radiation therapy with or without stereotactic radiosurgery boost for patients with one to three brain metastases: phase III results of the RTOG 9508 randomised trial. Lancet **363**, 1665–1672 (2004)

2. Ang, K.K., Byers, R.M., Peters, L.J., Maor, M.H., Wendt, C.D., Morrison, W.H., Hussey, D.H., Goepfert, H.: Regional radiotherapy as adjuvant treatment for head and neck malignant melanoma. Preliminary results. Arch Otolaryngol Head Neck Surg **116**, 169–172 (1990)

3. Ang, K.K., Peters, L.J., Weber, R.S., Morrison, W.H., Frankenthaler, R.A., Garden, A.S., Goepfert, H., Ha, C.S., Byers, R.M.: Postoperative radiotherapy for cutaneous melanoma of the head and neck region. Int J Radiat Oncol Biol Phys **30**, 795–798 (1994)

4. Ballo, M.T., Strom, E.A., Zagars, G.K., Bedikian, A.Y., Prieto, V.G., Mansfield, P.F., Lee, J.E., Gershenwald, J.E., Ross, M.I.: Adjuvant irradiation for axillary metastases from malignant melanoma. Int J Radiat Oncol Biol Phys **52**, 964–972 (2002)

5. Ballo, M.T., Bonnen, M.D., Garden, A.S., Myers, J.N., Gershenwald, J.E., Zagars, G.K., Schechter, N.R., Morrison, W.H., Ross, M.I., Kian Ang, K.: Adjuvant irradiation for cervical lymph node metastases from melanoma. Cancer **97**, 1789–1796 (2003)

6. Ballo, M.T., Zagars, G.K., Gershenwald, J.E., Lee, J.E., Mansfield, P.F., Kim, K.B., Camacho, L.H., Hwu, P., Ross, M.I.: A critical assessment of adjuvant radiotherapy for inguinal lymph node metastases from melanoma. Ann Surg Oncol **11**, 1079–1084 (2004)

7. Ballo, M.T., Garden, A.S., Myers, J.N., Lee, J.E., Diaz Jr., E.M., Sturgis, E.M., Morrison, W.H., Gershenwald, J.E., Ross, M.I., Weber, R.S., Ang, K.K.: Melanoma metastatic to cervical lymph nodes: can radiotherapy replace formal dissection after local excision of nodal disease? Head Neck **27**, 718–721 (2005)

8. Ballo, M.T., Ross, M.I., Cormier, J.N., Myers, J.N., Lee, J.E., Gershenwald, J.E., Hwu, P., Zagars, G.K.: Combined-modality therapy for patients with regional nodal metastases from melanoma. Int J Radiat Oncol Biol Phys **64**, 106–113 (2006)

9. Beadle, B.M., Guadagnolo, B.A., Ballo, M.T., Lee, J.E., Gershenwald, J.E., Cormier, J.N., Mansfield, P.F., Ross, M.I., Zagars, G.K.: Radiation therapy field extent for adjuvant treatment of axillary metastases from malignant melanoma. Int J Radiat Oncol Biol Phys **73**, 1376–1382 (2009)

10. Bonnen, M.D., Ballo, M.T., Myers, J.N., Garden, A.S., Diaz Jr., E.M., Gershenwald, J.E., Morrison, W.H., Lee, J.E., Oswald, M.J., Ross, M.I., Ang, K.K.: Elective radiotherapy provides regional control for patients with cutaneous melanoma of the head and neck. Cancer **100**, 383–389 (2004)

11. Burmeister, B.H., Smithers, B.M., Poulsen, M., McLeod, G.R., Bryant, G., Tripcony, L., Thorpe, C.: Radiation therapy for nodal disease in malignant melanoma. World J Surg **19**, 369–371 (1995)

12. Burmeister, B.H., Smithers, B.M., Davis, S., Spry, N., Johnson, C., Krawitz, H., Baumann, K.C.: Radiation therapy following nodal

surgery for melanoma: an analysis of late toxicity. ANZ J Surg **72**, 344–348 (2002)

13. Burmeister, B.H., Mark Smithers, B., Burmeister, E., Baumann, K., Davis, S., Krawitz, H., Johnson, C., Spry, N., Trans Tasman Radiation Oncology Group: A prospective phase II study of adjuvant postoperative radiation therapy following nodal surgery in malignant melanoma-Trans Tasman Radiation Oncology Group (TROG) Study 96.06. Radiother Oncol **81**, 136–142 (2006)

14. Chang, D.T., Amdur, R.J., Morris, C.G., Mendenhall, W.M.: Adjuvant radiotherapy for cutaneous melanoma: comparing hypofractionation to conventional fractionation. Int J Radiat Oncol Biol Phys **66**, 1051–1055 (2006)

15. Christie, D.R., Tiver, K.W.: Radiotherapy for melanotic freckles. Australas Radiol **40**, 331–333 (1996)

16. Cooper, J.S., Chang, W.S., Oratz, R., Shapiro, R.L., Roses, D.F.: Elective radiation therapy for high-risk malignant melanomas. Cancer J **7**, 498–502 (2001)

17. Corry, J., Smith, J.G., Bishop, M., Ainslie, J.: Nodal radiation therapy for metastatic melanoma. Int J Radiat Oncol Biol Phys **44**, 1065–1069 (1999)

18. Creagan, E.T., Cupps, R.E., Ivins, J.C., Pritchard, D.J., Sim, F.H., Soule, E.H., O'Fallon, J.R.: Adjuvant radiation therapy for regional nodal metastases from malignant melanoma: a randomized, prospective study. Cancer **42**, 2206–2210 (1978)

19. Dancuart, F., Harwood, A.R., Fitzpatrick, P.J.: Radiotherapy of lentigo maligna and lentigo maligna melanoma of the head and neck. Cancer **45**, 2279–2283 (1980)

20. Engin, K., Tupchong, L., Waterman, F.M., Moylan, D.J., Nerlinger, R.E., Leeper, D.B.: Hyperthermia and radiation in advanced malignant melanoma. Int J Radiat Oncol Biol Phys **25**, 87–94 (1993)

21. Farshad, A., Burg, G., Panizzon, R., Dummer, R.: A retrospective study of 150 patients with lentigo maligna and lentigo maligna melanoma and the efficacy of radiotherapy using Grenz or soft X-rays. Br J Dermatol **146**, 1042–1046 (2002)

22. Fenig, E., Eidelevich, E., Njuguna, E., Katz, A., Gutman, H., Sulkes, A., Schechter, J.: Role of radiation therapy in the management of cutaneous malignant melanoma. Am J Clin Oncol **22**, 184–186 (1999)

23. Fife, K.M., Colman, M.H., Stevens, G.N., Firth, I.C., Moon, D., Shannon, K.F., Harman, R., Petersen-Schaefer, K., Zacest, A.C., Besser, M., Milton, G.W., McCarthy, W.H., Thompson, J.F.: Determinants of outcome in melanoma patients with cerebral metastases. J Clin Oncol **22**, 1293–1300 (2004)

24. Foote, M.C., Burmeister, B., Burmeister, E., Bayley, G., Smithers, B.M.: Desmoplastic melanoma: the role of radiotherapy in improving local control. ANZ J Surg **78**, 273–276 (2008)

25. Fuhrmann, D., Lippold, A., Borrosch, F., Ellwanger, U., Garbe, C., Suter, L.: Should adjuvant radiotherapy be recommended following resection of regional lymph node metastases of malignant melanomas? Br J Dermatol **144**, 66–70 (2001)

26. Geara, F.B., Ang, K.K.: Radiation therapy for malignant melanoma. Surg Clin North Am **76**, 1383–1398 (1996)

27. Golden, D.W., Lamborn, K.R., McDermott, M.W., Kunwar, S., Wara, W.M., Nakamura, J.L., Sneed, P.K.: Prognostic factors and grading systems for overall survival in patients treated with radiosurgery for brain metastases: variation by primary site. J Neurosurg **109**(suppl), 77–86 (2008)

28. Harwood, A.R.: Conventional fractionated radiotherapy for 51 patients with lentigo maligna and lentigo maligna melanoma. Int J Radiat Oncol Biol Phys **9**, 1019–1021 (1983)

29. Harwood, A.R.: Radiotherapy of acral lentiginous melanoma of the foot. J La State Med Soc **151**(7), 373–376 (1999)

30. Harwood, A.R., Lawson, V.G.: Radiation therapy for melanomas of the head and neck. Head Neck Surg **4**(6), 468–474 (1982)

31. Harwood, A.R., Dancuart, F., Fitzpatrick, P.J., Brown, T.: Radiotherapy in nonlentiginous melanoma of the head and neck. Cancer **48**, 2599–2605 (1981)

32. Herbert, S.H., Solin, L.J., Rate, W.R., Schultz, D.J., Hanks, G.E.: The effect of palliative radiation therapy on epidural compression due to metastatic malignant melanoma. Cancer **67**, 2472–2476 (1991)

33. Lagerwaard, F.J., Levendag, P.C., Nowak, P.J., Eijkenboom, W.M., Hanssens, P.E., Schmitz, P.I.: Identification of prognostic factors in patients with brain metastases: a review of 1292 patients. Int J Radiat Oncol Biol Phys **43**, 795–803 (1999)

34. Lee, R.J., Gibbs, J.F., Proulx, G.M., Kollmorgen, D.R., Jia, C., Kraybill, W.G.: Nodal basin recurrence following lymph node dissection for melanoma: implications for adjuvant radiotherapy. Int J Radiat Oncol Biol Phys **46**, 467–474 (2000)

35. Miescher, G.: Erfolge der Karzinombehandlung an der dermatologischen Klinik Zürich. Einzeitige Höchstdosis und fraktionierte Behandlung. Strahlentherapie **49**, 65–81 (1934)

36. Moncrieff, M.D., Martin, R., O'Brien, C.J., Shannon, K.F., Clark, J.R., Gao, K., McCarthy, W.M., Thompson, J.F.: Adjuvant postoperative radiotherapy to the cervical lymph nodes in cutaneous melanoma: is there any benefit for high-risk patients? Ann Surg Oncol **15**, 3022–3027 (2008)

37. Morris, K.T., Marquez, C.M., Holland, J.M., Vetto, J.T.: Prevention of local recurrence after surgical debulking of nodal and subcutaneous melanoma deposits by hypofractionated radiation. Ann Surg Oncol **7**, 680–684 (2000)

38. Newlin, H.E., Morris, C.G., Amdur, R.J., Mendenhall, W.M.: Neurotropic melanoma of the head and neck with clinical perineural invasion. Am J Clin Oncol **28**, 399–402 (2005)

39. O'Brien, C.J., Petersen-Schaefer, K., Stevens, G.N., Bass, P.C., Tew, P., Gebski, V.J., Thompson, J.F., McCarthy, W.H.: Adjuvant radiotherapy following neck dissection and parotidectomy for metastatic malignant melanoma. Head Neck **19**, 589–594 (1997)

40. Overgaard, J., Overgaard, M.: Hyperthermia as an adjuvant to radiotherapy in the treatment of malignant melanoma. Int J Hyperthermia **3**, 483–501 (1987)

41. Overgaard, J., von der Maase, H., Overgaard, M.: A randomized study comparing two high-dose per fraction radiation schedules in recurrent or metastatic malignant melanoma. Int J Radiat Oncol Biol Phys **11**, 1837–1839 (1985)

42. Overgaard, J., Gonzalez Gonzalez, D., Hulshof, M.C., Arcangeli, G., Dahl, O., Mella, O., Bentzen, S.M.: Hyperthermia as an adjuvant to radiation therapy of recurrent or metastatic malignant melanoma. A multicentre randomized trial by the European Society for Hyperthermic Oncology. Int J Hyperthermia **12**, 3–20 (1996)

43. Rate, W.R., Solin, L.J., Turrisi, A.T.: Palliative radiotherapy for metastatic malignant melanoma: brain metastases, bone metastases, and spinal cord compression. Int J Radiat Oncol Biol Phys **15**, 859–864 (1988)

44. Richtig, E., Hoff, M., Rehak, P., Kapp, K., Hofmann-Wellenhof, R., Zalaudek, I., Poschauko, J., Uggowitzer, M., Kohek, P., Smolle, J.: Efficacy of superficial and deep regional hyperthermia combined with systemic chemotherapy and radiotherapy in metastatic melanoma. Dtsch Dermatol Ges **1**, 635–642 (2003)

45. Sampson, J.H., Carter Jr., J.H., Friedman, A.H., Seigler, H.F.: Demographics, prognosis, and therapy in 702 patients with brain metastases from malignant melanoma. J Neurosurg **88**, 11–20 (1998)

46. Sause, W.T., Cooper, J.S., Rush, S., Ago, C.T., Cosmatos, D., Coughlin, C.T., JanJan, N., Lipsett, J.: Fraction size in external beam radiation therapy in the treatment of melanoma. Int J Radiat Oncol Biol Phys **20**, 429–432 (1991)

47. Schmid-Wendtner, M.H., Brunner, B., Konz, B., Kaudewitz, P., Wendtner, C.M., Peter, R.U., Plewig, G., Volkenandt, M.: Fractionated radiotherapy of lentigo maligna and lentigo maligna melanoma in 64 patients. J Am Acad Dermatol **43**, 477–482 (2000)

48. Seegenschmiedt, M.H., Keilholz, L., Altendorf-Hofmann, A., Urban, A., Schell, H., Hohenberger, W., Sauer, R.: Palliative radiotherapy for recurrent and metastatic malignant melanoma:

prognostic factors for tumor response and long-term outcome: a 20-year experience. Int J Radiat Oncol Biol Phys **44**(3), 607–618 (1999)

49. Shidnia, H., Hornback, N.B., Shen, R.N., Shupe, R.E., Yune, M.: An overview of the role of radiation therapy and hyperthermia in treatment of malignant melanoma. Adv Exp Med Biol **267**, 531–545 (1990)

50. Stevens, G., Thompson, J.F., Firth, I., O'Brien, C.J., McCarthy, W.H., Quinn, M.J.: Locally advanced melanoma: results of postoperative hypofractionated radiation therapy. Cancer **88**, 88–94 (2000)

51. Stevens, G., McKay, M.J.: Dispelling the myths surrounding radiotherapy for treatment of cutaneous melanoma. Lancet Oncol **7**(7), 575–583 (2006)

52. Tsang, R.W., Liu, F.F., Wells, W., Payne DG, L.: Lentigo maligna of the head and neck. Results of treatment by radiotherapy. Arch Dermatol **130**, 1008–1012 (1994)

53. Tsao, M.N., Lloyd, N.S., Wong, R.K., Rakovitch, E., Chow, E., Laperriere, N., Supportive Care Guidelines Group of Cancer Care Ontario's Program in Evidence-based Care: Radiotherapeutic management of brain metastases: a systematic review and meta-analysis. Cancer Treat Rev **31**, 256–273 (2005)

54. von Essen, C.: Skin and lip. In: Fletcher, G.H. (ed.) Textbook of Radiotherapy, 3rd edn, pp. 271–285. Lea and Feibiger, Philadelphia (1980)

55. Vongtama, R., Safa, A., Gallardo, D., Calcaterra, T., Juillard, G.: Efficacy of radiation therapy in the local control of desmoplastic malignant melanoma. Head Neck **25**, 423–428 (2003)

Drug Therapy

1. Oblimersen: Augmerosen, BCL-2 antisense oligonucleotide – Genta, G 3139, GC 3139, oblimersen sodium. Drugs R. D. **8**, 321–334 (2007)

2. Amaravadi, R., Schuchter, L., McDermott, E.M.W., Kramer, A., Giles, L., Troxel, A.B., Medina, C.A., Nathanson, K.L., O'Dwyer, P.J., Flaherty, K.T.: Updated results of a randomized phase II study comparing two schedules of temozolomide in combination with sorafenib in patients with advanced melanoma. J. Clin. Oncol. **25**, ASCO Annual Meeting Proceedings Part I-Abstract No: 8527 (2007)

3. Atkins, M.B., Hsu, J., Lee, S., Cohen, G.I., Flaherty, L.E., Sosman, J.A., Sondak, V.K., Kirkwood, J.M.: Phase III trial comparing concurrent biochemotherapy with cisplatin, vinblastine, dacarbazine, interleukin-2, and interferon alfa-2b with cisplatin, vinblastine, and dacarbazine alone in patients with metastatic malignant melanoma (E3695): a trial coordinated by the Eastern Cooperative Oncology Group. J Clin Oncol **26**, 5748–5754 (2008)

4. Atkins, M.B., Lotze, M.T., Dutcher, J.P., Fisher, R.I., Weiss, G., Margolin, K., Abrams, J., Sznol, M., Parkinson, D., Hawkins, M., Paradise, C., Kunkel, L., Rosenberg, S.A.: High-dose recombinant interleukin 2 therapy for patients with metastatic melanoma: analysis of 270 patients treated between 1985 and 1993. J Clin Oncol **17**, 2105–2116 (1999)

5. Atkins, M.B.: Cytokine-based therapy and biochemotherapy for advanced melanoma. Clin Cancer Res **12**, 2353s–2358s (2006)

6. Attia, P., Phan, G.Q., Maker, A.V., Robinson, M.R., Quezado, M.M., Yang, J.C., Sherry, R.M., Topalian, S.L., Kammula, U.S., Royal, R.E., Restifo, N.P., Haworth, L.R., Levy, C., Mavroukakis, S.A., Nichol, G., Yellin, M.J., Rosenberg, S.A.: Autoimmunity correlates with tumor regression in patients with metastatic melanoma treated with anti-cytotoxic T-lymphocyte antigen-4. J Clin Oncol **23**, 6043–6053 (2005)

7. Avril, M.F., Aamdal, S., Grob, J.J., Hauschild, A., Mohr, P., Bonerandi, J.J., Weichenthal, M., Neuber, K., Bieber, T., Gilde, K., Guillem Porta, V., Fra, J., Bonneterre, J., Saïag, P., Kamanabrou, D., Pehamberger, H., Sufliarsky, J., Gonzalez Larriba, J.L., Scherrer, A., Menu, Y.: Fotemustine compared with dacarbazine in patients with disseminated malignant melanoma: a phase III study. J Clin Oncol **22**, 1118–1125 (2004)

8. Bajetta, E., Di Leo, A., Zampino, M.G., Sertoli, M.R., Comella, G., Barduagni, M., Giannotti, B., Queirolo, P., Tribbia, G., Bernengo, M.G.: Multicenter randomized trial of dacarbazine alone or in combination with two different doses and schedules of interferon alfa-2a in the treatment of advanced melanoma. J Clin Oncol **12**, 806–811 (1994)

9. Bedikian, A.Y., Millward, M., Pehamberger, H., Conry, R., Gore, M., Trefzer, U., Pavlick, A.C., DeConti, R., Hersh, E.M., Hersey, P., Kirkwood, J.M., Haluska, F.G.: Bcl-2 antisense (oblimersen sodium) plus dacarbazine in patients with advanced melanoma: the Oblimersen Melanoma Study Group. J Clin Oncol **24**, 4738–4745 (2006)

10. Bleehen, N.M., Newlands, E.S., Lee, S.M., Thatcher, N., Selby, P., Calvert, A.H., Rustin, G.J., Brampton, M., Stevens, M.F.: Cancer Research Campaign phase II trial of temozolomide in metastatic melanoma. J Clin Oncol **13**, 910–913 (1995)

11. Bong, A.B., Bonnekoh, B., Franke, I., Schon, M.P., Ulrich, J., Gollnick, H.: Imiquimod, a topical immune response modifier, in the treatment of cutaneous metastases of malignant melanoma. Dermatology **205**, 135–138 (2002)

12. Cameron, D.A., Cornbleet, M.C., Mackie, R.M., Hunter, J.A., Gore, M., Hancock, B., Smyth, J.F.: Adjuvant interferon alpha 2b in high risk melanoma – the Scottish study. Br J Cancer **84**, 1146–1149 (2001)

13. Carmichael, J., Atkinson, R.J., Calman, K.C., Mackie, R.M., Naysmith, A.M., Smyth, J.F.: A multicentre phase II trial of vindesine in malignant melanoma. Eur J Cancer Clin Oncol **18**, 1293–1295 (1982)

14. Carter, R.D., Krementz, E.T., Hill, G.J., Metter, G.E., Fletcher, W.S., Golomb, F.M., Grage, T.B., Minton, J.P., Sparks, F.C.: DTIC (nsc-45388) and combination therapy for melanoma. I. Studies with DTIC, BCNU (NSC-409962), CCNU (NSC-79037), vincristine (NSC-67574), and hydroxyurea (NSC-32065). Cancer Treat Rep **60**, 601–609 (1976)

15. Cascinelli, N., Belli, F., Mackie, R.M., Santinami, M., Bufalino, R., Morabito, A.: Effect of long-term adjuvant therapy with interferon alpha-2a in patients with regional node metastases from cutaneous melanoma: a randomised trial. Lancet **358**, 866–869 (2001)

16. Chapman, P.B., Einhorn, L.H., Meyers, M.L., Saxman, S., Destro, A.N., Panageas, K.S., Begg, C.B., Agarwala, S.S., Schuchter, L.M., Ernstoff, M.S., Houghton, A.N., Kirkwood, J.M.: Phase III multicenter randomized trial of the Dartmouth regimen versus dacarbazine in patients with metastatic melanoma. J Clin Oncol **17**, 2745–2751 (1999)

17. Chiarion-Sileni, V., Nortilli, R., Aversa, S.M., Paccagnella, A., Medici, M., Corti, L., Favaretto, A.G., Cetto, G.L., Monfardini, S.: Phase II randomized study of dacarbazine, carmustine, cisplatin and tamoxifen versus dacarbazine alone in advanced melanoma patients. Melanoma Res **11**, 189–196 (2001)

18. Chiarion-Sileni, V., Del Bianco, P., Romanini, A., Guida, M., Paccagnella, A., Dalla, P.M., Naglieri, E., Ridolfi, R., Silvestri, B., Michiara, M., De Salvo, G.L.: Tolerability of intensified intravenous interferon alfa-2b versus the ECOG 1684 schedule as adjuvant therapy for stage III melanoma: a randomized phase III Italian Melanoma Inter-group trial (IMI - Mel.A.) [ISRCTN75125874]. BMC Cancer **6**, 44 (2006)

19. Cornett, W.R., McCall, L.M., Petersen, R.P., Ross, M.I., Briele, H.A., Noyes, R.D., Sussman, J.J., Kraybill, W.G., Kane, J.M.I., Alexander, H.R., Lee, J.E., Mansfield, P.F., Pingpank, J.F.,

Winchester, D.J., RLJr, W., Chadaram, V., Herndon, J.E., Fraker, D.L., Tyler, D.S.: Randomized multicenter trial of hyperthermic isolated limb perfusion with melphalan alone compared with melphalan plus tumor necrosis factor: American College of Surgeons Oncology Group Trial Z0020. J Clin Oncol **24**, 4196–4201 (2006)

20. Costanzi, J.J., Al Sarraf, M., Groppe, C., Bottomley, R., Fabian, C., Neidhart, J., Dixon, D.: Combination chemotherapy plus BCG in the treatment of disseminated malignant melanoma: a Southwest Oncology Group Study. Med Pediatr Oncol **10**, 251–258 (1982)

21. Creagan, E.T., Ahmann, D.L., Frytak, S., Long, H.J., Chang, M.N., Itri, L.M.: Three consecutive phase II studies of recombinant interferon alfa-2a in advanced malignant melanoma. Updated analyses. Cancer **59**, 638–646 (1987)

22. Creagan, E.T., Dalton, R.J., Ahmann, D.L., Jung, S.H., Morton, R.F., Langdon Jr., R.M., Kugler, J., Rodrigue, L.J.: Randomized, surgical adjuvant clinical trial of recombinant interferon alfa-2a in selected patients with malignant melanoma. J Clin Oncol **13**, 2776–2783 (1995)

23. Creagan, E.T., Suman, V.J., Dalton, R.J., Pitot, H.C., Long, H.J., Veeder, M.H., Vukov, A.M., Rowland, K.M., Krook, J.E., Michalak, J.C.: Phase III clinical trial of the combination of cisplatin, dacarbazine, and carmustine with or without tamoxifen in patients with advanced malignant melanoma. J Clin Oncol **17**, 1884–1890 (1999)

24. Davies, B.R., Logie, A., McKay, J.S., Martin, P., Steele, S., Jenkins, R., Cockerill, M., Cartlidge, S., Smith, P.D.: AZD6244 (ARRY-142886), a potent inhibitor of mitogen-activated protein kinase/extracellular signal-regulated kinase kinase 1/2 kinases: mechanism of action in vivo, pharmacokinetic/pharmacodynamic relationship, and potential for combination in preclinical models. Mol Cancer Ther **6**, 2209–2219 (2007)

25. Dorval, T., Mathiot, C., Chosidow, O., Revuz, J., Avril, M.F., Guillaume, J.C., Tursz, T., Brandely, M., Pouillart, P., Fridman, W.H.: IL-2 phase II trial in metastatic melanoma: analysis of clinical and immunological parameters. Biotechnol Ther **3**, 63–79 (1992)

26. Egerer, G., Lehnert, T., Max, R., Naeher, H., Keilholz, U., Ho, A.D.: Pilot study of hepatic intraarterial fotemustine chemotherapy for liver metastases from uveal melanoma: a single-center experience with seven patients. Int J Clin Oncol **6**, 25–28 (2001)

27. Eggermont, A., Suciu, S., Ruka, W., Mardsen, J., Testori, A., Corrie, P.G., Aamdal, S., Ascierto, P., Patel, P., Spatz, A.: EORTC 18961: Post-operative adjuvant ganglioside GM2-KLH21 vaccination treatment vs observation in stage II (T3-T4N0M0) melanoma: 2nd interim analysis led to an early disclosure of the results. J. Clin. Oncol. **26**, abstract 9004 (2008)

28. Eggermont, A.M., Kirkwood, J.M.: Re-evaluating the role of dacarbazine in metastatic melanoma: what have we learned in 30 years? Eur J Cancer **40**, 1825–1836 (2004)

29. Eggermont, A.M., Suciu, S., Santinami, M., Testori, A., Kruit, W.H., Marsden, J., Punt, C.J., Sales, F., Gore, M., Mackie, R., Kusic, Z., Dummer, R., Hauschild, A., Musat, E., Spatz, A., Keilholz, U.: Adjuvant therapy with pegylated interferon alfa-2b versus observation alone in resected stage III melanoma: final results of EORTC 18991, a randomised phase III trial. Lancet **372**, 117–126 (2008)

30. Eggermont, A.M.M., Suciu, S., MacKie, R., Ruka, W., Testori, A., Kruit, W., Punt, C.J.A., Delauney, M., Fo, S., Groenewegen, G., Ruiter, D.J., Jagiello, I., Stoitchkov, K., Keilholz, U., Lienard, D.: Post-surgery adjuvant therapy with intermediate doses of interferon alfa 2b versus observation in patients with stage IIb/III melanoma (EORTC 18952): randomised controlled trial. Lancet **366**, 1189–1196 (2005)

31. Eigentler, T.K., Caroli, U.M., Radny, P., Garbe, C.: Palliative therapy of disseminated malignant melanoma: a systematic review of 41 randomised clinical trials. Lancet Oncol **4**, 748–759 (2003)

32. Eisen, T., Ahmad, T., Flaherty, K.T., Gore, M., Kaye, S., Marais, R., Gibbens, I., Hackett, S., James, M., Schuchter, L.M., Nathanson, K.L., Xia, C., Simantov, R., Schwartz, B., Poulin-Costello, M., O'Dwyer, P.J., Ratain, M.J.: Sorafenib in advanced melanoma: a phase II randomised discontinuation trial analysis. Br J Cancer **95**, 581–586 (2006)

33. Falkson, C.I., Ibrahim, J., Kirkwood, J.M., Coates, A.S., Atkins, M.B., Blum, R.H.: Phase III trial of dacarbazine versus dacarbazine with interferon alpha-2b versus dacarbazine with tamoxifen versus dacarbazine with interferon alpha-2b and tamoxifen in patients with metastatic malignant melanoma: an Eastern Cooperative Oncology Group study. J Clin Oncol **16**, 1743–1751 (1998)

34. Faries, M.B., Morton, D.L.: Therapeutic vaccines for melanoma: current status. Biodrugs **19**, 247–260 (2005)

35. Flaherty, K.T.: Chemotherapy and targeted therapy combinations in advanced melanoma. Clin Cancer Res **12**, 2366s–2370s (2006)

36. Flaherty, K.T., Brose, M.S., Schuchter, L.M., Tuveson, D., Lee, R., Schwartz, B., Lathia, C., Weber, B.L., O'Dwyer, P.J.: Phase I/II trial of BAY 43-9006, carboplatin (C) and paclitaxel (P) demonstrates preliminary antitumor activity in the expansion cohort of patients with metastatic melanoma. J. Clin. Oncol. **22**, ASCO Annual Meeting Proceedings (Post-Meeting Edition)-Abstract No: 7507 (2004)

37. Garaci, E.: Thymosin alpha1: a historical overview. Ann N Y Acad Sci **1112**, 14–20 (2007)

38. Garbe, C., Radny, P., Linse, R., Dummer, R., Gutzmer, R., Ulrich, J., Stadler, R., Weichenthal, M., Eigentler, T., Ellwanger, U., Hauschild, A.: Adjuvant low-dose interferon {alpha}2a with or without dacarbazine compared with surgery alone: a prospective-randomized phase III DeCOG trial in melanoma patients with regional lymph node metastasis. Ann Oncol **19**, 1195–1201 (2008)

39. Garbe, C., Eigentler, T.K.: Diagnosis and treatment of cutaneous melanoma: state of the art 2006. Melanoma Res **17**, 117–127 (2007)

40. Gimbel, M.I., Delman, K.A., Zager, J.S.: Therapy for unresectable recurrent and in-transit extremity melanoma. Cancer Control **15**, 225–232 (2008)

41. Gomez-Navarro, J., Antonia, S., Sosman, J.A., Kirkwood, J.M., Redman, B., Gajewski, T.F., Pavlov, D., Bulanhagui, C.A., Ribas, A., Camacho, L.H.: Survival of patients (pts) with metastatic melanoma treated with the anti-CTLA4 monoclonal antibody (mAb) CP-675,206 in a phase I/II study. J. Clin. Oncol. **25**, ASCO Annual Meeting Proceedings Part I. Abstract No: 8524 (2007)

42. Gonzalez, R., Hutchins, L., Nemunaitis, J., Atkins, M., Schwarzenberger, P.O.: Phase 2 trial of Allovectin-7 in advanced metastatic melanoma. Melanoma Res **16**, 521–526 (2006)

43. Green, D.S., Bodman-Smith, M.D., Dalgleish, A.G., Fischer, M.D.: Phase I/II study of topical imiquimod and intralesional interleukin-2 in the treatment of accessible metastases in malignant melanoma. Br J Dermatol **156**, 337–345 (2007)

44. Grob, J.J., Dreno, B., de la Salmonière, P., Delaunay, M., Cupissol, D., Guillot, B., Souteyrand, P., Sassolas, B., Cesarini, J.P., Lionnet, S., Lok, C., Chastang, C., Bonerandi, J.J.: Randomised trial of interferon alpha-2a as adjuvant therapy in resected primary melanoma thicker than 1.5 mm without clinically detectable node metastases. French Cooperative Group on Melanoma. Lancet **351**, 1905–1910 (1998)

45. Gundersen, S.: Dacarbazine, vindesine, and cisplatin combination chemotherapy in advanced malignant melanoma: a phase II study. Cancer Treat Rep **71**, 997–999 (1987)

46. Hamid, O., Urba, W., Yellin, M., Nichol, G., Weber, J.S., Hersh, E.M., Tchekmedyian, S., Hodi, F.S., Weber, S., O'Day, S.J.: Kinetics of response to ipilimumab (MDX-010) in patients with stage III/IV melanoma. J. Clin. Oncol. **25**, ASCO annual meeting proceedings part i-abstract no: 8525 (2007)

47. Hancock, B.W., Wheatley, K., Harris, S., Ives, N., Harrison, G., Horsman, J.M., Middleton, M.R., Thatcher, N., Lorigan, P.C.,

Marsden, J.R., Burrows, L., Gore, M.: Adjuvant interferon in high-risk melanoma: the AIM HIGH Study–United Kingdom Coordinating Committee on Cancer Research randomized study of adjuvant low-dose extended-duration interferon Alfa-2a in high-risk resected malignant melanoma. J Clin Oncol 22, 53–61 (2004)

48. Hayes, A.J., Clark, M.A., Harries, M., Thomas, J.M.: Management of in-transit metastases from cutaneous malignant melanoma. Br J Surg 91, 673–682 (2004)

49. Hersey, P.: Adjuvant therapy for high-risk primary and resected metastatic melanoma. Intern Med J 33, 33–43 (2003)

50. Ives, N.J., Stowe, R.L., Lorigan, P., Wheatley, K.: Chemotherapy compared with biochemotherapy for the treatment of metastatic melanoma: a meta-analysis of 18 trials involving 2,621 patients. J Clin Oncol 25, 5426–5434 (2007)

51. Jacquillat, C., Khayat, D., Banzet, P., Weil, M., Fumoleau, P., Avril, M.F., Namer, M., Bonneterre, J., Kerbrat, P., Bonerandi, J.J.: Final report of the French multicenter phase II study of the nitrosourea fotemustine in 153 evaluable patients with disseminated malignant melanoma including patients with cerebral metastases. Cancer 66, 1873–1878 (1990)

52. Jones, E.L., Oleson, J.R., Prosnitz, L.R., Samulski, T.V., Vujaskovic, Z., Yu, D., Sanders, L.L., Dewhirst, M.W.: Randomized trial of hyperthermia and radiation for superficial tumors. J Clin Oncol 23, 3079–3085 (2005)

53. Jungnelius, U., Ringborg, U., Aamdal, S., Mattsson, J., Stierner, U., Ingvar, C., Malmstrom, P., Andersson, R., Karlsson, M., Willman, K., Wist, E., Bjelkengren, G., Westberg, R.: Dacarbazine-vindesine versus dacarbazine-vindesine-cisplatin in disseminated malignant melanoma. A randomised phase III trial. Eur J Cancer 34, 1368–1374 (1998)

54. Kamin, A., Eigentler, T.K., Radny, P., Bauer, J., Weide, B., Garbe, C.: Imiquimod in the treatment of extensive recurrent lentigo maligna. J Am Acad Dermatol 52, 51–52 (2005)

55. Kaufmann, R., Spieth, K., Leiter, U., Mauch, C., von den, D.P., Vogt, T., Linse, R., Tilgen, W., Schadendorf, D., Becker, J.C., Sebastian, G., Krengel, S., Kretschmer, L., Garbe, C., Dummer, R.: Temozolomide in combination with interferon-alfa versus temozolomide alone in patients with advanced metastatic melanoma: a randomized, phase III, multicenter study from the Dermatologic Cooperative Oncology Group. J Clin Oncol 23, 9001–9007 (2005)

56. Kavanagh, D., Hill, A.D.K., Djikstra, B., Kennelly, R., McDermott, E.M.W., O'Higgins, N.J.: Adjuvant therapies in the treatment of stage II and III malignant melanoma. Surgeon 3, 245–256 (2005)

57. Keilholz, U., Stoter, G., Punt, C.J., Scheibenbogen, C., Lejeune, F., Eggermont, A.M.: Recombinant interleukin-2-based treatments for advanced melanoma: the experience of the European Organization for Research and Treatment of Cancer Melanoma Cooperative Group. Cancer J Sci Am 3(suppl 1), S22–S28 (1997)

58. Keilholz, U., Punt, C.J.A., Gore, M., Kruit, W., Patel, P., Lienard, D., Thomas, J., Proebstle, T.M., Schmittel, A., Schadendorf, D., Velu, T., Negrier, S., Kleeberg, U., Lehman, F., Suciu, S., Eggermont, A.M.M.: Dacarbazine, cisplatin, and interferon-alfa-2b with or without interleukin-2 in metastatic melanoma: a randomized phase III trial (18951) of the European Organisation for Research and Treatment of Cancer Melanoma Group. J Clin Oncol 23, 6747–6755 (2005)

59. Kim, C.J., Dessureault, S., Gabrilovich, D., Reintgen, D.S., Slingluff, C.L.: Immunotherapy for melanoma. Cancer Control 9, 22–30 (2002)

60. Kim, K.B., Legha, S.S., Gonzalez, R., Anderson, C., Papadopoulos, N.E., Eton, O., Plager, C., Roe, A., Liu, P., Bedikian, A.Y.: A phase III randomized trial of adjuvant biochemotherapy (BC) versus interferon-alpha-2b (IFN) in patients (pts) with high risk for melanoma recurrence. J. Clin. Oncol. 24, 8003 (2006)

61. Kirkwood, J.M., Ibrahim, J.G., Sondak, V.K., Richards, J., Flaherty, L.E., Ernstoff, M.S., Smith, T.J., Rao, U., Steele, M., Blum, R.H.: High- and low-dose interferon alfa-2b in high-risk melanoma: first analysis of intergroup trial E1690/S9111/C9190. J Clin Oncol 18, 2444–2458 (2000)

62. Kirkwood, J.M., Ibrahim, J.G., Sosman, J.A., Sondak, V.K., Agarwala, S.S., Ernstoff, M.S., Rao, U.: High-dose interferon alfa-2b significantly prolongs relapse-free and overall survival compared with the GM2-KLH/QS-21 vaccine in patients with resected stage IIB-III melanoma: results of intergroup trial E1694/S9512/C509801. J Clin Oncol 19, 2370–2380 (2001)

63. Kirkwood, J.M., Strawderman, M.H., Ernstoff, M.S., Smith, T.J., Borden, E.C., Blum, R.H.: Interferon alfa-2b adjuvant therapy of high-risk resected cutaneous melanoma: the Eastern Cooperative Oncology Group Trial EST 1684. J Clin Oncol 14, 7–17 (1996)

64. Kirkwood, J.M., Bender, C., Agarwala, S., Tarhini, A., Shipe-Spotloe, J., Smelko, B., Donnelly, S., Stover, L.: Mechanisms and management of toxicities associated with high-dose interferon alfa-2b therapy. J Clin Oncol 20, 3703–3718 (2002)

65. Knutson, K.L.: GMK (Progenics Pharmaceuticals). Curr Opin Investig Drugs 3, 159–164 (2002)

66. Legha, S.S., Gianan, M.A., Plager, C., Eton, O.E., Papadopoulous, N.E.: Evaluation of interleukin-2 administered by continuous infusion in patients with metastatic melanoma. Cancer 77, 89–96 (1996)

67. Lens, M.B., Dawes, M.: Interferon alfa therapy for malignant melanoma: a systematic review of randomized controlled trials. J Clin Oncol 20, 1818–1825 (2002)

68. Lens, M.B., Eisen, T.G.: Systemic chemotherapy in the treatment of malignant melanoma. Expert Opin Pharmacother 4, 2205–2211 (2003)

69. Leyvraz, S., Spataro, V., Bauer, J., Pampallona, S., Salmon, R., Dorval, T., Meuli, R., Gillet, M., Lejeune, F., Zografos, L.: Treatment of ocular melanoma metastatic to the liver by hepatic arterial chemotherapy. J Clin Oncol 15, 2589–2595 (1997)

70. Malek-Mansour, S.: Remission of melanoma with D.N.C.B. treatment. Lancet 2, 503–504 (1973)

71. McClay, E.F., Mastrangelo, M.J., Bellet, R.E., Berd, D.: Combination chemotherapy and hormonal therapy in the treatment of malignant melanoma. Cancer Treat Rep 71, 465–469 (1987)

72. McDermott, E.M.W., Sosman, J.A., Hodi, F.S., Gonzalez, R., Linette, G., Richards, J., Jakub, J.K., Beerem, M., Patel, K., Kramner, C.: Randomized phase II study of dacarbazine with or without sorafenib in patients with advanced melanoma. J. Clin. Oncol. 25, ASCO Annual Meeting Proceedings Part I-Abstract No: 8511 (2007)

73. Middleton, M.R., Grob, J.J., Aaronson, N., Fierlbeck, G., Tilgen, W., Seiter, S., Gore, M., Aamdal, S., Cebon, J., Coates, A., Dreno, B., Henz, M., Schadendorf, D., Kapp, A., Weiss, J., Fraass, U., Statkevich, P., Muller, M., Thatcher, N.: Randomized phase III study of temozolomide versus dacarbazine in the treatment of patients with advanced metastatic malignant melanoma. J Clin Oncol 18, 158–166 (2000)

74. Miller, R.L., Steis, R.G., Clark, J.W., Smith, J.W., Crum, E., McKnight, J.E., Hawkins, M.J., Jones, M.J., Longo, D.L., Urba, W.J.: Randomized trial of recombinant alpha 2b-interferon with or without indomethacin in patients with metastatic malignant melanoma. Cancer Res 49, 1871–1876 (1989)

75. Millward, M., Bedikian, A.Y., Conry, R,. Gore, M., Pehamberger, H., Sterry, W., Pavlick, A., De Conti, R., Gordon, D., Itri, L.M.: Randomized multinational phase 3 trial of dacarbazine (DTIC) with or without Bcl-2 antisense (oblimersen sodium) in patients (pts) with advanced malignant melanoma (MM): Analysis of long-term survival. J. Clin. Oncol. 22, ASCO Annual Meeting Proceedings (Post-Meeting Edition)-Abstract No: 7505 (2004)

76. Mornex, F., Thomas, L., Mohr, P., Hauschild, A., Delaunay, M.M., Lesimple, T., Tilgen, W., Bui, B.N., Guillot, B., Ulrich, J., Bourdin, S., Mousseau, M., Cupissol, D., Bonneterre, M.E., De Gislain, C., Bensadoun, R.J., Clavel, M.: A prospective randomized multicentre phase III trial of fotemustine plus whole brain irradiation versus

fotemustine alone in cerebral metastases of malignant melanoma. Melanoma Res **13**, 97–103 (2003)

77. Morton, D., Mozzillo, N., Thompson, J.A., Kelly, M., Faries, M., Wagner, J., Schneebaum, S., Schuchter, L., Gammon, G., Elashoff, R.: An international, randomized, phase III trial of bacillus Calmette-Guerin (BCG) plus allogeneic melanoma vaccine (MCV) or placebo after complete resection of melanoma metastatic to regional or distant sites. J. Clin. Oncol. **25**, ASCO Annual Meeting Proceedings Part I-Abstract No: 8508 (2007)

78. Naylor, M.F., Crowson, N., Kuwahara, R., Teague, K., Garcia, C., Mackinnis, C., Haque, R., Odom, C., Jankey, C., Cornelison, R.L.: Treatment of lentigo maligna with topical imiquimod. Br J Dermatol **149**, 66–70 (2003)

79. Neefe, J.R., Legha, S.S., Markowitz, A., Salmon, S., Meyskens, F., Groopman, J., Campion, M., Evans, L.: Phase II study of recombinant alpha-interferon in malignant melanoma. Am J Clin Oncol **13**, 472–476 (1990)

80. Nelimark, R.A., Peterson, B.A., Vosika, G.J., Conroy, J.A.: Vindesine for metastatic malignant melanoma. A phase II trial. Am J Clin Oncol **6**, 561–564 (1983)

81. O'Day, S.J., Hamid, O., Urba, W.J.: Targeting cytotoxic T-lymphocyte antigen-4 (CTLA-4): a novel strategy for the treatment of melanoma and other malignancies. Cancer **110**, 2614–2627 (2007)

82. O'Day, S.J., Gonzalez, R., Lawson, L., Weber, R., Hutchins, L., Anderson, C., McLeod, M., Hurwitz, C., Haddad, J., Jacobson, E.: Subgroup analysis of efficacy and safety analysis of a randomized, double-blinded controlled phase II study of STA-4783 in combination with paclitaxel in patients with metastatic melanoma. J. Clin. Oncol. **25**, ASCO Annual Meeting Proceedings Part I-Abstract No: 8528 (2007)

83. Pectasides, D., Alevizakos, N., Bafaloukos, D., Tzonou, A., Asimakopoulos, G., Varthalitis, I., Dimitriadis, M., Athanassiou, A.: Adjuvant chemotherapy with dacarbazine, vindesine, and cisplatin in pathological stage II malignant melanoma. Am J Clin Oncol **17**, 55–59 (1994)

84. Pehamberger, H., Soyer, H.P., Steiner, A., Kofler, R., Binder, M., Mischer, P., Pachinger, W., Aubock, J., Fritsch, P., Kerl, H., Wolff, K.: Adjuvant interferon alfa-2a treatment in resected primary stage II cutaneous melanoma. Austrian Malignant Melanoma Cooperative Group. J Clin Oncol **16**, 1425–1429 (1998)

85. Pföhler, C., Cree, I.A., Ugurel, S., Kuwert, C., Haass, N., Neuber, K., Hengge, U., Corrie, P.G., Zutt, M., Tilgen, W., Reinhold, U.: Treosulfan and gemcitabine in metastatic uveal melanoma patients: results of a multicenter feasibility study. Anticancer Drugs **14**, 337–340 (2003)

86. Powell, A.M., Russell-Jones, R., Barlow, R.J.: Topical imiquimod immunotherapy in the management of lentigo maligna. Clin Exp Dermatol **29**, 15–21 (2004)

87. Prins, R.M., Craft, N., Bruhn, K.W., Khan-Farooqi, H., Koya, R.C., Stripecke, R., Miller, J.F., Liau, L.M.: The TLR-7 agonist, imiquimod, enhances dendritic cell survival and promotes tumor antigen-specific T cell priming: relation to central nervous system antitumor immunity. J Immunol **176**, 157–164 (2006)

88. Quaglino, P., Mortera, C., Osella-Abate, S., Barberis, M., Illengo, M., Rissone, M., Savoia, P., Bernengo, M.G.: Electrochemotherapy with intravenous bleomycin in the local treatment of skin melanoma metastases. Ann Surg Oncol **15**, 2215–2222 (2008)

89. Radny, P., Caroli, U.M., Bauer, J., Paul, T., Schlegel, C., Eigentler, T.K., Weide, B., Schwarz, M., Garbe, C.: Phase II trial of intralesional therapy with interleukin-2 in soft-tissue melanoma metastases. Br J Cancer **89**, 1620–1626 (2003)

90. Rao, R.D., Holtan, S.G., Ingle, J.N., Croghan, G.A., Kottschade, L.A., Creagan, E.T., Kaur, J.S., Pitot, H.C., Markovic, S.N.: Combination of paclitaxel and carboplatin as second-line therapy for patients with metastatic melanoma. Cancer **106**, 375–382 (2006)

91. Rasi, G., Terzoli, E., Izzo, F., Pierimarchi, P., Ranuzzi, M., Sinibaldi-Vallebona, P., Tuthill, C., Garaci, E.: Combined treatment with thymosin-alpha1 and low dose interferon-alpha after dacarbazine in advanced melanoma. Melanoma Res **10**, 189–192 (2000)

92. Ribas, A.: Update on immunotherapy for melanoma. J Natl Compr Canc Netw **4**, 687–694 (2006)

93. Ribas, A., Antonia, S., Sosman, J.A., Kirkwood, J.M., Redman, B., Gajewski, T.F., Pavlov, D., Bulanhagui, C.A., Gomez-Navarro, J., Camacho, L.H.: Results of a phase II clinical trial of 2 doses and schedules of CP-675,206, an anti-CTLA4 monoclonal antibody, in patients (pts) with advanced melanoma. J. Clin. Oncol. **25**, ASCO Annual Meeting Proceedings Part I-Abstract No: 3000 (2007)

94. Ribas, A., Hanson, D.C., Noe, D.A., Millham, R., Guyot, D.J., Bernstein, S.H., Canniff, P.C., Sharma, A., Gomez-Navarro, J.: Tremelimumab (CP-675, 206), a cytotoxic T lymphocyte associated antigen 4 blocking monoclonal antibody in clinical development for patients with cancer. Oncologist **12**, 873–883 (2007)

95. Ringborg, U., Rudenstam, C.M., Hansson, J., Hafstrom, L., Stenstam, B., Strander, H.: Dacarbazine versus dacarbazine-vindesine in disseminated malignant melanoma: a randomized phase II study. Med Oncol Tumor Pharmacother **6**, 285–289 (1989)

96. Robinson, W.A., Mughal, T.I., Thomas, M.R., Johnson, M., Spiegel, R.J.: Treatment of metastatic malignant melanoma with recombinant interferon alpha 2. Immunobiology **172**, 275–282 (1986)

97. Satyamoorthy, K., Li, G., Gerrero, M.R., Brose, M.S., Volpe, P., Weber, B.L., Van Belle, P., Elder, D.E., Herlyn, M.: Constitutive mitogen-activated protein kinase activation in melanoma is mediated by both BRAF mutations and autocrine growth factor stimulation. Cancer Res **63**, 756–759 (2003)

98. Schadendorf, D., Ugurel, S., Schuler-Thurner, B., Nestle, F.O., Enk, A., Bröcker, E.B., Grabbe, S., Rittgen, W., Edler, L., Sucker, A., Zimpfer-Rechner, C., Berger, T., Kamarashev, J., Burg, G., Jonuleit, H., Tuttenberg, A., Becker, J.C., Keikavoussi, P., Kämpgen, E., Schuler, G.: Dacarbazine (DTIC) versus vaccination with autologous peptide-pulsed dendritic cells (DC) in first-line treatment of patients with metastatic melanoma: a randomized phase III trial of the DC study group of the DeCOG. Ann Oncol **17**, 563–570 (2006)

99. Seegenschmiedt, M.H., Keilholz, L., Altendorf-Hofmann, A., Urban, A., Schell, H., Hohenberger, W., Sauer, R.: Palliative radiotherapy for recurrent and metastatic malignant melanoma: prognostic factors for tumor response and long-term outcome: a 20-year experience. Int J Radiat Oncol Biol Phys **44**, 607–618 (1999)

100. Seigler, H.F., Lucas Jr., V.S., Pickett, N.J., Huang, A.T.: DTIC, CCNU, bleomycin and vincristine (BOLD) in metastatic melanoma. Cancer **46**, 2346–2348 (1980)

101. Senzer, N.N., Kaufman, H.L., Amatruda, T.T., Nemunaitis, M., Reid, T.R., Love, C., Marshall, T., Goldsweig, H., Coffin, R.S., Nemunaitis, J.: Phase II clinical trial with a second generation, GM-CSF encoding, oncolytic herpesvirus in unresectable metastatic melanoma. J. Clin. Oncol. **26**(suppl), Abstract No: 9008 (2008)

102. Siegel, R., Hauschild, A., Kettelhack, C., Kahler, K.C., Bembenek, A., Schlag, P.M.: Hepatic arterial Fotemustine chemotherapy in patients with liver metastases from cutaneous melanoma is as effective as in ocular melanoma. Eur J Surg Oncol **33**, 627–632 (2007)

103. Smith, K.A., Green, J.A., Eccles, J.M.: Interferon alpha 2a and vindesine in the treatment of advanced malignant melanoma. Eur J Cancer **28**, 438–441 (1992)

104. Sondak, V.K.: Adjuvant therapy for melanoma. Cancer J **7**(suppl 1), S24–S27 (2001)

105. Stadler, R., Luger, T., Bieber, T., Köhler, U., Linse, R., Technau, K., Schubert, R., Schroth, K., Vakilzadeh, F., Volkenandt, M., Gollnick, H., Von Eick, H., Thoren, F., Strannegård, O.: Long-term

survival benefit after adjuvant treatment of cutaneous melanoma with dacarbazine and low dose natural interferon alpha: A controlled, randomised multicentre trial. Acta Oncol **45**, 389–399 (2006)

106. Tarhini, A.A., Kirkwood, J.M.: Oblimersen in the treatment of metastatic melanoma. Future Oncol **3**, 263–271 (2007)

107. Terheyden, P., Kortum, A.K., Schulze, H.J., Durani, B., Remling, R., Mauch, C., Junghans, V., Schadendorf, D., Beiteke, U., Junger, M., Becker, J.C., Bröcker, E.B.: Chemoimmunotherapy for cutaneous melanoma with dacarbazine and epifocal contact sensitizers: results of a nationwide survey of the German Dermatologic Co-operative Oncology Group. J Cancer Res Clin Oncol **133**, 437–444 (2007)

108. Thompson, J.F., Kam, P.C., Waugh, R.C., Harman, C.R.: Isolated limb infusion with cytotoxic agents: a simple alternative to isolated limb perfusion. Semin Surg Oncol **14**, 238–247 (1998)

109. Verschraegen, C.F., Kleeberg, U.R., Mulder, J., Rumke, P., Truchetet, F., Czarnetzki, B., Rozencweig, M., Thomas, D., Suciu, S.: Combination of cisplatin, vindesine, and dacarbazine in advanced malignant melanoma. A Phase II Study of the EORTC Malignant Melanoma Cooperative Group. Cancer **62**, 1061–1065 (1988)

110. Wack, C., Kirst, A., Becker, J.C., Lutz, W.K., Brocker, E.B., Fischer, W.H.: Chemoimmunotherapy for melanoma with dacarbazine and 2, 4-dinitrochlorobenzene elicits a specific T cell-dependent immune response. Cancer Immunol Immunother **51**, 431–439 (2002)

111. Weber, J.S., Hersh, E.M., Yellin, M., Nichol, G., Urba, W., Powderly, W., O'Day, S.J.: The efficacy and safety of ipilimumab (MDX-010) in patients with unresectable stage III or stage IV malignant melanoma. J. Clin. Oncol. **25**, ASCO Annual Meeting Proceedings Part I-Abstract No: 8523 (2007)

112. Wheatley, K., Ives, N., Eggermont, A.: Interferon-alpha as adjuvant therapy for melanoma: An individual patient data meta-analysis of randomised trials. J. Clin. Oncol. **25**, ASCO Annual Meeting Proceedings Part I-Abstract No: 8526 (2007)

113. Wheatley, K., Ives, N., Hancock, B., Gore, M., Eggermont, A., Suciu, S.: Does adjuvant interferon-alpha for high-risk melanoma provide a worthwhile benefit? A meta-analysis of the randomised trials. Cancer Treat Rev **29**, 241–252 (2003)

114. Wolf, I.H., Richtig, E., Kopera, D., Kerl, H.: Locoregional cutaneous metastases of malignant melanoma and their management. Dermatol Surg **30**, 244–247 (2004)

115. Wolf, I.H., Smolle, J., Binder, B., Cerroni, L., Richtig, E., Kerl, H.: Topical imiquimod in the treatment of metastatic melanoma to skin. Arch Dermatol **139**, 273–276 (2003)

116. York, R.M., Foltz, A.T.: Bleomycin, vincristine, lomustine, and DTIC chemotherapy for metastatic melanoma. Cancer **61**, 2183–2186 (1988)

117. Young, A.M., Marsden, J., Goodman, A., Burton, A., Dunn, J.A.: Prospective randomized comparison of dacarbazine (DTIC) versus DTIC plus interferon-alpha (IFN-alpha) in metastatic melanoma. Clin Oncol (R Coll Radiol) **13**, 458–465 (2001)

118. Zarour, H.M., Kirkwood, J.M.: Melanoma vaccines: early progress and future promises. Semin Cutan Med Surg **22**, 68–75 (2003)

Adjuvant Immunotherapy in Melanoma: Pegylated Interferons: A New Perspective

1. Isaacs, A., Lindenmann, J.: Virus Interference. I The interferon. Proc R Soc London Ser B **147**, 258 (1957)

2. Kerr, I.M., Stark, G.R.: The antiviral effects of the interferons and their inhibition. J Interferon Res **12**, 237–240 (1992)

3. Samuel, C.E.: Antiviral actions of interferons. Clin Microbiol Rev **14**, 778–809 (2001)

4. Sen, G.C., Lengyel, P.: The interferon system. A bird's eye view of its biochemistry. J Biol Chem **267**, 5017–5020 (1992)

5. Nathan, C.: Interferon and inflammation. In: Gallin, J.I., Goldstein, I.M., Schnyder, R. (eds.) Inflammation: Basic Principles and Clinical Correlates, pp. 265–290. Raven, New York (1992)

6. Beattie, E., Tartaglia, J.: PaolettiE: Vaccinia virus-encoded elF-2a homolog abbrogates the anitiviral effect of interferon. Virology **183**, 419–422 (1991)

7. Bandyopadhyay, S., Perussia, B., Trinchieri, G., et al.: Requirement for HLA-DR+ accessory cells in natural killing of cytomegalovirus-infected fibroblasts. J Exp Med **164**, 180–195 (1986)

8. Siegal, F.P., Kadowaki, N., Shodell, M., et al.: The nature of the principal type 1 interferon-producing cells in human blood. Science **284**, 1835–1837 (1999)

9. Cella, M., Jarrossay, D., Facchetti, F., et al.: Plasmacytoid monocytes migrate to inflamed lymph nodes and produce large amounts of type I interferon. Nat Med **5**, 919–923 (1999)

10. Colonna, M., Trinchieri, G., Liu, Y.J.: Plasmacytoid dendritic cells in immunity. Nat Immunol **5**, 1219–1226 (2004)

11. McKenna, K., Beignon, A.S., Bhardwaj, N.: Plasmacytoid dendritic cells: linking innate and adaptive immunity. J Virol **79**, 17–27 (2005)

12. Iwasaki, A., Medzhitov, R.: Toll-like receptor control of the adaptive immune responses. Nat Immunol **5**, 987–995 (2004)

13. Bell, D., Chomarat, P., Broyles, D., et al.: In breast carcinoma tissue, immature dendritic cells reside within the tumor, whereas mature dendritic cells are located in peritumoral areas. J Exp Med **190**, 1417–1426 (1999)

14. Vermi, W., Bonecchi, R., Facchetti, F., et al.: Recruitment of immature plasmacytoid dendritic cells (plasmacytoid monocytes) and myeloid dendritic cells in primary cutaneous melanomas. J Pathol **200**, 255–268 (2003)

15. Liu, C., Lou, Y., Lizee, G., et al.: Plasmacytoid dendritic cells induce NK cell-dependent, tumor antigen-specific T cell cross-priming and tumor regression in mice. J Clin Invest **118**, 1165–1175 (2008)

16. Pestka, S., Langer, J.A., Zoon, K.C., et al.: Interferons and their actions. Annu Rev Biochem **56**, 727–777 (1987)

17. Kaplan, D.H., Shankaran, V., Dighe, A.S., et al.: Demonstration of an interferon gamma-dependent tumor surveillance system in immunocompetent mice. Proc Natl Acad Sci U S A **95**, 7556–7561 (1998)

18. Dunn, G.P., Bruce, A.T., Sheehan, K.C., et al.: A critical function for type I interferons in cancer immunoediting. Nat Immunol **6**, 722–729 (2005)

19. Paredes, J., Krown, S.E.: Interferon-alpha therapy in patients with Kaposi's sarcoma and the acquired immunodeficiency syndrome. Int J Immunopharmacol **13**(suppl 1), 77–81 (1991)

20. Baron, S., Tyring, S.K., Fleischmann Jr., W.R., et al.: The interferons. Mechanisms of action and clinical applications. JAMA **266**, 1375–1383 (1991)

21. Borden, E.C.: Interferons. In: Holland, J.F., Frei, I.I.I., Bast, J.R., Kufe, D.W., Morton, D.L., Wechselbaum, R.R. (eds.) Cancer Medicine, pp. 1119–1212. Lippincott Wiliams & Wilkins, Philadelphia (1997)

22. Gutterman, J.U.: Cytokine therapeutics: lessons from interferon alpha. Proc Natl Acad Sci U S A **91**, 1198–1205 (1994)

23. Buzaid, A.C., Robertone, A., Kisala, C., et al.: Phase II study of interferon alfa-2a, recombinant (Roferon-A) in metastatic renal cell carcinoma. J Clin Oncol **5**, 1083–1089 (1987)

24. Krown, S.E.: Interferon treatment of renal cell carcinoma. Current status and future prospects. Cancer **59**, 647–651 (1987)

25. Interferon nomenclature. Nature **286**, 110 (1980)

26. Platanias, L.C.: Mechanisms of type-I- and type-II-interferon-mediated signalling. Nat Rev Immunol **5**, 375–386 (2005)

27. Pestka, S.: The human interferon-alpha species and hybrid proteins. Semin Oncol **24**, S9-4–S9-17 (1997)
28. LaFleur, D.W., Nardelli, B., Tsareva, T., et al.: Interferon-kappa, a novel type I interferon expressed in human keratinocytes. J Biol Chem **276**, 39765–39771 (2001)
29. Conklin, D., Grant, F., Rixon, M., et al: Interferon-epsilon. US Patent 6329175, 2002
30. Kotenko, S.V., Gallagher, G., Baurin, V.V., et al.: IFN-lambdas mediate antiviral protection through a distinct class II cytokine receptor complex. Nat Immunol **4**, 69–77 (2003)
31. Weiss, K.: Safety profile of interferon-alpha therapy. Semin Oncol **25**, 9–13 (1998)
32. Domanski, P., Colamonici, O.R.: The type-I interferon receptor. The long and short of it. Cytokine Growth Factor Rev **7**, 143–151 (1996)
33. Pestka, S.: The human interferon alpha species and receptors. Biopolymers **55**, 254–287 (2000)
34. Schindler, C., Shuai, K., Prezioso, V.R., et al.: Interferon-dependent tyrosine phosphorylation of a latent cytoplasmic transcription factor. Science **257**, 809–813 (1992)
35. Fu, X.Y., Schindler, C., Improta, T., et al.: The proteins of ISGF-3, the interferon alpha-induced transcriptional activator, define a gene family involved in signal transduction. Proc Natl Acad Sci U S A **89**, 7840–7843 (1992)
36. Shuai, K., Schindler, C., Prezioso, V.R., et al.: Activation of transcription by IFN-gamma: tyrosine phosphorylation of a 91-kD DNA binding protein. Science **258**, 1808–1812 (1992)
37. Chen, J., Baig, E., Fish, N.E.: Diversity and relatedness among the type I interferons. J Interferon Cytokine Res **24**, 687-9-698 (2004)
38. Darnell Jr., J.E., Kerr, I.M., Stark, G.R.: Jak-STAT pathways and transcriptional activation in response to IFNs and other extracellular signaling proteins. Science **264**, 1415–1421 (1994)
39. Ihle, J.N.: The Janus protein tyrosine kinase family and its role in cytokine signaling. Adv Immunol **60**, 1–35 (1995)
40. Parmar, S., Platanias, L.C.: Interferons: mechanisms of action and clinical applications. Curr Opin Oncol **15**, 431–439 (2003)
41. Horvath, C.M., Darnell Jr., J.E.: The antiviral state induced by alpha interferon and gamma interferon requires transcriptionally active Stat1 protein. J Virol **70**, 647–650 (1996)
42. Darnell Jr., J.E.: STATs and gene regulation. Science **277**, 1630–1635 (1997)
43. Aaronson, D.S., Horvath, C.M.: A road map for those who don't know JAK-STAT. Science **296**, 1653–1655 (2002)
44. Meinke, A., Barahmand-Pour, F., Wohrl, S., et al.: Activation of different Stat5 isoforms contributes to cell-type-restricted signaling in response to interferons. Mol Cell Biol **16**, 6937–6944 (1996)
45. Farrar, J.D., Smith, J.D., Murphy, T.L., et al.: Recruitment of Stat4 to the human interferon-alpha/beta receptor requires activated Stat2. J Biol Chem **275**, 2693–2697 (2000)
46. Torpey, N., Maher, S.E., Bothwell, A.L., et al.: Interferon alpha but not interleukin 12 activates STAT4 signaling in human vascular endothelial cells. J Biol Chem **279**, 26789–26796 (2004)
47. Matikainen, S., Sareneva, T., Ronni, T., et al.: Interferon-alpha activates multiple STAT proteins and upregulates proliferation-associated IL-2Ralpha, c-myc, and pim-1 genes in human T cells. Blood **93**, 1980–1991 (1999)
48. Fasler-Kan, E., Pansky, A., Wiederkehr, M., et al.: Interferon-alpha activates signal transducers and activators of transcription 5 and 6 in Daudi cells. Eur J Biochem **254**, 514–519 (1998)
49. Uddin, S., Majchrzak, B., Woodson, J., et al.: Activation of the p38 mitogen-activated protein kinase by type I interferons. J Biol Chem **274**, 30127–30131 (1999)
50. Goh, K.C., Haque, S.J., Williams, B.R.: p38 MAP kinase is required for STAT1 serine phosphorylation and transcriptional activation induced by interferons. EMBO J **18**, 5601–5608 (1999)
51. Li, Y., Sassano, A., Majchrzak, B., et al.: Role of p38a Map kinase in type I interferon signaling. J Biol Chem **279**, 970–979 (2004)
52. Uddin, S., Yenush, L., Sun, X.J., et al.: Interferon-alpha engages the insulin receptor substrate-1 to associate with the phosphatidylinositol 3′-kinase. J Biol Chem **270**, 15938–15941 (1995)
53. Ahmad, S., Alsayed, Y.M., Druker, B.J., et al.: The type I interferon receptor mediates tyrosine phosphorylation of the CrkL adaptor protein. J Biol Chem **272**, 29991–29994 (1997)
54. Pestka, S., Krause, C.D., Walter, M.R.: Interferons, interferon-like cytokines, and their receptors. Immunol Rev **202**, 8–32 (2004)
55. Dummer, R., Cozzio, A., Urosevic, M.: Interferons in cutaneous T-cell Lymphomas. Hematol Rep **2**(13), 71–74 (2006)
56. Creasey, A.A., Eppstein, D.A., Marsh, Y.V., et al.: Growth regulation of melanoma cells by interferon and (2′–5′)oligoadenylate synthetase. Mol Cell Biol **3**, 780–786 (1983)
57. Buzaid, A.C., Grimm, E.A., Ali-Osman, F., et al.: Mechanism of the anti-tumor effect of biochemotherapy in melanoma: preliminary results. Melanoma Res **4**, 327–330 (1994)
58. Anderson, C.M., Buzaid, A.C., Sussman, J., et al.: Nitric oxide and neopterin levels and clinical response in stage III melanoma patients receiving concurrent biochemotherapy. Melanoma Res **8**, 149–155 (1998)
59. Bernengo, M.G., Quaglino, P., Cappello, N., et al.: Macrophage-mediated immunostimulation modulates therapeutic efficacy of interleukin-2 based chemoimmunotherapy in advanced metastatic melanoma patients. Melanoma Res **10**, 55–65 (2000)
60. Haller, O., Arnheiter, H., Lindenmann, J., et al.: Host gene influences sensitivity to interferon action selectively for influenza virus. Nature **283**, 660–662 (1980)
61. Sadler, A.J., Williams, B.R.: Interferon-inducible antiviral effectors. Nat Rev Immunol **8**, 559–568 (2008)
62. Aebi, M., Fah, J., Hurt, N., et al.: cDNA structures and regulation of two interferon-induced human Mx proteins. Mol Cell Biol **9**, 5062–5072 (1989)
63. Horisberger, M.A., McMaster, G.K., Zeller, H., et al.: Cloning and sequence analyses of cDNAs for interferon- and virus-induced human Mx proteins reveal that they contain putative guanine nucleotide-binding sites: functional study of the corresponding gene promoter. J Virol **64**, 1171–1181 (1990)
64. Holzinger, D., Jorns, C., Stertz, S., et al.: Induction of MxA gene expression by influenza A virus requires type I or type III interferon signaling. J Virol **81**, 7776–7785 (2007)
65. Gilli, F., Marnetto, F., Caldano, M., et al.: Biological markers of interferon-beta therapy: comparison among interferon-stimulated genes MxA, TRAIL and XAF-1. Mult Scler **12**, 47–57 (2006)
66. Jakschies, D., Hochkeppel, H.K., Horisberger, M.A., et al.: Correlation of the antiproliferative effect and the Mx-homologous protein induction by IFN in patients with malignant melanoma. J Invest Dermatol **95**, 238S–241S (1990)
67. Ralph, S.J., Wines, B.D., Payne, M.J., et al.: Resistance of melanoma cell lines to interferons correlates with reduction of IFN-induced tyrosine phosphorylation. Induction of the anti-viral state by IFN is prevented by tyrosine kinase inhibitors. J Immunol **154**, 2248–2256 (1995)
68. Yurkovetsky, Z.R., Kirkwood, J.M., Edington, H.D., et al.: Multiplex analysis of serum cytokines in melanoma patients treated with interferon-alpha2b. Clin Cancer Res **13**, 2422–2428 (2007)
69. Critchley-Thorne, R.J., Yan, N., Nacu, S., et al.: Down-regulation of the interferon signaling pathway in T lymphocytes from patients with metastatic melanoma. PLoS Med **4**, e176 (2007)
70. Takahashi, Y., Kaneda, H., Takasuka, N., et al.: Enhancement of antiproliferative activity of interferons by RNA interference-mediated silencing of SOCS gene expression in tumor cells. Cancer Sci **99**, 1650–1655 (2008)
71. Hanada, T., Yoshimura, A.: Regulation of cytokine signaling and inflammation. Cytokine Growth Factor Rev **13**, 413–421 (2002)
72. Sakai, I., Takeuchi, K., Yamauchi, H., et al.: Constitutive expression of SOCS3 confers resistance to IFN-alpha in chronic myelogenous leukemia cells. Blood **100**, 2926–2931 (2002)

73. Gogas, H., Ioannovich, J., Dafni, U., et al.: Prognostic significance of autoimmunity during treatment of melanoma with interferon. N Engl J Med **354**, 709–718 (2006)

74. Bouwhuis, M., Suciu, S., Kruit, W., et al.: Prognostic value of autoantibodies (auto-AB) in melanoma patients (pts) in the EORTC 18952 trial of adjuvant interferon (IFN) vs Observation (Obs). Proc Am Soc Clin Oncol **25**, 8507 (2007). Abstract

75. Nordlung, J., Kirkwood, J., Milton, B.F.G., et al.: Vitiligo in patients with metastatic melanoma: a good prognostic sign. J. Am. Acad. Dermatol. **9**, 689–696; Abstract (1983)

76. Zeuzem, S., Welsch, C., Herrmann, E.: Pharmacokinetics of peginterferons. Semin Liver Dis **23**(suppl 1), 23–28 (2003)

77. Wang, Y.S., Youngster, S., Bausch, J., et al.: Identification of the major positional isomer of pegylated interferon alpha-2b. Biochemistry **39**, 10634–10640 (2000)

78. PEG-Intron: Drug Information, Schering Corporation

79. Peg-INFa-2a, Pegasus: Drug Information

80. Balch, C.M., Buzaid, A.C., Soong, S.J., et al.: Final version of the American Joint Committee on Cancer staging system for cutaneous melanoma. J Clin Oncol **19**, 3635–3648 (2001)

81. Dummer, R., Panizzon, R., Bloch, P.H., et al.: Updated Swiss guidelines for the treatment and follow up of cutaneous melanoma. Dermatology **210**, 39–44 (2005)

82. Kirkwood, J.M., Ibrahim, J.G., Sondak, V.K., et al.: High- and low-dose interferon alfa-2b in high-risk melanoma: first analysis of intergroup trial E1690/S9111/C9190. J Clin Oncol **18**, 2444–2458 (2000)

83. Kirkwood, J.M., Manola, J., Ibrahim, J., et al.: A pooled analysis of eastern cooperative oncology group and intergroup trials of adjuvant high-dose interferon for melanoma. Clin Cancer Res **10**, 1670–1677 (2004)

84. Eggermont, A.M., Suciu, S., MacKie, R., et al.: Post-surgery adjuvant therapy with intermediate doses of interferon alfa 2b versus observation in patients with stage IIb/III melanoma (EORTC 18952): randomised controlled trial. Lancet **366**, 1189–1196 (2005)

85. Kirkwood, J.M., Strawderman, M.H., Ernstoff, M.S., et al.: Interferon alfa-2b adjuvant therapy of high-risk resected cutaneous melanoma: the Eastern Cooperative Oncology Group Trial EST 1684. J Clin Oncol **14**, 7–17 (1996)

86. Eggermont, A.M., Suciu, S., Santinami, M., et al.: Adjuvant therapy with pegylated interferon alfa-2b versus observation alone in resected stage III melanoma: final results of EORTC 18991, a randomised phase III trial. Lancet **372**, 117–126 (2008)

87. Dummer, R., Garbe, C., Thompson, J.A., et al.: Randomized dose-escalation study evaluating peginterferon alfa-2a in patients with metastatic malignant melanoma. J Clin Oncol **24**, 1188–1194 (2006)

88. Millwald, M.J., Bedikian, A.Y., Conry, R.M., et al.: Randomized multinational phase III trial of dacarbazine(DTIC) with or without Bcl-2 antisense (oblimersen sodium) in patients with advnced maligannt melanoma (MM). Analysis of long-term survival. ASCO Annual Meeting:Abstract No 7505 (2004)

89. Schadendorf, D., Ugurel, S., Schuler-Thurner, B., et al.: Dacarbazine (DTIC) versus vaccination with autologous peptide-pulsed dendritic cells (DC) in first-line treatment of patients with metastatic melanoma: a randomized phase III trial of the DC study group of the DeCOG. Ann Oncol **17**, 563–570 (2006)

90. Kurokohchi, K., Takaguchi, K., Kita, K., et al.: Successful treatment of advanced hepatocellular carcinoma by combined administration of 5-fluorouracil and pegylated interferon-alpha. World J Gastroenterol **11**, 5401–5403 (2005)

91. Son, M.J., Song, H.S., Kim, M.H., et al.: Synergistic effect and condition of pegylated interferon alpha with paclitaxel on glioblastoma. Int J Oncol **28**, 1385–1392 (2006)

92. Hwu, W.J., Panageas, K.S., Menell, J.H., et al.: Phase II study of temozolomide plus pegylated interferon-alpha-2b for metastatic melanoma. Cancer **106**, 2445–2451 (2006)

93. Middleton, M.R., Grob, J.J., Aaronson, N., et al.: Randomized phase III study of temozolomide versus dacarbazine in the treatment of patients with advanced metastatic malignant melanoma. J Clin Oncol **18**, 158–166 (2000)

94. Spieth, K., Kaufmann, R., Dummer, R., et al.: Temozolomide plus pegylated interferon alfa-2b as first-line treatment for stage IV melanoma: a multicenter phase II trial of the Dermatologic Cooperative Oncology Group (DeCOG). Ann Oncol **19**, 801–806 (2008)

95. Kaufmann, R., Spieth, K., Leiter, U., et al.: Temozolomide in combination with interferon-alfa versus temozolomide alone in patients with advanced metastatic melanoma: a randomized, phase III, multicenter study from the Dermatologic Cooperative Oncology Group. J Clin Oncol **23**, 9001–9007 (2005)

96. Hauschild, A., Dummer, R., Ugurel, S., et al.: Combined treatment with pegylated interferon-alpha-2a and dacarbazine in patients with advanced metastatic melanoma: a phase 2 study. Cancer **113**, 1404–1411 (2008)

97. Vaishampayan, U.N., Heilbrun, L.K., Marsack, C., et al.: Phase II trial of pegylated interferon and thalidomide in malignant metastatic melanoma. Anticancer Drugs **18**, 1221–1226 (2007)

98. Medwatch: What is a serious adverse effect? www.fda.gov. Retrieved on 18 Sep 2007

99. Hauschild, A., Gogas, H., Tarhini, A., et al.: Practical guidelines for the management of interferon-alpha-2b side effects in patients receiving adjuvant treatment for melanoma: expert opinion. Cancer **112**, 982–994 (2008)

100. Malik, U.R., Makower, D.F., Wadler, S.: Interferon-mediated fatigue. Cancer **92**, 1664–1668 (2001)

Cutaneous Lymphoma

Reinhard Dummer, Kazuhiro Kawai, and Marie C. Zipser

4.3.1 Surgery

Reinhard Dummer

Cutaneous lymphomas, like other lymphomas, are systemic diseases by definition. Therefore, surgery has limited indications.

However, primary cutaneous B-cell lymphomas (CBCL), such as follicle center lymphomas and large cell primary cutaneous CD30+ T-cell lymphomas, may present as a single nodule in the skin. In these cases, because investigation on tumor material is necessary, an excision biopsy might be a good alternative to an incisional biopsy.

In the case of surgical treatment of a nodule in primary cutaneous lymphomas, a safety margin of at least 1 cm should be applied, although there are no supporting clinical trials.

In B-cell lymphomas but also in other lymphomas, there is often a relapse very close to the scar, indicating that the excision did not remove the entire tumor. Therefore, in case of narrow safety margins, postoperative irradiation therapy must be considered.

4.3.2 Phototherapy and Radiation

4.3.2.1 Indication

Phototherapy is a powerful treatment option for different types of cutaneous lymphomas.

Narrow band UVB therapy is recommended for patch-stage mycosis fungoides (MF). If the patient has thicker lesions, systemic psoralen plus UVA (PUVA) therapy is preferred.

PUVA therapy can also be used in other types of cutaneous lymphomas, such as CD30+ and cutaneous T-cell lymphoma (CTCL), as well as in erythrodermic patients.

Alternatively, high dose UVA is an option. However, there are few studies available.

Photopheresis is one of the first-line treatment options for Sézary syndrome [1].

4.3.2.2 Technique

Narrow band UVB is typically applied three times per week [2, 3]. The initial dose depends on the skin type and is generally around 0.4 J/cm². There is no agreement on how long the phototherapy should be continued. Typically, the treating physician makes this decision on individual basis [1].

4.3.2.2.1 PUVA Therapy

Before initiating PUVA therapy, a phototoxicity assay is recommended in order to determine the initial dose. The treatment is performed three times per week. Especially in erythrodermic patients, dose enhancement should be done very carefully as to avoid solar erythema. Treatment should last at least 3 months. PUVA therapy can be combined with interferon alpha [4] or targretin [1].

Photopheresis is a complex technique. It causes apheresis of lymphocytes by applying UVA irradiation in the presence of psoralens. Thereafter, the irradiated lymphocytes are re-infused, thus resulting in immune modifications.

R. Dummer (✉)
Department of Dermatology, University Hospital of Zürich,
Gloriastrasse 31, 8091 Zürich,
Switzerland
e-mail: reinhard.dummer@usz.ch

K. Kawai
Department of Dermatology, Kagoshima University Graduate
School of Medical and Dental Sciences, 8-35-1 Sakuragaoka,
Kagoshima, 890-8544, Japan
e-mail: kazkawai@m2.kufm.kagoshima-u.ac.jp

M.C. Zipser
University Hospital of Zürich, Department of Dermatology F2,
Gloriastrasse 31, 8091 Zürich,
Switzerland
e-mail: marie.zipser@usz.ch

R. Dummer et al. (eds.), *Skin Cancer – A World-Wide Perspective*,
DOI: 10.1007/978-3-642-05072-5_4.3, © Springer-Verlag Berlin Heidelberg 2011

The typical indication for extracorporeal photopheresis is Sézary syndrome. It is performed on 2 days every 2 weeks in the beginning; later, the intervals are decreased to four times every 6 weeks.

4.3.2.3 Outcome

For early MF, the response rates are between 50 and 80% for narrow band UVB; some patients achieve complete remission [2].

PUVA therapy reveals similar results in MF.

Extracorporeal photopheresis in Sézary syndrome has a response rate of 50% and higher [5].

4.3.3 Radiation Indication

4.3.3.1 Indication

Radiation with electrons or orthovolt therapy (X-rays) is an excellent treatment option for localized manifestations. It is often combined with the systemic therapy in MF and can effectively eliminate tumors.

Irradiation is the treatment of choice in cases of localized manifestations, for example, in large CD30+ CTCL that present with one lesion or localized disease.

All types of B-cell lymphomas can be successfully treated. For b-cell lymphomas, radiation therapy is the first-line treatment option [6].

4.3.3.2 Technique

Orthovolt therapy is an excellent treatment option for localized disease. Electron beam irradiation is a rather complex procedure. The description of the techniques can be found in the chapter (Baumert et al. Radiation of melanoma 4.2.2).

4.3.3.3 Outcome

For primary CBCL (especially marginal zone lymphomas), low-dose radiotherapy with soft X-rays may result in complete clearance in 80-90% of cases [6]. Typically, less than 20 Gy can be used. Tumor manifestations in MF are typically irradiated with higher dosages.

Unfortunately, there is no evidence that MF or Sézary syndrome can be cured with irradiation therapy [7].

4.3.4 Topical Therapy (CTCL)

Kazuhiro Kawai

4.3.4.1 Indication

Sequential skin-directed local therapies (topical therapy, phototherapy, and radiation therapy), with the choice of therapy depending on the extent of cutaneous disease and plaque thickness, are appropriate treatment options for early stages (IA–IIA) of mycosis fungoides (MF), as in a randomized controlled trial, aggressive systemic chemotherapy combined with total skin electron beam therapy (TSEBT) failed to demonstrate improved survival of patients with MF [11]. Because superficial disease is easily accessible with topically applied agents, topical therapy is the preferred first-line treatment for early patch/plaque-stage MF.

Indolent types of CTCL other than MF, particularly lymphomatoid papulosis and primary cutaneous anaplastic large cell lymphoma, may be treated with topical therapy. However, thick tumors tend to be resistant to topical therapy and usually require surgical excision or radiation therapy.

Patients with aggressive CTCL are treated primarily with systemic chemotherapy, but in some epidermotropic CTCL, such as subtypes of adult T-cell leukemia/lymphoma mainly affecting the skin, topical therapy may be used as palliative therapy. Topical therapy is also used as an adjuvant therapy for patients with CTCL after remissions have been obtained with the use of TSEBT.

Currently used topical therapies for CTCL include topical corticosteroids, topical chemotherapy with alkylating agents such as mechlorethamine (nitrogen mustard, HN_2) and carmustine (BCNU), and topical retinoids such as bexarotene. Another promising topical therapeutic agent for CTCL is topical immune response modifier imiquimod.

4.3.5 Technique

4.3.5.1 Topical Corticosteroids

Superpotent topical corticosteroids such as 0.05% clobetasol propionate and 0.05% diflorasone diacetate, as either cream or ointment, are applied twice daily to the individual lesions. Response to topical corticosteroids is usually evident within the first 3 months [16]. Patients with responsive disease continue maintenance therapy for as long as required and tolerated after the lesions are cleared [1].

4.3.5.2 Topical HN$_2$

Topical HN$_2$ is used as either an aqueous solution or ointment-based preparation, and both preparations appear to have equivalent efficacy [2, 9, 26]. The aqueous solution is made by dissolving HN$_2$ at 0.01–0.02% in water. For 0.01% (10 mg/100 mL) concentration, one vial of 10 mg of HN$_2$ is dissolved in 100 mL of tap water. The aqueous solution is unstable and must be prepared immediately before use [2]. HN$_2$ ointment prepared in Aquaphor or an equivalent base at a concentration of 0.01–0.02% is stable for at least a few months.

The 0.01–0.02% HN$_2$ solution or ointment is applied once daily to the entire skin for patients with diffuse skin involvement. Alternatively, HN$_2$ solution or ointment is applied only to involved skin if the skin disease is limited. For patients with a slow response to treatment, concentration of HN$_2$ may be increased to 0.03–0.04%, or the frequency of application may be increased to twice daily. Therapy is usually continued for 2–6 months after complete clearance of skin lesions [2, 12]. There is no evidence that more prolonged maintenance therapy is beneficial [2, 12, 26].

4.3.5.3 Topical BCNU

Topical BCNU is also used as either an aqueous solution or ointment-based preparation [3, 14]. The 0.2% alcoholic stock solution is prepared by dissolving one vial of 100 mg of BCNU in 50 mL of 95% ethanol, which is stable in a refrigerator for at least 3 months [3]. Aqueous solution of 0.01–0.02% BCNU is made from the 0.2% stock solution before use. For total body application, 5 mL (10 mg BCNU) of the 0.2% stock solution is diluted in 60 mL of tap water. The BCNU solution (approximately 0.017%) is applied once daily only to the involved skin with a brush or gauze pad. In patients with very limited disease, the undiluted 0.2% solution may be applied once daily using a cotton-tipped applicator stick [3]. BCNU ointment 0.01–0.02% (10–20 mg/100 g) in petrolatum is stable at room temperature [3] and can be applied once daily only to the involved skin. Due to systemic absorption that results in bone marrow suppression, duration of topical BCNU therapy is usually limited to 6 months, and maintenance therapy is not recommended.

4.3.5.4 Topical Bexarotene

Bexarotene belongs to a new class of retinoids called 'rexinoids' that bind selectively to the retinoid X receptors. A phase I/II dose-ranging trial of topical bexarotene gel 0.01–1% demonstrated that bexarotene gel 1% applied twice daily is well-tolerated and effective in patients with stage IA–IIA MF [21]. Bexarotene gel 1% has been approved for topical therapy in patients with stage IA–IB MF who are resistant or intolerant to other therapies.

Bexarotene gel 1% is applied to the individual lesions every other day with increasing frequency up to four times per day as tolerated.

4.3.6 Outcome

4.3.6.1 Topical Corticosteroids

Zackheim et al. [16] evaluated the effects of topical corticosteroids on early-stage (IA/IB) MF in a prospective study. Of 79 patients, 95% had patch-stage disease, and most patients were treated with superpotent corticosteroids (predominantly 0.05% clobetasol propionate) [16]. Of 51 patients with T1 (stage IA) disease, 63% achieved complete response (CR) and 31% achieved partial response (PR) for an overall response rate (ORR) of 94% [16]. Of 28 patients with T2 (stage IB) disease, 25% achieved CR and 57% achieved PR for an ORR of 82% [16]. At a median follow-up period of 9 months, 80% of T1 patients and 68% of T2 patients were in CR or PR [16]. Reversible depression of serum cortisol occurred in 13% of the patients, but none of the patients showed clinical signs of adrenal insufficiency [16]. Minor skin irritation and purpura were seen in approximately 10–20% of the patients [1], but localized reversible skin atrophy and striae were seen in only a small number of patients [16].

4.3.6.2 Topical HN$_2$

In a cohort of 107 patients with stage IA/IB MF, Ramsay et al. [10] reported that the probability of achieving CR within 2 years was 63% with the use of topical HN$_2$ therapy. The CR rate for patients with patch-stage disease was 76% and 45% for patients with plaque-stage disease [10]. Vonderheid et al [12] reported a 72% CR rate in 201 patients with stage IA–IIA MF treated with topical HN$_2$. CR rates were 80% for stage IA, 68% for IB, and 61% for IIA [12]. In some patients, long-lasting responses for more than 8 years after discontinuing maintenance therapy were documented [12]. In the updated long-term analysis of the Stanford experience of topical HN$_2$ therapy, 195 patients with stage IA–IIA MF received topical HN$_2$ as initial therapy [26]. CR rates were 69% for stage IA, 35% for IB, 28% for IIA, and 51% for IA-IIA [26]. Most of the patients achieving CR received only topical HN$_2$ therapy throughout the follow-up period [26]. In a prospective study conducted by the French Study Group of Cutaneous Lymphomas, effects of twice-weekly applications of 0.02% HN$_2$ solution and topical corticosteroid (betamethasone dipropionate cream) on early-stage MF were determined [32]. At 6 months, CR rate for the 64 patients with stage IA–IIA MF was 58%: 61% for IA, 58% for IB, and 40% for IIA [32]. Severe cutaneous intolerance that forced discontinuation of treatment occurred in 28% of the patients [32]. These studies showed that with topical HN$_2$ monotherapy, CR rates of 51–78% can be achieved in patients with stage IA–IIA MF [7, 10, 12, 26]. CR rates are usually low (less than 50%) in patients with tumors and erythrodermic disease [7, 9, 10, 12, 17, 26].

Although TSEBT has been shown to have higher CR rates than topical HN$_2$ therapy, there were no differences in overall survival between the therapies in patients with early-stage MF [7, 15, 17, 19]. Topical HN$_2$ therapy is a useful adjuvant therapy in patients with stage T2 (IB–IIA) MF for prolonging remissions after TSEBT [6, 7, 17].

Reported incidence of cutaneous hypersensitivity reactions to aqueous HN$_2$ solution varies from 35% to two-thirds [9, 10, 12, 18], but it can be reduced to less than 10% with the use of the ointment-based preparation [8, 9, 26]. Options for patients with cutaneous intolerance include changing from an aqueous solution to an ointment, reducing the frequency of application or the concentration of HN$_2$, applying concomitant topical corticosteroids, and attempting desensitization [2]. Other cutaneous complications of topical HN$_2$ therapy include xerosis, hyperpigmentation, and rarely, urticaria [14]. Reported incidence of secondary cutaneous malignancies was 4–11%, but this may not be directly due to topical HN$_2$ therapy [9, 26]. Combination of topical HN$_2$ with phototherapy or radiation therapy may increase the risk of non-melanoma skin cancers. Bone marrow suppression is not a potential complication because of the minimal systemic absorption of topically applied HN$_2$.

4.3.6.3 Topical BCNU

Most of the previous reports of topical BCNU therapy for early-stage MF are from the University of California at San Francisco [13, 14]. Zackheim et al. [13] reported the outcome of the retrospective cohort of 143 patients with MF (including 109 patients with stage IA–IIA disease) treated with topical BCNU over a 15-year period. Of 49 patients with stage IA disease, 86% achieved CR and 12% achieved PR for an ORR of 98%. Of 38 patients with stage IB disease, 47% achieved CR and 37% achieved PR for an ORR of 84%. CR in 55% and PR in 36% for an ORR of 91% were achieved in 22 patients with stage IIA disease [13]. Long-term analysis of 188 patients revealed that, at 36 months, 91% of patients with T1 disease and 62% of patients with T2 disease were still in CR or PR [14].

The majority of patients experienced some degree of erythematous reactions following topical BCNU therapy, which may leave persistent telangiectasia [3, 14]. Hypersensitivity reactions occurred less often (less than 10%) than with topical HN$_2$ therapy, and no secondary cutaneous malignancies occurred [3, 14]. Mild leukocytopenia occurred in 3.7% of the 188 patients and in 5% of those treating the total body surface, but was not serious enough to cause discontinuation of treatment [14]. Complete blood counts should be performed regularly during topical BCNU therapy to monitor for bone marrow suppression.

4.3.6.4 Topical Bexarotene

Phase I–II trial of topical bexarotene gel 0.01–1% involving 66 patients with stage IA–IIA MF demonstrated CR in 21% and PR in 42% for an ORR of 63% [21]. A dose–response effect was observed with greater efficacy at higher concentrations and frequencies of application [21]. Median time to response was 20 weeks, and median response duration was 25 months [21]. Patients who had not previously received other skin-directed therapies had a higher ORR (75%) than those who had (67%) [21]. In the phase III trial of 49 patients with refractory stage IA–IIA MF, topical bexarotene gel 1% demonstrated a 44% ORR with an 8% CR rate [25]. The predominant adverse events were mild-to-moderate local irritation restricted to the site of application [21, 25]. Local irritation can be reduced by gradual increase in the frequency of application or concomitant use of topical corticosteroids. Favorable responses to topical bexarotene gel 1% were also demonstrated in a small case series of lymphomatoid papulosis [27].

4.3.7 Experimental Topical Therapies for CTCL

4.3.7.1 Topical Tazarotene

Tazarotene, a retinoid A receptor-selective retinoid, has been used as a topical agent for the treatment of psoriasis. In a pilot study of 20 patients with stage IA–IB MF with less than

20% skin involvement, tazarotene gel 0.1% was applied daily for 6 months [28]. The ORR was similar to topical bexarotene [28]. Local irritation could be controlled in most patients with topical corticosteroids or by reducing the frequency of application [28].

4.3.7.2 Topical Imiquimod

Imiquimod, a low molecular weight synthetic compound of the imidazoquinoline family, is an immune response modifier with potent antiviral and antitumor activity in vivo [5]. Imiquimod directly activates cells of the innate immune system, including plasmacytoid dendritic cells though Toll-like receptor 7, and induces production of IFN-α, inflammatory cytokines such as IL-12 and TNF-α, and chemokines that results in activation of innate as well as Th1-type acquired immunity [5, 34]. Topical imiquimod (5% imiquimod cream) has been approved for actinic keratosis, superficial basal cell carcinoma, and external genital warts.

There are several case reports and small case series that suggest beneficial effects of 5% imiquimod cream on patients with CTCL. Topical imiquimod was successfully used in patch/plaque-stage MF [22, 24, 29, 33, 35, 39]. Topical imiquimod may also be useful for patients with primary cutaneous anaplastic large cell lymphoma [30, 35, 38]. In most studies, 5% imiquimod cream was applied to the individual lesions three times per week to daily as tolerated until the treated lesions were cleared. Local skin reactions at the treated site were common. The treated site should be washed with mild soap and water 6–10 h following topical imiquimod application.

4.3.7.3 Topical Methotrexate

Beneficial effects of topical methotrexate (MTX) on patients with early-stage (IA–IB) MF have been demonstrated in a phase I–II trial [23]. There is one case report of a patient with lymphomatoid papulosis who was successfully treated with topical MTX [4].

4.3.7.4 Topical Romidepsin

Histone deacetylase inhibitors represent a new class of anticancer drugs [31]. Histone deacetylase inhibitors, romidepsin (depsipeptide) and vorinostat, have shown notable clinical responses in patients with CTCL when administered systemically [20, 36, 37]. Topical romidepsin is being tested for patients with early-stage CTCL in a clinical trial.

4.3.8 Topical Therapy (CBCL)

Reinhard Dummer and Marie C. Zipser

4.3.8.1 Indication

First-line treatment approaches for primary cutaneous B-cell lymphomas (CBCL) include surgical excision (enabling histological confirmation of the diagnosis) and radiation (see other chapters).

In case of multiple lesions, alternative treatment applications might be useful. This is of special relevance for young patients suffering from marginal zone lymphoma.

4.3.8.2 Technique

4.3.8.2.1 Intralesional Corticosteroids

A 1:1 dilution of lidocaine with synthetic corticosteroids in suspension such as triamcinolone acetonide (Kenacort®-A 40) can be used for direct intralesional application. This may result in regressions (complete or partial regressions) within a few weeks after application. This treatment can be repeated every 4–8 weeks.

4.3.8.2.2 Intralesional Interferone α2a

Intralesional application of Interferone α2a has been found to lead to complete clinical regression of injected tumors in patients with primary cutaneous marginal zone lymphomas. Eight patients with primary cutaneous marginal zone lymphomas were injected with three million units of recombinant Interferone α2a (Roferon-A1; Roche, Switzerland) intralesionally three times weekly [1]. All patients experienced complete clinical regression of injected tumors after a mean of 8.5 weeks; complete responses are ongoing in six out of eight patients for 1–9 years. [1].

4.3.8.2.3 Topical BCNU

Topical BCNU is also used as either an aqueous solution or ointment-based preparation [5, 6]. The 0.2% alcoholic stock solution is prepared by dissolving one vial of 100 mg of BCNU in 50 ml of 95% ethanol, which is stable in a refrigerator for at least 3 months [6]. Aqueous solution of 0.01–0.02% BCNU is made from the 0.2% stock solution before use. For total body application, 5 mL (10 mg BCNU) of the 0.2% stock solution is diluted in 60 mL of tap water. The

BCNU solution (approximately 0.017%) is applied once daily only to the involved skin with a brush or gauze pad. In patients with very limited disease, the undiluted 0.2% solution may be applied once daily using a cotton-tipped applicator stick. BCNU ointment 0.01–0.02% (10–20 mg/100 g) in petrolatum is stable at room temperature [6] and can be applied once daily only to the involved skin. Due to systemic absorption that results in bone marrow suppression, duration of topical BCNU therapy is usually limited to 6 months, and maintenance therapy is not recommended.

4.3.8.2.4 Topical Imiquimod

Imiquimod cream 5% (Aldara®) is reported to induce regressions, especially in very superficial small CBCL lesions, for example, in patients with papules of marginal zone lymphoma. However, clinical experiences are very limited [3].

4.3.8.2.5 Rituximab

Rituximab (chimeric monoclonal anti-CD20 antibody) is typically used systemically. However, in order to reduce costs, intralesional applications are also successful. It has to be stated that the intralesional application also results in systemic effects, reflected by reduced circulating B-lymphocytes [4].

4.3.9 Experimental Topical Therapies for CBCL

4.3.9.1 Adeno Interferon-Gamma

Adeno interferon-gamma has been used in the context of clinical trials for patients with primary CBCL [2]. Actually, all injected lesions have responded to the therapy. There are also reports on regression of non-injected lesions associated with a formation of systemic immune activation such as antibody formation and induction of cytokines [2].

4.3.10 Systemic Therapy

Reinhard Dummer

4.3.10.1 Indication

Most cutaneous lymphomas (CL) are indolent neoplasms with a very wide variety of clinical presentations. In early stages, they affect quality of life, due to their impact on skin appearance and annoying symptoms such as pruritus. In some cases, depending on the quality of skin involvement and areas involved, they can be disfiguring even in early disease stages. In advanced stages, local skin problems are accompanied by systemic deviations in the immune reaction pattern, which result in an increased risk of infections and secondary malignancies. It is important to note that some of the late stage problems in CL patients might be aggravated by earlier therapeutic interventions. For example, radiotherapy or phototherapy may contribute to mutations that increase the proliferative and invasive capacity of tumor cell populations. Cytotoxic drugs favor infectious complications. Most patients with advanced disease do not die due to lymphoma manifestations but secondary problems such as infections.

The patient population suffering from CL is of advanced age. Those patients may have many comorbidities such as hypertension, heart failure, diabetes, and other diseases. Since current literature does not offer any curative treatment options for CL, a realistic goal for treatment will be to achieve long-lasting remissions in a significant percentage of patients, with drugs that can be safely used over a period of time, without long-term toxicity. Many clinical studies dealing with the treatment of CL are difficult, if not impossible, to evaluate and to compare because of changing classification schemes and staging systems. For these reasons, high quality, prospective randomized therapeutic trials, using the accepted diagnostic criteria for assessment of skin involvement and staging, are urgently needed [1].

Based on current knowledge, initial therapy should be skin-directed. If the disease is not sufficiently controlled, systemic biological therapy can be added. Aggressive polychemotherapy is only justified for advanced disease.

4.3.11 Technique and Outcome

4.3.11.1 Therapy of CTCL

4.3.11.1.1 Mycosis Fungoides, Follicular Mucinosis, and Pagetoid Reticulosis

A stage-adjusted, conservative, therapeutic approach is recommended for MF and its variants. In a prospective study,

103 patients with mycosis fungoides (MF) were randomized to receive either total skin electron beam therapy (TSEBT), in a dosage of 30 Gy, combined with chemotherapy or various topical treatments, adjusted to the stage of disease, including phototherapy and mechlorethamine (nitrogen mustard). In more advanced stages, both radiation therapy and methotrexate (MTX) were employed. This study showed, as expected, a higher response rate in the group treated with TSEBT and chemotherapy but also identified serious side effects and showed no difference in the overall survival rate [54].

In earlier studies, favored treatments were topical measures such as topical corticosteroids, Psoralen plus UVA (PUVA), topical cytostatic agents such as mechlorethamine (HN2) and BCNU or radiation therapy with electron beam or soft X-rays. The topical cytostatic agents are popular in the USA and Scandinavia but not often used in central Europe, where PUVA is the favored option [55].

In more advanced stages, combined topical and systemic therapy is often employed, for example, a combination of PUVA and systemic retinoids or recombinant interferon-α (IFN-α) (Table 4.3.1).

In another randomized multicenter study, patients with Stage I and II MF and pleomorphic CTCL were treated with IFN-α (9 million units three times weekly) combined with PUVA or acitretin (Neotigason) (25 mg daily in the first week, then 50 mg daily). Both rate of complete remission (70%) and duration of remission were better in the IFN-α and PUVA group. The IFN-α and acitretin groups achieved 38% complete remission [56] (Table 4.3.1). In the follow-up randomized study, PUVA plus IFN-α was compared to PUVA alone. The group receiving retinoids required

significantly less UVA and had longer remission times. The response rate for Stage I–IIa CTCL was around 80%. While the combination of PUVA with IFN-α did not increase the remission rate, it produced quicker healing and a longer remission times.

Localized forms of MF such as pagetoid reticulosis are best treated with radiation therapy — soft X-rays (12–20 Gy total dose 2 Gy two times weekly for 3–5 weeks) or electron beam (30–40 Gy) (Table 4.3.1).

4.3.11.1.2 Lymphomatoid Papulosis and Large Cell CD30+ CTCL

Primary cutaneous CD30+ lymphoproliferative disorders have an excellent prognosis, in contrast to nodal CD30+ lymphomas [57]. Both lymphomatoid papulosis and the nodules of large cell CD30+ CTCL often spontaneously regress, healing with scarring. The therapeutic recommendations are given in Tables 4.3.2 and 4.3.3. Although the use of PUVA in these disorders has not been examined in a large study, various centers have had success with small numbers of patients using this modality.

4.3.11.1.3 Sézary Syndrome

Many retrospective studies on the treatment of Sézary syndrome (SS) contain inadequate information on the diagnostic criteria and staging of the disease [6], making a comparison of the therapeutic options impossible (Table 4.3.4).

Table 4.3.1 Therapy recommendations for MF, MF variants, and pagetoid reticulosis [53]

Stage	Recommended therapy First line	Recommended therapy Second line	Comments
I A	Watch and wait PUVA Topical corticosteroids; class III-IV Topical HN2/BCNU UVB/UVB narrow band	Bexarotene gel Hexadecyphosphocholine solution	PUVA favored in Europe
Unilesional MF Pagetoid reticulosis	Radiation therapy (soft X-rays or electron beam, total dose 30–40; 2 Gy 5 times weekly)	Topical PUVA Intralesional IFN Topical corticosteroids; class III-IV Bexarotene gel	These disorders represent special presentations of CTCL in Stage IA
IB–IIA	PUVA Topical HN2/BCNU	PUVA+IFN-α Oral bexarotene	
IIB	PUVA+IFN-α and radiation therapy for tumors Topical HN2/BCNU	Low-dose methotrexate Oral Bexarotene Total body electron beam Denileukin diftitox	Consider maintenance therapy with PUVA+IFN-α or bexarotene when remission is achieved
III[a]	PUVA+IFN-α Topical HN2/BCNU Extracorporeal photopheresis	Low-dose methotrexate Oral bexarotene Total body electron beam Chlorambucil/corticosteroids Low-dose long distance (2m) soft X-rays Vorinostat	Consider maintenance therapy with PUVA+IFN-α or bexarotene when remission is achieved
IV A	PUVA+IFN-α Extracorporeal photopheresis Evetually combined with IFN or methotrexate	Low-dose methotrexate Oral bexarotene Total body electron beam Chlorambucil /corticosteroids, Vorinostat Low-dose long distance (2m) soft X-rays	Consider maintenance therapy with PUVA+IFN-α or bexarotene when remission is achieved
IV B	PUVA+IFN-α chlorambucil/corticosteroids, liposomal doxorubicin Soft X-rays or electron beam for tumors	Oral bexarotene CHOP polychemotherapy Denileukin diftitox, Cladribine (2-chlorodeoxyadenosine), Gemcitabine Vorinostat alemtuzumab (anti-CD52)	Consider maintenance therapy with PUVA+IFN-α or bexarotene when remission is achieved

[a]Erythrodermic MF

Table 4.3.2 Therapy recommendations for lymphomatoid papulosis [53]

Degree of involvement	First-line therapy	Second-line therapy
Solitary or localized lesions	Excision	
	Observation	
Multifocal lesions	Observation	IFN
	PUVA	IFN + retinoid
	Methotrexate up to 20 mg/weekly	Bexarotene

Table 4.3.3 Therapy recommendations for large cell CD30+ CTCL [53]

Degree of involvement	First-line therapy	Second-line therapy
Solitary or localized lesions	Excision	Methotrexate
	Radiation therapy	perhaps IFN
Multifocal lesions without spontaneous remission	Methotrexate	Radiation therapy, perhaps IFN

Table 4.3.4 Therapy recommendations for Sézary syndrome [1]

First-line therapy	Second-line therapy
PUVA + IFN	Bexarotene
Extracorporeal photopheresis	Chlorambucil/corticosteroids
HN2	Low-dose methotrexate
	CHOP polychemotherapy
	Denileukin diftitox
	Vorinostat
	Total skin electron beam therapy

Table 4.3.5 Therapy recommendations for low-grade primary cutaneous B-cell lymphoma (follicular lymphoma, marginal zone lymphoma) [1]

Degree of involvement	First-line therapy	Second-line therapy
Solitary lesions	Excision	Intralesional rituximab
	Antibiotics	Intralesional corticosteroids
	Radiation therapy	
Multiple lesions	Antibiotics	Intralesional IFN-α
	Radiation therapy	Intralesional rituximab
		Intravenous rituximab

Table 4.3.6 Therapy recommendations for large cell CBCL

Degree of involvement	First-line therapy	Second-line therapy
Solitary or localized lesions	Radiation therapy	
	Excision	
Multiple lesions	Monochemotherapy (e.g., liposomal doxorubicin)	Chemotherapy + rituximab
	Polychemotherapy (e.g., CHOP)	

4.3.12 Therapy of CBCL

4.3.12.1 *Low-Grade Primary Cutaneous B-Cell Lymphoma (Follicular Lymphoma, Marginal Zone Lymphoma)*

The low-grade CBCLs are morphologically similar to mucosa-associated lymphoid tissue (MALT) lymphomas and therefore described by some authors as SALT (skin-associated lymphoid tissue) lymphomas. The prognosis of these tumors is in general very favorable [7–9]. In those cases in which infectious agents (such as *Borrelia burgdorferi* DNA) can be identified, an initial treatment with broad-spectrum antibiotics is recommended [10, 11]. Since the

identification of borrelial DNA can give false-negative results and is very time-consuming, we recommend giving each patient in this group a course of doxycycline (100 mg b.i.d. for 3 weeks) and assessing the clinical response. Distinguishing between low-grade CBCL and reactive B-cell pseudolymphomas can be quite difficult; even clonality studies cannot separate the two entities with certainty. The therapeutic recommendations are given in Table 4.3.5. Rituximab should only be employed in those cases in which CD20 expression has been proven histologically.

4.3.12.2 *Large Cell B-Cell Lymphoma*

This group of CBCL has a worse prognosis than those with follicular differentiation [12]. There are no large studies dealing with these tumors, making the formulation of guidelines difficult. Our suggestions are given in Table 4.3.6.

4.3.13 Therapy of Non-CD4+/CD56+ Hematodermic Neoplasm

In general, aggressive polychemotherapy regimens are recommended in these neoplasms of plasmacytoid dendritic cells and other rare unclassified CL [13], although no large studies or therapeutic comparisons are available (Table 4.3.7) [14].

Table 4.3.7 Therapy recommendations for CD4+/CD56+ hematodermic neoplasm

Degree of involvement	First-line therapy	Second-line therapy
Solitary or localized lesions	Radiation therapy	Monochemotherapy (e.g., liposomal doxorubicin)
	Excision	Polychemotherapy (e.g., CHOP)
Multiple lesions	Radiation therapy	Polychemotherapy
	Monochemotherapy (e.g., liposomal doxorubicin)	

References

Phototherapy

1. Dummer, R., Dreyling, M.: Primary cutaneous lymphoma: ESMO clinical recommendations for diagnosis, treatment and follow-up. Ann Oncol 19(suppl. 2), ii72–ii76 (2008)
2. Pavlotsky, F., Barzilai, A., Kasem, R., Shpiro, D., Trau, H.: UVB in the management of early stage mycosis fungoides. J Eur Acad Dermatol Venereol 20(5), 565–572 (2006)
3. Hofer, A., Cerroni, L., Kerl, H., Wolf, P.: Narrowband (311-nm) UV-B therapy for small plaque parapsoriasis and early-stage mycosis fungoides. Arch Dermatol 135(11), 1377–1380 (1999)
4. Stadler, R., Otte, H.G., Luger, T., Henz, B.M., Kuhl, P., Zwingers, T., et al.: Prospective randomized multicenter clinical trial on the use of interferon -2a plus acitretin versus interferon -2a plus PUVA in patients with cutaneous T-cell lymphoma stages I and II. Blood 92(10), 3578–3581 (1998)
5. Fraser Andrews, E., Seed, P., Whittaker, S., Russell Jones, R.: Extracorporeal photopheresis in Sezary syndrome. No significant effect in the survival of 44 patients with a peripheral blood T-cell clone. Arch Dermatol 134(8), 1001–1005 (1998)
6. Senff, N.J., Noordijk, E.M., Kim, Y.H., Bagot, M., Berti, E., Cerroni, L., et al.: European Organization for Research and Treatment of Cancer and International Society for Cutaneous Lymphoma consensus recommendations for the management of cutaneous B-cell lymphomas. Blood 112(5), 1600–1609 (2008)
7. Kaye, F.J., Bunn Jr., P.A., Steinberg, S.M., Stocker, J.L., Ihde, D.C., Fischmann, A.B., et al.: A randomized trial comparing combination electron-beam radiation and chemotherapy with topical therapy in the initial treatment of mycosis fungoides. N Engl J Med 321(26), 1784–1790 (1989)

Topical Therapy (CTCL)

1. Zackheim, H.S.: Treatment of patch-stage mycosis fungoides with topical corticosteroids. Dermatol Ther 16, 283–287 (2003)
2. Kim, Y.H.: Management with topical nitrogen mustard in mycosis fungoides. Dermatol Ther 16, 288–298 (2003)
3. Zackheim, H.S.: Topical carmustine (BCNU) in the treatment of mycosis fungoides. Dermatol Ther 16, 299–302 (2003)
4. Bergstrom, J.S., Jaworsky, C.: Topical methotrexate for lymphomatoid papulosis. J Am Acad Dermatol 49, 937–939 (2003)
5. Schon, M.P., Schon, M.: Imiquimod: mode of action. Br J Dermatol 157(suppl. 2), 8–13 (2007)
6. Price, N.M., Hoppe, R.T., Constantine, V.S., et al.: The treatment of mycosis fungoides: adjuvant topical mechlorethamine after electron beam therapy. Cancer 40, 2851–2853 (1977)
7. Hamminga, B., Noordijk, E.M., van Vloten, W.A.: Treatment of mycosis fungoides: total-skin electron-beam irradiation vs topical mechlorethamine therapy. Arch Dermatol 118, 150–153 (1982)
8. Price, N.M., Hoppe, R.T., Deneau, D.G.: Ointment-based echlorethamine treatment for mycosis fungoides. Cancer 52, 2214–2219 (1983)
9. Hoppe, R.T., Abel, E.A., Deneau, D.G., et al.: Mycosis fungoides: management with topical nitrogen mustard. J Clin Oncol 5, 1796–1803 (1987)
10. Ramsay, D.L., Halperin, P.S., Zeleniuch-Jacquotte, A.: Topical mechlorethamine therapy for early stage mycosis fungoides. J Am Acad Dermatol 19, 684–691 (1988)
11. Kaye, F.J., Bunn Jr., P.A., Steinberg, S.M., et al.: A randomized trial comparing combination electron-beam radiation and chemotherapy with topical therapy in the initial treatment of mycosis fungoides. N Engl J Med 321, 1784–1790 (1989)
12. Vonderheid, E.C., Tan, E.T., Kantor, A.F., et al.: Long-term efficacy, curative potential, and carcinogenicity of topical mechlorethamine chemotherapy in cutaneous T cell lymphoma. J Am Acad Dermatol 20, 416–428 (1989)
13. Zackheim, H.S., Epstein Jr., E.H., Crain, W.R.: Topical carmustine (BCNU) for cutaneous T cell lymphoma: a 15-year experience in 143 patients. J Am Acad Dermatol 22, 802–810 (1990)
14. Ramsay, D.L., Meller, J.A., Zackheim, H.S.: Topical treatment of early cutaneous T-cell lymphoma. Hematol Oncol Clin North Am 9, 1031–1056 (1995)
15. Kim, Y.H., Jensen, R.A., Watanabe, G.L., et al.: Clinical stage IA (limited patch and plaque) mycosis fungoides. A long-term outcome analysis. Arch Dermatol 132, 1309–1313 (1996)
16. Zackheim, H.S., Kashani-Sabet, M., Amin, S.: Topical corticosteroids for mycosis fungoides. Experience in 79 patients. Arch Dermatol 134, 949–954 (1998)
17. Chinn, D.M., Chow, S., Kim, Y.H., et al.: Total skin electron beam therapy with or without adjuvant topical nitrogen mustard or nitrogen mustard alone as initial treatment of T2 and T3 mycosis fungoides. Int J Radiat Oncol Biol Phys 43, 951–958 (1999)
18. Esteve, E., Bagot, M., Joly, P., et al.: A prospective study of cutaneous intolerance to topical mechlorethamine therapy in patients with cutaneous T-cell lymphomas. French Study Group of Cutaneous Lymphomas. Arch Dermatol 135, 1349–1353 (1999)
19. Kim, Y.H., Chow, S., Varghese, A., et al.: Clinical characteristics and long-term outcome of patients with generalized patch and/or plaque (T2) mycosis fungoides. Arch Dermatol 135, 26–32 (1999)
20. Piekarz, R.L., Robey, R., Sandor, V., et al.: Inhibitor of histone deacetylation, depsipeptide (FR901228), in the treatment of peripheral and cutaneous T-cell lymphoma: a case report. Blood 98, 2865–2868 (2001)
21. Breneman, D., Duvic, M., Kuzel, T., et al.: Phase 1 and 2 trial of bexarotene gel for skin-directed treatment of patients with cutaneous T-cell lymphoma. Arch Dermatol 138, 325–332 (2002)

22. Suchin, K.R., Junkins-Hopkins, J.M., Rook, A.H.: Treatment of stage IA cutaneous T-Cell lymphoma with topical application of the immune response modifier imiquimod. Arch Dermatol **138**, 1137–1139 (2002)

23. Demierre, M.F., Vachon, L., Ho, V., et al.: Phase 1/2 pilot study of methotrexate-laurocapram topical gel for the treatment of patients with early-stage mycosis fungoides. Arch Dermatol **139**, 624–628 (2003)

24. Dummer, R., Urosevic, M., Kempf, W., et al.: Imiquimod induces complete clearance of a PUVA-resistant plaque in mycosis fungoides. Dermatology **207**, 116–118 (2003)

25. Heald, P., Mehlmauer, M., Martin, A.G., et al.: Topical bexarotene therapy for patients with refractory or persistent early-stage cutaneous T-cell lymphoma: results of the phase III clinical trial. J Am Acad Dermatol **49**, 801–815 (2003)

26. Kim, Y.H., Martinez, G., Varghese, A., et al.: Topical nitrogen mustard in the management of mycosis fungoides: update of the Stanford experience. Arch Dermatol **139**, 165–173 (2003)

27. Krathen, R.A., Ward, S., Duvic, M.: Bexarotene is a new treatment option for lymphomatoid papulosis. Dermatology **206**, 142–147 (2003)

28. Apisarnthanarax, N., Talpur, R., Ward, S., et al.: Tazarotene 0.1% gel for refractory mycosis fungoides lesions: an open-label pilot study. J Am Acad Dermatol **50**, 600–607 (2004)

29. Chong, A., Loo, W.J., Banney, L., et al.: Imiquimod 5% cream in the treatment of mycosis fungoides-a pilot study. J Dermatolog Treat **15**, 118–119 (2004)

30. Didona, B., Benucci, R., Amerio, P., et al.: Primary cutaneous CD30+ T-cell lymphoma responsive to topical imiquimod (Aldara). Br J Dermatol **150**, 1198–1201 (2004)

31. Marks, P.A., Richon, V.M., Miller, T., et al.: Histone deacetylase inhibitors. Adv Cancer Res **91**, 137–168 (2004)

32. de Quatrebarbes, J., Esteve, E., Bagot, M., et al.: Treatment of early-stage mycosis fungoides with twice-weekly applications of mechlorethamine and topical corticosteroids: a prospective study. Arch Dermatol **141**, 1117–1120 (2005)

33. Deeths, M.J., Chapman, J.T., Dellavalle, R.P., et al.: Treatment of patch and plaque stage mycosis fungoides with imiquimod 5% cream. J Am Acad Dermatol **52**, 275–280 (2005)

34. Akira, S., Uematsu, S., Takeuchi, O.: Pathogen recognition and innate immunity. Cell **124**, 783–801 (2006)

35. Coors, E.A., Schuler, G., Von Den, D.P.: Topical imiquimod as treatment for different kinds of cutaneous lymphoma. Eur J Dermatol **16**, 391–393 (2006)

36. Duvic, M., Talpur, R., Ni, X., et al.: Phase 2 trial of oral vorinostat (suberoylanilide hydroxamic acid, SAHA) for refractory cutaneous T-cell lymphoma (CTCL). Blood **109**, 31–39 (2007)

37. Olsen, E.A., Kim, Y.H., Kuzel, T.M., et al.: Phase IIb multicenter trial of vorinostat in patients with persistent, progressive, or treatment refractory cutaneous T-cell lymphoma. J Clin Oncol **25**, 3109–3115 (2007)

38. Ehst, B.D., Dreno, B., Vonderheid, E.C.: Primary cutaneous CD30 + anaplastic large cell lymphoma responds to imiquimod cream. Eur J Dermatol **18**, 467–468 (2008)

39. Martinez-Gonzalez, M.C., Verea-Hernando, M.M., Yebra-Pimentel, M.T., et al.: Imiquimod in mycosis fungoides. Eur J Dermatol **18**, 148–152 (2008)

Topical Therapy (CBCL)

1. Cozzio, A., Kempf, W., et al.: Intra-lesional low-dose interferon alpha2a therapy for primary cutaneous marginal zone B-cell lymphoma. Leuk Lymphoma **47**(5), 865–869 (2006)

2. Dummer, R., Hassel, J.C., et al.: Adenovirus-mediated intralesional interferon-gamma gene transfer induces tumor regressions in cutaneous lymphomas. Blood **104**(6), 1631–1638 (2004)

3. Farkas, A., Kemeny, L., et al.: New and experimental skin-directed therapies for cutaneous lymphomas. Skin Pharmacol Physiol **22**(6), 322–334 (2009)

4. Heinzerling, L., Dummer, R., et al.: Intralesional therapy with anti-CD20 monoclonal antibody rituximab in primary cutaneous B-cell lymphoma. Arch Dermatol **136**(3), 374–378 (2000)

5. Ramsay, D.L., Meller, J.A., et al.: Topical treatment of early cutaneous T-cell lymphoma. Hematol Oncol Clin North Am **9**(5), 1031–1056 (1995)

6. Zackheim, H.S.: Topical carmustine (BCNU) in the treatment of mycosis fungoides. Dermatol Ther **16**(4), 299–302 (2003)

Systemic Therapy

1. Dummer, R., Dreyling, M.: Primary cutaneous lymphoma: ESMO clinical recommendations for diagnosis, treatment and follow-up. Ann Oncol **19**(suppl. 2), ii72–ii76 (2008)

2. Kaye, F.J., Bunn, P.J., Steinberg, S.M., Stocker, J.L., Ihde, D.C., Fischmann, A.B., et al.: A randomized trial comparing combination electron-beam radiation and chemotherapy with topical therapy in the initial treatment of mycosis fungoides. N Engl J Med **321**(26), 1784–1790 (1989)

3. Trautinger, F., Knobler, R., Willemze, R., Peris, K., Stadler, R., Laroche, L., et al.: EORTC consensus recommendations for the treatment of mycosis fungoides/Sezary syndrome. Eur J Cancer **42**(8), 1014–1030 (2006)

4. Stadler, R., Otte, H.G., Luger, T., Henz, B.M., Kuhl, P., Zwingers, T., et al.: Prospective randomized multicenter clinical trial on the use of interferon -2a plus acitretin versus interferon-2a plus PUVA in patients with cutaneous T-cell lymphoma stages I and II. Blood **92**(10), 3578–3581 (1998)

5. Willemze, R., Kerl, H., Sterry, W., Berti, E., Cerroni, L., Chimenti, S., et al.: EORTC classification for primary cutaneous lymphomas: a proposal from the Cutaneous Lymphoma Study Group of the European Organization for Research and Treatment of Cancer. Blood **90**(1), 354–371 (1997)

6. Vonderheid, E.C., Bernengo, M.G., Burg, G., Duvic, M., Heald, P., Laroche, L., et al.: Update on erythrodermic cutaneous T-cell lymphoma: report of the International Society for Cutaneous Lymphomas. J Am Acad Dermatol **46**(1), 95–106 (2002)

7. Berti, E., Alessi, E., Caputo, R., Gianotti, R., Delia, D., Vezzoni, P.: Reticulohistiocytoma of the dorsum. J Am Acad Dermatol **19**, 259–272 (1988)

8. Burg, G., Hess, M., Küng, E., Dommann, S., Dummer, R.: Semimalignant ("pseudolymphomatous") cutaneous B-cell lymphomas. Dermatol Clin **12**, 399–407 (1994)

9. Zinzani, P.L., Quaglino, P., Pimpinelli, N., Berti, E., Baliva, G., Rupoli, S., et al.: Prognostic factors in primary cutaneous B-cell lymphoma: the Italian Study Group for Cutaneous Lymphomas. J Clin Oncol **24**(9), 1376–1382 (2006)

10. Cerroni, L., Zochling, N., Putz, B., Kerl, H.: Infection by *Borrelia burgdorferi* and cutaneous B-cell lymphoma. J Cutan Pathol **24**(8), 457–461 (1997)

11. Bogle, M.A., Riddle, C.C., Triana, E.M., Jones, D., Duvic, M.: Primary cutaneous B-cell lymphoma. J Am Acad Dermatol **53**(3), 479–484 (2005)

12. Grange, F., Bekkenk, M.W., Wechsler, J., Meijer, C.J., Cerroni, L., Bernengo, M., et al.: Prognostic factors in primary cutaneous large

B-cell lymphomas: a European multicenter study. J Clin Oncol **19**(16), 3602–3610 (2001)

13. Urosevic, M., Conrad, C., Kamarashev, J., Asagoe, K., Cozzio, A., Burg, G., et al.: CD4+CD56+ hematodermic neoplasms bear a plasmacytoid dendritic cell phenotype. Hum Pathol **36**(9), 1020–1024 (2005)

14. Petrella, T., Bagot, M., Willemze, R., Beylot-Barry, M., Vergier, B., Delaunay, M., et al.: Blastic NK-cell lymphomas (agranular CD4+CD56+ hematodermic neoplasms): a review. Am J Clin Pathol **123**(5), 662–675 (2005)

Other Therapies

Keiji Iwatsuki, Naohito Hatta, Nagwa M. Elwan, Selma Ugurel, Lauren L. Lockwood, and Jürgen C. Becker

4.4.1 Histiocytoses

Keiji Iwatsuki

4.4.1.1 Langerhans Histiocytosis

Prognostic factors for Langerhans cell histiocytosis (LCH) or class I histiocytosis may include: (1) the number of organs involved, (2) the severity of organ failure, and (3) the age of the patients. Complications such as hemophagocytic syndrome and thrombocytopenia also affect the prognosis [1–4]. In general, younger patients with widely disseminated disease and organ dysfunction have a high risk of mortality. In a series of 101 children with LCH [2], the overall survival rate was 79% at 1 year, 74% at 3 years, and 71% at 5 years; however, in patients with liver or spleen involvement, 1-year survival was 33% and 5-year survival was only 25%. In adult LCH [3], the probability of survival 5 years post diagnosis was 92.3% overall: 100% for patients with single-system disease, 87.8% for isolated pulmonary disease, and 91.7% for multisystem disease.

K. Iwatsuki (✉)
Department of Dermatology, Okayama University Graduate School
of Medicine, Dentistry and Pharmaceutical Sciences,
2-5-1 Shikata-cho, Okayama, 700-8558, Japan
e-mail: keijiiwa@cc.okayama-u.ac.jp

N. Hatta
Division of Dermatology, Toyama Prefectural Central Hospital,
2-2-78 Nishinagae, Toyama, 930-8550, Japan
e-mail: hattanao@tch.pref.toyama.jp

N.M. Elwan
Department of Medicine, Tanta University,
Tanta-Egypt
e-mail: elwan2egy@yahoo.com

S. Ugurel and J.C. Becker
Department of General Dermatology, Medical university of Graz,
Auenbruggerplatz 8, A-8010 Graz, Austria,
97080 Würzburg, Germany
e-mail: selma.ugurel@medunigraz.at; juergen.becker@medunigraz.at

L.L. Lockwood
Department of Dermatology, University Hospital Zurich,
Gloriastrasse 31, 8091 Zurich, Switzerland

4.4.1.1.1 Solitary LCH or Single-System Involvement

A localized or single-organ disease involving skin or bone usually shows a good prognosis and requires minimal treatment (Table 4.4.1) [1–4]. Watchful waiting may be the best choice for cases of solitary cutaneous LCH because of possible spontaneous regression. A solitary lytic lesion of the long bone (eosinophilic granuloma) is curable by curettage. Patients with LCH in the orbit or middle cranial fossa may present with diabetes insipidus and other endocrine abnormalities. Multiple cutaneous lesions have successfully been treated with topical steroid, topical nitrogen mustard [5], PUVA [6] (Fig. 4.4.1), and thalidomide [7]. In infants with Hashimoto-Pritzker disease, even though the lesions are multiple, observation may be the best option.

4.4.1.1.2 LCH with Multisystem Involvement

Infants with multisystem involvement have higher rates of mortality and morbidity. Corticosteroids have been effective initially, but recurrence is frequent. Monochemotherapy using vinblastine or etoposide is an option for therapy. Patients with multisystem involvement and organ dysfunction should be treated with polychemotherapy including corticosteroid, vincristine, cyclophosphamide, cytosine arabinoside, and methotrexate. Previous protocols designated DAL-HX [8], LCH-I [9], and JLSG-96 [10] as providing similarly beneficial therapeutic results. The LCH-III protocol is ongoing. Patients who respond to chemotherapy have an 88–91% survival rate, but for patients who do not demonstrate an early response, the survival rate drops to 17–34% [1]. Recent reports suggest that 2-chlorodeoxy-adenosine (2-CdA) appears to be useful in LCH treatment, but it cannot yet be recommended as first-line therapy [11].

4.4.1.2 Non-Langerhans Cell Histiocytosis

4.4.1.2.1 Juvenile Xanthogranuloma

Juvenile xanthogranuloma (JXG), a representative disorder of non-LC histiocytosis, is generally a benign, self-limiting

R. Dummer et al. (eds.), *Skin Cancer – A World-Wide Perspective*,
DOI: 10.1007/978-3-642-05072-5_4.4, © Springer-Verlag Berlin Heidelberg 2011

histiocytic disorder of the skin, and requires no treatment. Both generalized eruptive histiocytosis and benign cephalic histiocytosis also disappear months to years after onset (Fig. 4.4.2). In the Kiel Pediatric Tumor Registry, cutaneous JXG showed a generally favorable prognosis with a low

relapse rate (7.0%) and even complete involution after incomplete resection [12]. In contrast to the cutaneous form, systemic JXG with organ involvement and xanthoma disseminatum may be associated with significant complications requiring aggressive medical care, although visceral lesions may regress spontaneously. When feasible, surgical excision of the lesions may be curative. Disseminated, multisystem JXG needs LCH-based polychemotherapy including cytarabine, vincristine, methotrexate, and prednisolone [13, 14]. Therapeutic approaches should be decided while taking into account the risks and uncertain efficacy of anti-JXG therapy and the possibility of spontaneous regression of the disease [13].

Table 4.4.1 Therapy of choice for LCH and prognosis

Prognostic factors	
The number of organs involved, organ dysfunction	
Age (if multiorgan involvement exists)	
Response to the initial chemotherapy	
Complications (hemophagocytosis, thrombocytopenia)	
Single organ involvement	*(Therapy)*
Limited cutaneous	Observation, topical steroid, CO_2 laser topical nitrogen mustard [5], PUVA [6], thalidomide [7]
Localized bone	Curettage or excision, intralesional steroid, radiotherapy
Multiple	The same as above, systemic steroid, interferon α2 monochemotherapy (vinblastine, etoposide)
Multiorgan involvement	
No organ dysfunction	Monochemotherapy (vinblastine, etoposide) with or without systemic steroid
Organ dysfunction	Polychemotherapy (vincristine, doxorubicin, cyclophosphamide, chlorambucil) DAL-HX [8], JLSG-96 [9], LCH-III (ongoing)
Refractory case	2-chlorodeoxyadenosine [10]

4.4.1.2.2 Systemic and Progressive Forms of XG Family

This category may include progressive nodular histiocytosis (PNH), necrobiotic xanthogranuloma (NXH) and Erdheim-Chester disease. Patients with PNH may present with continuous development of new lesions but remain in good health without any treatment [15].

NXG is a chronic and progressive disease associated with systemic involvement such as thorax and granulomatous myocarditis. The prognosis is closely related to the underlying disorders including plasma cell dyscrasia, multiple myeloma and POEMS syndrome. Some cases were successfully treated with a low dose of chlorambucil, combination therapy of melphalan and prednisone, or methotrexate followed by corticosteroid [15].

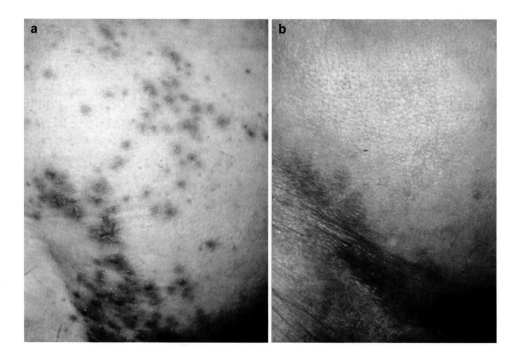

Fig. 4.4.1 PUVA treatment for adult LCH. Cutaneous manifestations before (**a**) and after (**b**) topical PUVA treatments [6]

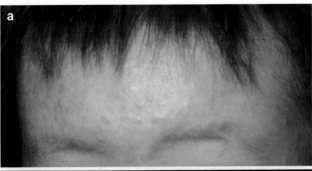
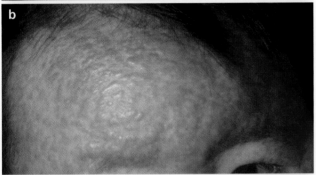
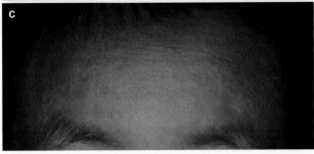

Fig. 4.4.2 Spontaneous regression of benign cephalic histiocytosis (BCH)/generalized eruptive histiocytosis (GEH). A 14-month-old boy had multiple reddish papules on the forehead mimicking BCH (**a**), which increased in number a month later, and expanded on the trunk symmetrically, the feature of which was consistent with GEH (**b**), and spontaneously regressed at the age of 4. During the clinical course, no apparent xanthomatous yellowish change was observed clinically

Erdheim-Chester disease has been treated with systemic steroids, radiation, LCH-based chemotherapy, interferon α and surgery, although the efficacy of these treatments has not fully been evaluated.

In the previous report, 22 (59%) of 37 patients died of the disease, and 8 (36%) died in less than 6 months [15, 16]. The mean survival duration was less than 3 years.

4.4.1.3 Multicentric Reticulohistiocytosis (MCRH)

Prior to treatment, underlying diseases such as tuberculosis, autoimmune diseases, and malignancies should be ruled out. Although nonsteroidal antiinflammatory drugs and

corticosteroids have been used for arthritis, they do not improve the clinical course. There were some cases where polyarthritis was successfully treated with methotrexate, cyclophosphamide, chlorambucil, anti-TNF-α agents, and alendronate [17].

4.4.1.4 Rosai–Dorfman Disease

Spontaneous regression is common, but various treatments have been tried with some benefits: corticosteroids, thalidomide, liquid nitrogen, surgical excision, and radiotherapy [18].

4.4.2 Mastocytosis

Naohito Hatta

4.4.2.1 Cutaneous Involvement

In contrast to children, most adult-onset patients do not show spontaneous regression of skin lesions. Psoralen-Photochemotherapy (PUVA) shows a benefit for the skin lesions treatment [31]. However, most patients require repeated treatment, and long-term adverse effects should be considered. Local use of corticosteroid can lead to the clearance of skin lesions[20].

4.4.2.2 Mediator-Related Symptoms

Mediator-related symptoms such as flushing and urticaria can be evoked by physical stimuli. Thus, temperature extremes, friction, massage, hot bathing, and alcohol should be avoided [8]. The severest form of these symptoms is anaphylactic shock. For these patients, carrying an epinephrine pen for self-injection may be considered [14]. The use of antimediator drugs such as antihistamines (including third generation ones) for urticaria, flushing, and itching is the mainstay of therapy. H_2 antihistamines or a proton pump inhibitor are used for gastrointestinal symptoms [8]. Acetyl salicylic acid (aspirin) and other NSAIDs are reported to be useful for prostaglandin-mediated flushing, tachycardia, and syncope [9]. Short-term oral glucocorticoids may be required for patients with severe systemic symptoms [14].

4.4.2.3 Systemic Mastocytosis

Cytoreductive agents such as interferon-alfa (INF-α) and cladribine are the mainstay of therapy. INF-α is considered to affect growth of early myeloid progenitor cells and to produce clinical responses in about 35–40% of patients with aggressive systemic mastocytosis (SM) [3, 6]. Cladribine effectively reduces the mast cell burden in some patients with aggressive systemic mastocytosis (ASM) (slow-progressing type). Glucocorticoids have an inhibitory effect on mast cell growth. In systemic mastocytosis, glucocorticoids are usually used in combination with cytoreductive drugs and polychemotherapy. These drugs have a potential risk for disease progression and development of secondary leukemia; thus, they should be administered only to patients with "C" findings (Table 4.4.2) [11] due to impaired organ function caused by mast cell infiltration.

Table 4.4.2 "B" and "C" findings in systemic mastocytosis

"B" findings
Bone marrow biopsy showing >30% infiltration by mast cells (focal, dense aggregates) and/or serum total tryptase levels >200 ng/mL
Signs of dysplasia or myeloproliferation in the nonmast cell lineage, but insufficient criteria for definitive diagnosis of a hematopoietic neoplasm by WHO, with normal or only slightly abnormal blood counts
Hepatomegaly without impairment of liver function, and/or palpable splenomegaly without hypersplenism, and/or palpable or visceral lymphadenopathy
"C" findings
Bone marrow dysfunction manifested by one or more cytopenia (absolute neutrophil count <1,000/μL, or hemoglobin <10 g/dL, or platelets <100,000/μL), but no frank nonmast cell hematopoietic malignancy
Palpable hepatomegaly with impairment of liver function, ascites, and/or portal hypertension
Skeletal involvement with large-sized osteolysis and/or pathological fractures
Palpable splenomegaly with hypersplenism
Malabsorption with weight loss due to GI mast cell infiltrates

1. Indolent systemic mastocytosis (ISM)

In ISM, cytoreductive therapy is not usually required because it exhibits a prolonged clinical course. In smoldering SM, if clinical and laboratory signs suggest significant proliferation of neoplastic mastocytes, cytoreductive therapy is considered.

2. Aggressive systemic mastocytosis (ASM)

Although no curative therapy is available for this group of patients, cytoreductive agents are the mainstay of therapy. For patients who do not respond to INF-α, polychemotherapy or bone marrow transplantation is considered. Patients with mast cell leukemia (MCL) have been treated with chemotherapy regimens similar to those employed in patients with acute myeloid leukemia [14].

In patients with systemic mastocytosis with associated clonal hematologic nonmast cell lineage disease (SM-AHNMD), treatment plans for the SM and for the AHNMD should be established separately. When splenomegaly and resulting thrombocytopenia prohibit performing treatment, splenectomy may be considered [4].

4.4.2.4 Molecularly Targeted Drugs

Recent investigation showed that gain-of-functional mutations in the Kit proto-oncogene resulted in ligand-independent constitutive activation of Kit signaling, leading to uncontrolled mast cell proliferation. More than 80% of SM patients carry the Kit D816V mutation, and other Kit mutations were reported in sporadic cases of SM. New drugs that inhibit this target have been developed and some have entered clinical trials. Imatinib is an inhibitor of various protein kinases, including Kit, and has been employed to treat gastrointestinal stromal tumors and myeloid leukemia. However, imatinib failed to inhibit the growth of mast cells from patients with the Kit D816V mutation, because the site of the mutation interfered with the binding of the drug to the enzymatic site of Kit. Recently, a novel point mutation within the Kit transmembrane domain, F522C was identified in a patient with SM. After therapy with imatinib, the patient showed dramatic improvement in mast cell burden and clinical symptoms [1]. With regard to the D816V mutation, the potential efficacy of PKC412 has been reported [5, 10].

4.4.3 Therapy of Cutaneous Angiosarcoma

4.4.3.1 Surgery

Radical surgical excision of the tumor is the *conditio sine qua non* in the treatment of every angiosarcoma; however, the histological extension of the tumor often exceeds the clinically recognizable size. Preoperative magnetic resonance imaging can be helpful in quantifying the infiltrative growth, and the execution of (punch) biopsies all around the optically evident lesion can bring more clues about tangential spreading. Unfortunately, even with accurate preoperative local staging and extensive radical ablation, surgical margins are too often not tumor-free. A study by Pawlik et al. [6] demonstrated that intraoperative frozen sectioning is not a reliable tool, with a sensitivity of 64.7%, a positive predictive value of 100%, but a poor negative predictive value of 33%. Wound healing should be achieved with primary suture or, in cases of larger defects, using mesh grafts; rotation flaps or other plastic surgery techniques should be avoided because of the consequent diagnostic and therapeutic difficulties in cases of local recurrence.

4.4.3.2 Radiotherapy

Usually, angiosarcomas respond very well to radiation. Mark et al. [16] analyzed a large series of patients with cutaneous and extracutaneous angiosarcoma, reporting a significantly better 5-year disease-free-survival in patients receiving surgery and radiotherapy (43%) than patients undergoing surgery alone or in combination with adjuvant chemotherapy as a first-line treatment (17%). Thus, aggressive postsurgical adjuvant radiation is strongly recommended, with wide margins and a cumulative dose of 55–75 Gy (e.g., 2–3 Gy per

fraction, 5 days per week, over 5–8 weeks). Radiotherapy can also represent a palliative alternative in patients with inoperable disease and/or those refusing radical, disfiguring surgery.

4.4.3.3 Chemotherapy

Chemotherapy is reported in the literature as a neoadjuvant option, but mostly as a palliative treatment in cases of nonresectable or metastatic angiosarcoma. Many agents have been described to lead to partial or complete response, namely methotrexate, ifosfamide, dacarbazine, and cisplatin. The most positive results have been demonstrated with two substances: pegylated liposomal doxorubicin and paclitaxel (or docetaxel).

- Pegylated liposomal doxorubicin (Caelyx®) mostly shows high effectiveness against soft tissue sarcomas and is highly active in Kaposi's sarcoma as well as angiosarcoma. It acts by interfering with DNA and RNA synthesis in tumor cells and by interacting with the cytochrome P-450 system, thus producing intracellular toxic superoxides. Encapsulation in pegylated liposomes ensures neoplastic tissue concentrations three times higher than in plasma. Extravasation at disease sites is facilitated and circulation time is significantly prolonged, allowing for lower plasma peak concentrations and leading to reduced cardiotoxicity and nephrotoxicity. Pegylated liposomal doxorubicin is administered intravenously with two alternative schemes, 50 mg/m^2 every 4 weeks or 20 mg/m^2 every week. Both schemes have shown comparable results, with some case reports showing complete remission of both primary tumors and lymph node metastases, while larger series indicate progression-free survival between 3.7 and 6 months.

- Taxanes mostly have limited activity in soft tissue sarcomas, but, surprisingly, they have proven to be highly active against angiosarcoma. Paclitaxel (Taxol®) demonstrates antimitotic activity by inhibiting microtubular depolymerization and dynamic reorganization, both necessary for interphase and other steps of mitosis. Paclitaxel is administered as a continuous infusion; many treatment protocols have been proposed, ranging from 250 mg/m^2 over 24 h every 3 weeks to 80 mg/m^2 over 1 h on a weekly basis. In a well documented study by Skubitz and Haddad [15], paclitaxel was administered 140 mg/m^2 over 7 days every 4 weeks, with 5 out of the 8 patients showing major responses (3 partial responses, 2 complete responses). The same study reported progression-free survival between 2 and 20 months. A recent study by Nagano et al. [7] demonstrated that another taxane, docetaxel

(Taxotere®, administered 25 mg/m² as an infusion over 1 h every week), showed comparable results, with 6 out of the 9 treated patients having major responses (4 partial responses, 2 complete responses) and an average progression-free survival of 9.5 months.

- Other, recently investigated regimens include Anti-VEGF-antibodies like Bevacizumab (Avastin®), tyrosine kinase inhibitors such as Imatinib (Glivec®), and the RAF-kinase inhibitor Sorafenib (Nexavar®), which also possesses antiproliferative and antiangiogenic characteristics, inhibiting VEGFR-2 and -3. Presently, knowledge of angiosarcoma treatment with these substances is limited to isolated cases.

4.4.3.4 Immunotherapy

Recent advances in angiosarcoma therapy include the use of interferon-α (intravenous or intralesional) to potentiate the effects of pegylated liposomal doxorubicin and other classical chemotherapeutics. Interleukin-2 could represent a valid treatment alternative in the near future; IL-2 activates natural killer (NK) cells, induces inflammatory cytokines and cytotoxic T-cells, and also exhibits a direct effect on tumor cells. In 2005, Inaba et al. [2] reported a complete remission in a patient with angiosarcoma treated with radiotherapy and a combination of recombinant human IL-2 and OK-432, a penicillin- and heat-inactivated lyophilized powder of a *Streptococcus pyogenes* A3 substrain which boosts the inflammatory response on IL-2 by activating Toll-like receptor 4, thus stimulating the production of IL-12, interferon-γ, and TNF-α by dendritic cells. IL-12 itself could be an interesting therapeutic option thanks to its antiangiogenetic and immune-stimulating characteristics, but further preclinical trials in this direction are still needed.

4.4.4 Therapy of Kaposi Sarcoma

Nagwa M. Elwan

Both the clinical presentation and disease progression of Kaposi sarcoma (KS) are variable, ranging from a localized, solitary lesion up to disseminated cutaneous lesions with or without multicentric lesions affecting internal organs. Accordingly, different therapeutic modalities have been proposed to fit the variable clinical presentations and stages of KS. In spite of all these therapeutic modalities, a challenge still remains regarding complete remission of the disease.

4.4.4.1 Local Therapy of KS

4.4.4.1.1 Surgical Excision

Surgical excision may be considered in cases of localized nodular lesion of KS and to alleviate severe affection of the organs such as the extremities or gut [45].

4.4.4.1.2 Cryotherapy

Cryotherapy can be considered as a local therapy for various cutaneous forms of KS, but the lesions tend to recur after weeks or months due to the deep localization of KS lesions [47].

4.4.4.1.3 Laser Therapy

Laser therapy may be used in early-stage disease confined to the skin or mucosa with a favorable response, using 585-nm pulsed dye laser or high energy pulsed carbon dioxide laser [12, 33].

4.4.4.1.4 Radiotherapy

Radiotherapy may be considered a therapeutic option in patients with single lesions, usually localized on the skin, especially the feet, or mucosa [22, 38]. In a study conducted in 36 patients affected by epidemic KS localized on the feet, 80% complete remission was achieved after radiotherapy, but the side effects of radiotherapy often caused patients to stop the treatment [22]. Electron-beam radiotherapy, which has limited penetration beyond the dermis, may be a good modality for superficial lesions. Deeper or unresponsive KS may be treated using standard nonelectron beam radiation. Radiotherapy may be more effective on new rather than chronic lesions and may provide local control in patients with AIDS- related KS [40]. Hypofractionated radiation therapy was composed of a conventional fractionation regimen in the treatment of epidemic KS, but equivalent results in terms of treatment response and recurrence were reported [42].

4.4.4.1.5 Intralesional Chemotherapy

Intralesional chemotherapy is indicated for KS confined to the skin or mucosa. Intralesional vinblastine and vincristine have been reported to result in complete remission (CR) in 60–88% of AIDS – associated KS as well as other forms of KS. Recurrences may occur in 40% of patients within 4–6 months. Side effects include postinflammatory hyperpigmentation, pain, and transient mononeuropathy when injected near nerves [8, 47].

4.4.4.1.6 Local Immunotherapy

Topical Imiquimod 5% Cream

Topical imiquimod is an immune response modifier capable of inducing interferon-alfa secretion in situ and regression of vascular neoplasms including those of KS [4]. In a study of 17 patients with classic and endemic KS treated with topical imiquimod 5% cream for their HIV negative skin lesions, imiquimod 5% cream demonstrated antitumor activity in about half of the patients and was generally well tolerated [11]. It may also be beneficial in the management of cutaneous AIDS- related KS [36].

Intralesional Interferon-Alfa (INF- α)

Intralesional INF- α showed complete or partial remission rates of 20% and 70%, respectively, in ten patients with classic sporadic KS, injected with three million u INF- α three times per week for 1 month and variable doses for an additional month [43]. Also, complete or partial remission was reported in 85% of the lesions in 14 patients with AIDS associated KS receiving systemic therapy with azidothymidine (AZT) combined with intralesional INF- α [17].

Intralesional Tumor Necrosis Factor- Alfa (TNF- α)

TNF – α has antiangiogenic effect, which in one study resulted in a clinical response in 15 of 16 patients with AIDS – associated KS but was accompanied with severe side effects such as fever, rigors, pain, nausea, and vomiting [24].

Topical Retinoids

Topical 0.1% alitretinoin gel was approved by the FDA in 1999 for the treatment of localized cutaneous KS. This naturally occurring endogenous retinoid inhibits KS cell proliferation by binding to retinoid receptors. It should be applied generously to the affected cutaneous lesions twice a day initially, increasing up to 4 times a day [21].

Other trials, including the treatment of classical Kaposi sarcoma with a nicotine dermal patch, showed no demonstrable effect on nodular KS lesions or HHV-8 levels [20]. On the other hand, intralesional human chorionic gonadotropin was reported to be effective in the treatment of KS [41].

4.4.4.2 Systemic Therapy of KS

4.4.4.2.1 Systemic Chemotherapy

Chemotherapeutic agents are often reserved for disseminated KS. They attack both cutaneous and visceral KS lesions, inhibiting cell growth and proliferation. Combination chemotherapy is indicated for disseminated aggressive KS [15].

Vinblastine is an important vinca alkaloid. Systemic vinblastine 3.5–10 mg intravenously (IV) weekly with, at times, one intralesional injection, is mostly used in cases of disseminated classic KS and AIDS–related KS [44]. Vinblastine 0.1 mg/kg IV alternating with vincristine 2 mg IV every week can also be beneficial, especially in patients with AIDS-KS, but leukopenia and opportunistic infections may limit its use [25]. The combination of vinblastine and bleomycin is recommended as a first-line combination chemotherapy for advanced classic KS, as it achieves a high rate of objective responses without considerable toxicity [9].

Etoposide is an inhibitor of the enzyme topoisomerase II. It has been used in the treatment of a wide variety of neoplasms including KS. Its current therapeutic use is limited by myelosuppression, particularly neutropenia [27].

Liposomal anthracyclines are the best option for most patients with disseminated AIDS-related KS. They include pegylated liposomal doxorubicin (PLD), daunorubicin citrate liposome (DNX), and nonpegylated liposomal doxorubicin (NPLD) [16]. In general, PLD treatment was well tolerated with no toxic deaths, but neutropenia and thrombocytopenia have been reported [15].

Toxanes (paclitaxel and docetaxel) are microtubule-stabilizing agents that have demonstrated effectiveness against KS associated with AIDS. If multiple chemotherapeutic agents or liposomal anthracyclines fail, taxanes should be considered. Docetaxel is a new chemotherapeutic option for the treatment of advanced- stage KS. It is well tolerated; neutropenia but no neutropenic fever has been reported [10, 31].

4.4.4.2.2 Systemic Immunotherapy

The efficacy of immunotherapy may often depend upon the pretreatment immune status of the patient, specifically the degree of reduction in the helper-inducer T cell (T4) sub-population [5]. *Interferon – alfa* (INF- α) is a protein product manufactured by recombinant DNA technology [26]. It induces antitumor activity through direct inhibition of KS cell proliferation and nodulation of host immune response. It is approved by the FDA for systemic administration in KS [2]. Contraindications include autoimmune hepatitis and hypersensitivity to mouse immunoglobulin G, egg protein, or neomycin. Cimetidine may increase its antitumor effects, while zidovudine and vinblastine may increase its toxicity. Severe side effects may occur such as chills, fever, fatigue, and depression. In spite of the barriers limiting its use in AIDS- associated KS, including its adverse effects and the decrease in KS incidence among HIV–infected patients due to highly active antiretroviral therapy (HAART), IFN- α has proven to be one of the more effective agents in the treatment of KS, inducing sustained and sometimes dramatic tumor regression. The possibility of using IFN in combination with other pathogenesis-directed agents remains [28].

Thalidomide is an immunomodulating agent that has been noted to have anticancer activity. Two recent studies have reported encouraging results with the use of thalidomide in non- AIDS- related KS, but grade I sensory neuropathy and vertigo were reported as side effects [6, 37].

Vascular endothelial growth factor (VEGF) type-2 receptor inhibitor was reported to induce disease regression in patients with AIDS-related KS [3]. *Sirolimus* is a new immunosuppressive agent that also acts as a VEGF inhibitor, providing prospective therapeutic benefits and possible prevention of KS [23, 39].

Interleukin- 12 (IL-12) activities against KS has been reported. It enhances type I immunity, induces production of IFN-gamma, and mediates antiangiogenic effects [46]. KS treatment trials included new matrix metalloproteinase – 2 inhibitors, such as tetracycline analogs without antibiotic activity [14], green tea flavonoids [18], and IL-4 receptor – directed cytotoxin [5].

4.4.4.2.3 Antiangiogenic Therapy

A novel antiangiogenic systemic therapy consisting of the biomodulator pioglitazone hydrochloride and rofecoxib combined with trofosfamide has recently been reported for the treatment of endemic KS, with no significant toxic effects. It has the potential to become a cheap, practical, and feasible alternative treatment for endemic KS [13].

4.4.4.2.4 Anti-HHV-8 Drugs

Antiviral drugs may play a role in the prevention and treatment of KSHV- associated disease. HHV-8 is quite sensitive to cidofovir, moderately sensitive to foscarnet and ganciclovir, and relatively unaffected by acyclovir [19]. Complete clearing of cutaneous KS associated with cidofovir treatment has been reported [34], but another pilot study showed conflicting results [32].

4.4.4.2.5 Highly Active Antiretroviral Therapy (HAART)

In some patients, AIDS-KS may resolve clinically with the use of HAART. Protease inhibitor-based HAART favorably affects survival in HIV-associated advanced KS patients treated with chemotherapy [30]. In a few HIV sero-positive patients, HAART- induced improvements in immune status paradoxically resulted in cutaneous and / or visceral KS attributed to immune reconstitution inflammatory syndrome (IRIS). This flare may produce life-threatening visceral progression even if cutaneous nodules regress, leading to death from pulmonary KS [29]. Although HAART and chemotherapy showed significant clinical responses in KS, only half of the patients achieved complete resolution of the disease [35].

4.4.4.2.6 Systemic Retinoids

Systemic retinoids may be employed in the treatment of KS. Oral 9- *cis*-retinoic in capsule form has shown moderate efficacy in AIDS- related KS patients, but its toxic effects limit its therapeutic value [1]. IV liposomal tretinoin remains another option [7].

4.4.5 Treatment of Dermatofibrosarcoma Protuberans

Selma Ugurel and Lauren L. Lockwood

4.4.5.1 Surgical Therapy

The therapy of choice for operable DFSP is complete surgical excision. In the current literature, recommendations for margin size vary greatly between 1 and 5 cm. One centimeter margins are adequate for excision using micrographic surgery, as it allows for complete histological visualization of surgical margins (3D-Histology of paraffin sections). Increased recurrence rate is associated with conventional excision and histopathological evaluation, making larger *margins of 2–3 cm* reasonable in these cases [1]. Because of the subclinical undercutting growth pattern of DFSP, taking multiple measures to ensure adequate safety margins on all sides is necessary in many cases. Utilization of immunohistochemical techniques, particularly CD34-staining, can be helpful in the evaluation of the excised tumor's borders. Because problematic localizations are common, of the mostly stammnahen localization, particularly in the presternal region as well as on the head and neck, surgery as the first-line DFSP therapy can often be accompanied by extensive scarring.

4.4.5.2 Targeted Molecular Therapy

The development of a molecularly controlled DFSP therapy that disrupts the continuous, PDGF-controlled growth stimulus appears reasonable. In 2002, a patient with metastatic DFSP was treated with orally administrated *Tyrosinkinase-inhibitor Imatinib* (Glivec®), an inhibitor of PDGF-receptor as well as many other kinases; in this case, extensive remission of tumors was observed [2]. Imatinib has already proven highly effective in the treatment of other tumors, and it has also been approved for the treatment of chronic myelogenous leukemia (CML) and gastrointestinal stromal tumors (GIST). In two clinical studies of Imatinib, totaling 25 cases, an average *therapeutic response rate of approximately 70%* was observed in cases of extensive primary, locally recurring, and metastatic DFSP [3, 4]. Because of the lack of systemic treatment alternatives for these tumors, Imatinib was, based on these studies, approved for the treatment of nonoperable primary, locally recurring, and metastatic DFSP, using fast-track-procedures, by the Food and Drug Administration (FDA) in the US as well as in Europe (EMEA), at the end of 2006. Hereby, the rare DFSP became the first dermatological tumor to be approved for treatment with a signal transduction inhibitor.

Imatinib therapy can be used in large tumors to reduce preoperative tumor size, allowing for improved surgical results. A single dose of 600 mg Imatinib is considered to be reasonable for presurgical treatment. Generally, low doses do not produce the desired result, while higher doses clearly produce adverse side effects, particularly an intense itching rash. As early as 4 weeks, no later than 8, after initiation of the therapy, a decrease in lesion size should be detectable upon clinical inspection and palpation; for an objective assessment, MRI may be used. In the absence of a response to therapy after this period of time, a therapeutic result should no longer be awaited. With Imatinib treatment, destruction of tumor cells is revealed upon histological evaluation through a hyaline transformation within the tumor. Clinically, there is nearly no change in tumor size (Fig. 4.4.3); it is, however, because of the reduced vitality of the remaining tumor cells after Imatinib pretreatment that a small margin is sufficient for the final excision. Therefore, through pretreatment with Imatinib, less scarring of the tumor region can be achieved after surgery. Whether or not this procedure eventually results in higher rates of local recurrence must be explored in a clinical study. Also, successful Imatinib treatment of DFSP in infancy has been reported; treatment of an 18-month-old with widespread DFSP on the lower leg was effective and without complications [5]. Additionally, R1 and R2 resected DFSP, DFSP excised with narrow safety margins, and cases of multiple recurrences may be treated with Imatinib. However, there has been no approval for these indications; clinical trials are anticipated.

The adverse side effects of this treatment are of concern. These are common, but usually mild and include nausea, Völlegefühl, peripheral edema, fatigue, and rash. Even in cases of successful Imatinib treatment, surgical excision of residual tumors and histological confirmation of tumor cell destruction is recommended, to reduce chances of local recurrence. It is uncertain whether pretreatment with Imatinib could complicate later excision by fragmenting residual tumor. Primary as well as secondary *resistance to Imatinib* in DFSP has been reported [4, 6]. Molecular-diagnostic method of predicting potential resistance to Imatinib remains unknown.

Theoretically, there are other PDGFβ-signaling pathway inhibitors applicable to the treatment of DFSP such as, e.g., Sunitinib (Sutent®) and Dasatinib (Sprycel®), multikinase inhibitors which feature a high binding affinity to PDGFβ. Additionally, Nilotinib (Tasigna®), a successor of Imatinib, is approved for use in CML exhibiting secondary resistance to Imatinib. Clinical studies of these agents for the treatment of DFSP are anticipated. The application of these treatments in cases of secondary resistance to Imatinib is, however, conceivable.

Fig. 4.4.3 (a) Dermatofibrosarcoma protuberans on the right
shoulder of a 48-year-old man. It
presents as a plaque-like tumor
with multiple nodules up to 1 cm
in diameter presenting at the
lesion border. (b) State before
therapy, and (c) after 3 months of
treatment with Imatinib 600 mg/
day. The extent of the tumors
remains unchanged; the nodules
(*arrow*) are clearly remissive

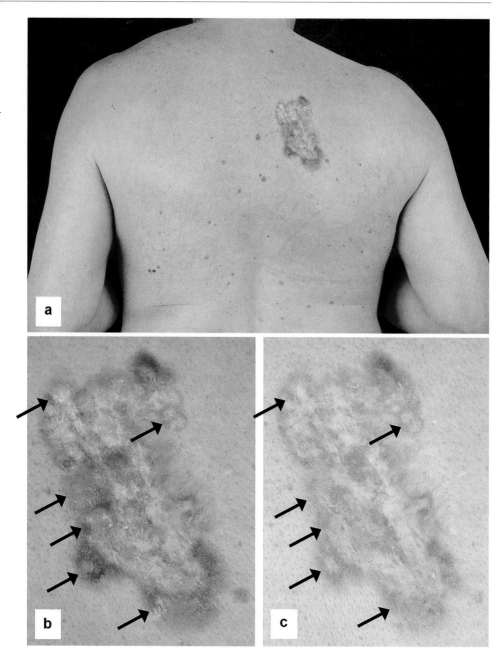

4.4.5.3 Other Therapeutic Possibilities

DFSP is considered to be, in principle, a radiation sensitive
tumor, so use of *Radiation* in inoperable primary tumors as
well as upon presentation of metastases seems reasonable
[7]. Never the less, adjuvant post operative irradiation is
generally not recommended. Retrospective analyses evidence a likely decrease in local recurrence with adjuvant
irradiation [8]; prospective studies, however, have not yet
been conducted. Irradiation therapy proved particularly
effective in cases of primary inoperable lesions, multiple
recurrence, R1- and R2-resected tumors or resection with
narrow margins, and in difficult localizations [9]. In cases
of curative intention, the target volume should encompass
the primary tumor localization with a safety margin of
approximately 3–5 cm with single doses of 2 Gy, fractionation of 5 per week and a cumulative dose from 60 to
70 Gy. In palliative treatment and dependent upon the
localization and sensitivity of surrounding structures to
radiation (e.g., eyes), one should aim for a cumulative dose
of 50 Gy.

In cases of inoperable distant DFSP metastases, particularly in internal organs, *Chemotherapy* may be considered in
addition to targeted molecular therapy. Unfortunately, to date
the reported results are very limited. The therapy schemata in
most cases orient themselves to the schemata for malignant
soft tissue sarcoma; a standardized therapy for metastatic
DFSP does not exist.

4.4.6 Merkel Cell Carcinoma – Therapy

Jürgen C. Becker and Selma Ugurel

Management of Merkel Cell Carcinoma (MCC) is controversial. To date there have been no controlled therapeutic trials in this disease. For primary tumors without indications of the presence of organ metastases, complete surgical excision is the basic therapy [1, 4, 6, 14].

Although the relationship between extent of surgery and locoregional control has not always proven correlative, a complete wide local excision with at least 2–3 cm margins along with the resection of any pathologic nodes when possible is mostly recommended [9, 22]. The safety margin seems necessary due to the otherwise high rate of local metastases which can be attributed to subclinical satellite metastases. In special locations where balancing the entire situation necessitates a smaller safety margin, this should be compensated by a complete histologic examination of the excision margins including immunohistology to detect CK 20 and perhaps a radiation therapy intervention [10, 28]. O'Connor et al. performed a retrospective analysis of 86 patients to assess the effectiveness of Mohs surgery [19]. Indeed, their analysis indicates that Mohs surgery with postoperative radiation therapy substantially reduces regional metastatic disease. When micrometastases are found in the sentinel lymph node, this should be followed by complete lymphadenectomy [7].

MCC are usually radiosensitive [2, 10]; however, most MCC cell lines are more radioresistant than other small cell carcinomas. Retrospective analyses show that the high local recurrence rate after R0 surgery of the primary tumor alone can be reduced significantly by a combined locoregional adjuvant radiation therapy (surgical scar with 3 cm safety margin as well as regional lymph node basin) [8, 21, 29]. These reports are in contrast to the study of Allen at al [1]. They reviewed 251 patients with MCC and did not find an improvement in local control with adjuvant radiation therapy. However, most clinical studies demonstrated better local control rates with adjuvant radiation therapy after surgery. A recent query of the SEER data on 1,665 cases of MCC from 1973 through 2002 from the National Cancer Institute showed that the median survival was 63 vs. 45 months for those treated with and without adjuvant radiation therapy, respectively [18]. Patients with larger tumors (>2 cm) benefited even more in terms of survival improvement. Thus, for primary MCCs and local recurrences an adjuvant radiation therapy of the tumor region and the regional lymphatic draining basin is recommended [4]. The required total dose is considered to be 50 Gy with a single dose of 2 Gy five times weekly. For MCC, in the stage of distant metastases radiation therapy is employed in a multimodal therapy concept in addition to surgical excision and/or systemic chemotherapy [2]. This approach, however, must be adapted to the individual case.

Traditionally, the role of chemotherapy in the management of MCC has been for palliation, and salvage of recurrent, locally advanced, or metastatic disease; even though MCC is considered a chemosensitive tumor, an evidence-based standardized chemotherapy does not yet exist.

Due to morphological similarities in the past, schemes that are established for small cell lung cancer have often been chosen; these include anthracyclines, antimetabolites, bleomycin, cyclophosphamide, etoposide, and platinum derivatives singly or in combination [2, 11, 20, 27]. With administration of these, in part, highly toxic regimens, relatively high remission rates of up to 70% are achieved, but due to the generally short duration of remission this does not lead to a significant increase in survival time. It appears that complete healing is not achieved in this stage of the disease. It is further significant that there is obviously no correlation between intensity of therapy and response. Therefore, systemic chemotherapy is indicated as a palliative measure when distant metastases are present, but, especially due to the high degree of toxicity of most chemotherapeutic agents for elderly patients (limited hepatic and renal function as well as hematopoiesis), it must be adapted to the individual case. Well-tolerated monotherapies include etoposide or anthracyclines, e. g, liposomal encapsulated doxorubicin [4].

The description of Merkel cell polyomavirus by Feng et al. and the confirmation of their findings by others render viral oncogenesis of MCC possible [3, 12, 13, 15]; thereby, new therapeutic avenues such as, e. g., use of interferons with their antiviral effects or the development of immuno-therapeutic strategies are opened [16]. For the latter, target antigens include not only viral proteins but also proteins induced by polyomaviruses such as survivin. To date, only sporadic case reports exist where immunotherapy agents have been used in MCC. Anecdotal case reports exist on the successful use of tumor necrosis factor α (TNF α), antiCD56 antibodies, or vaccines.

Imatinib is a tyrosine kinase inhibitor successfully used in the treatment of chronic myelogenous leukemia, gastrointestinal stroma tumors and dermatofibrosarcoma protuberans. The rationale for administering imatinib for MCC is based on the observation that the receptor tyrosine kinase Kit is often expressed in tumor tissue [24, 25], while normal Merkel cells are predominantly Kit-negative. Activating Kit mutations have indeed not yet been found in MCC. A recent study to test the clinical efficacy of imatinib therapy in advanced MCC had to be discontinued due to the lack of efficacy (Wolf Samlowski; personal communication). Oblimersen is an antisense oligonucleotide which inhibits the expression of the antiapoptotic protein bcl-2. A series of studies had demonstrated the expression of bcl-2 in MCC, and the successful treatment of MCC xenotransplants with bcl-2 antisense oligonucleotides in the naked mouse model [26] provides the most important rationale for a clinical study. First results that show good tolerability but no objective response as of yet were recently presented at a meeting of the AACR [23]. The recruitment of further patients was suspended. The role of treatment with somatostatin analogs per so or coupled to radio isotopes (octreotide, pasireotide) was reported controversial; however, only small case series or case reports have been reported so far [5, 17].

References

Histiocytoses

1. Satter, E.K., High, W.A.: Langerhans cell histiocytosis: a review of the current recommendations of the Histiocyte Society. Pediatr. Dermatol. **3**, 291–295 (2008)
2. Alston, R.D., Tatevossian, R.G., McNally, R.J., Kelsey, A., Birch, J.M., Eden, T.O.B.: Incidence and survival of childhood Langerhans cell histiocytosis in Northwest England from 1954 to 1998. Pediatr. Blood Cancer **48**, 555–560 (2007)
3. Arico, M., Girschikofsky, M., Genereau, T., Klersy, C., McClain, K., Grois, N., Emile, J.F., Lukina, E., DeJuki, E., Danesino, C.: Langerhans cell histiocytosis in adults. Report from the International Registry of the Histiocyte Society. Eur. J. Cancer **39**, 2341–2348 (2003)
4. Stockschlaeder, M., Sucker, C.: Adult Langerhans cell histiocytosis. Adult Langerhans cell histiocytosis. Eur. J. Haematol. **76**, 363–368 (2006)
5. Hoeger, P.H., Nanduri, V.R., Harper, J.I., Atherton, D.A., Preitchard, J.: Long term follow up of topical mustine treatment for cutaneous Langerhans cell histiocytosis. Arch. Dis. Child. **82**, 483–487 (2000)
6. Iwatsuki, K., Tsugiki, M., Yoshizawa, N., Takigawa, M., Yamada, M., Shamoto, M.: The effect of phtotherapies on cutaneous lesions of histiocytosis X in the elderly. Cancer **57**, 1931–1936 (1986)
7. Wu, J.J., Huang, D.B., Pang, K.R., Hsu, S., Tyring, S.K.: Thalidomide: dermatological indications, mechanisms of action and side-effects. Br. J. Dermatol. **153**, 254–273 (2005)
8. Minkov, M., Grois, N., Heitger, A., Potschger, U., Westermeier, T., Gadner, H.: Treatment of multisystem Langerhans cell histiocytosis. Results of the DAL-HX 83 and DAL-HX 90 studies. DAL-HX Study Group. Klin. Pädiatr. **212**, 139–144 (2000)
9. Gadner, H., Grois, N., Arico, M., Society, H., et al.: A randomized trial of treatment for multisystem Langerhans' cell histiocytosis. J. Pediatr. **138**, 728–734 (2001)
10. Morimoto, A., Ikushima, S., Kinugawa, N., Japan Langerhans Cell Histiocytosis Study Group: Improved outcome in the treatment of pediatric multifocal Langerhans cell histiocytosis. Results from the Japan Langerhans Cell Histiocytosis Study Group-96 protocol stisy. Cancer **107**, 613–619 (2006)
11. Weitzman, S., Wayne, A.S., Arceci, R., Lipton, J.M., Whitlock, J.A., Rossi, G.D., Society, H.: Nucleoside analogues in the therapy of Langerhans cell histiocytosis: a Survey of Members of the Histiocyte Society and Review of the Literature. Med. Pediatr. Oncol. **33**, 476–481 (1999)
12. Janssen, D., Harms, D.: Juvenile xanthogranuloma in childhood and adolescence: a clinicopathologic study of 129 patients from the Kiel Pediatric Tumor Registry. Am. J. Surg. Pathol. **29**, 21–28 (2005)
13. Freyer, D.R., Kennedy, R., Bostrom, B.C., Kohut, G., Dehner, L.P.: Juvenile xanthogranuloma: Forms of systemic disease and their clinical implications. J. Pediatr. **129**, 227–237 (1996)
14. Stover, D.G., Alapati, S., Regueira, O., Tumer, C., Whitlock, J.A.: Treatment of juvenile xanthogranuloma. Pediatr. Blood Cancer **51**, 130–133 (2008)
15. Caputo, R., Marzano, A.V., Passoni, E., Berti, E.: Unsual varinats of non-Langerhans cell histiocytosis. J. Am. Acad. Dermatol. **57**, 1031–1045 (2007)
16. Veyssier-Belot, C., Cacoub, P., Caparros-Lefebvre, D., Wechsler, J., Brun, B., Remy, M., et al.: Erdheim-Chester disease: clinical and radiologic characteristics of 59 cases. Medicine (Baltimore) **75**, 157–169 (1996)
17. Newman, B., Hu, W., Nigro, K., Gilliam, A.C.: Aggressive histiocytic disorders that can involve the skin. J. Am. Acad. Dermatol. **56**, 302–316 (2007)
18. Wang, K.H., Chen, W.Y., Liu, H.N., Huang, C.C., Lee, W.R., Hu, C.H.: Cutaneous Rosa-Dorfman disease: clinicopathological profiles, spectrum and evolution of 21 lesions in six patients. Br. J. Dermatol. **154**, 277–286 (2006)

Mastocytosis

1. Akin, C., Fumo, G., Yavuz, A.S., et al.: A novel form of mastocytosis associated with a transmembrane c-kit mutation and response to imatinib. Blood **103**, 3222–3225 (2004)
2. Barton, J., Lavker, R.M., Schechter, N.M., et al.: Treatment of urticaria pigmentosa with corticosteroids. Arch. Dermatol. **121**, 1516–1523 (1985)
3. Casassus, P., Caillat-Vigneron, N., Martin, A., et al.: Treatment of adult systemic mastocytosis with interferon-alpha: results of a multicentre phase II trial on 20 patients. Br. J. Haematol. **119**, 1090–1097 (2002)
4. Friedman, B., Darling, G., Norton, J., et al.: Splenectomy in the management of systemic mast cell disease. Surgery **107**, 94–100 (1990)
5. Gleixner, K.V., Mayerhofer, M., Aichberger, K.J., et al.: PKC412 inhibits in vitro growth of neoplastic human mast cells expressing the D816V-mutated variant of KIT: comparison with AMN107, imatinib, and cladribine (2CdA) and evaluation of cooperative drug effects. Blood **107**, 752–759 (2006)
6. Hauswirth, A.W., Simonitsch-Klupp, I., Uffmann, M., et al.: Response to therapy with interferon alpha-2b and prednisolone in aggressive systemic mastocytosis: report of five cases and review of the literature. Leuk. Res. **28**, 249–257 (2004)
7. Horny, H.P., Sotlar, K., Valent, P.: Mastocytosis: state of the art. Pathobiology **74**, 121–132 (2007)
8. Marone, G., Spadaro, G., Granata, F., et al.: Treatment of mastocytosis: pharmacologic basis and current concepts. Leuk. Res. **25**, 583–594 (2001)
9. Roberts 2nd, L.J., Fields, J.P., Oates, J.A.: Mastocytosis without urticaria pigmentosa: a frequently unrecognized cause of recurrent syncope. Trans. Assoc. Am. Physicians **95**, 36–41 (1982)
10. Shah, N.P., Lee, F.Y., Luo, R., et al.: Dasatinib (BMS-354825) inhibits KITD816V, an imatinib-resistant activating mutation that triggers neoplastic growth in most patients with systemic mastocytosis. Blood **108**, 286–291 (2006)
11. Valent, P., Horny, H.P., Li, C.Y., et al.: Mastocytosis (mast cell disease). In: Jaffe, E.S., Harris, N.L., Stein, H. (eds.) World Health Organization Classification of Tumors, pp. 291–302. IARC, Geneva (2001)
12. Valent, P., Akin, C., Sperr, W.R., et al.: Diagnosis and treatment of systemic mastocytosis: state of the art. Br. J. Haematol. **122**, 695–717 (2003)
13. Vella Briffa, D., Eady, R.A., James, M.P., et al.: Photochemotherapy (PUVA) in the treatment of urticaria pigmentosa. Br. J. Dermatol. **109**, 67–75 (1983)
14. Worobec, A.S.: Treatment of systemic mast cell disorders. Hematol. Oncol. Clin. North Am. **14**, 659–687 (2000)

Therapy of Cutaneous Angiosarcoma

1. Maddox, J.C., Evans, H.L.: Angiosarcoma of skin and soft tissue: a study of forty-four cases. Cancer **48**(8), 1907–1921 (1981)
2. Inaba, T., Yamanaka, K., Asahi, K., Omoto, Y., Isoda, K., Hurwitz, D., Kupper, T.S., Mizutani, H.: Complete remission in a patient with angiosarcoma by the combination of OK-432, rhIL-2, and radiotherapy. Eur. J. Dermatol. **15**(5), 411–413 (2005)
3. Cannavò, S.P., Lentini, M., Magliolo, E., Guarneri, C.: Cutaneous angiosarcoma of the face. JEADV **17**, 594–595 (2003)
4. Eiling, S., Lischner, S., Busch, J.-O., Rothaupt, D., Christophers, E., Hauschild, A.: Complete remission of a radio-resistant cutaneous angiosarcoma of the scalp by systemic treatment with liposomal doxorubicin. Br. J. Dermatol. **147**, 150–153 (2002)
5. Folpe, A.L., Veikkola, T., Valtola, R., Weiss, S.W.: Vascular endothelial growth factor receptor-3 (VEGFR-3): a marker of vascular tumors with presumed lymphatic differentiation, including Kaposi's sarcoma, Kaposiform and dabska-type hemangioendotheliomas, and a subset of angiosarcomas. Mod. Pathol. **13**(2), 180–185 (2000)
6. Pawlik, T.M., Paulino, A.F., Mcginn, C.J., Baker, L.H., Cohen, D.S., Morris, J.S., Rees, R., Sondak, V.K.: Cutaneous angiosarcoma of the scalp. Cancer **98**, 1716–1726 (2003)
7. Nagano, T., Yamada, Y., Ikeda, T., Kanki, H., Kamo, T., Nishigori, C.: Docetaxel: a therapeutic option in the treatment of cutaneous angiosarcoma. Cancer **110**, 648–651 (2007)
8. Pestoni, C., Paredes-Suarez, C., Peteiro, C., Toribio, J.: Early detection of cutaneous angiosarcoma of the face and scalp and tratment with paclitaxel. J. Eur. Acad. Dermatol. Venereol. **19**, 357–359 (2005)
9. Morgan, M.B., Swann, M., Somach, S., Eng, W., Smoller, B.: Cutaneous angiosarcoma: a case series with prognostic correlation. J. Am. Acad. Dermatol. **50**, 867–874 (2004)
10. Mendenhall, W.M., Mendenhall, C.M., Werning, J.W., Reith, J.D., Mendenhall, N.P.: Cutaneous angiosarcoma. Am. J. Clin. Oncol. **29**, 524–528 (2006)
11. Fayette, J., et al.: Angiosarcomas, a heterogeneous group of sarcomas with specific behavior depending on primary site: a retrospective study of 161 cases. Ann. Oncol. **18**(12), 2030–2036 (2007)
12. Vogt, T.: Angiosarkom. Hautarzt **59**, 237–251 (2008)
13. DeMartelaere, S.L., Roberts, D., Burgess, M.A., et al.: Neoadjuvant Chemotherapy-specific and overall treatment outcomes in patients with cutaneous angiosarcoma of the face with periorbital involvement. Head Neck **30**(5), 639–646 (2008)
14. Abraham, J.A., Hornicek, F.J., Kaufman, A.M., Harmon, D.C., et al.: Treatment and outcome of 82 patients with angiosarcoma. Ann. Surg. Oncol. **14**(6), 1953–1967 (2007). Epub 2007 Mar 14
15. Skubitz, K.M., Haddad, P.A.: Paclitaxel and pegylated-liposomal Doxorubicin are both active in angiosarcoma. Cancer **104**(2), 361–366 (2005)
16. Mark, R.J., Poen, J.C., Tran, L.M., Fu, Y.S., Juillard, G.F.: Angiosarcoma. A report of 67 patients and a review of the literature. Cancer **77**(11), 2400–2406 (1996)
17. Fury, M.G., Antonescu, C.R., Van Zee, K.J., Brennan, M.F., Maki, R.G.: A 14-year retrospective review of angiosarcoma: clinical characteristics, prognostic factors, and treatment outcomes with surgery and chemotherapy. Cancer J. **11**(3), 241–247 (2005)

Therapy of Kaposi Sarcoma

1. Aboulafia, D.M., Norris, D., Henry, D., et al.: 9-cis-retinoic acid capsules in the treatment of AIDS-related Kaposi sarcoma: results of a phase 2 multicenter clinical trial. Arch. Dermatol. **139**, 178–186 (2003)
2. Aldenhoven, M., Barlo, N.P., Sanders, C.J.: Therapeutic strategies for epidemic Kaposi's sarcoma. Int. J. STD AIDS **17**, 571–578 (2006)
3. Arastéh, K., Hannah, A.: The role of vascular endothelial growth factor (VEGF) in AIDS-related Kaposi's sarcoma. Oncologist **5 suppl 1**, 28–31 (2000)
4. Babel, N., Eibl, N., Ulrich, C., et al.: Development of Kaposi's sarcoma under sirolimus-based immunosuppression and successful treatment with imiquimod. Transpl. Infect. Dis. **10**, 59–62 (2008)
5. Bagnato, A., Rosanò, L.: The endothelin axis in cancer. Int. J. Biochem. Cell Biol. **40**, 1443–1451 (2008)
6. Ben M'barek, L., Fardet, L., Mebazaa, A., et al.: A retrospective analysis of thalidomide therapy in non-HIV-related Kaposi's sarcoma. Dermatology **215**, 202–205 (2007)
7. Bernstein, Z.P., Chanan-Khan, A., Miller, K.C., et al.: A multicenter phase II study of the intravenous administration of liposomal tretinoin in patients with acquired immunodeficiency syndrome-associated Kaposi's sarcoma. Cancer **95**, 2555–2561 (2002)
8. Boudreaux, A.A., Smith, L.L., Cosby, C.D., et al.: Intralesional vinblastine for cutaneous Kaposi's sarcoma associated with acquired immunodeficiency syndrome. A clinical trial to evaluate efficacy and discomfort associated with infection. J. Am. Acad. Dermatol. **28**, 61–65 (1993)
9. Brambilla, L., Miedico, A., Ferrucci, S., et al.: Combination of vinblastine and bleomycin as first line therapy in advanced classic Kaposi's sarcoma. J. Eur. Acad. Dermatol. Venereol. **20**, 1090–1094 (2006)
10. Brambilla, L., Romanelli, A., Bellinvia, M., et al.: Weekly paclitaxel for advanced aggressive classic Kaposi sarcoma: experience in 17 cases. Br. J. Dermatol. **158**, 1339–1344 (2008)
11. Célestin Schartz, N.E., Chevret, S., Paz, C., et al.: Imiquimod 5% cream for treatment of HIV-negative Kaposi's sarcoma skin lesions: A phase I to II, open-label trial in 17 patients. J. Am. Acad. Dermatol. **58**, 585–591 (2008)
12. Chun, Y.S., Chang, S.N., Park, W.H.: A case of classical Kaposi's sarcoma of the penis showing a good response to high-energy pulsed carbon dioxide laser therapy. J. Dermatol. **26**, 240–243 (1999)
13. Coras, B., Hafner, C., Reichle, A., Hohenleutner, U., et al.: Antiangiogenic therapy with pioglitazone, rofecoxib, and trofosfamide in a patient with endemic kaposi sarcoma. Arch. Dermatol. **140**, 1504–1507 (2004)
14. Dezube, B.J., Krown, S.E., Lee, J.Y., et al.: Randomized phase II trial of matrix metalloproteinase inhibitor COL-3 in AIDS-related Kaposi's sarcoma: an AIDS Malignancy Consortium Study. J. Clin. Oncol. **24**, 1389–1394 (2006)
15. Di Lorenzo, G., Di Trolio, R., Montesarchio, V., et al.: Pegylated liposomal doxorubicin as second-line therapy in the treatment of patients with advanced classic Kaposi sarcoma: a retrospective study. Cancer **112**, 1147–1152 (2008)
16. Di Trolio, R., Di Lorenzo, G., Delfino, M., et al.: Role of pegylated lyposomal doxorubicin (PLD) in systemic Kaposi's sarcoma: a systematic review. Int. J. Immunopathol. Pharmacol. **19**, 253–263 (2006)
17. Dupuy, J., Price, M., Lynch, G., et al.: Intralesional interferon-alpha and zidovudine in epidemic Kaposi's sarcoma. J. Am. Acad. Dermatol. **28**, 966–972 (1993)
18. Garbisa, S., Sartor, L., Biggin, S., et al.: Tumor gelatinases and invasion inhibited by the green tea flavanol epigallocatechin-3-gallate. Cancer **91**, 822–832 (2001)
19. Glesby, M.J., Hoover, D.R., Weng, S., et al.: Use of antiherpes drugs and the risk of Kaposi's sarcoma: data from the Multicenter AIDS Cohort Study. J. Infect. Dis. **173**, 1477–1480 (1996)
20. Goedert, J.J., Scoppio, B.M., Pfeiffer, R., et al.: Treatment of classic Kaposi sarcoma with a nicotine dermal patch: a phase II clinical trial. J. Eur. Acad. Dermatol. Venereol. **22**, 1101–1109 (2008)
21. de González, Arriba A., Pérez-Gala, S., Goiriz-Valdés, R., et al.: Kaposi's sarcoma treated with topical alitretinoin. Actas Dermosifiliogr. **98**, 50–53 (2007)

22. Gressen, E.L., Rosenstock, J.G., Xie, Y., et al.: Palliative treatment of epidemic Kaposi sarcoma of the feet. Am. J. Clin. Oncol. **22**, 286–290 (1999)

23. Guenova, E., Metzler, G., Hoetzenecker, W., et al.: Classic Mediterranean Kaposi's sarcoma regression with sirolimus treatment. Arch. Dermatol. **144**, 692–693 (2008)

24. Kahn, J.O., Kaplan, L.D., Volberding, P.A., et al.: Intralesional recombinant tumor necrosis factor-alpha for AIDS-associated Kaposi's sarcoma: a randomized, double-blind trial. J. Acquir. Immune Defic. Syndr. **2**, 217–223 (1989)

25. Kaplan, L., Abrams, D., Volberding, P.: Treatment of Kaposi's sarcoma in acquired immunodeficiency syndrome with an alternating vincristine-vinblastine regimen. Cancer Treat. Rep. **70**, 1121–1122 (1986)

26. Kirkwood, J.: Cancer immunotherapy: the interferon-alpha experience. Semin. Oncol. **29**, 18–26 (2002)

27. Kobayashi, K., Ratain, M.J.: Pharmacodynamics and long-term toxicity of etoposide. Cancer Chemother. Pharmacol. **34**, 564–568 (1994)

28. Krown, S.E.: AIDS-associated Kaposi's sarcoma: is there still a role for interferon alfa? Cytokine Growth Factor Rev. **18**, 395–402 (2007)

29. Leidner, R.S., Aboulafia, D.M.: Recrudescent Kaposi's sarcoma after initiation of HAART: a manifestation of immune reconstitution syndrome. AIDS Patient Care STDs **19**, 635–644 (2005)

30. Leitch, H., Trudeau, M., Routy, J.P.: Effect of protease inhibitor-based highly active antiretroviral therapy on survival in HIV-associated advanced Kaposi's sarcoma patients treated with chemotherapy. HIV Clin. Trials **4**, 107–114 (2003)

31. Lim, S.T., Tupule, A., Espina, B.M., et al.: Weekly docetaxel is safe and effective in the treatment of advanced-stage acquired immunodeficiency syndrome-related Kaposi sarcoma. Cancer **103**, 417–421 (2005)

32. Little, R.F., Merced-Galindez, F., Staskus, K., et al.: A pilot study of cidofovir in patients with kaposi sarcoma. J. Infect. Dis. **187**, 149–153 (2003)

33. Marchell, N., Alster, T.S.: Successful treatment of cutaneous Kaposi's sarcoma by the 585-nm pulsed dye laser. Dermatol. Surg. **23**, 973–975 (1997)

34. Mazzi, R., Parisi, S.G., Sarmati, L., et al.: Efficacy of cidofovir on human herpesvirus 8 viraemia and Kaposi's sarcoma progression in two patients with AIDS. AIDS **15**, 2061–2062 (2001)

35. Nguyen, H.Q., Magaret, A.S., Kitahata, M.M., et al.: Persistent Kaposi sarcoma in the era of highly active antiretroviral therapy: characterizing the predictors of clinical response. AIDS **22**, 937–945 (2008)

36. Rosen, T.: Limited extent AIDS-related cutaneous Kaposi's sarcoma responsive to imiquimod 5% cream. Int. J. Dermatol. **45**, 854–856 (2006)

37. Rubegni, P., Sbano, P., De Aloe, G., et al.: Thalidomide in the treatment of Kaposi's sarcoma. Dermatology **215**, 240–244 (2007)

38. Ruszczak, Z., Stadler, R., Schwartz, R.A.: Kaposi's sarcoma limited to penis treated with cobalt-60 radiotherapy. J. Med. **27**, 211–220 (1996)

39. Saggar, S., Zeichner, J.A., Brown, T.T., et al.: Kaposi's sarcoma resolves after sirolimus therapy in a patient with pemphigus vulgaris. Arch. Dermatol. **144**, 654–657 (2008)

40. Schwartz, R.A., Micali, G., Nasca, M.R., et al.: Kaposi sarcoma: a continuing conundrum. J. Am. Acad. Dermatol. **59**, 179–206 (2008)

41. Simonart, T., Van Vooren, J.P., Meuris, S.: Treatment of Kaposi's sarcoma with human chorionic gonadotropin. Dermatology **204**, 330–333 (2002)

42. Singh, N.B., Lakier, R.H., Donde, B.: Hypofractionated radiation therapy in the treatment of epidemic Kaposi sarcoma - A prospective randomized trial. Radiother. Oncol. **88**, 211–216 (2008)

43. Trattner, A., Reizis, Z., David, M., et al.: The therapeutic effect of intralesional interferon in classical Kaposi's sarcoma. Br. J. Dermatol. **129**, 590–593 (1993)

44. Turk, H.M., Buyukberber, S., Camci, C., et al.: Chemotherapy of disseminated cutaneous classic Kaposi's sarcoma with vinblastine. J. Dermatol. **29**, 657–660 (2002)

45. Weintraub, C.M., Skudowitz, R.B.: Excision of 1, 674 classic Kaposi's sarcomas. S. Afr. J. Surg. **40**, 80 (2002)

46. Yarchoan, R., Pluda, J.M., Wyvill, K.M., et al.: Treatment of AIDS-related Kaposi's sarcoma with interleukin-12: rationale and preliminary evidence of clinical activity. Crit. Rev. Immunol. **27**, 401–414 (2007)

47. Zalla, M.J.: Kaposi's sarcoma. An Update. Dermatol. Surg. **22**, 274–287 (1996)

Treatment of Dermatofibrosarcoma Protuberans

1. Khatri, V.P., Galante, J.M., et al.: Dermatofibrosarcoma protuberans: reappraisal of wide local excision and impact of inadequate initial treatment. Ann. Surg. Oncol. **10**, 1118–1122 (2003)

2. Rubin, B.P., Schuetze, S.M., et al.: Molecular targeting of platelet-derived growth factor B by imatinib mesylate in a patient with metastatic dermatofibrosarcoma protuberans. J. Clin. Oncol. **20**, 3586–3591 (2002)

3. McArthur, G.A., Demetri, G.D., et al.: Molecular and clinical analysis of locally advanced dermatofibrosarcoma protuberans treated with imatinib: imatinib target exploration consortium study B2225. J. Clin. Oncol. **23**, 866–873 (2005)

4. Ugurel, S., Utikal, J., et al.: Imatinib in locally advanced dermatofibrosarcoma protuberans (DFSP): a phase II trial of the Dermatologic Cooperative Oncology Group (DeCOG). J. Clin. Oncol. **24**(Suppl), 535s (2006). Abstract 9561

5. Price, V.E., Fletcher, J.A., et al.: Imatinib mesylate: an attractive alternative in young children with large, surgically challenging dermatofibrosarcoma protuberans. Pediatr. Blood Cancer **44**, 511–515 (2005)

6. Maki, R.G., Awan, R.A., et al.: Differential sensitivity to imatinib of 2 patients with metastatic sarcoma arising from dermatofibrosarcoma protuberans. Int. J. Cancer **100**, 623–626 (2002)

7. Ballo, M.T., Zagars, G.K., et al.: The role of radiation therapy in the management of dermatofibrosarcoma protuberans. Int. J. Radiat. Oncol. Biol. Phys. **40**, 823–827 (1998)

8. Sun, L.M., Wang, C.J., et al.: Dermatofibrosarcoma protuberans: treatment results of 35 cases. Radiother. Oncol. **57**, 175–181 (2000)

9. Suit, H., Spiro, I., et al.: Radiation in management of patients with dermatofibrosarcoma protuberans. J. Clin. Oncol. **14**, 2365–2369 (1996)

Merkel Cell Carcinoma – Therapy

1. Allen, P.J., Bowne, W.B., Jaques, D.P., Brennan, M.F., Busam, K., Coit, D.G.: Merkel cell carcinoma: prognosis and treatment of patients from a single institution. J. Clin. Oncol. **23**, 2300–2309 (2005)

2. Becker, G., Bottke, D.: Potential of radiation therapy in the multimodal management of merkel cell carcinoma. Front. Radiat. Ther. Oncol. **39**, 87–95 (2006)

3. Becker, J.C., Houben, R., Ugurel, S., Trefzer, U., Pfohler, C., Schrama, D.: MC polyomavirus is frequently present in merkel cell carcinoma of european patients. J. Invest. Dermatol. **129**, 248–250 (2009)

4. Becker, J.C., Mauch, C., Kortmann, R.D., Keilholz, U., Bootz, F., Garbe, C., Hauschild, A., Moll, I.: Short German guidelines: merkel cell carcinoma. J. Dtsch. Dermatol. Ges. **6**(S1), 15–16 (2008)

5. Ben Shlomo, A., Melmed, S.: Pasireotide - a somatostatin analog for the potential treatment of acromegaly, neuroendocrine tumors and Cushing's disease. IDrugs **10**, 885–895 (2007)

6. Bichakjian, C.K., Lowe, L., Lao, C.D., Sandler, H.M., Bradford, C.R., Johnson, T.M., Wong, S.L.: Merkel cell carcinoma: critical review with guidelines for multidisciplinary management. Cancer **110**, 1–12 (2007)

7. Civantos, F.J., Moffat, F.L., Goodwin, W.J.: Lymphatic mapping and sentinel lymphadenectomy for 106 head and neck lesions: contrasts between oral cavity and cutaneous malignancy. Laryngoscope **112**, 1–15 (2006)

8. Clark, J.R., Veness, M.J., Gilbert, R., O'Brien, C.J., Gullane, P.J.: Merkel cell carcinoma of the head and neck: is adjuvant radiotherapy necessary? Head Neck **29**, 249–257 (2007)

9. Dancey, A.L., Rayatt, S.S., Soon, C., Ilchshyn, A., Brown, I., Srivastava, S.: Merkel cell carcinoma: a report of 34 cases and literature review. J. Plast. Reconstr. Aesthet. Surg. **59**, 1294–1299 (2006)

10. Decker, R.H., Wilson, L.D.: Role of radiotherapy in the management of merkel cell carcinoma of the skin. J. Natl. Compr. Canc. Netw. **4**, 713–718 (2006)

11. Eng, T.Y., Boersma, M.G., Fuller, C.D., Goytia, V., Jones III, W.E., Joyner, M., Nguyen, D.D.: A comprehensive review of the treatment of Merkel cell carcinoma. Am. J. Clin. Oncol. **30**, 624–636 (2007)

12. Feng, H., Shuda, M., Chang, Y., Moore, P.S.: Clonal integration of a polyomavirus in human Merkel cell carcinoma. Science **319**, 1096–1100 (2008)

13. Garneski, K.M., Warcola, A.H., Feng, Q., Kiviat, N.B., Leonard, J.H., Nghiem, P.: Merkel cell polyomavirus is more frequently present in North American than Australian Merkel cell carcinoma tumors. J. Invest. Dermatol. **129**, 246–248 (2008)

14. Henness, S., Vereecken, P.: Management of Merkel tumors: an evidence-based review. Curr. Opin. Oncol. **20**, 280–286 (2008)

15. Kassem, A., Schopflin, A., Diaz, C., Weyers, W., Stickeler, E., Werner, M., Zur, H.A.: Frequent detection of Merkel cell polyomavirus in human Merkel cell carcinomas and identification of a unique deletion in the VP1 gene. Cancer Res. **68**, 5009–5013 (2008)

16. Krasagakis, K., Kruger-Krasagakis, S., Tzanakakis, G.N., Darivianaki, K., Stathopoulos, E.N., Tosca, A.D.: Interferon-alpha inhibits proliferation and induces apoptosis of merkel cell carcinoma in vitro. Cancer Invest. **26**, 562–568 (2008)

17. Meier, G., Waldherr, C., Herrmann, R., Maecke, H., Mueller-Brand, J., Pless, M.: Successful targeted radiotherapy with 90Y-DOTATOC in a patient with Merkel cell carcinoma. A Case Report. Oncology **66**, 160–163 (2004)

18. Mojica, P., Smith, D., Ellenhorn, J.D.: Adjuvant radiation therapy is associated with improved survival in Merkel cell carcinoma of the skin. J. Clin. Oncol. **25**, 1043–1047 (2007)

19. O'Connor, W.J., Roenigk, R.K., Brodland, D.G.: Merkel cell carcinoma. Comparison of Mohs micrographic surgery and wide excision in eighty-six patients. Dermatol. Surg. **23**, 929–933 (1997)

20. Pectasides, D., Pectasides, M., Psyrri, A., Koumarianou, A., Xiros, N., Pectasides, E., Gaglia, A., Lianos, E., Papaxoinis, G., Lampadiari, V., Economopoulos, T.: Cisplatin-based chemotherapy for merkel cell carcinoma of the skin. Cancer Invest. **24**, 780–785 (2006)

21. Poulsen, M., Rischin, D., Walpole, E., Harvey, J., Mackintosh, J., Ainslie, J., Hamilton, C., Keller, J., Tripcony, L.: High-risk Merkel cell carcinoma of the skin treated with synchronous carboplatin/etoposide and radiation: a Trans-Tasman Radiation Oncology Group Study-TROG 96:07. J. Clin. Oncol. **21**, 4371–4376 (2003)

22. Senchenkov, A., Barnes, S.A., Moran, S.L.: Predictors of survival and recurrence in the surgical treatment of merkel cell carcinoma of the extremities. J. Surg. Oncol. **95**, 229–234 (2007)

23. Shah, M.H., Varker, K.A., Collamore, M., Zwiebel, J.A., Chung, K.Y., Coit, D., Kelsen, D.: Multicenter phase II trial of bcl-2 antisense therapy (Genasense®) in patients with advanced Merkel cell carcinoma. AACR abstract (2007)

24. Su, L.D., Fullen, D.R., Lowe, L., Uherova, P., Schnitzer, B., Valdez, R.: CD117 (KIT receptor) expression in Merkel cell carcinoma. Am. J. Dermatopathol. **24**, 289–293 (2002)

25. Swick, B.L., Ravdel, L., Fitzpatrick, J.E., Robinson, W.A.: Merkel cell carcinoma: evaluation of KIT (CD117) expression and ww to demonstrate activating mutations in the C-KIT proto-oncogene - implications for treatment with imatinib mesylate. J. Cutan. Pathol. **34**, 324–329 (2007)

26. Tai, P.: Merkel cell cancer: update on biology and treatment. Curr. Opin. Oncol. **20**, 196–200 (2008)

27. Tai, P.T., Yu, E., Winquist, E., Hammond, A., Stitt, L., Tonita, J., Gilchrist, J.: Chemotherapy in neuroendocrine/Merkel cell carcinoma of the skin: case series and review of 204 cases. J. Clin. Oncol. **18**, 2493–2499 (2000)

28. Thomas, C.J., Wood, G.C., Marks, V.J.: Mohs micrographic surgery in the treatment of rare aggressive cutaneous tumors: the Geisinger experience. Dermatol. Surg. **33**, 333–339 (2007)

29. Weller, K., Vetter-Kauzcok, C., Kähler, K., Hauschild, A., Eigentler, T., Pföhler, C., Neuber, K., Moll, I., Krause, M., Kneisel, L., Nashan, D., Thoelke, A., Letsch, B., Näher, H., Becker, J.C.: Umsetzung von Leitlinien bei seltenen Erkrankungen am Beispiel des Merkelzellkarzinoms [Guideline implementation in Merkel cell carcinoma: an example of a rare disease.]. Dtsch. Arztebl. **103**, 2791–2796 (2006)

Part **V**

Diagnostics

Dermoscopy

Isabel Kolm, Reinhard Dummer, and Ralph Peter Braun

5.1.1 Introduction

Because melanoma in advanced stages is still incurable, early detection is indispensable to reduce mortality. With the introduction of dermoscopy into the clinical practice, the diagnostic accuracy of pigmented skin lesions can be improved. Dermoscopy is a noninvasive diagnostic technique for the in vivo observation in dermatology. This technique enables the clinician to visualize pigmented structures of the epidermis, dermo–epidermal junction, and papillary dermis, which are not visible to the naked eye. The structures observed by dermoscopy correlate with histopathological findings. Dermoscopy opens a new dimension in the clinical morphology of pigmented skin lesions but diagnostic accuracy depends significantly on the experience of the examiner.

5.1.2 Physical Aspects

Light is either reflected, dispersed, or absorbed by the stratum corneum due to its refraction index and its optical density, which are different from that of air. Thus, deeper underlying structures cannot be adequately visualized. However, when various immersion liquids are used, they render the skin surface translucent and reduce the reflection, so that underlying structures are readily visible. The application of a glass plate flattens the skin surface and provides an even surface. Optical magnification is used for examination. Taken together, these optical means allow the visualization of certain epidermal, dermo–epidermal, and dermal structures.

I. Kolm, R. Dummer (✉) and R.P. Braun
Department of Dermatology, University Hospital of Zürich,
Gloriastrasse 31, 8091 Zürich,
Switzerland
e-mail: reinhard.dummer@usz.ch

5.1.3 Instrumentation for Dermoscopy

Dermoscopy requires optical magnification and liquid immersion. Specially designed handheld devices are commercially available (Dermatoscope Delta 20®, (Heine AG); DermoGenius Basic® (Biocam); Dermlite II pro HR® (3GenLLC)).

5.1.4 Dermoscopic Criteria

The use of dermoscopy allows the identification of many different structures and colors, not seen by the naked eye [1–5].

5.1.5 Colors

Colors play an important role in dermoscopy. Common colors are light brown, dark brown, black, blue, blue-gray, red, yellow, and white. The most important chromophore in melanocytic neoplasms is melanin. The color of melanin essentially depends on its localization in the skin. Melanin appears black in the stratum corneum and the upper epidermis, light to dark brown in the epidermis, gray to gray-blue in the papillary dermis, and steel blue in the reticular dermis.

5.1.6 Dermoscopic Structures

5.1.6.1 Pigment Network

The pigment network is a grid-like (honeycomb-like) network consisting of pigmented "lines" and hypopigmented "holes." The anatomic basis of the pigment network is melanin pigment either in keratinocytes or in melanocytes along the dermo–epidermal junction. The reticulation (network) represents the rete ridge pattern of the epidermis. The relatively hypomelanotic holes in the network correspond to tips

R. Dummer et al. (eds.), *Skin Cancer – A World-Wide Perspective*,
DOI: 10.1007/978-3-642-05072-5_5.1, © Springer-Verlag Berlin Heidelberg 2011

373

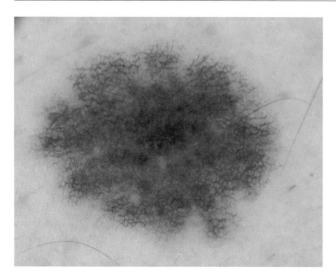

Fig. 5.1.1 Typical network pattern in a junctional nevus. Relatively uniform network, regularly meshed, homogeneous in color, and fading out at the periphery

of the dermal papillae and the overlying supra-papillary plates of the epidermis.

The pigment network can be either typical or atypical. A typical network is relatively uniform, regularly meshed, homogeneous in color, and usually thinning out at the periphery (Fig. 5.1.1). An atypical network is nonuniform, with darker and/or broadened lines and "holes" that are heterogeneous in area and shape. The lines are often hyperpigmented and may end abruptly at the periphery.

If the rete ridges are short or less pigmented the pigment network may not be visible. Areas devoid of any network (but without signs of regression) are called "structureless areas."

5.1.6.2 Dots

Dots are small, round structures of less than 0.1 mm in diameter which may be black, brown, gray, or blue-gray. Black dots are due to pigment accumulation in the stratum corneum and in the upper part of the epidermis. Brown dots represent focal melanin accumulations at the dermo–epidermal junction. Gray-blue granules are due to tiny melanin structures in the papillary dermis. Gray-blue or blue granules are due to loose melanin, fine melanin particles, or melanin "dust" in melanophages or free in the deep papillary or reticular dermis.

5.1.6.3 Globules

Globules are symmetrical, round to oval, well-demarcated structures that may be brown, black, or red. They have a

diameter which is usually larger than 0.1 mm and correspond to nests of pigmented benign or malignant melanocytes, clumps of melanin, and/or melanophages situated usually in the lower epidermis, at the dermo–epidermal junction, or in the papillary dermis.

Both dots and globules may occur in benign as well as in malignant melanocytic proliferations. In benign lesions, they are rather regular in size and shape and quite evenly distributed (frequently in the center of a lesion). In melanomas they tend to vary in size and shape and are frequently found in the periphery of lesions.

5.1.6.4 Branched Streaks

Branched streaks are an expression of an altered, perturbed pigment network in which the network becomes broken up. Their pathological correlation is remnants of pigmented rete ridges and bridging nests of melanocytic cells within the epidermis and papillary dermis.

5.1.6.5 Radial Streaming

Radial streaming appears as radially and asymmetrically arranged parallel linear extensions at the periphery of a lesion. Histologically, they represent confluent pigmented junctional nests of pigmented melanocytes.

5.1.7 Pseudopods

Pseudopods represent fingerlike projections of dark pigment (brown to black) at the periphery of the lesion. They may have small knobs at their tips, and are either connected to the pigment network or directly connected to the tumor body. They correspond as well to intraepidermal or junctional confluent radial nests of melanocytes. Menzies et al. found pseudopods to be one of the most specific features of superficial spreading melanoma [6].

5.1.7.1 Streaks

"Streaks" is a term used by some authors interchangeably with radial streaming or pseudopods. This is because both these structures have the same histopathological correlation. Streaks can be irregular, when they are unevenly distributed (malignant melanoma), or regular (symmetrical radial arrangement over the entire lesion). The latter is particularly found in the pigmented spindle cell nevi (Reed's nevi).

5.1.7.2 Structureless Areas

Structureless areas represent areas devoid of any discernible structures (globules, network, etc.). They tend to be hypopigmented, which is due to the absence of pigment or diminution of pigment intensity within a pigmented skin lesion.

5.1.7.3 Blotches

Blotches (also called black lamellas) are due to a large concentration of melanin pigment localized throughout the epidermis and/or dermis visually obscuring the underlying structures. Black dots and blotches can be removed by placing cellophane tape on the stratum corneum and then quickly removing the tape [7]. This procedure should be repeated several times to allow better visualization of the underlying pigmented network. The "stripping procedure" may avoid unnecessary biopsies.

5.1.7.4 Regression Pattern

Regression appears as white scar-like depigmentation (lighter than the surrounding skin) or "peppering" (speckled multiple blue-gray granules within a hypopigmented area) [8]. Histologically, regression shows fibrosis, loss of pigmentation, epidermal thinning, effacement of the rete ridges, and melanin granules free in the dermis or in melanophages scattered in the papillary dermis.

5.1.7.5 Blue–White Veil

Blue–white veil is an irregular, indistinct, confluent blue pigmentation with an overlying white ground-glass haze. The pigmentation cannot occupy the entire lesion. Histopathologically this corresponds to an aggregation of heavily pigmented cells or melanin in the dermis (blue

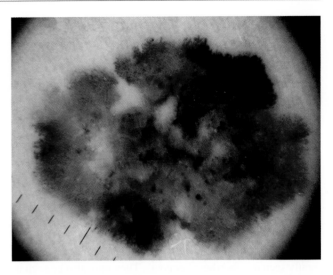

Fig. 5.1.2 Superficial spreading melanoma. Breslow 1.5 mm, Clark IV. This melanoma has all dermoscopy criteria for malignancy: *Blue–white* veil, atypical network, streaks and pseudopods at the periphery, irregularly distributed *dots* and *globules*

color) in combination with a compact orthokeratosis (Fig. 5.1.2).

5.1.7.6 Vascular Pattern

Pigmented skin lesions may have dermoscopically visible vascular patterns which include "comma vessels," "point vessels," "tree-like vessels," "wreath-like vessels," and "hairpin-like vessels." Atypical vascular patterns may include linear, dotted, or globular red structures irregularly distributed within the lesion. Some of the vascular patterns may be due to neo-vascularization. For the evaluation of vascular patterns, there has to be as little pressure as possible on the lesion during examination because otherwise the vessels are simply compressed and will not be visible. The use of ultrasound gel for immersion helps to reduce the pressure necessary for the best evaluation of the skin lesion.

5.1.7.7 Milia-Like Cysts

Milia-like cysts are round whitish or yellowish structures which are mainly seen in seborrheic keratosis. They correspond to intraepidermal keratin-filled cysts and may also be seen in congenital nevi as well as in some papillomatous melanocytic nevi. At times, milia-like cysts are pigmented, and thus can resemble globules.

5.1.7.8 Comedo-Like Openings (Crypts, Pseudofollicular Openings)

Comedo-like openings (with "blackhead-like plugs") are mainly seen in seborrheic keratosis or in some rare cases in papillomatous melanocytic nevi. The keratin-filled invaginations of the epidermis correspond to the comedo-like structures histopathologically.

5.1.7.9 Fissures and Ridges

Fissures are irregular, linear keratin-filled depressions, commonly seen in seborrheic keratosis. They may also be seen in melanocytic nevi with congenital patterns and in some dermal melanocytic nevi. Multiple fissures might give a "brain-like appearance" to the lesion (Fig. 5.1.3).

5.1.7.10 Fingerprint-Like Structures

Some flat seborrheic keratoses can show tiny ridges running in parallel and producing a pattern that resembles fingerprints.

5.1.7.11 Moth-Eaten Border

Some flat seborrheic keratoses (mainly on the face) have a concave border so that the pigment ends with a curved structure, which has been compared to a moth-eaten garment.

5.1.7.12 Leaf-Like Areas

Leaf-like areas (maple-leaf-like areas) are seen as brown to gray-blue discrete bulbous blobs, sometimes forming a leaf-like pattern. Their distribution reminds one of the shape of finger pads. In absence of a pigment network, they are suggestive of pigmented basal cell carcinomas.

5.1.7.13 Spoke-Wheel-Like Structures

Spoke-wheel-like structures are well-circumscribed brown to gray-blue-brown radial projections meeting at a darker brown central hub. In absence of a pigment network, they are highly suggestive of basal-cell carcinoma.

5.1.7.14 Large Blue–Gray Ovoid Nests

Ovoid nests are large, well-circumscribed, confluent or near-confluent pigmented ovoid areas, larger than globules, and not intimately connected to a pigmented tumor body. When a network is absent, ovoid nests are highly suggestive of basal-cell carcinoma (Fig. 5.1.4).

5.1.7.15 Multiple Blue–Gray Globules

Multiple blue-gray globules are round, well-circumscribed structures, which are in the absence of a pigment network

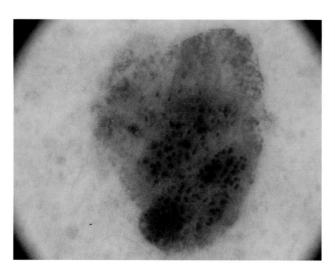

Fig. 5.1.3 Pigmented seborrheic keratosis. Wedge-shaped clefts of epidermis and keratin-filled depressions resemble gyri and sulci of the brain. That is the reason why this pattern is also called "brain-like pattern"

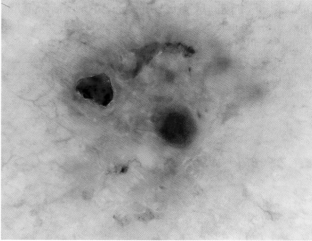

Fig. 5.1.4 Pigmented basal cell carcinoma. This lesion shows no criteria for melanocytic lesion but a large *gray-blue* globule in the center, ulcerations, and fine, in-focus, telangiectatic vessels

highly suggestive of a basal-cell carcinoma. They have to be differentiated from multiple blue-gray dots (which correspond to melanophages and melanin dust).

5.1.8 Differential Diagnosis of Pigmented Lesions of the Skin

There are many publications on the subject of the differential diagnosis of pigmented lesions of the skin. The five algorithms most commonly used are pattern analysis, the Menzies method, the ABCD rule of dermoscopy, the 7-point checklist, and the revised pattern analysis [1, 5, 9–11].

The Board of the Consensus Net meeting [12] agreed on a two-step procedure for the classification of pigmented lesions of the skin (Tables 5.1.1 and 5.1.2) [13].

Table 5.1.1 Two-step procedure for the classification of pigmented skin lesions (modified)

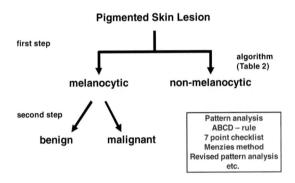

The first step is the differentiation between a melanocytic and a nonmelanocytic lesion. For this decision, the following algorithm is used:

Are aggregated globules, pigment network, branched streaks, homogeneous blue pigmentation, or a parallel pattern (palms, soles, and mucosa) visualized? If this is the case, the lesion should be considered as a melanocytic lesion. If not, the lesion should be evaluated for the presence of comedo-like plugs, multiple milia-like cysts, and comedo-like openings, irregular crypts, light brown fingerprint-like structures, or "fissures and ridges" (brain-like appearance) pattern. If so, the lesion is suggestive of a seborrheic keratosis. If not, the lesion has to be evaluated for the presence of arborising blood vessels (telangiectasias), leaf-like areas, large blue-gray ovoid nests, multiple blue-gray globules, spoke-wheel areas, or ulceration. If present, the lesion is suggestive of basal-cell carcinoma. If not, one has to look for red or red-blue (to black) lagoons. If these structures are present, the lesion should be considered a hemangioma or an angiokeratoma.

If all the preceding questions are answered with a "no," the lesion should still be considered as a melanocytic lesion.

Once the lesion is identified to be of melanocytic origin, the decision has to be made if the melanocytic lesion is benign, suspect, or malignant (Table 5.1.3).

The most commonly used algorithm is the 7-point checklist (Table 5.1.4). In 1998 Argenziano and colleagues described a 7-point checklist based on the analysis of 342 pigmented skin lesions [10]. They distinguish three major criteria and four minor criteria. Each major criterion has a

Table 5.1.2 Algorithm for the decision of melanocytic vs. nonmelanocytic lesion according to the proposition of the board of the Consensus Net meeting (modified)

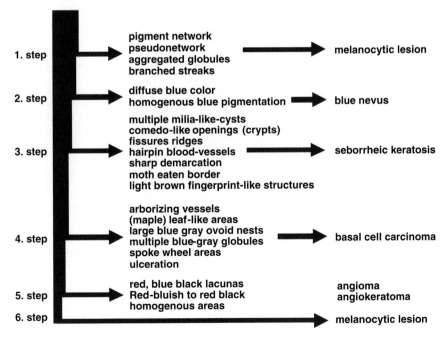

Table 5.1.3 Pattern of benign and malignant melanocytic lesions

	Benign melanocytic lesions	Malignant melanocytic lesions
Dots	Centrally located or situated right on the network	Unevenly distributed and scattered focally at the periphery
Globules	Uniform in size, shape, and color symmetrically located at the periphery, centrally located, or uniform throughout the lesion as in a cobblestone pattern	Globules which are unevenly distributed and when reddish in color are highly suggestive of melanoma
Streaks	Radial streaming or pseudopods tend to be symmetrical and uniform at the periphery	Radial streaming or pseudopods tend to be focal and irregular at the periphery
Blue–white veil	Tends to be centrally located	Tends to be asymmetrically located or diffuse almost over the entire lesion
Blotch	Centrally located or may be a diffuse hyper pigmented area that extends almost to the periphery of the lesion	Asymmetrically located or there are often multiple asymmetrical blotches
Network	Typical network that consists of light to dark uniform pigmented lines and hypo pigmented holes	Atypical network which may be non-uniform with black/brown or gray thickened lines and holes of different sizes and shapes
Network borders	Either fades into the periphery or is symmetrically sharp	Focally sharp

Table 5.1.4 The 7-point checklist according to Argenziano et al. [10]

Criteria	7-Point score
Major criteria	
Atypical pigment network	2
Blue–whitish veil	2
Atypical vascular pattern	2
Minor criteria	
Irregular streaks	1
Irregular pigmentation	1
Irregular dots/globules	1
Regression structures	1

score of 2 points while each minor criterion has a score of 1 point. A minimum total score of 3 is required for the diagnosis of malignant melanoma.

Dermoscopy can significantly increase the diagnostic performance of differentiating melanocytic and nonmelanocytic pigmented lesions. A recent meta-analysis showed that dermoscopy used for the diagnosis of primary melanoma revealed a 16% improvement compared to naked eye examination [14]. But only physicians who are experienced in dermoscopy can achieve this improvement in the diagnosis of pigmented lesions; therefore formal training in dermoscopy is crucial.

References

1. Pehamberger, H., Steiner, A., Wolff, K.: In vivo epiluminescence microscopy of pigmented skin lesions. I. Pattern analysis of pigmented skin lesions. J Am Acad Dermatol 17(4), 571–83 (1987)
2. Carli, P., De Giorgi, V., Soyer, H.P., Stante, M., Mannone, F., Giannotti, B.: Dermatoscopy in the diagnosis of pigmented skin lesions: a new semiology for the dermatologist. JEADV 14, 353–69 (2000)
3. Binder, M., Braun, R.P.: Principles of dermoscopy. In: Marghoob, A.A., Braun, R.P., Kopf, A.W. (eds.) Atlas of dermoscopy, pp. 7–10. Taylor & Francis, London (2005)
4. Kreusch, J.F.: Vascular patterns in melanocytic and non-melanocytic lesions. In: Malvehy, J., Puig, S. (eds.) Principles of dermoscopy, pp. 155–73. CEGE, Barcelona (2002)
5. Menzies, S.W., Ingvar, C., McCarthy, W.H.: A sensitivity and specificity analysis of the surface microscopy features of invasive melanoma. Melanoma Res 6, 55–62 (1996)
6. Menzies, S., Crotty, K., McCarthy, W.: The morphologic criteria of the pseudopod in surface microscopy. Arch Dermatol 131, 436–40 (1995)
7. Guillod, J.F., Skaria, A.M., Salomon, D., Saurat, J.H.: Epiluminiscence videomicroscopy: black dots and brown globules revisited by stripping the stratum corneum. J Am Acad Dermatol 36, 371–7 (1997)
8. Braun, R.P., Gaide, O., Oliviero, M., et al.: The significance of multiple blue-grey dots (granularity) for the dermoscopic diagnosis of melanoma. Br J Dermatol. 157(5), 907–13 (2007)
9. Stolz, W., Riemann, A., Cognetta, A.B., et al.: ABCD rule of dermoscopy: a new practical method for early recognition of malignant melanoma. Eur J Dermatol 4, 521–7 (1994)
10. Argenziano, G., Fabbrocini, G., Carli, P., de Giorgi, V., Sammaro, E., Delfino, M.: Epiluminiscence microscopy for the diagnosis of doubtful melanocytic skin lesions. Comparision of the ABCD rule of dermatoscopy and a new 7-point checklist based on pattern analysis. Arch Dermatol 134, 1563–70 (1998)
11. Kittler, H., Seltenheim, M., Dawid, M., Pehamberger, H., Wolff, K., Binder, M.: Morphologic changes of pigmented lesions: a useful extension of the ABCD rule for dermatoscopy. J Am Acad Dermatol 43, 467–76 (1999)
12. Argenziano, G., Soyer, H.P., Chimenti, S., et al.: Dermoscopy of pigmented skin lesions: results of a consensus net meeting via the Internet. J Am Acad Dermatol 48, 679–93 (2003)
13. Braun, R.P., Rabinovitz, H.S., Oliviero, M., et al.: Pattern analysis: a two-step procedure for the dermoscopic classification of melanoma. Clin Dermatol 20, 236–9 (2002)
14. Vestergaard, M.E., Macaskill, P., Holt, P.E., Menzies, S.W.: Dermoscopy compared with naked eye examination for the diagnosis of primary melanoma: a meta-analysis of studies performed in a clinical setting. Br J Dermatol. 159(3), 669–76 (2008)

PET and PET/CT of Malignant Melanoma

Hans C. Steinert

Malignant melanoma is the most aggressive cancer of the skin. The 5-year survival is 99% for localized disease but drops off rapidly to 65% for patients with regional metastases, and declines further to 15% for patients with distant metastases at the time of diagnosis [3]. This dramatic reduction in survival of patients with disseminated disease requires the accurate identification of metastases at the time of initial diagnosis and during follow-up. This chapter reviews the role of positron emission tomography (PET) and combined positron emission tomography with computed tomography (PET/CT) in the management of patients with malignant melanoma.

Any pigmented lesion with a change in size, configuration, or color should be considered a potential melanoma, and an excisional biopsy should be performed. Fortunately, in most developed countries, patients are generally diagnosed early, and thus melanoma can usually be cured with surgical excision of the lesion. Nevertheless, late diagnoses in locations that are not visible to the patient such as the scalp, neck, back, and plantar areas are fairly common. The widely varying mortality reports in the literature depend more on the stage at diagnosis than on variations in surgical and treatment technique.

Histologic verification and accurate microstaging of tumor thickness are essential for treatment decisions and to predict the risk of metastases. It has been demonstrated that the Breslow tumor thickness is the most important prognostic factor in clinically localized melanoma and is a highly reproducible parameter [4].

The American Joint Committee on Cancer (AJCC) has developed a four-stage system that allows subclassification of primary localized melanomas according to their malignant potential [5]. Stages I and II refer to localized melanoma and negative lymph nodes. Early malignant melanoma is curable by means of surgical excision. Stage III melanoma includes patients with lymph node metastases, either in regional nodes or as satellite or in-transit metastases. Patients with distant metastases represent stage IV.

The Breslow tumor thickness is an important prognostic factor in melanoma for guiding treatment decisions. Patients with a Breslow tumor thickness up to 1 mm have an excellent prognosis not differing significantly from that of the general population. Patients with thin melanomas less than 1 mm are usually cured by excision of the primary lesion. Melanomas with a size of 1–2 mm are generally treated with wide local excision and are nowadays also commonly evaluated with sentinel lymph node scintigraphy. Patients with an indeterminate melanoma thickness of 2–4 mm have an increased risk of occult regional nodal metastases but have a relatively low risk (less than 20%) of distant metastases and are often staged using sentinel node detection methods. Melanomas greater than 4 mm in thickness have a 10-year survival of less than 40%. Once patients develop metastases, other prognostic factors have to be considered. The number of metastatic nodes has a significant prognostic value. Surgical excision of metastatic nodes is the only effective treatment for cure or locoregional disease control. These patients are generally treated with radical lymphadenectomy. High-risk patients with resected regional lymph-node metastases may be candidates for various adjuvant chemo- or immunotherapies.

The high mortality of patients with melanoma is due to the early hematogenous spread. The mechanism of hematogenous spread and implantation of melanoma cells is poorly understood, and the location of metastases is unpredictable. The skin, subcutaneous tissue, and distant lymph nodes are the most common sites of distant metastases, but melanoma can metastasize to all organs. Early detection and surgical excision of single distant metastases are important in improving the prognosis. As soon as distant metastases are diagnosed, the prognosis is poor. Significant factors predicting survival in patients with distant metastases are the number of metastatic sites and the remission duration (less than 12 months vs. more than 12 months). The results of vaccine therapies for melanoma suggest that immune and clinical responses are promising in patients with metastatic disease.

For unknown primary melanomas, the distribution of metastases localized to a region or multiple sites at

H.C. Steinert
Department of Medical Radiology, University Hospital of Zurich, Zurich, Switzerland
e-mail: hans.steinert@usz.ch

R. Dummer et al. (eds.), *Skin Cancer – A World-Wide Perspective*,
DOI: 10.1007/978-3-642-05072-5_5.2, © Springer-Verlag Berlin Heidelberg 2011

presentation is 43% and 57%, respectively. One must assume that the predominant origins of these unknown primary melanomas arise from a cutaneous melanoma that spontaneously regressed. Spontaneous regression is observed in up to 0.4% of melanomas and is likely mediated by an immune mechanism. The 5-year survival rate is similar to that of stage III disease (49%). Several reports have shown that the surgical management of patients with lymph-node disease from unknown primary melanomas fared as well as patients with known cutaneous primary sites.

The clinical course of melanoma can be characterized by the risk of recurrent disease and death well beyond 10 years after the initial diagnosis. Twenty-five percent of the patients who survive more than 10 years will experience recurrence. Among patients with stage III disease, about 70% relapse, of which two thirds occur at distant locations. Therefore, lifetime annual follow-up has been recommended and imaging studies are a key to this follow-up.

5.2.1 Staging of Malignant Melanoma

Proper tumor staging is a key prerequisite to choosing the appropriate treatment strategy in melanoma. After resection of the primary melanoma, the analysis of Breslow tumor thickness gives an immediate estimate of the likelihood of regional lymph node metastases and distant metastases. In patients with thin melanomas (Breslow thickness <1 mm), the likelihood of metastases is so small that staging with imaging modalities is not cost-effective.

Patients having melanomas with a Breslow thickness of 1–4 mm have an increased risk of occult regional nodal metastases but have a relatively low risk of distant metastases. Hafner et al. demonstrated that sentinel lymph node scintigraphy and biopsy is the most effective examination for staging these patients at baseline [20]. One hundred consecutive patients with malignant melanoma and a tumor thickness greater than 1 mm were enrolled in the study. The patients underwent extensive baseline staging including physical examination, ultrasonography (US) of the regional lymph nodes and abdomen, sentinel lymph node scintigraphy and biopsy, chest X-ray film, and whole-body 2[^{18}F] fluoro-2-deoxy-D-glucose (FDG) PET. Twenty-six percent of patients had a positive sentinel lymph node among 90% with microscopic disease. The macroscopic nodal metastases could be detected by physical examination, US, or PET. Therefore, at the author's institution, a sentinel lymph node scintigraphy is performed at baseline for microscopic staging. A whole-body PET scan is performed to screen for distant metastases only when metastatic sentinel lymph node is found. This observation of higher sensitivity of sentinel node imaging combined with histological assessment as

compared to PET for small tumors has been shown by several groups.

Patients with melanomas over 4 mm have a high risk (greater than 30%) of developing distant metastases. Due to the erratic pattern of distant metastases, whole-body staging is recommended. In the past, a combination of conventional imaging modalities were used for staging of malignant melanoma, such as chest X-ray, US, CT, magnetic resonance imaging (MRI), and bone scintigraphy. However, specific identification of tumor tissue is difficult with these methods. Cross-sectional imaging methods are generally used to evaluate a specific region, rather than the entire body. Diagnosis of a lymph node metastasis with cross-sectional imaging modalities is mainly based on size, choosing 1–1.5 cm in short-axis nodal diameter as a cutoff value between benign and pathologic lymph nodes. However, using these criteria, metastases in small nodes can be missed and reactively enlarged nodes can cause false-positive results, limiting the value of the methods. CT often misses small metastases, particularly those in bowel and bone. CT is known to have a high rate of false-positive findings if applied as a screening method in patients with malignant melanoma [9].

Due to the limitations of morphological imaging modalities, several radiopharmaceuticals have been used in nuclear medicine to visualize metastases of melanoma. These include gallium-67-citrate [25], immunoscintigraphy with monoclonal antibodies [8], indium-111-pentetreotide [22], technetium-99m-methoxyisobutylisonitrile [2], iodine-123-methyltyrosine [37], fluorine-18-fluoroethyltyrosine [33], iodine-123-iodobenzufuran [38], fluorine-18-fluoro-dopa [28], bromine-76-bromodeoxyuridine [7], and fluorine-18-fluorodesoxyuridine [46]. However, these radiotracers did not offer any significant advantage in diagnostic sensitivity in screening for metastases of malignant melanoma. False-negative scan results were common because of the poor sensitivity. These radiotracers were found to be suitable for screening of melanoma only in exceptional cases. Several carbon-11-labeled radiopharmaceuticals have been used for experimental studies in malignant melanoma. Due to the short half-life of carbon-11, the clinical use of these tracers for whole-body staging remains limited.

5.2.2 Whole-Body PET and PET/CT Imaging with FDG

Today, FDG is the most widely used radiopharmaceutical for staging of malignant melanoma. In vitro and in vivo experiments with tumor cells demonstrated higher FDG accumulation in melanoma than in any other tumors [49]. Whole-body PET and integrated PET with CT (PET/CT) with FDG have been proven to be highly effective and cost-effective modalities to screen for metastases of malignant melanoma throughout the body [11, 13, 19, 23, 24, 30–32, 39, 44] (Figs. 5.2.1 and 5.2.2). With the exception of the brain, whole-body FDG PET and PET/CT scan largely replace the standard battery of imaging tests currently performed on high-risk patients.

Due to the erratic pattern of metastases of malignant melanoma, whole-body FDG PET scanning or PET/CT scanning is required. At the author's institution, only combined PET/CT systems are available. A whole-body PET/CT scan is routinely performed from the head to the knees. If the primary tumor was located in a lower limb, additional PET/CT scanning is performed from the knees to the feet for the detection of satellite lesions or in-transit metastases (N3 stage).

At the author's institution, whole-body PET/CT with FDG is restricted to patients with high-risk malignant melanoma (Breslow tumor thickness >4 mm or known metastasis). The preselection of patients ensures the high effectiveness of PET/CT imaging. According to the guidelines of the Swiss Society of Dermatology PET or PET/CT scanning is annually recommended in the first 5 years after the diagnosis of a high-risk melanoma [12]. For baseline staging, sentinel lymph node scintigraphy and biopsy are routinely performed in patients with a Breslow tumor thickness from 1 to 4 mm. In cases of microscopic tumor spread to a sentinel lymph node, an additional whole-body PET/CT for screening of distant metastases will be performed.

Whole-body FDG PET or PET/CT should be used to exclude unsuspected occult metastases in patients in whom surgery of a known metastasis is planned. If multiple metastases are present, chemotherapy is the therapy of choice. In extended disease, only palliative therapy is indicated. Whole-body FDG PET or PET/CT plays an important role in the evaluation of patients when immunotherapy is considered. Adjuvant treatment with recombinant interferon alpha is only indicated in disease-free patients after resection of high-risk melanoma. FDG PET or PET/CT is also useful in evaluating the treatment response.

As early as in 1993, Gritters et al. described promising results of FDG PET imaging in melanoma [19]. In this initial study, the sensitivity of PET was 100% for intraabdominal visceral and lymph node metastases, but it enrolled only 12 patients in the study with known metastatic melanoma on conventional staging. This study clearly demonstrated that melanoma generally has a high FDG accumulation, that PET can detect most lesions seen by conventional imaging with the exception of pulmonary nodules, and that PET also detects occult disease originally missed by CT while correctly excluding morphological false-positive lesions.

Steinert et al. reported, in a study of 33 patients, a sensitivity of 92% with a specificity of 77% for reading the PET images without clinical information [39]. Specificity improved to 100% when clinical information such as location of biopsy sites or subcutaneous injections of interferon was obtained. PET was also highly accurate in differentiating benign from

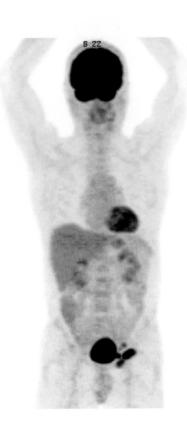
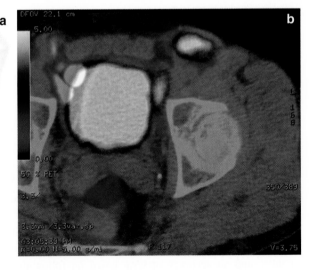

Fig 5.2.1 A 63-year-old man with malignant melanoma of the left leg excised 6 years ago. There was a suspicion on lymph node metastases in the left inguinal. PET/CT imaging with FDG was performed staging. (**a**) Maximum intensity projection (MIP) PET scan demonstrated multiple lymph node metastases in the left inguinal. No further lesions. (**b**) Axial co-registered PET/CT scan showed exact anatomic localization of the inguinal lymph node metastases

Fig 5.2.2 A 78-year-old
man with a with malignant
melanoma temporal right.
Surgery of the primary was
performed 3 weeks before.
PET/CT imaging with FDG
was performed for staging.
(**a**) Maximum intensity
projection (MIP) PET scan,
(**b, c**) axial co-registered
PET/CT scans showed 2
cervical lymph node
metastases on the right
side. No distant metastases
were detected.

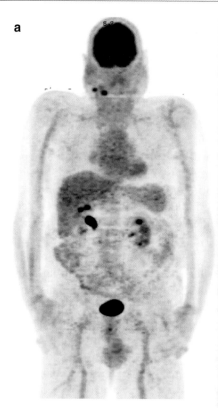

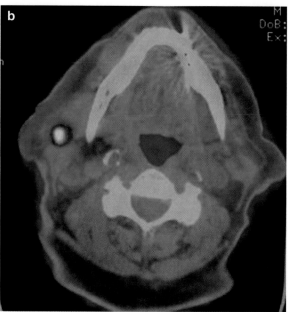

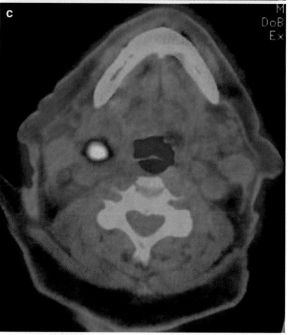

malignant lesions. In six patients (20%), whole-body PET depicted previously unknown metastases. In four of these six patients, the metastases were surgically removed.

A study by Rinne et al. [32] described lesion sensitivity in primary staging of high-risk melanoma of 100%, a specificity of 94%, and an accuracy of 95% based on follow-up and biopsy, compared to an accuracy of only 68% for conventional imaging. Importantly, different sensitivities of PET compared to conventional imaging by body region were observed. Lesion detection was substantially higher with PET in the neck nodes and abdomen but substantially lower in the lung.

The excellent results in staging high-risk melanoma patients with whole-body FDG PET were confirmed in large patient studies in different PET centers worldwide [11, 13, 23, 24, 30, 44] (Fig. 5.2.3). PET demonstrated high FDG accumulation in melanoma metastases in the lymph nodes and viscera. Due to the results, whole-body FDG PET and PET/CT are reimbursed by insurance and by government health-care agencies for patients with high-risk melanoma in many countries.

Steinert et al. performed a meta-analysis of the literature for staging of high-risk melanoma with FDG PET [41]. In this study, a quality assessment of all articles was applied. PET studies for the microscopic tumor involvement of SLN were excluded. Only PET studies with the definitive confirmation of lesions were included. These pooled data were used for the

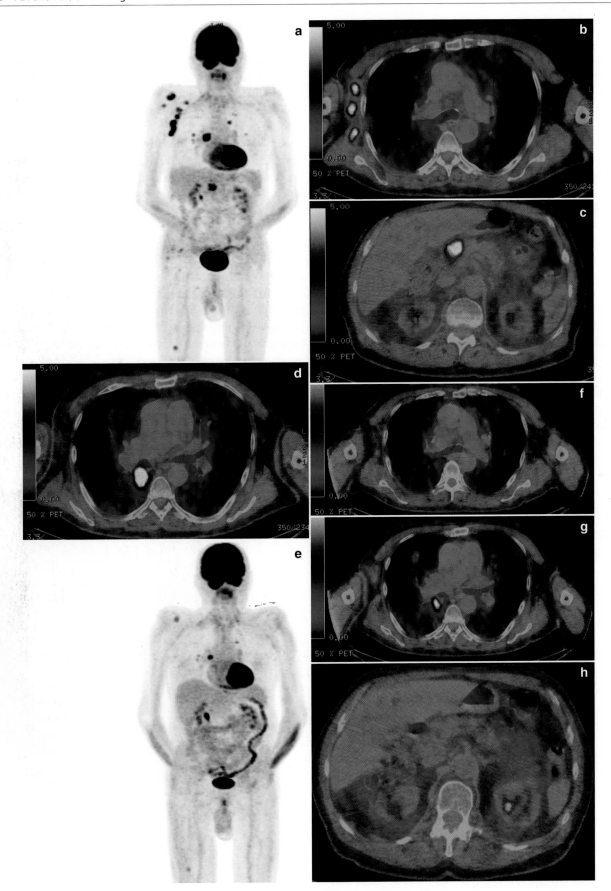

Fig 5.2.3 A 75-year-old man with malignant melanoma stage IV. PET/CT imaging with FDG was performed at baseline (**a-d**) and for treatment response after 6 weeks chemotherapy (**e-h**). (**a**) Maximum intensity projection (MIP) PET scan showed multiple metastases throughout the body, (**b-d**) axial co-registered PET/CT scans showed metastases in the right axilla, right lung, and the hepatic portal. (**e-h**) The corresponding images after chemotherapy showed good treatment response.

meta-analysis. A total of 323 lesions could be included for the meta-analysis. An overall sensitivity of 90% (95% confidence level, 86–94%) and an overall specificity of 87% (95% confidence level, 79–95%) were determined. Other reviews of the FDG PET literature have been published. Since studies for the detection of microscopic tumor involvement of lymph nodes were included in these analyses, the accuracy of FDG PET was lower than our results [17, 27]. It is clear that lesion size is important in detecting tumor foci with PET and PET/CT, hence those studies involving small tumor-related nodes are more likely to produce false-negative results.

It has been demonstrated that FDG PET is superior to CT in detecting melanoma metastases throughout the body. Buzaid et al. analyzed the value of CT in the staging of patients with locoregional metastases of melanoma [9]. The records of 99 patients were recorded. False-positive findings were observed in 22% of patients. Holder et al. compared FDG PET with CT in 76 patients with metastatic melanoma [23]. For the detection of melanoma metastases, PET scanning had a sensitivity of 94% compared with 55% for CT scanning. The four false-negative FDG PET scan results were due to smaller lesions (less than 0.3 mm).

FDG PET and PET/CT play a large role in the evaluation of patients with clinical recurrence. The superiority of PET over conventional staging has been reported [35]. In a study by Fuster et al. 156 patients with recurrent melanoma were examined with both PET and CT [16]. The overall

accuracy of PET was 81% compared with 52% for other methods.

However, limitations of FDG PET imaging have been recognized. A number of factors may interfere with the accuracy of PET scanning for metastases. It is well known that FDG is not a tumor-specific substance. False-positive results may be caused by an increased FDG accumulation in inflammatory lesions or postoperative changes [34, 42] (Figs. 5.2.4 and 5.2.5). Therefore, the clinical correlation of lesions with increased FDG accumulation is obligatory to exclude tracer uptake in recent sites of surgery or infected or inflamed lesions or at injection sites, for example. In most cases, these benign causes of FDG uptake can be specifically recognized and properly categorized. Other common benign lesions with a focal FDG uptake are colonic adenomas, inflammatory changes such as villonodular synovitis and tendinits, Warthin's tumors, and acute fractures [36] (Fig. 5.2.6). Sarcoid-like lesions may mimic generalized metastatic melanoma. Therefore, histological confirmation of lesions is recommended, particularly when PET or PET/CT findings might result in a change of treatment.

False-negative results may occur in patients with slow-growing metastases or in metastases with a large necrotic component. Due to the physiological FDG uptake in the cortex, CT and MRI are generally superior to FDG PET in the detection of brain metastases. However, in our institution the brain is always included in the whole-body PET/CT

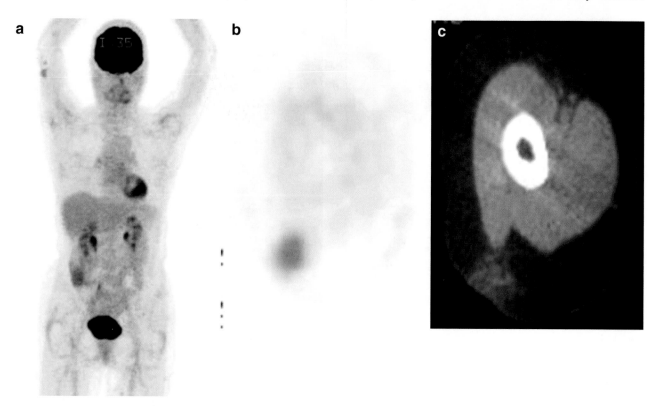

a   b   c

Fig 5.2.4 A 70-year-old woman with a malignant melanoma stage of her left upper led with stage IV. PET/CT imaging with FDG was performed after interferon treatment. (**a**) Maximum intensity projection (MIP) PET scan, (**b**, **c**) axial PET and CT scans of the right arm. The images show a lesion with slighty increased FDG activity in the right arm. This lesion was caused by an inflammatory reaction after subcutaneous interferon injection.

Fig 5.2.5 A 44-year-old
man with a malignant
melanoma of the right
scapula excised 4 years
ago (Breslow tumor
thickness 5.5mm). PET/
CT imaging with FDG
was performed staging.
(**a**) Maximum intensity
projection (MIP) PET
scan and (**b**) axial
co-registered PET/CT
scan showed bilateral
hilar and mediastinal
FDG-active lymph
nodes. The distribution
of the lymph nodes is
typical for a granuloma-
tous disease
(sarcoidosis). No
metastases.

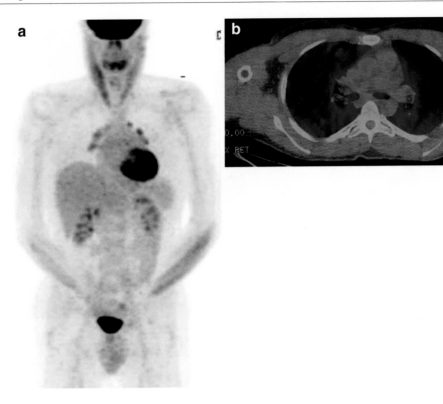

Fig 5.2.6 A 72-year-old
man with a malignant
melanoma lumbal
excised 2 years ago.
PET/CT imaging with
FDG was performed
staging. (**a**) Maximum
intensity projection
(MIP) PET scan and
(**b**) axial co-registered
PET/CT scan showed
inguinal lymph node
metastasis on the left.
(**c**) In addition, three
FDG-active lesions in
the right basal rips were
detected. The patient fell
some weeks ago on the
right side. The lesions of
the rips arepresent
fractures.

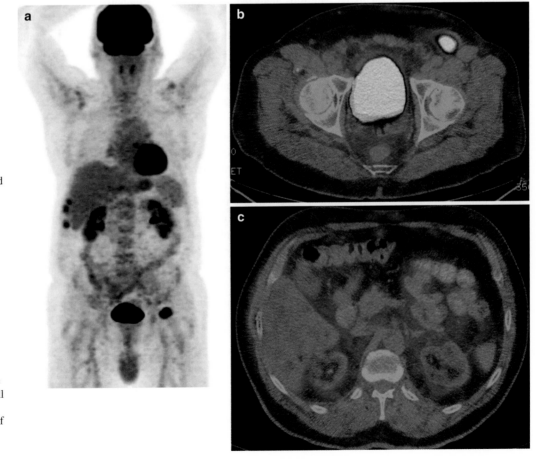

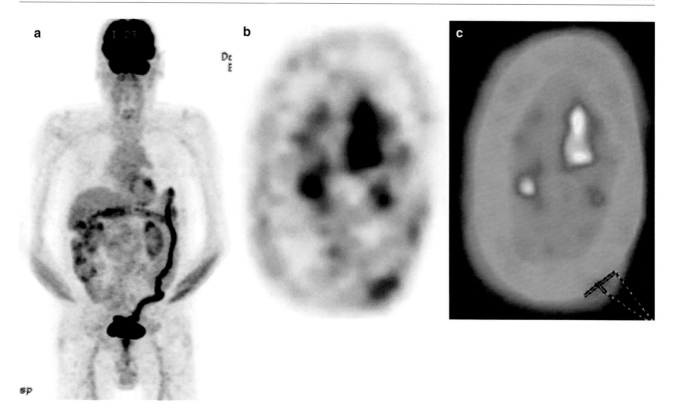

Fig 5.2.7 A 77-year-old man with a malignant melanoma temporal excised 2 years ago. PET/CT imaging with FDG was performed staging. (a) Maximum intensity projection (MIP) PET scan revealed no FDG-active lesions. (b, c) However, with different scaling axial PET scan and co-registered PET/CT scan showed multiple FDG-active brain metastases.

examination and images have to be carefully analyzed in search of metastases. In some cases, clinically occult brain metastases have been detected (Fig. 5.2.7). In patients with neurological symptoms, MRI of the brain is the reference method to diagnose or exclude brain metastases. Due to the small tumor volume, cutaneous and subcutaneous lesions can be missed with PET imaging [39]. Therefore, thorough clinical examination of the patients is mandatory.

In the assessment of pulmonary metastases of melanoma, FDG PET shows a higher specificity but lower sensitivity than CT [29, 32]. In a more recent study, the sensitivity of CT and PET were 93% and 57%, respectively, in the evaluation of lung nodules [35]. In the author's experience, this limitation of PET imaging can be overcome with the use of integrated PET/CT imaging [43]. FDG-inactive but solid pulmonary nodules without calcification are highly suspicious for lung metastases. Since the author's institute implemented integrated PET/CT scanning in staging of melanoma patients, it has encountered cases with FDG-inactive lung metastases (Fig. 5.2.8). An explanation might be the slow proliferation rate of these lesions. Therefore, dedicated CT analysis is strongly recommended to improve the sensitivity and the accuracy of the integrated PET/CT imaging in the staging of the patients with high-risk melanoma.

Recently, it was shown that the diagnostic performance of whole-body PET/CT for staging of distant metastases was significantly superior to CT alone and PET alone [31]. In the

study by Reinhard et al., 250 consecutive patients were included. The most significant advantage of combined PET/CT imaging in comparison to the single modalities was the improved detection and differentiation of visceral metastases. The accurate anatomic correlation of areas with increased FDG uptake resulted in a significant reduction of false-positive and false-negative findings by PET/CT. The specificity of PET/CT compared to PET alone was clearly superior for the detection of distant lymph node metastases (97% and 90%, respectively) and visceral metastases (95% and 88%, respectively). As other studies reported, a significant contribution of CT was the detection of pulmonary metastases, where PET is highly specific but has a limited sensitivity. Even the specificity of CT for the differentiation of pulmonary metastases increased after image fusion with PET from 86% to 96%.

Although malignant melanoma is one of the most highly FDG-accumulating tumors, the spatial resolution of 5 mm of dedicated PET scanners is limited. Resolution is further degraded near the edges of the scanner field of view and with the filtering methods typically applied to smooth the PET images for interpretation. The smallest metastases detected with dedicated PET scanners were 4–5 mm. Micrometastatic disease cannot be detected with any imaging modality. Sentinel lymph node scintigraphy and biopsy is the most effective examination for microscopic staging. It has been shown that FDG accumulation in nodal metastasis is dependent on nodal tumor involvement of greater than 50% or

Fig 5.2.8 A 63-year-old man with a malignant melanoma and regional lymph node metastasis of the left leg excised 4 years ago. PET/CT imaging with FDG was performed restaging. **(a)** Maximum intensity projection (MIP) PET scan revealed no FDG-active lesions. **(b)** Axial CT scan demonstrated a new lesion in the left lung with an irregular margin highly suspicious for a lung metastasis. **(c)** Corresponding axial co-registered PET/CT scan showed no FDG accumulation in the lesion. The nodule was resected and a metasta-sis of a malignant melanoma was confirmed.

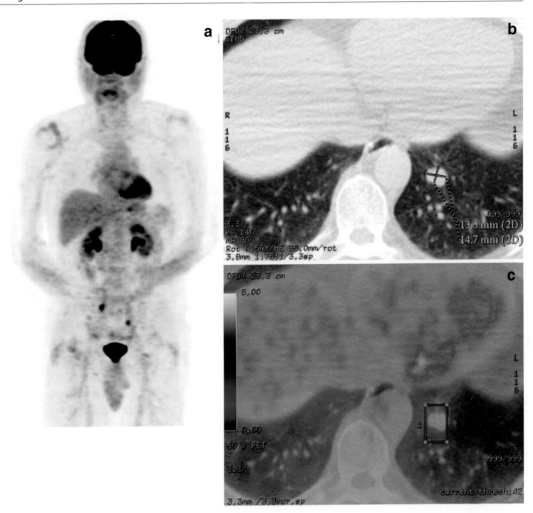

capsular infiltration and on the size of the metastasis. In a study by Crippa et al., FDG PET detected 100% of metasta-ses 10 mm and larger, 83% of metastases 6–10 mm, but only 23% of metastases 5 mm or smaller [10]. Steinert et al. dem-onstrated the importance of image acquisition and process-ing in relation to lesion detectability in a study comparing whole-body PET with planar coincidence imaging [40]. The sensitivities were 89% and 18%, respectively. Detection of lesions smaller than 22 mm in diameter showed a reduced sensitivity with coincidence imaging. Therefore, only dedi-cated PET scanners can be recommended for whole-body staging of malignant melanoma, as the goal is to detect both large and small tumor foci.

5.2.2.1 FDG PET and Prognosis

The intensity of FDG uptake with primary tumors or metas-tases has become an area of interest in the assessment of

the prognosis. Typically, increasingly FDG-avid tumors tend to behave in a more aggressive fashion and carry a worse prognosis. Recently, Bastiaannet et al. measured the FDG uptake in local lymph node metastases and found that individuals with higher standardized uptake values (SUV) had a shorter duration of disease-free survival [6]. However, for lymph node metastases, size will also affect the SUV. It is possible that the higher-SUV lesions were larger and thus possibly represented more advanced disease. Overall survival was not affected by the SUV in this study.

5.2.2.2 Treatment Response Evaluation

Measurement of early metabolic treatment response before the onset of changes in tumor morphology is a promising area of research within PET. There are limited data examin-ing the utility of PET in this regard for patients with mela-noma. In 2001, changes on sequential FDG PET studies were found to be predictive of response to isolated limb perfusion therapy in patients with locally advanced melanoma [21]. Others have demonstrated the use of FDG PET for monitoring treatment response to radiation therapy for neurotropic desmoplastic melanoma [1].

5.2.2.3 Effectiveness of Whole-Body FDG PET

Patients with stage I melanoma (Breslow tumor thickness <1.0 mm) are cured with surgery. Since most malignant melanomas develop in the cutis, these lesions are simply visible through clinical examination and amenable to diagnostic biopsy. In addition, the size of most primary melanomas is far below the spatial resolution of PET and PET/CT imaging. The likelihood of metastases is so small that staging with radiographic or PET and PET/CT imaging is not effective.

In melanoma patients with a Breslow thickness from 1.0 to 4.0 mm, sentinel lymph node scintigraphy and biopsy is the most effective examination for staging at baseline [20]. Dedicated PET scanners have a spatial resolution of 5–6 mm. Therefore, PET and PET/CT imaging are not useful in determining subclinical microscopic tumor spread to lymph nodes [1, 14, 21, 26, 48]. Additionally, the risk for distant metastases is low in this patient group.

Patients with a melanoma Breslow thickness >4.0 mm or known nodal metastases, have a high risk, about 30%, of developing distant metastases. The early detection of metastases is crucial for the optimal management of patients. Several studies have demonstrated that whole-body FDG PET imaging is an accurate method for staging and in the follow-up of high-risk patients and in the restaging of patients with known distant metastases to evaluate tumor response. Surgical excision of metastases is recommended if only one or a few sites of disease are apparent [15]. Therefore, the number and the location of metastases should be exactly defined. Today, whole-body integrated PET/CT imaging is the best single examination to identify and to localize the metastases.

Several studies have explored the cost effectiveness of whole-body FDG PET in melanoma patients. Our group [47] reviewed treatment records of 100 patients with newly diagnosed high-risk malignant melanoma. In patients with known metastatic disease, all metastases had been removed. Two staging procedures were defined: (a) Conventional staging consisting physical examination, chest X-ray, and US of lymph nodes and abdomen. Any suspicious lesion after conventional staging resulted in additional CT scans and histopathologic correlation. (b) Staging with whole-body PET and inspection of the skin. Suspicious lesions were confirmed with a biopsy or another imaging modality. The

review found 172 staging protocols that could be analyzed for cost comparison. The total cost of conventional staging was approximately $170,000, compared to approximately $173,000 for PET, thus only around 2% more. Among the 72 patients with metastatic disease, conventional staging costs were $145,000 while PET staging costs were $130,000. In this subset, the PET protocol cost approximately 11% less than conventional staging.

Gambhir et al. [18] compared the cost-effectiveness of the imaging strategies using conventional staging alone, including body CT and brain MRI vs. conventional staging with whole-body FDG PET. Sixty patients with suspected recurrence from malignant melanoma were included in this study. The study also evaluated predicted survival, using measures of life expectancy based on the literature, and savings due to changes in patient management resulting from the use of PET. The incremental cost-effectiveness ratio of the FDG PET strategy, compared with the conventional staging strategy, was $3,000–8,000 per year of life saved, a figure far below the standard of $50,000 per year of life saved used by US health economists to characterize a cost-effective intervention.

In another study, the impact of FDG PET on patient stage and management has been evaluated from the referring physician's perspective [50]. Referring physicians indicated that whole-body FDG PET changed the clinical stage in 29% of patients. Twenty percent of patients were up-staged and 10% of patients were down-staged. The PET findings resulted in inter-modality management changes in 29% of patients. Intra-modality management change occurred in 18% of patients. This survey-based study of referring physicians demonstrated that FDG PET has a major impact on the management of melanoma patients.

In the author's experience, PET changes the treatment in 20% of patients with high-risk melanoma. Other groups reported an even higher influence of FDG PET on the diagnostic and therapeutic management of patients. In one study, PET resulted in a change in surgical management in 16 of 45 patients (36%). The addition of FDG PET to the diagnostic algorithm resulted in a savings to cost ratio of 2:1 because of the avoidance of unnecessary procedures [45]. In a study of patients with recurrent melanoma, PET results changed the clinical management of 36% of patients in comparison to conventional staging [27].

5.2.3 Summary

Whole-body FDG PET is a very effective imaging modality to screen for metastases in patients with malignant melanoma and a high risk for metastases (Breslow thickness

>4.00 mm or already known metastases). The preselection of patients ensures high effectiveness of PET imaging and PET/CT imaging. The advantage of PET and PET/CT, particularly in melanoma with its unpredictable spread of metastases, is that the whole body can easily be examined. Limitations of FDG PET in the early detection of lung and brain metastases have been recognized. Recently it has been shown that integrated PET/CT is superior to conventional CT in lesion detection. Dedicated interpretation of the CT part of integrated PET/CT imaging improves the early detection of lung metastases. Due to the clear advantages of integrated PET/CT scanning it is not surprising that worldwide many conventional PET scanners are replaced by combined PET/CT devices. Whole-body FDG PET and PET/CT have a major impact on the management of patients with melanoma.

Surgical resection is the treatment of choice for regional lymph node metastases or single distant metastases. Whole-body FDG PET or PET/CT should be used to exclude unsuspected occult metastases in patients in whom surgery is planned. If multiple metastases are present, patients are referred to chemo- and/or immunotherapy. In extended metastatic disease, only palliative therapy is indicated. Whole-body FDG PET and PET/CT are also helpful in treatment follow-up. Assessment of the efficacy of treatments with PET is also becoming more common as the therapeutic options for systemic metastatic disease continue to grow.

References

1. Acland, K.M., Healy, C., Calonje, E., et al.: Comparison of positron emission tomography scanning and sentinel node biopsy in the detection of micrometastases of primary cutaneous malignant melanoma. J. Clin. Oncol. 19, 2674–2678 (2001)
2. Alonso, O., Martinez, M., Mut, F., et al.: Detection of recurrent malignant melanoma with 99mTc-MIBI scintigraphy. Melanoma Res. 8, 355 (1998)
3. American Cancer Society: Cancer Facts and Figures 2007. American cancer Society, Atlanta (2007)
4. Balch, C.M., Murad, T.M., Soong, S.-J., Ingalls, A.L., Halpern, N.B., Maddox, W.A.: A multifactorial analysis of melanoma: prognostic histopathological features comparing Clark's and Breslow's staging methods. Ann. Surg. 188, 732–742 (1978)
5. Balch, C.M., Sober, A.J., Soong, S.-J., Gershenwald, J.E.: AJCC Melanoma Staging Committee. The new melanoma staging system. Semin. Cutan. Med. Surg. 22, 42–51 (2004)
6. Bastaiaannet, E., Hoekstra, O.S., Oyen, W.J., Jager, P.L., Wobbes, T., Hoekstar, H.J.: Level of fluorodeoxyglucose uptake predicts risk for recurrence in melanoma patients presenting with lymph node metastases. Ann. Surg. Oncol. 13, 919–926 (2006)
7. Böni, R., Bläuenstein, P., Dummer, R., von Schulthess, G.K., Schubiger, P.A., Steinert, H.C.: Non-invasive assessment of tumor cell proliferation with positron emission tomography and ^{76}Br-bromodeoxyuridine. Melanoma Res. 9, 569–573 (1999)
8. Böni, R., Huch-Böni, R., Steinert, H.C., Dummer, R., Burg, G., von Schulthess, G.K.: Antimlenoma monoclonal antibody 225.28S immunoscintigraphy in metastatic melanoma. Dermatology 191, 119–123 (1995)
9. Buzaid, A.D., Sandler, A.B., Mani, S., et al.: Role of computed tomography in the staging of primary melanoma. J. Clin. Oncol. 19, 2674–2678 (2001)
10. Crippa, F., Leutner, M., Belli, F., et al.: Which kinds of lymph node metastases can FDG PET detect? A clinical study in melanoma. J. Nucl. Med. 41, 1491–1494 (2000)
11. Damian, D.L., Fulham, M.J., Thompson, E., Thompson, J.F.: Positron emission tomography in the detection and mangement of metastatic melanoma. Melanoma Res. 6, 325–329 (1996)
12. Dummer, R., Panizzon, R., Bloch, P.H., Burg, G.: Updated Swiss guidelines for the treatment and follow-up of cutaneous melanoma. Dermatology 210, 39–44 (2005)
13. Eigtved, A., Andersson, A.P., Dahlstrom, K., et al.: Use of fluorine-18 fluorodeoxyglucose positron emission tomography in the detection of silent metastases from malignant melanoma. Eur. J. Nucl. Med. 27, 70–75 (2000)
14. Fink, A.M., Holle-Robatsch, S., Herzog, N., et al.: Positron emission tomography is not useful in detecting metastasis in the sentinel lymph node in patients with primary malignant melanoma stage I and II. Melanoma Res. 14, 141–145 (2004)
15. Finkelstein, S.E., Carrasquillo, J.A., Hoffmann, J.M., et al.: A prospective analysis of positron emission tomography and conventional imaging for detection of stage IV metastatic melanoma in patients undergoing metastasectomy. Ann. Surg. Oncol. 11, 731–738 (2004)
16. Fuster, D., Chiang, S., Johnson, G., et al.: Is 18F-FDG PET more accurate than standard diagnostic procedures in the detection of suspected recurrent melanoma? J. Nucl. Med. 45, 1323–1327 (2004)
17. Gambhir, S.S., Czernin, J., Schwimmer, J., Silverman, D.H.S., Coleman, R.E., Phelps, M.E.: A tabulated summary of the FDG PET literature. Oncologic applications: Melanoma. J. Nucl. Med. 42(suppl 1), 13S–15S (2001)
18. Gambhir, S.S., Hoh, C.K., Essner, R., et al.: A decision analysis model for the role of whole body FDG PET in the management of patients with recurrent melanoma. J. Nucl. Med. 39(suppl), 94P (1998)
19. Gritters, L.S., Francis, I.R., Zasadny, K.R., Wahl, R.: Initial assessment of positron emission tomography using 2-fluorine-18-fluoro-2-deoxy-D-glucose in the imaging of malignant melanoma. J. Nucl. Med. 34, 1420–1427 (1993)
20. Hafner, J., Schmid, M.H., Kempf, W., et al.: Baseline staging in cutaneous malignant melanoma. Br. J. Dermatol. 150, 677–686 (2004)
21. Hannah, A., Feigen, M., Quong, G., et al.: Useof[F]-fluorodeoxyglucose positron emission tomography in monitoring response to recurrent neurotropic desmoplastic melanoma to radiotherapy. Otolaryngol. Head neck Surg. 122, 304–306 (2000)
22. Hoefnagel, C.A., Rankin, E.M., Valdes Olmos, R.A., Israels, S.P., Pavel, S., Janssen, A.G.M.: Sensitivity versus specificity in melanoma using iodine-123 iodobenzamide and indium-111 pentetreotide. Eur. J .Nucl. Med. 21, 587–588 (1994)
23. Holder Jr., W.D., White Jr., R.L., Zuger, J.H., Easton Jr., E.J., Greene, F.L.: Effectiveness of positron emission tomography for the detection of melanoma metastases. Ann. Surg. 227, 764–769 (1998)
24. Hsueh, E.C., Gupta, R.K., Glass, E.C., Yee, R., Qi, K., Morton, D.L.: Positron emission tomography plus serum TA90 immune complex assay for detection of occult metastatic melanoma. J. Am. Coll. Surg. 187, 191–197 (1998)
25. Kalff, V., Hicks, R.J., Ware, R.E., Greer, B., Binns, D.S., Hogg, A.: Evaluation of high-risk melanoma: comparison of [18F]FDG PET and high-dose 67Ga SPET. Eur. J. Nucl. Med. 29, 506–515 (2002)
26. Mercier, G.A., Alavi, A., Farker, D.L.: FDG positron emission tomography in isolated limb perfusion therapy in patients with locally advanced melanoma: preliminary results. Clin. Nucl. Med. 26, 832–836 (2001)

27. Mijnhout, G.S., Hoekstra, O.S., van Tulder, M.W., Teule, G.J.J., Devillé, W.L.J.M.: Systematic review of the diagnostic accuracy of 18F-fluorodeoxyglucose positron emission tomography in melanoma patients. Cancer **91**, 1530–1542 (2001)

28. Mishima, Y., Imahori, Y., Honda, C., Hiratsuka, J., Ueda, S., Ido, T.: In vivo diagnosis of human malignant melanoma with PET using specific melanoma seeking fluorine-18-DOPA analogue. J. Neurooncol. **33**, 163–169 (1997)

29. Nguyen, A.T., Akhurst, T., Larson, S.M., et al.: PET scanning with FDG in patients with melanoma: benefits and limitations. Clin. Positron Imaging **2**, 93–98 (1999)

30. Paquet, P., Henry, F., Belhocine, T., et al.: An appraisal of 18-fluorodeoxyglucose positron emission tomography for melanoma staging. Dermatology **200**, 167–169 (2000)

31. Reinhardt, M.J., Joe, A.Y., Huber, A., et al.: Diagnostic performance of whole body dual modality ¹⁸F-FDG PET/CT imaging for N- and M-staging of malignant melanoma: experience with 250 consecutive patients. J. Clin. Oncol. **24**, 1178–1187 (2006)

32. Rinne, D., Baum, R.P., Hör, G., Kaufmann, R.: Primary staging and follow-up of high risk melanoma patients with whole-body ¹⁸F-fluorodeoxyglucose positron emission tomography. Cancer **82**, 1664–1671 (1998)

33. Schreckenberger, M., Kadalie, C., Enk, A., et al.: First results of 18F-fluoroethyl-tyrosine PET for imaging of metastatic malignant melanoma. J. Nucl. Med. **42**(suppl), 30P (2001)

34. Shreve, P.D., Anzai, Y., Wahl, R.L.: Pitfalls in oncologic diagnosis with FDG PET imaging: physiologic and benign variants. Radiographics **19**, 61–77 (1999)

35. Stas, M., Stroobants, S., Dupont, P., et al.: 18-FDG PET scan in the staging of recurrent melanoma: additional value and therapeutic impact. Melanoma Res. **12**, 479–490 (2002)

36. Steinert, H.C., Bode, B., Boeni, R., Griff, M., Pfaltz, M., Dummer, R.: Malignant melanoma: non-malignant "hot spots" in whole-body FDG PET with radiologic pathologic correlation. Radiology **217**(suppl), 359 (2000)

37. Steinert, H.C., Böni, R., Huch-Böni, R., Capaul, R., von Schulthess, G.K., Westera, G.: Jod-123-Methyltyrosin-Szintigraphie beim malignen Melanom. Nuklearmedizin **36**, 36–41 (1997)

38. Steinert, H.C., Huch-Böni, R., Böni, R., Westera, G., Buck, A.: Dopamin-D2-Rezeptorszintigraphie mit Jod-123-Jodbenzofuran beim malignen Melanom. Nuklearmedizin **34**, 146–150 (1995)

39. Steinert, H.C., Huch-Böni, R.A., Buck, A., et al.: Malignant melanoma: staging with whole-body positron emission tomography and 2-[F-18]-fluoro-2-deoxy-D-glucose. Radiology **195**, 705–709 (1995)

40. Steinert, H.C., Voellmy, D.R., Trachsel, C., et al.: Planar coincidence scintigraphy and PET in staging malignant melanoma. J. Nucl. Med. **39**, 1892–1897 (1998)

41. Steinert, H.C., von Schulthess, G.K., Reuland, P., Peter, R.U., Sterry, W., Kaufmann, R., Reske, S.N.: A meta-analysis of the literature for staging of malignant melanoma with whole-body FDG PET. J. Nucl. Med. **42**(suppl), 307P (2001)

42. Strauss, L.G.: Fluorine-18 deoxyglucose and false-positive results: a major problem in the diagnostics of oncological patients. Eur. J. Nucl. Med. **23**, 1409–1415 (1996)

43. Strobel, K., Dummer, R., Husarik, D.B, Pérez Lago, M., Hany, T.F., Steinert, H.C.: Staging of high-risk melanoma with integrated PET/CT: the additional value of CT for detection of metastases. Radiology (2007)

44. Tyler, D.S., Onaitis, M., Kherani, A., et al.: Positron emission tomography scanning in malignant melanoma. Clinical utility in patients with stage III disease. Cancer **89**, 1019–1025 (2000)

45. Valk, P.E., Pounds, T.R., Tesar, R.D., et al.: Cost-effectiveness of PET imaging in clinical oncology. Nucl. Med. Biol. **23**, 737–743 (1996)

46. Vogg, A.T., Glatting, G., Möller, P., et al.: ¹⁸F5-fluoro-2′-desoxyuridine as PET-tracer for imaging of solid malignomas. J. Nucl. Med. **42**(suppl), 30P (2001)

47. Von Schulthess, G.K., Steinert, H.C., Dummer, R., Weder, W.: Cost effectiveness of whole-body FDG imaging in non-small cell lung cancer and malignant melanoma. Acad. Radiol. **5**(suppl 2), S300–S302 (1998)

48. Wagner, J.D., Schauwecker, D.S., Davidson, D., et al.: FDG-PET sensitivity for melanoma lymph node metastases is dependent on tumor volume. J. Surg. Oncol. **77**, 237–242 (2001)

49. Wahl, R.L., Hutchins, G.D., Buchsbaum, D.J., et al.: 18F-2-deoxy-2-fluoro-D-glucose uptake into human tumor xenografts. Cancer **67**, 1544–1550 (1991)

50. Wong, C., Silverman, D.H., Seltzre, M., et al.: The impact of 2-deoxy-2[18F]fluoro-D-glucose whole body positron emission tomography for managing patients with melanoma: the referring physician's perspective. Mol. Imaging Biol. **4**, 185–190 (2002)

Index

R. Dummer et al. (eds.), *Skin Cancer – A World-Wide Perspective*,
DOI: 10.1007/978-3-642-05072-5, © Springer-Verlag Berlin Heidelberg 2011